Surgical Foundations: Essentials of Surgical Oncology

Surgical Foundations: Essentials of Surgical Oncology

Michael S. Sabel, MD
Assistant Professor
Department of Surgery
University of Michigan Comprehensive Cancer Center
Ann Arbor, Michigan

Vernon K. Sondak, MD
Chief
Division of Cutaneous Oncology;
Director of Surgical Education
H. Lee Moffitt Cancer Center and Research Institute;
Professor
Departments of Interdisciplinary Oncology and Surgery
University of South Florida College of Medicine
Tampa, Florida

Jeffrey J. Sussman, MD
Assistant Professor
Division of Surgical Oncology
University of Cincinnati & VAMC
Cincinnati, Ohio

Series Editor: Larry R. Kaiser, MD
The John Rhea Barton Professor and Chairman
Department of Surgery
University of Pennsylvania School of Medicine
Philadelphia, Pennsylvania

MOSBY
ELSEVIER

MOSBY
ELSEVIER

1600 John F. Kennedy Blvd.
Ste 1800
Philadelphia, PA 19103-2899

ISBN: 0-8151-4385-0
ISBN-13: 978-0-8151-4385-7

Notice

Knowledge and best practice in this field are constantly changing. As new research and experience broaden our knowledge, changes in practice, treatment and drug therapy may become necessary or appropriate. Readers are advised to check the most current information provided (i) on procedures featured or (ii) by the manufacturer of each product to be administered, to verify the recommended dose or formula, the method and duration of administration, and contraindications. It is the responsibility of the practitioner, relying on their own experience and knowledge of the patient, to make diagnoses, to determine dosages and the best treatment for each individual patient, and to take all appropriate safety precautions. To the fullest extent of the law, neither the Publisher nor the Editors assumes any liability for any injury and/or damage to persons or property arising out or related to any use of the material contained in this book.

The Publisher

Library of Congress Cataloging-in-Publication Data

Essentials of surgical oncology: surgical foundations / [edited by] Michael S. Sabel, Vernon K. Sondak, Jeffrey J. Sussman.
p. ; cm.
ISBN 0-8151-4385-0
1. Cancer–Surgery. I. Sabel, Michael S. II. Sondak, Vernon K., 1957- III. Sussman, Jeffrey J.
[DNLM: 1. Neoplasms–surgery. QZ 268 E787 2007]
RD651.E87 2007
616.99'4059–dc22 2006044954

Acquisitions Editor: Judy Fletcher
Editorial Assistant: Ryan Creed
Project Manager: Bryan Hayward

Printed in The United States of America

Last digit is the print number: 9 8 7 6 5 4 3 2 1

Much effort and more than a little angst goes into the development of a textbook like *Surgical Foundations: Essentials of Surgical Oncology*. This textbook is certainly no exception. The motivation to persevere in the effort has been provided by the residents and fellows we've had the privilege to work with over the years, and the angst has been shared with and mitigated by our families who have supported us through thick and thin. But this particular textbook owes its very existence to one person—Michael Sabel—who kept the process of preparation moving through the doldrums and kept his fellow editors focused in the face of the many distractions and competing priorities we face on a daily basis. Because of his dedication to the completion of this textbook, we in turn dedicate this textbook to him.

Vernon K. Sondak, MD
Tampa, Florida

Contributors

Alisha Arora, MD
Formerly of University of Michigan Hospitals
Ann Arbor, Michigan

Syed A. Ahmad, MD
Assistant Professor
Department of Surgery
University of Cincinnati Cancer Center
Cincinnati, Ohio

Charles E. Binkley, MD
Attending Surgeon
Department of Surgery
Kaiser-Permanente Medical Center
Hayward, California

William M. Burke, MD

Alfred E. Chang, MD
Hugh Cabot Professor of Surgery;
Chief
Division of Surgical Oncology
Department of Surgery
University of Michigan Comprehensive
Cancer Center
Ann Arbor, Michigan

Vincent M. Cimmino, MD
Clinical Professor
University of Michigan Comprehensive
Cancer Center and Hospitals
Ann Arbor, Michigan

Kathleen M. Diehl, MD
Assistant Professor
Department of Surgery
University of Michigan Comprehensive
Cancer Center
Ann Arbor, Michigan

Gerard M. Doherty, MD
Norman W. Thompson Professor of Surgery
Department of Surgery
University of Michigan Hospitals
Ann Arbor, Michigan

Derek A. DuBay, MD
Fellow, Hepatobiliary Surgery and Liver
Transplant
Department of Surgery
University of Toronto
Toronto, Ontario, Canada

Elaina M. Gartner, MD
Assistant Professor
Division of Hematology/Oncology
Wayne State University;
Barbara Ann Karmanos Cancer Institute
Detroit, Michigan

Paul G. Gauger, MD
Associate Professor
Departments of Surgery and Medical Education
University of Michigan Hospitals
Ann Arbor, Michigan

James D. Geiger, MD
Associate Professor
Section of Pediatric Surgery;
Director
Minimally Invasive Surgery Program
Department of Surgery
University of Michigan Hospitals
Ann Arbor, Michigan

Scott D. Gitlin, MD
Associate Professor
Division of Hematology/Oncology
Department of Internal Medicine
University of Michigan Comprehensive
Cancer Center
Ann Arbor, Michigan

Kathleen Graziano, MD
Formerly of University of Michigan Hospitals
Ann Arbor, Michigan

Pamela J. Hodul, MD
Assistant Professor
Department of Surgery
University of South Florida College of Medicine;
Assistant Professor
Department of Interdisciplinary Oncology
H. Lee Moffitt Cancer Center and Research Institute
Tampa, Florida

Emina H. Huang, MD
Assistant Professor
Department of Surgery
University of Michigan Hospitals
Ann Arbor, Michigan

Mark D. Iannettoni, MD
Formerly of University of Iowa Hospitals
Iowa City, Iowa

Kathleen M. Woods Ignatoski, PhD
Research Investigator
Department of Urology
University of Michigan Comprehensive Cancer Center
Ann Arbor, Michigan

Carolyn Johnston, MD
Associate Professor
Department Obstetrics and Gynecology
University of Michigan Comprehensive Cancer Center
Ann Arbor, Michigan

Joseph Kim, MD
Formerly of University of Cincinnati Cancer Center
Cincinnati, Ohio

Jules Lin, MD
Formerly of University of Michigan Hospitals
Ann Arbor, Michigan

Quan P. Ly, MD

Erika A. Newman, MD
Resident Surgeon
Department of Surgery
University of Michigan Hospitals
Ann Arbor, Michigan

Julio M. Pow-Sang, MD
Formerly of H. Lee Moffitt Cancer Center and Research Institute
Tampa, Florida

Michael E. Ray, MD, PhD
Assistant Professor
Department of Radiation Oncology
University of Michigan Comprehensive Cancer Center
Ann Arbor, Michigan

Alejandro Rodriguez, MD

Dana E. Rollison, PhD
Assistant Professor
Department of Interdisciplinary Oncology
University of South Florida College of Medicine;
Assistant Professor
Department of Cancer Prevention and Control
H. Lee Moffitt Cancer Center and Research Institute
Tampa, Florida

Michael S. Sabel, MD
Assistant Professor
Department of Surgery
University of Michigan Comprehensive Cancer Center
Ann Arbor, Michigan

Elizabeth A. Shaughnessy, MD, PhD
Assistant Professor
Department of Surgery
University of Cincinnati Cancer Center;
Surgeon
Department of Surgery
University of Cincinnati Hospital
The Christ Hospital
Cincinnati, Ohio

Diane M. Simeone, MD
Associate Professor
Department of Surgery
University of Michigan Comprehensive Cancer Center
Ann Arbor, Michigan

Vernon K. Sondak, MD
Chief,
Division of Cutaneous Oncology
Director of Surgical Education
H. Lee Moffitt Cancer Center and Research Institute;
Professor
Departments of Interdisciplinary Oncology and Surgery
University of South Florida College of Medicine
Tampa, Florida

Sonia L. Sugg, MD
Formerly of Medical College of Wisconsin
Milwaukee, Wisconsin

Jeffrey J. Sussman, MD
Assistant Professor
Division of Surgical Oncology
University of Cincinnati & VAMC
Cincinnati, Ohio

Susan Tsai, MD
Formerly of University of Michigan Hospitals
Ann Arbor, Michigan

Candace Y. Williams-Covington, MD
Formerly of Baylor College of Medicine
Houston, Texas

Keith Wilson, MD
Formerly of University of Cincinnati Cancer Center
Cincinnati, Ohio

Michael J. Wolfe, MD

Derek T. Woodrum, MD
Resident
Department of Anesthesiology
University of Michigan Hospitals
Ann Arbor, Michigan

Preface

For the first half of the 20th century, cancer was essentially a surgical disease. The major medical centers boasted large staffs of "cancer surgeons," and the few dedicated cancer centers that existed were staffed almost entirely by surgeons. By the mid-20th century, with the development of radiation therapy subsequent to the discovery of x-rays and chemotherapy beginning with nitrogen mustard (derived from a World War I chemical warfare agent) and folic acid antagonists, the treatment of cancer changed dramatically. The fields of medical oncology and radiation oncology grew rapidly as it became evident that cancer could, and should, be treated by more than one modality. In the mid 1960s, the term *surgical oncology* first arose, primarily to differentiate between medical oncologists and surgeons who specialized in the treatment of cancer. Although many general surgeons felt comfortable performing cancer operations, it became increasingly apparent that to best serve their patients, the cancer surgeon had to have a strong knowledge of and familiarity with multimodality therapy. In 1975, the Society of Surgical Oncology was formed, and in conjunction with the National Cancer Institute, defined a surgical oncologist as a fully qualified general surgeon who has had additional training and experience in all aspects of oncology, is capable of collaborating well with other oncology disciplines, has a full-time commitment to oncology, and serves the important role of leader of his fellow general surgeons in the care of the cancer patient.

Today, the surgical oncologist is often called upon to not only diagnose, stage, and treat cancer but also to coordinate the care of the patient among the multiple disciplines within oncology. The treatment of cancer is constantly changing as new technologies and therapies emerge, so the surgical oncologist is increasingly in need of a strong grasp of chemotherapy, radiation therapy, cancer biology, genetics, immunology, and epidemiology. It is with this in mind that we present *Surgical Foundations: Essentials of Surgical Oncology*. Because the study of oncology covers such a wide array of topics, many textbooks are too overwhelming for the surgeon in training. We therefore sought to capture the true "essentials" of cancer surgery in an easily readable and absorbable format. The book covers the basics of tumor biology and cancer epidemiology, the principles of multimodality therapy, and the work-up, staging, and therapy for a wide array of malignancies, all from a surgical perspective. Each chapter begins with a list of key topics that should focus the reader on the most important topics in each category. Liberal use of tables, text boxes, and figures help reinforce the information in each chapter. Our goal is to present a textbook that surgeons in training can lean heavily upon as they develop their own experience with all aspects of oncology, and our hope is that this textbook will inspire a new generation of leaders in the care of future cancer patients.

Michael S. Sabel, MD

Jeffrey J. Sussman, MD

Vernon K. Sondak, MD

Foreword

As I write this foreword, I am reminded of how long ago we began this effort and am thrilled that the second volume in the series has come to fruition. What has come to be called the "Surgical Foundations" series evolved from a set of topics in radiology, each produced as a single volume and at the time called "The Requisites." Like that series, the original intent of the current series was to address the major areas of surgery, each in a single volume written in a concise format that would be readily accessible to trainees at all levels, including medical students, nurses, and the practicing surgeon alike. To accomplish this goal, we adopted a format used in the Radiology series that called for the liberal use of tables, graphics, and the clear articulation of Key Points to make the pertinent information all the more accessible. We also used boxes to display summaries of important material at multiple points throughout each chapter. The first book completed in the "Surgical Foundation" series, though not intended to be the first, was the volume on thoracic surgery that I did along with Sunil Singhal. Vern Sondak along with his co-editors, Michael Sabel and Jeffrey Sussman, has produced an outstanding volume that uses all of the hallmarks that distinguish these volumes from others dealing with similar topics and makes for a more compelling read.

Though our initial plan called for each volume to have a single author with perhaps one collaborator, we concluded that the breadth of the topics in *Surgical Oncology* was better served using a multiple author format but with a consistent chapter plan. The editors have worked diligently to create a work with a single voice while taking advantage of the expertise of multiple authors. I believe it works extremely well here. The book is packed with the most up-to-date information written in a style that is eminently readable and approachable. I anticipate that this volume will appeal to surgeons and nonsurgeons alike who work in multiple specialties that deal with malignant disease. I also believe the volume will appeal to those providers who work alongside physician partners specifically nurses and nurse practitioners. I am especially impressed with the introductory chapters dealing with molecular and cellular biologic principles that are key to understanding malignancy. The chapter on epidemiologic methods for cancer investigations nicely sets the stage for the interpretation of clinical trials, a major issue for anyone who takes care of cancer patients.

Overall this is a comprehensive volume that covers the entire field of surgical oncology including aspects of endocrine surgery in a format that all will find useful. This volume is a major accomplishment and I congratulate Dr. Sondak and his colleagues. It truly sets the stage for the additional volumes that will follow in this series.

Larry R. Kaiser, MD
Philadelphia, Pennsylvania

Contents

1

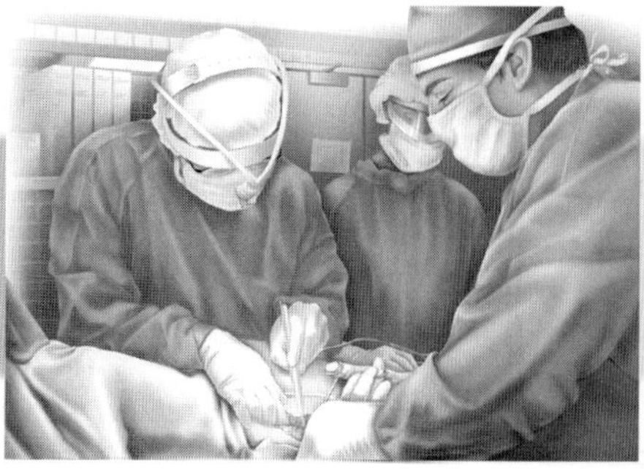

Molecular Biology: Oncogenes and Tumor Suppressor Genes

Kathleen M. Diehl and Kathleen M. Woods Ignatoski

Molecular Biology: Oncogenes and Tumor Suppressor Genes: Key Points

- Explain the progression from normal tissue to cancer.
- Compare the roles of oncogenes and tumor suppressor genes in carcinogenesis.
- Relate the molecular biology and behavior of cancer to targeted treatments.

In 1911, when Peyton Rous injected healthy chickens with a filtrate of chicken tumors and saw new tumors form at those sites, the field of viral oncology was born. This discovery ultimately led molecular biologists to study other viral oncogenes and the role of their human counterparts in cancer, and it led to the current understanding of cancer being the phenotype resulting from underlying genetic alterations in the involved cell. These alterations can arise from multiple factors; some are environmental, some are inherited, and all lead to changes at a cellular level (Figure 1-1). These changes lead to the hallmarks of malignant transformation, such as loss of contact inhibition of cells or anchorage- and growth-factor–independent growth. Combine these altered cells with an environment with

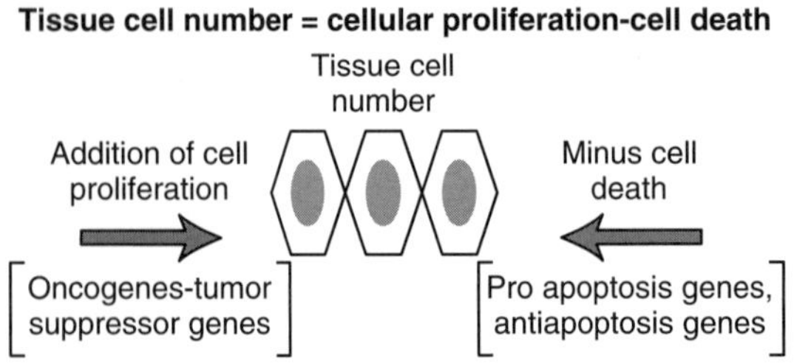

Figure 1-1. The total cell number in tissue is a sum of cellular proliferation factors acting on the cell minus factors encouraging or contributing to cellular death.

supportive hormonal or growth-factor changes and one sees growth, proliferation, and, sometimes, metastasis leading to the clinical disease that is commonly recognized as cancer. This is a multifactorial, multistep process. This chapter focuses on the underlying genetic changes that lead to the transformation of normal cells into cancer cells; Chapter 2 focuses on tumor growth on a larger level.

Background

Tumors are generally thought of as a clonal population of cells with karyotypic or genetic abnormalities. Mutations that alter cells and contribute to transformation can be inherited germline mutations, such as deletion of the retinoblastoma *(Rb)* gene, or they may be somatic mutations that are acquired during a patient's lifetime. Inherited tendencies in cancer are most often found in tumor suppressor genes, and they are most often inherited in an autosomal-dominant fashion. Factors known to contribute to somatic mutations include environmental factors, such as radiation, chemical exposure, or chronic inflammation. Viruses such as the Rous sarcoma virus (RSV) have been shown to cause cancer in animals and to transform cells in culture. Some viruses have been associated with a higher risk of cancer in humans, such as hepatitis C and hepatocellular cancer (Table 1-1).

Mutations can be characterized as follows: (1) gain of an entire chromosome (e.g., trisomy); (2) loss of an entire chromosome (e.g., monosomy); (3) deletion of a portion of a chromosome; (4) inversion, amplification, or translocation of a portion of a chromosome; or (5) intragenic mutations. Most cancers, when analyzed, will show multiple genetic abnormalities, which reinforces the idea that the development of cancer is a multistep process. A good example is found in the progression of a colon polyp to an invasive cancer (Figure 1-2). It is estimated that the average cell divides 10^{16} times in a person's lifetime and that the average gene is mutated 10^{10} times in a lifetime. Given the low incidence of cancer in comparison, there obviously exist numerous mechanisms of DNA repair and redundancy in cellular processes to overcome these mutations and to provide cellular homeostasis.

Oncogenes

Building on Peyton Rous's work with the RSV, Duesberg and Vogt showed that the virulent form of RSV contained an extra sequence of DNA, which they termed *SARC* (for sarcoma;

TABLE 1-1 • *Viruses Associated with Human Cancers*

Virus	Type	Cancer
Human T-lymphotropic virus 1 (HTLV-I)	RNA retrovirus	T cell leukemia
Human T-lymphotropic virus 2 (HTLV-II)	RNA retrovirus	Hairy cell leukemia
Hepatitis B virus (HBV)	DNA hepadnavirus	Hepatocellular carcinoma
Hepatitis C virus (HBC)	RNA flavivirus	Hepatocellular carcinoma
Human papilloma virus (HPV)	DNA papillomavirus	Cervical cancer, anogenital cancers, skin cancer
Epstein-Barr virus (EBV)	DNA herpesvirus	Burkitt's lymphoma, immunoblastic lymphoma, nasopharyngeal carcinoma
KS-associated herpesvirus/human herpesvirus-8 (KSHV/HHV-8)	DNA herpesvirus	Kaposi's sarcoma, Castleman's disease

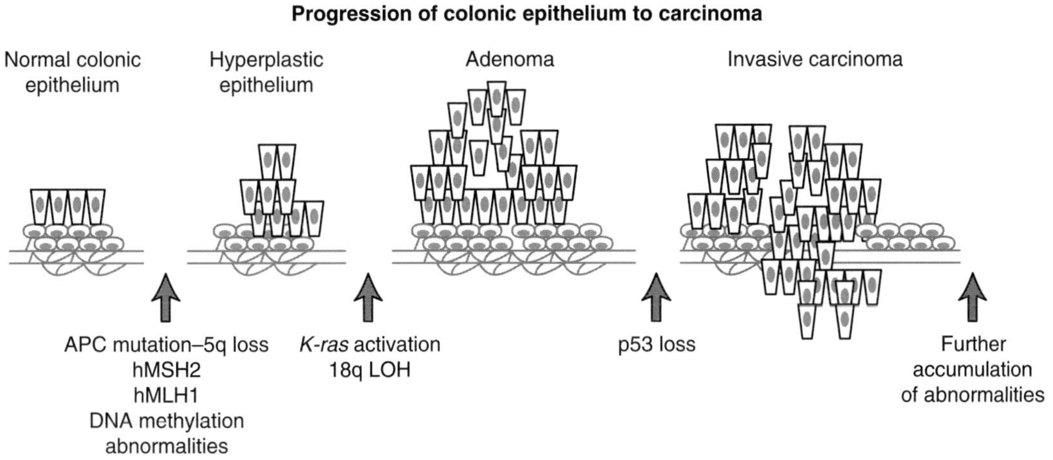

Figure 1–2. Progression of colonic epithelium to carcinoma. As colonic epithelium accumulates additional genetic abnormalities, there is a progression from a hyperplastic polyp to an adenoma to frank carcinoma. (From Fearon ER, Vogelstein BA. A genetic model for colorectal tumorigenesis, *Cell* 1990;61: 759-767.)

this was later shortened to SRC). The extra sequence was called an *oncogene,* meaning that it was a cancer-causing gene. In their Nobel-Prize–winning work, Stehelin and colleagues demonstrated that viral oncogenes were normal cellular genes with protein products that controlled cellular proliferation and that were incorporated into viruses and moved to other cells (Table 1-2). Subsequently, in 1981, Weinberg and colleagues demonstrated that the human homologue of the viral oncogene v-*ras* was a cause of bladder cancer (Figure 1-3). This confirmed the concept of cancer being caused by the mutation of preexisting normal cellular genes.

Normal cellular genes become oncogenic by somatic mutations (e.g., amplification) whereby extra copies of chromosomal DNA are transcribed, thus leading to overexpression of a protein that contributes to the malignant phenotype (Table 1-3). For example, amplification of the *ERBB-2* gene in breast cancer leads to the overexpression of numerous ERBB-2 receptors on the cell surface. The ERBB-2 receptor is a growth-factor receptor; in normal circumstances, this responds to growth factors in the environment signaling to the cell for increased growth and proliferation. When overexpressed, however, this leads to unrestrained signaling for growth and proliferation and the inhibition of apoptosis; in addition, when this is involved with other mutations, it contributes to growth independent of outside factors and the transformed phenotype. Somatic mutations can also occur by translocation, transposition, or transfer of one chromosomal segment to a new position. This is usually a result of the abnormal breakage and refusion of segments of chromosomes. For example, the Philadelphia chromosome involves translocation between chromosomes 9 and 23; this results in the production of a hybrid BCR-ABL fusion protein and leads to chronic myelogenous leukemia (CML). Oncogenes can also be a result of something as simple as a single base substitution. For example, *H-ras* consists of a single missense mutation, which has been cloned and found to be an oncogene in human bladder cancer.

TABLE 1–2 • *Tumor Virus Oncogenes*

Virus	Oncogene	Human Oncogene
Rous sarcoma	v-*SRC*	*SRC*
Maloney murine sarcoma	v-*mos*	*Mos*
Harvey murine sarcoma	v-*Ha-ras*	H-*ras*
Simian sarcoma virus	v-*sis*	*PDGFB*
Avian erythroblastosis	v-*erbB*	*EGFR*

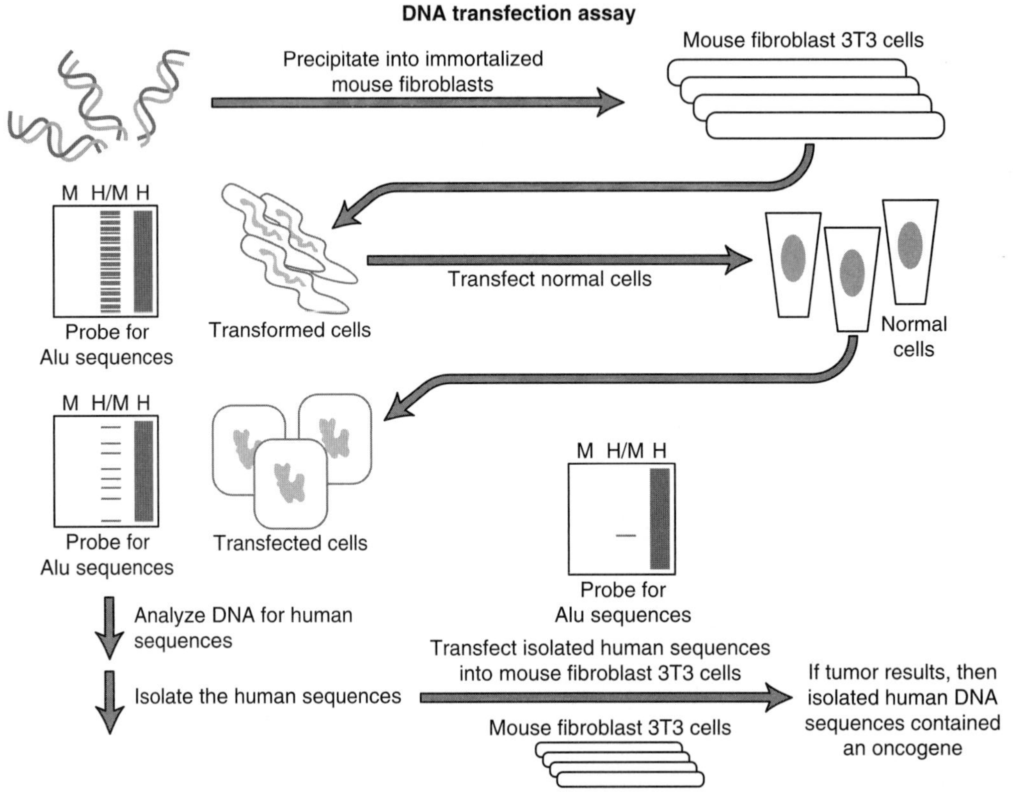

Figure 1–3. In the Weinberg experiments, DNA was isolated from a human bladder cancer and transfected into mouse cells. The DNA isolated from resulting transformed mouse cells was transfected into new mouse cells, and the procedure was repeated, each time taking some of the DNA for Southern blot analysis. Probing the DNA on the blots for the human *alu* sequence indicated how much human DNA was present. This procedure was repeated until only one *alu* band was seen in the transformed cells. This band was probed with a variety of known oncogenes, eventually leading to the identification of *ras* as the gene that played a role in transformation.

Oncogenes tend to be associated with mutations in growth-factor pathways that will lead to changes that accelerate the growth and proliferation of the cells involved and that can be categorized into many different protein classes based on function.

Because oncogenes are mutations of preexisting normal cellular genes that contribute to transformation of the cell, usually only one copy of the gene needs to be altered, with the result being an abnormal stimulatory effect on the cell. The classic analogy is that oncogenes work in the same way as "stepping on the accelerator of a car." In other words, there is an abnormal gain of function (Table 1-4). Although a single oncogene (such as is seen in the example of the Philadelphia chromosome given above) can result in transformation of the cell, normally two or more mutant oncogenes that collaborate or potentiate each other will be found in a tumor type. The result must provide a selective advantage to the cell to contribute to the malignant process. Other mutations, such as mutations in tumor suppressor genes, can potentiate transformation of the cell.

TABLE 1–3 • *Example of Oncogenes Amplified in Human Cancer*

Tumor Type	Amplified Gene
Neuroblastoma	*N-myc*
Glial brain tumor	*EGFR*
Breast cancer	*ERBB-2*
Ovarian cancer	*ERBB-2*

Tumor Suppressor Genes

Tumor suppressor genes are also referred to as *antioncogenes* and *recessive oncogenes.* As

TABLE 1–4 • *Examples of Oncogenes Found in Human Cancers*

Oncogene	Gene	Alteration
Growth-Factor Receptors	*ERBB-2*	Amplification
	EGFR	Amplification, point mutation
	MET	Missense mutation, fusion translocation
	RET	Missense mutation, fusion translocation
Signal Transducers		
Guanosine-triphosphate–binding proteins	*K-Ras*	Missense mutation
	H-Ras	Missense mutation
	N-Ras	Missense mutation
Tyrosine kinases	*ABL*	Fusion protein
Nuclear Oncoproteins		
Transcriptional control	*C-Myc*	Amplification, promoter translocation
	N-Myc	Amplification
	L-Myc	Amplification
Cell-cycle control	Cyclin D1	Amplification, promoter translocation
	CDK4	Amplification, missense mutation
Antagonists of Apoptosis	*BCL2*	Promoter translocation
Antagonists of Tumor Suppression	*MDM2*	Amplification

opposed to oncogenes, usually both copies of the gene must be deleted or mutated to alter the function of the gene in the cell. This can be the result of somatic mutations or a combination of germline and somatic mutations. The classic example used in oncology is the *Rb* gene. The Rb protein negatively regulates the entry of cells into the cell cycle. Without it, there can be failure to arrest during mitosis. Patients who inherit a deletion of the portion of the long arm of chromosome 13 (known as 13q14) are predisposed to malignant transformation. A somatic mutation of the second copy of the gene will result in retinoblastoma. Although retinoblastoma can occur during a patient's lifetime as a result of mutations in both copies of the *Rb* gene, the probability of this "double hit" is much less likely; rather, those who inherit a germline mutation of one copy are much more likely to develop the disease, and they will be more likely to develop the disease at a young age. This is a hallmark of hereditary cancer syndromes, which are often associated with germline mutations of tumor suppressor genes, namely the tendency of clustering a cancer type and the development of cancer at a young age, or the development of bilateral disease (Figure 1-4).

Tumor suppressor genes can be inactivated by mutation or by methylation of the promoter of the gene, thereby leading to decreased transcription and an effective loss of the protein and its function. The typical analogy of tumor suppressor genes is that they act as "the brakes on a car." In other words, there is an abnormal loss of function of the gene product meant to regulate cell division, growth, or apoptosis. Tumor suppressor genes tend to code for proteins that control proliferation in a negative way; their loss allows uncontrolled proliferation to proceed, which is a hallmark of the tumor phenotype.

BOX 1–1 CLASSES OF TUMOR SUPPRESSORS (NEGATIVE REGULATORS OF CELL PROLIFERATION)

- Cell cycle regulation/apoptosis (e.g., p53)
- Signal transduction (e.g., GTPase-activating protein)
- Cytoskeletal proteins
- Cell matrix proteins

Additional Changes that Contribute to Cell Transformation

DNA Repair and Cancer

Because it is estimated that the cells in the body undergo an average of 10^{16} divisions during a lifetime, there will be occasional mistakes in DNA replication. The cells contain enzyme systems that identify and repair mistakes in DNA replication. Patients who inherit or develop

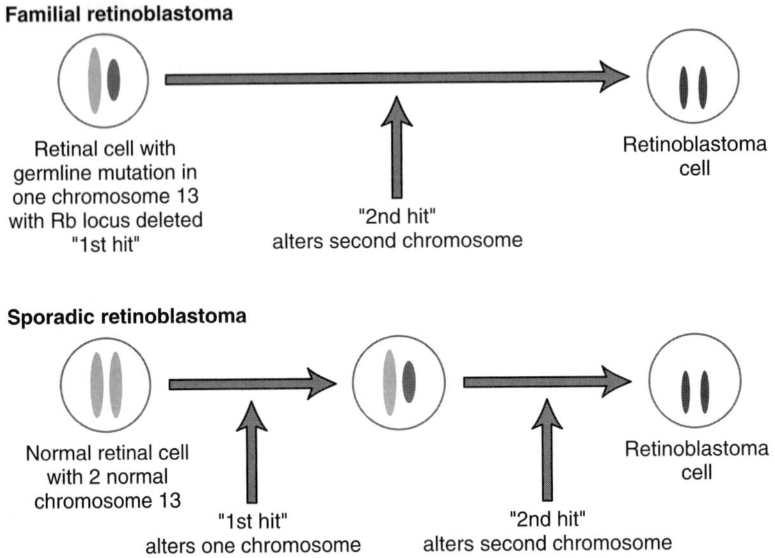

Figure 1–4. The retinoblastoma tumor suppressor gene. In familial retinoblastoma, there is a germline mutation in chromosome 13, and the additional second hit leads to retinoblastoma, usually at a young age. In sporadic retinoblastoma, cells start with two normal chromosomes. The accumulation of two hits to chromosome 13 to lead to retinoblastoma occurs less frequently and at a later age in life.

mutations in DNA repair genes will be susceptible to an accumulation of mutations that ultimately may lead to cell transformation. An example is hereditary nonpolyposis colon cancer, a disease in which mutations in the *MSH2, PMS2, MSH6,* or *MLH1* genes lead to deficiencies in the mismatch repair apparatus and genomic instability.

Epigenetic Changes in Cancer

Changes in cell behavior without an underlying change in the genetic makeup of the cell that contributes to transformation are referred to as *epigenetic changes*. The methylation of cell promoters that inhibit the binding of transcription factors—and, therefore, the transcription of the protein—can have the same result as the loss or deletion of the gene. This happens when methyl groups are added to cytosines in the DNA, which often happens in stretches of C-G-C-G repeats.

Clinical Applications of Molecular Biology

Traditionally, chemotherapy agents have been nonspecific agents that interfere with the ability of cells to replicate and grow. They affect all replicating cells, and they result in the need to balance the desired effect on cancer cells with the undesired effect on normal replicating cells. As knowledge about the underlying molecular biology and behavior of cancer has grown, so has the desire to be able to tailor treatments to individual patients. If changes unique to the cancer cell can be identified and a treatment targeted to that unique change developed, then treatment for the cancer with minimal side effects on normal cells can be performed.

One of the best-known examples of targeted therapy is the use of imatinib (Gleevec) for the treatment of CML and gastrointestinal stromal tumors (GISTs). CML is caused by a translocation between the long arms of chromosomes 9 and 22 [t(9;22)(q34;q11)] called the *Philadelphia chromosome.* The chimeric protein formed by the chromosomal joining contains a region called the breakpoint cluster region (Bcr), which is fused to the c-*abl* tyrosine kinase to create *BCR-ABL*. The *BCR-ABL* protein has deregulated kinase activity as compared with wild-type *Abl,* and it has been shown to play a causative role in CML. Imatinib binds in the kinase domain of the *Abl* portion of the protein and blocks its activity with inhibitory activity toward BCR-ABL. Imatinib also has inhibitory activity toward platelet-derived growth-factor receptor and c-*KIT*. A majority of GISTs contain activating c-*KIT* mutations. Imatinib has been a breakthrough treatment for both CML and GIST;

however, drug resistance has been a problem. It appears that the most common method of resistance is a point mutation in the kinase domain, which blocks the binding of the inhibitor but does not block kinase activity. Also, in a small subset, the genomic amplification of *BCR-ACL* is seen. This implies that the amount of protein increases to a point at which its combined kinase activity overwhelms the inhibitory effects of the drug. Improved versions of imatinib are being developed to circumvent the problem of mutation-directed resistance.

The small-molecule inhibitors can inhibit a molecule thought to be a causative agent in tumorigenesis by inhibiting kinase activities, fatty-acid additions, growth-factor actions, DNA unwinding, proteosome degradation, or other enzymatic activities. For example, inhibitors have been developed that target the ERBB family of tyrosine kinase receptors (Figure 1-5). These inhibitors block the adenosine-triphosphate–binding site in the kinase domain of the receptor. Blocking adenosine triphosphate binding stops the transfer of phosphate groups to molecules that are downstream of the receptors in signaling cascades, thus blocking the growth and survival signals from the receptors. Examples include gefitinib (Iressa), which mainly blocks epidermal growth-factor receptor (EGFR), but it can also block ERBB-2; PKI-166, and EKB-569 (all of which block EGFR specifically); GW-2016 (which blocks both EGFR and ERBB-2); and lapatinib (which blocks all ERBB receptors). All of these drugs have been in at least Phase I clinical trials with favorable toxicity profiles. However, these drugs—along with other targeted therapies—appear only to work in a subset of patients, which indicates that the mechanistic action of these drugs is complex and that it may involve more than the inactivation of ERBB kinases. Many new targeted therapies are currently being evaluated (Table 1-5), and much work is needed to identify the subsets of patients that would benefit most from the use of these drugs.

Finding New Targets

In the past, genes involved in tumorigenesis were identified by their homology to known oncogenes. Then, as advancements in molecular biology grew, tumorigenesis-related genes were identified, because they were amplified in a number of cancers; these genes were isolated and expressed in non-transformed cells. In vitro assays on the cells

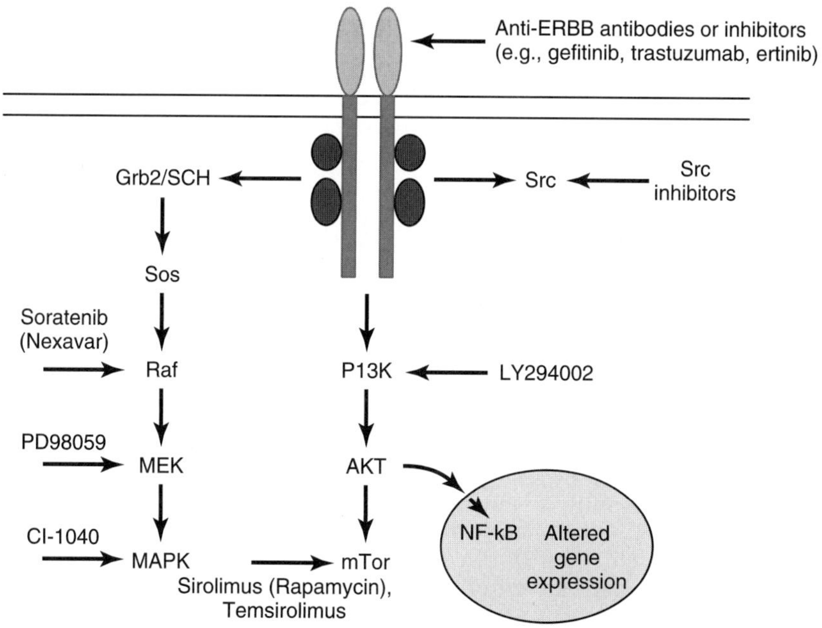

Figure 1–5. Targets for tyrosine kinase receptors. Dimerization of the tyrosine kinase receptor leads to phosphorylation and activation of the receptor-activating cell signal cascades involved in cellular growth, proliferation, and anti-apoptosis. At each step in the cascade, targeted inhibitors are being developed to disrupt the oncogenic signaling from the amplified receptors.

TABLE 1–5 • *Examples of Targeted Therapies in Clinical Use/Evaluation*

Agent	Mechanism of Action
AG2037	GAR transformylase inhibitor
Bevacizumab (Avastin)	Anti-VEGF antibody
Bortezomib (Velcade)	Proteasome inhibitor
Cetuximab (Erbitux)	Anti-EGFR antibody
EKB-569	EGFR inhibitor
Gefitinib (Iressa)	EGFR inhibitor
HMN214	Polo kinase inhibitor
Lapatinib	EGFR, ERBB-2 antagonist
Lurtotecan	Liposomal Topo I inhibitor
NM-3	VEGF inhibitor
Oblimersen (Genesense)	Antisense to bcl2
PKC412	Tyrosine kinase inhibitor
PKI-166	EGFR inhibitor
Px-12	Thioredoxin reductase inhibitor
SAHA	Histone deacetylase inhibitor
SCH 66334	Farnesyl transferase inhibitor
Sorafenib (Nexavar)	Raf kinase inhibitor
Tipifamib (Zarnestra)	Farnesyl transferase inhibitor

EGFR, Epidermal growth-factor receptor; *GAR,* glycinamide ribonucleotide; *VEGF,* vascular endothelial growth factor.

expressing the genes were performed to determine motility, invasion, and anchorage-independent growth, all of which are phenotypes of transformed cells. If the cells became transformed, they were placed in mice to see if they grew into tumors. These processes were tedious because only one gene could be analyzed at a time.

Today, multiple genes can be examined simultaneously for their transformation potential. For example, all of the expressed genes from a cancer cell or genes from a region of amplification that is common among cancers are cloned into viruses. These viruses are used to infect non-transformed cells. Transformed cells are then selected by various criteria, including the ability to grow without anchorage to a substrate or to grow without growth factors. The genes responsible for the transformation are then isolated. This approach is called *expression cloning.*

Another multigene approach is via microarrays. With this technique, expressed RNA is isolated from a normal cell and a cancer cell, labeled with different colors, and used to probe a glass slide (a "chip") that contains fragments of as many as 64,000 genes. The intensity of the different colors, or of a combined color indicates whether a gene is overexpressed or under-expressed in the cancer cells. Recently, protein microarrays have been developed with which antibodies are spotted on a glass slide and proteins from normal and tumor cells are labeled. Again, color intensity indicates what proteins are overexpressed or underexpressed in the cancer cells.

Conclusion

Although oncogenes and their transformation mechanisms have been known of for almost 30 years, we are just now understanding how to abrogate the function of these genes to block cancer growth. The advent of specific small-molecule inhibitors has been a tremendous step in the fight against cancer. The potential of these agents is best exemplified by imatinib (Gleevec). During the early 1990s, treatment of CML (primarily with interferon-α) resulted in a response rate of about 33%. Today, with Gleevec, the response rate among CML patients is 95%, with 89% progression-free survival at 18 months. There are still drawbacks to the new therapies, such as drug resistance after a period of treatment, but new drugs and combination therapies are being designed that will hopefully bypass the resistance mechanisms. It is foreseeable that the future of cancer therapy will include the molecular profiling of a tumor, which will allow for the targeting of therapy to an individual patient's tumor.

Key Selected Reading

Mendelsohn J, Howley PM, Israel MA, Liotta LA. *The molecular basis of cancer,* ed 2, Philadelphia: WB Saunders, 2001.

Selected Readings

Deininger M, Druker B. Specific targeted therapy of chronic myelogenous leukemia with imatinib, *Pharmacol Rev* 2003; 55:401-423.

Downward J. Control of ras activation, *Cancer Surv* 1996; 27:87-100.

Esteller M. Epigenetics provides a new generation of oncogenes and tumour-suppressor genes. *Br J Cancer* 2006;94:179–183.

Gomparts BD, Kramer IM, Tatham PER. *Signal transduction.* New York: Academic Press, 2002.

Hardie G, Hanks S. *The protein kinase facts book: protein-serine kinases,* vol 1, New York: Academic Press, 1995.

Hardie G, Hanks S. *The protein kinase facts book: protein-tyrosine kinases,* vol 2, New York: Academic Press, 1995.

Heeg S, Doebele M, von Werder A, Opitz OG. In vitro transformation models: modeling human cancer. *Cell Cycle* 2006;5:630–634.

Hesketh R. *The oncogene facts book,* ed 2, New York: Academic Press, 1997.

Krause DS, Van Etten RA. Tyrosine kinases as targets for cancer therapy. *N Engl J Med* 2005;353:172–187.

Normanno N, Maiello M, DeLuca A. Epidermal growth factor receptor tyrosine kinase inhibitors (EGFR-TKIs): simple drugs with a complex mechanism of action?, *J Cell Physiol* 2003;194:13-19.

Pegram MD, Pietras R, Bajamonde A, *et al.* Targeted therapy: wave of the future. *J Clin Oncol* 2005;23:1776–1781.

Quackenbush J. Microarray analysis and tumor classification. *N Engl J Med* 2006;354:2463–2472.

Rous P. A sarcoma of the fowl transmissible by an agent separable from the tumor cells, *J Exp Med* 1911;13: 397-411.

Steel M. Molecular biology and surgical practice. *Surgeon* 2005;3:145–149.

Venkitaraman AR. A growing network of cancer-susceptibility genes. *N Engl J Med* 2003;348:1917–1919.

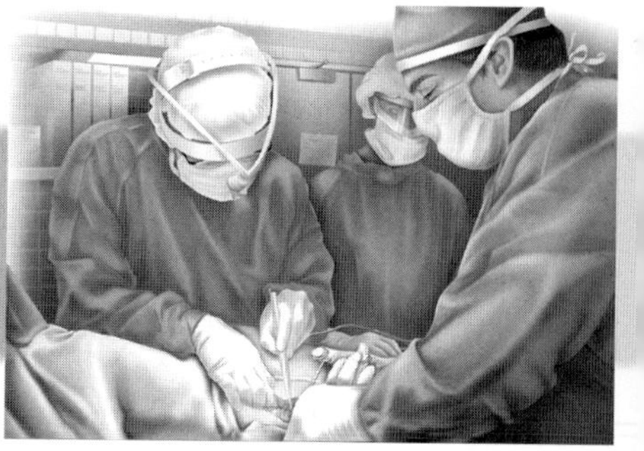

2

Cellular Biology: Tumor Growth and Metastasis

Michael S. Sabel

MECHANISMS OF TUMOR GROWTH AND METASTASES

HOST DEFENSES AGAINST METASTASES

APPLYING PRINCIPLES OF CELLULAR BIOLOGY TO CANCER TREATMENT

Cellular Biology: Tumor Growth and Metastasis: Key Points

- Understand the factors that contribute to the development of metastasis.
- Identify processes that prevent metastasis formation.
- Describe the contribution made by angiogenesis to tumor growth and metastasis.
- Discuss how motility enhances the tumor's invasive nature.
- Define *intravasation, arrest,* and *extravasation.*
- Identify factors that influence tumor cell proliferation.
- Discuss the "seed and soil" concept with respect to tumor metastasis.

The majority of cancer-related deaths ultimately result from distant metastases. Despite improvements in adjuvant therapies, surgery and other local therapies are effective for treating cancer only if metastases have not been seeded at the time that treatment is initiated. Unfortunately, the presence of these metastatic deposits is rarely detectable at the time of surgical therapy, leaving both the patient and the physician with the uncertainty relating to the likelihood of distant recurrence.

Metastatic dissemination does not occur by purely mechanical factors, with the site of metastasis determined solely by the anatomy of the surrounding vessels. Instead, the process by which a cancer cell can leave the primary site, travel to a distant site via the circulatory system, and establish a secondary tumor is the cumulative result of a series of complex genetic and epigenetic events. More than a century ago, Paget documented that metastases occurred in a nonrandom pattern, suggesting that certain tumor cells had a specific affinity for certain organs: the "seed and soil" theory. Since that time, knowledge about the molecular and cellular mechanisms involved in the regulation of tumor metastasis has dramatically increased. Several interdependent steps are necessary, and the failure to complete any of the steps prevents the formation of distant tumors (Figure 2-1). These essential steps consist of the following:

1. After neoplastic transformation, tumor growth depends on neovascularization or angiogenesis if the tumor is to grow beyond 1 to 2 mm in diameter. As the tumor grows, it becomes biologically heterogeneous, containing subpopulations of cells with different properties.
2. The cancer cell gains the ability to break free of the surrounding cells (dissociatiation) and to actively migrate (motility).
3. The cells must invade through the host stroma, into the vessels, and then detach and embolize.
4. If these cells survive in the circulation, they must then adhere to capillary endothelial cells (arrest).
5. Although the tumor cells may proliferate within the lumen of the vessel, in most cases, they will need to extravasate into the organ parenchyma and then proliferate within the new environment.
6. Finally, the cycle returns to step 1. The cells must develop a vascular supply (angiogenesis) in order to grow beyond just 1 to 2 mm. The cycle can then repeat itself, with the metastases giving rise to additional metastases.

Metastasis formation will only be successful if at least one tumor cell is capable of surviving every single step of the metastatic cascade. This is a rare event. Although millions of tumor cells can be delivered to the circulation by even small primary tumors, less than 0.05% of circulating tumor cells successfully establish metastatic deposits. Several host responses,

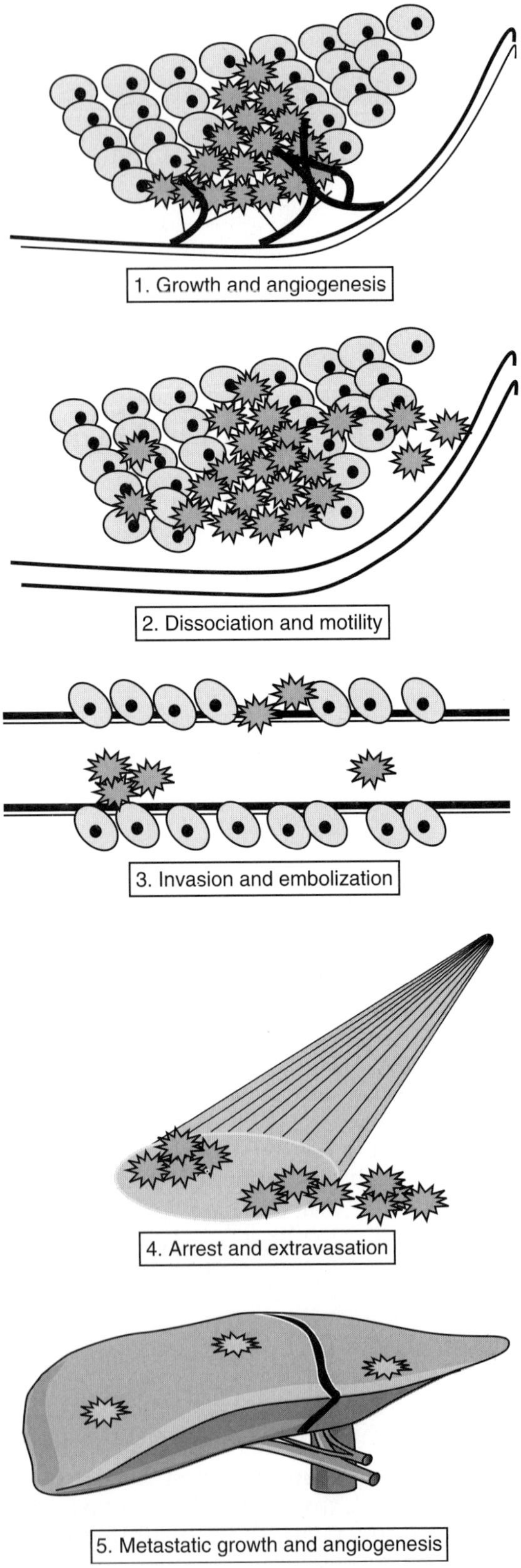

Figure 2-1. Multiple steps are necessary for tumor cells to be able to metastasize.

BOX 2–1 STEPS NECESSARY FOR TUMOR PROGRESSION

- Neoplastic transformation
- Angiogenesis and neovascularization
- Dissociation
- Motility
- Invasion
- Detachment and embolization
- Adherence and arrest
- Extravasation

including nitric oxide production, antiangiogenic and antiproteolytic factors, specific and nonspecific immune responses, and organ-specific factors (e.g., pH, nutrient availability, inhibitory cytokines), can prevent the development of metastases. This chapter will review the most recent understanding of the mechanisms behind tumor growth and metastases, and it will address how this information is being used to design novel anticancer therapies.

Mechanisms of Tumor Growth and Metastases

Angiogenesis

Within organs, oxygen is able to diffuse radially from the capillaries for only 150 to 200 µm. If a tumor grows larger than 2 mm in diameter without an adequate blood supply, cell death occurs. Thus, if the tumor is going to grow, it is imperative that angiogenesis (the process by which new blood vessels grow out of an existing vascular bed into a developing avascular organ) occur. Many molecules are responsible for the induction of angiogenesis. These are released by both the tumor cells and the host cells; some stimulate vessel formation, whereas others are inhibitory (Table 2-1). The ultimate fate of any tumor is determined by the balance between these factors. The process by which new vessels grow into a tumor is somewhat similar to the way that cancer cells invade. First, the proliferation of endothelial cells occurs. This is then followed by the breakdown of the extracellular matrix and finally by the migration of the endothelial cells into the tumor mass.

BOX 2–2 HOST FACTORS PREVENTING TUMOR METASTASES

- Antiangiogenesis factors
- Antiproteolytic factors
- Nitrous oxide
- Immune responses (specific and non-specific)
- Seed versus soil (i.e., p, nutrient availability, waste accumulation)

TABLE 2–1 • *Molecules Affecting Angiogenesis*

Stimulatory	Angiogenin
	Angiotropin
	Epidermal growth factor
	Basic fibroblast growth factor (bFGF)
	Fibronectin
	Interleukin-8 (IL-8)
	Nicotinamide
	Platelet-derived endothelial growth factor
	Prostaglandins E1 and E2
	Transforming growth factor (TGF-α, TGF-β)
	Tumor necrosis factor (TNF-α)
	Vascular endothelial growth factor
Inhibitory	Angiopoietin-1
	Angiostatin
	Canstatin
	Cartilage-derived inhibitor
	Endostatin
	Interferon-α
	Interferon-β
	Interleukins-1, 4, and 12
	Platelet factor-4
	Prolactin
	Retinoids
	Thrombospondin-1 (TSP-1)
	Vasostatin

One of the most-studied inducers of angiogenesis is vascular endothelial growth factor (VEGF). VEGF is produced by tumor cells; the binding of VEGF to VEGF receptors belonging to the tyrosine kinase family on endothelial cells induces their proliferation and migration. The production of VEGF is often stimulated by hypoxia, but it can also be upregulated by some of the most common activated oncogenes found in human tumors, such as the *ras* and *raf* oncogenes. It also appears as though the tumor cell does not need to produce VEGF

BOX 2–3 VASCULAR ENDOTHELIAL GROWTH FACTOR

- Production stimulated by hypoxia in both normal (stromal) cells and cancer cells; can also be stimulated by growth factors and cytokines (PDGF, bFGF, TNF-α, IL-8)
- Upregulated by oncogenes *(ras, raf)*
- Inhibition can be suppressed (mutant p53)
- Induces proliferation and migration of endothelial cells and permeabilization of blood vessels

itself, but rather that it can stimulate the surrounding nontransformed stromal tissues to produce VEGF. On the other hand, there are factors that inhibit the expression of VEGF, such as wild-type p53. Mutated p53, however, can enhance VEGF expression, which is why inactivating mutations in p53 are often associated with increased VEGF-induced tumor angiogenesis and poor prognosis.

In addition to stimulating endothelial cells to proliferate, VEGF induces the permeabilization of blood vessels, which leads to the extravasation of plasma proteins; this permeabilization is inhibited by angiopoietin-1. The extravasated plasma proteins then form a new provisional extracellular matrix that is rich in fibrin and adhesive proteins. This matrix enhances the invasion of stromal cells and more blood vessels into the tumor. This invasion is assisted by the production of proteases by the endothelial cells. The blood vessels created by this pathway are not normal, but rather they appear to be locked in a partially immature state. They are distributed unevenly, they have a serpentine morphology, and they remain hyperpermeable to plasma proteins.

Looking at the similarities between how new blood vessels form and invade the tumor and how tumors invade and metastasize, one can now see how the process of angiogenesis not only provides the oxygen and nutrients necessary for the tumor mass to grow but also assists in the next crucial steps involved in metastasis. The proteases produced by the invading endothelial cells enhance the migration of tumor cells, and the hyperpermeability of the new vessels encourages entrance into the vascular system. Thus, it is not surprising that an increase in microvessel density correlates with the probability that tumor cells will metastasize. One can measure the number of microvessels in a tumor by immunohistochemical staining with antibodies against factor VIII, which is a protein that is expressed only on the surface of endothelial cells. This "angiogenic index" has been reported to be an independent prognostic variable in many cancers.

Tumor Growth

The tumor doubling time (T_D) is the time it takes for a tumor to double its mass. Solid tumors tend to have a much longer T_D than hematologic cancers. Theoretically, it might be expected that tumor growth would follow a straightforward exponential growth curve, with each cell doubling at the same rate over the tumor's entire life span; however, this is not the case. It is actually a sigmoid curve (Figure 2-2), referred to as Gompertzian kinetics, with initial slow growth followed by rapid expansion and, finally, a progressive slowing. Tumor growth is initially slow before angiogenesis, and it is limited by the diffusion gradient for oxygen and essential nutrients. Immunosurveillance and other host factors may also play a role during this early lag phase. However, after angiogenesis occurs and blood vessels grow into the tumor, there is a rapid exponential growth of the tumor. The vast majority of this tumor growth occurs before the tumor is clinically recognizable. A tumor is generally not detectable until it is at least 1 gram (10^9 cells); this requires roughly 30 doublings. Only another 10 doublings are required for the tumor to reach 10^{12} cells, or 1 kg of tumor, which is usually a lethal tumor burden. However, there is a reduction in growth rate as the tumor size increases, and there are many factors responsible for this. T_D can vary between different regions of the

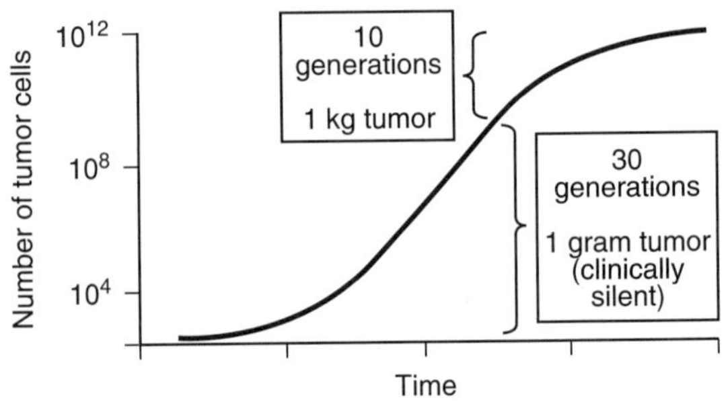

Figure 2–2. Gompertzian growth (a reduction in growth rate as tumor size increases). This reduction is thought to be due to intratumoral heterogeneity, limited oxygen and nutrients, and immunosuppressive factors.

same tumor. As the tumor cells divide, genetic alterations occur; this results in different subpopulations, all with different growth kinetics (Figure 2-3). Not all cells are actively proliferating, nor do they all have equivalent cell-cycle phase durations (Figure 2-4). The more cells within a subpopulation that enter the G_0 phase, the slower the T_D. In addition, differences in the vascular distribution, space restrictions, and the presence of other cell populations may influence the growth of the tumor.

In the absence of any further mutations, the tumor is still clinically benign, and it is unable to invade into surrounding tissues or to metastasize to other organs. However, as the cells continue to divide rapidly, increased genetic instability increases the possibility of further genetic alterations. These genetic alterations lead to new subpopulations of cells with a greater tendency toward malignant behavior. Many will be incompatible with survival, but, ultimately, the tumor microenvironment (i.e., blood supply, growth factors, immune surveillance, and even therapeutic interventions) provides a selective advantage to specific subclones. This natural selection will lead to more aggressive subclones becoming dominant, with an accelerated growth potential. In addition, many mutations will confer upon the cells the ability to produce proteins that predispose toward invasion and metastases.

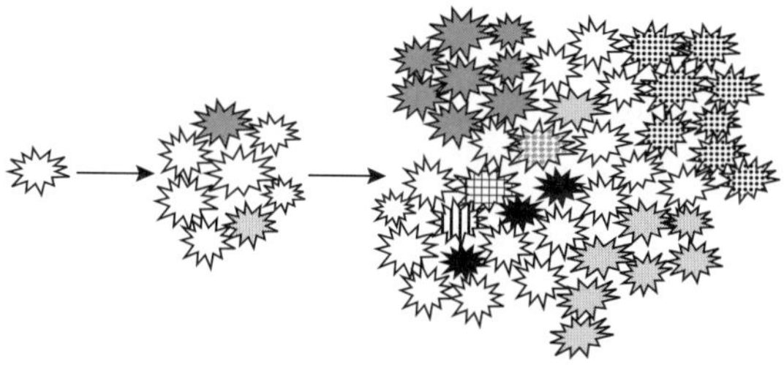

Figure 2–3. Heterogeneity of cells within a tumor. Subpopulations of cells arise from mutations, resulting in a heterogeneous population. Some are lethal, whereas others result in properties associated with tumor progression.

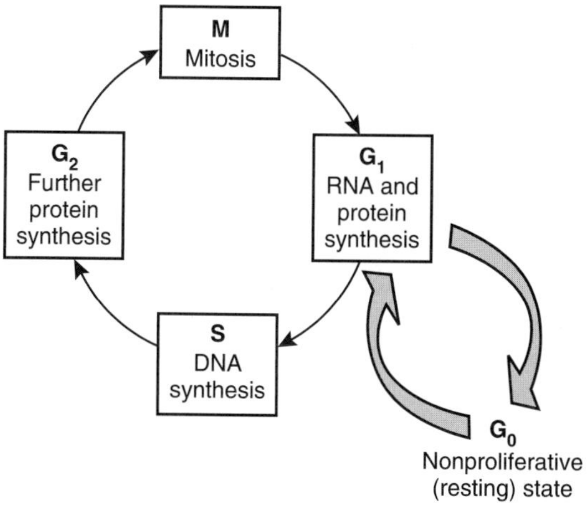

Figure 2–4. The normal cell cycle. Not all cells are actively proliferating, nor do they all have equivalent cell-cycle phase durations. Cells in the nonproliferative G_0 phase are dormant, although they maintain their ability to divide. The more cells within a subpopulation that enter the G_0 phase, the slower the tumor doubling time.

Motility and Invasion

With its newfound blood supply, the tumor is able to grow. However, if it is to spread to other parts of the body, it must invade into the surrounding tissue and, more importantly, into the vessels. As the tumor grows, mechanical pressure on the surrounding tissue helps this process, but it plays only a minor role. When one looks at a tumor histologically, there are often tumor cells that are discontinuous with the main mass; this is because the cells have gained the tools necessary for *dissociation* and *motility*. To do so, they must first lose their dependence on cell-to-cell adhesion, which is regulated by two groups of molecules: the calcium-independent immunoglobulin superfamily (N-CAM, CEA, DCC, MUC-18) and the calcium-dependent cadherins (primarily E-cadherin). E-cadherin is a cell-surface glycoprotein located at the epithelial junction complex, and it is responsible for the organization of epithelial tissues. Downregulation of E-cadherin is often a crucial step in the transition

BOX 2–4 E-CADHERIN

- Cell-surface glycoprotein involved in calcium-dependent cell-to-cell adhesion
- Located at the epithelial junction complex
- Responsible for the organization of epithelial tissues
- Reduced levels found with decreased differentiation and increasing tumor grade
- Mutations associated with transition from noninvasive to invasive phenotype

of tumor cells from noninvasive to invasive. After these cell-to-cell adhesions are lost, the cell is free to move.

Movement, however, is no small feat. Active locomotion is a multistep process by which a leading edge adheres to the extracellular matrix (ECM), and this edge is pulled forward, thus forming pseudopodia. The cell then contracts at the same time that the adhesion receptors at the back of the cell release. The expansion and contraction of the cell cytoskeleton results from actin polymerization, which is largely mediated by the Rho-like GTPases such as Rac1, RhoA, and Cdc42. These can be induced by many growth factors, such as platelet-derived growth factor (PDGF), epidermal growth factor (EGF), scatter factor/hepatocyte growth factor (SF/HGF), insulin, and autocrine motility factor. Equally important to the cell's motility is its ability to establish temporary cell contacts with the ECM. Integrins play a pivotal role in this process, and they make up more than 20 varieties of transmembrane heterodimers, which are composed of α and β subunits. These interact with multiple components of the ECM, including laminin, collagen, and fibronectin. They not only provide mechanical linkers to the surrounding matrix, but they also participate in signal transduction and influence migration, proliferation, and apoptosis.

The cancer cell is now able to dissociate from the tumor mass and to move toward the vessels, but there are still several obstacles within the interstitial matrix, including proteoglycans, glycoproteins, and filament proteins. The cell must be able to break these down to successfully invade through tissues. This is known as *proteolysis,* and four major groups of proteases play an important role: (1) matrix metalloproteinases (MMPs); (2) serine proteinases; (3) cysteine proteinases; and (4) aspartate proteinases (Table 2-2).

BOX 2–5 STEPS IN ACTIVE LOCOMOTION

- Protrusion of a cellular projection (pseudopodia)
- Organization of the adhesion receptors at the front, with binding to the extracellular matrix
  - Mediated by integrins
- Adhesion receptors at the back of the cell release
- Traction force is generated by the contraction and reinforcement of the actin cytoskeleton
  - Actin polymerization mediated by Rho-like guanosine triphosphatases

Matrix metalloproteinases are a family of zinc-binding enzymes that are secreted as proenzymes. After they have been activated in the extracellular matrix, they cleave components of the ECM. It is not surprising that the increased expression of MMPs correlates strongly with the invasiveness of the tumor. Urokinase plasminogen activator (uPA), which is a serine protease, is also secreted as an inactive proenzyme (pro-uPA). Upon binding to its receptor, uPAR, it becomes an active enzyme that catalyses plasminogen to plasmin. Plasmin then degrades tissue proteins, and it is also capable of activating the MMPs. Inhibitors to proteolysis exist as well. Tissue inhibitors of metalloproteinases prevent the subsequent activation of the MMP proenzymes, and plasminogen activator inhibitors regulate uPA. These molecules serve as important regulators of invasiveness and the metastatic process.

Embolization, Arrest, and Extravasation

Tumor cells that have broken free and moved through the surrounding tissue now need to successfully invade into the vasculature. The process by which this occurs is called *intravasation,* and it requires coordinated proteolysis and locomotion. However, the mere presence of tumor cells in the blood does not constitute metastasis, and the vast majority of circulating tumor cells do not lead to the formation of metastases. Tumor cells are much more likely to survive in the circulation if they form

TABLE 2–2 • *Molecules Causing Degradation of the Extracellular Matrix*

Type	Specific Molecules
Matrix metalloproteinases	Interstitial collagenases Stromelysins (stromelysins-1, 2, and 3; matrilysin) Gelatinases (type IV collagenases)
Serine proteinases	Urokinase plasminogen activator Tissue-type plasminogen activator Elastase Cathepsin G
Cysteine proteinases	Cathepsin B Cathepsin L
Aspartate proteinases	Cathepsin D

aggregates. Cells that enter the vasculature through intravasation and that travel as tumor emboli are less prone to succumb to mechanical trauma or the immune system and more likely to arrest in capillary beds and survive. These emboli are formed from fibrin deposits and platelet aggregation around the tumor cells. This process is assisted by the production of procoagulant factors such as thromboplastin and procoagulant-A, and it may be associated with the increased coagulability observed among cancer patients.

These tumor emboli must then *arrest* somewhere. Large tumor cell aggregates, which are composed of either tumor cells alone (homotypic) or combined with lymphocytes and platelets (heterotypic), are likely to be trapped in small-diameter vessels by a simple wedging process. This is not the only process by which tumor cell arrest occurs. Tumor emboli attach firmly to the internal layer of the intima of a vessel. This may be aided in heterotypic emboli by the platelets and lymphocytes clumped together with the tumor cells in the tumor emboli and regulated by mechanisms similar to the way these cells normally attach to the intima. After they have been arrested, however, the cells must *extravasate* through the vessel wall to grow in the extravascular tissue. This is assisted by the presence of temporary gaps in the basement membrane, which are exposed through the typical wear and tear of endothelium or by the retraction of endothelial cells in response to the tumor cells. After being exposed to the ECM, the tumor cell can invade into the extravascular tissue using the same process of proteolysis and motility that allowed it to invade into the vessels in the first place.

Metastatic Growth and Proliferation

Finally, the tumor cells, having successfully relocated, need to proliferate in their new environment. This may be the most difficult part of their journey (Figure 2-5). Although the overwhelming majority of cancer cells released into the vasculature are eliminated, a significant percentage survive the journey intact and even successfully extravasate. This suggests that the metastatic inefficiency of circulating tumor cells may be more related to postextravasation growth than intravascular tumor cell destruction.

Tumor cell proliferation in foreign tissue is either stimulated or inhibited by a complex combination of autocrine, paracrine, and endocrine signals. The presence of stimulatory or inhibitory growth factors in a particular tissue correlates with the site-specific pattern of metastasis. For example, stromal cells in bone produce a growth factor that stimulates prostate cancer cells. Human colon cancer cells respond to certain growth factors that regulate tissue repair in the liver (e.g., hepatocyte growth factors). These may explain these cancers' predilection for those sites. Finally, for the deposits to grow beyond 2 mm in size, they must again initiate angiogenesis to develop a vascular network.

Tumor cells may successfully metastasize but fail to grow, instead remaining viable with full tumorigenic potential; this phenomenon is referred to as *tumor dormancy*. Clinically, this may lead to the recurrence of disease many years after the successful removal of the primary tumor. The mechanisms by which this occurs, however, remain a mystery. One possibility is that the cells are nonproliferative, remaining in the G_0 phase of the cell cycle and thus protected from the host's defenses. Alternatively, the cells may be dividing, but this is offset by a high rate of cell death. Another possibility is that the cells do not possess the capability to promote angiogenesis in the new tissue and so cannot grow beyond 2 mm in size. What triggers these cells to exit the dormant phase and to develop into clinically relevant metastases is an area of active investigation.

Host Defenses Against Metastases

As stated, the majority of cells that enter the vasculature will not successfully establish metastatic deposits. In many cases, this is because they lack one of the essential components of successful metastasis described. However, even if the cell has all the necessary machinery to metastasize, there are other factors that may regulate this process. Much of this regulation is organ specific, which goes back to the original "seed and soil" concept. Tumor cells can reach the microvasculature of many organs, but extravasation and growth can only occur in some organs. In part, this is related to tissue-specific differences between the organ of origin and the site of metastases, such as gradients of pH, oxygen, nutrients, and cell waste products. Differences in the stroma and the ECM of organs may result in tumors that may be able to invade through the stroma of one

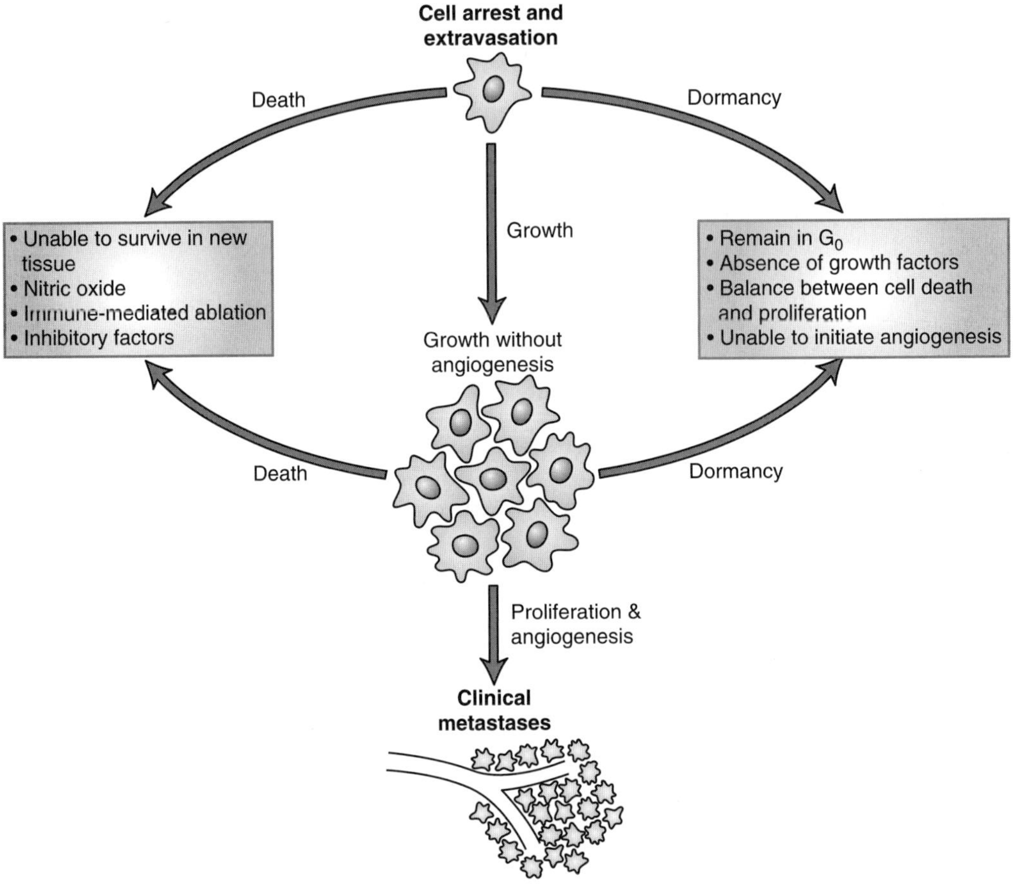

Figure 2–5. Potential fates of metastatic cells that have successfully relocated.

organ but that are not able to invade through the ECM of a different organ. On top of this, different organs may produce higher levels of metastasis-inhibitory factors. These include antiproteolysis factors, such as tissue inhibitors of metalloproteinases or plasminogen activator inhibitors, or antiangiogenic factors, such as angiostatin, platelet factor-4, IFN-α, IFN-β, or prolactin.

Another defense against metastasis is nitric oxide (NO), which is a highly reactive free radical. The terminal guanido-nitrogen of L-arginine is catalyzed into NO by the enzyme nitric oxide synthase (NOS). This enzyme is constitutively expressed in neuronal and endothelial cells (cNOS) and can be induced in several cells (particularly macrophages) by inflammatory cytokines, endotoxin, hypoxia, and oxidative stress (iNOS).There are many effects of NO that can be detrimental to metastasis, including the regulation of vasodilation and platelet aggregation (which affect tumor cell arrest), the destruction of tumor cells, and the induction of apoptosis.

BOX 2–6 NITRIC OXIDE

- Derived from the terminal nitrogen of L-arginine
- L-arginine is catalyzed by constitutive nitric oxide synthase or inducible nitric oxide synthase
- Regulates vasodilation and platelet aggregation, thus preventing tumor cell arrest
- Capable of destroying tumor cells passing through capillary beds

Finally, the immune system has a possible role in the ability of a tumor to metastasize. It is well documented that tumor cells are susceptible to destruction by antibody-dependent cellular cytotoxicity, natural killer cells, and cytotoxic T cells. However, the role that the immune system plays in the prevention of metastasis is unclear. Cancer cells are extremely heterogeneous in their antigenicity, immunogenicity, and susceptibility to immune-mediated death. In patients with certain cancers, immune suppression increases the incidence of metastasis, whereas, in patients with other cancers, depression of host immunity has no effect on metastatic potential. The immune system can both inhibit and stimulate tumor growth, and the factors that determine this are not fully elucidated. Even when tumors are highly antigenic, and even if the host recognizes these antigens, metastases may not be able to be eliminated by immunologic means (see Chapter 7: Principles of Immunotherapy).

Applying Principles of Cellular Biology to Cancer Treatment

Clinically, a significant percentage of patients who undergo successful treatment of their primary tumor will develop recurrence with metastatic disease as a result of the presence of undetectable micrometastases at the time of therapy. The use of adjuvant chemotherapy will improve these odds for many types of cancers, but the commonly used methods for predicting the likelihood of recurrence (tumor size, grade, nodal status) do not sufficiently identify those patients most likely to benefit from chemotherapy. One result of this is that many patients whose tumors did not spread and who were cured by surgery alone are unnecessarily subjected to the morbidity of chemotherapy. Predicting the metastatic potential of an individual patient's tumor would allow clinicians to better select patients to receive adjuvant therapy. Many of the factors described in this chapter correlate with prognosis, but they have not been specific enough to significantly influence clinical management for an individual patient. The development of metastasis requires multiple steps, each of which is regulated by the activation or deactivation of many specific genes. Microarray gene analysis is a new technique that can rapidly examine thousands of genes within a tumor and determine which genes are overexpressed or underexpressed. This provides a profile that may predict a tumor's ability to metastasize and that may allow for the better selection of which patients may benefit from adjuvant therapy.

In addition to better selecting patients to receive present adjuvant therapies, increased understanding of the pathways involved in metastasis will identify areas for new, targeted therapies. For example, targeting vascular endothelial growth factor may prevent metastases (Figure 2-6). Bevacizumab (Avastin) is an antibody that targets and inhibits vascular endothelial growth factor. When VEGF is targeted and bound to Avastin, it cannot stimulate the growth of blood vessels, thus denying tumors blood, oxygen and other nutrients needed for growth. Avastin has been approved for the treatment of colorectal cancer. Other examples of ways the steps of invasion and metastasis may be specifically targeted for therapy are described in Box 2-7.

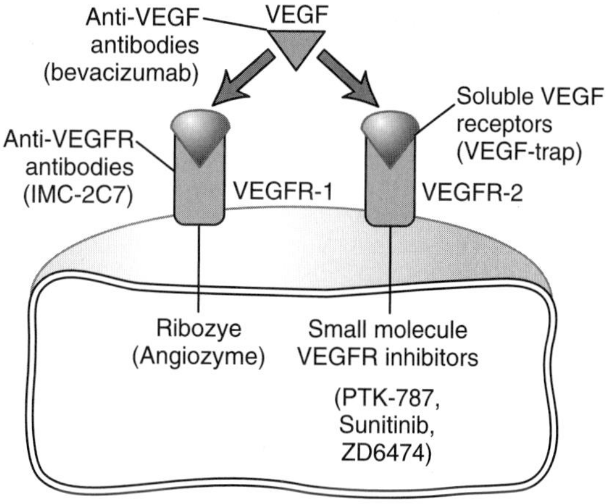

Figure 2-6. Possible methods for targeting vascular endothelial growth factor and vascular endothelial growth factor receptors as anticancer therapy.

BOX 2-7 POTENTIAL THERAPIES TARGETED AT TUMOR METASTASES

- Using anticoagulation and antiplatelet agents to prevent tumor cell embolization and arrest
- Using antiangiogenic factors to prevent tumor angiogenesis and growth
- Inducing the expression of inducible nitric oxide synthase to produce nitric oxide and prevent tumor cell arrest
- Preventing membrane degradation by matrix metalloproteinases (e.g., blocking activation of the proenzyme)
- In vivo transfection of tumor cells with E-cadherin to suppress invasion
- Using inhibitors of proteolysis (tissue inhibitors of metalloproteinases or plasminogen activator inhibitors)

Key Suggested Reading

Brodt P., (ed.) *Surgical Oncology Clinics of N.A.: Cancer Metastasis: Biological and Clinical Aspects,* Philadelphia: WB Saunders, 2001.

Suggested Readings

Bogenrieder T, Herlyn M. Axis of evil: molecular mechanisms of cancer metastasis, *Oncogene* 2003;22: 6524–6536.

Cavallaro U, Christofori G. Cell adhesion and signaling by cadherins and Ig-CAMs in cancer, *Nat Rev Cancer* 4:118–122, 2004.

Chirco R, Liu XW, Jung KK, Kim HR. Novel functions of TIMPs in cell signaling. *Cancer Metastasis Rev* 2006;25:99–113.

Coussens LM, Fingleton B, Martrisian LM. Matrix metalloproteinase inhibitors and cancer: trials and tribulations, *Science* 2002;295:2387–2392.

Deryugina EI, Quigley JP. Matrix metalloproteinases and tumor metastasis. *Cancer Metastasis Rev* 2006;25:9–34.

Dvorak HF. Vascular permeability factor/vascular endothelial growth factor: a critical cytokine in tumor angiogenesis and a potential target for diagnosis and therapy, *J Clin Oncol* 2002;20:4368–4380.

Eschrich S, Yeatman TJ. DNA microarrays and data analysis: an overview. *Surgery* 2004;136:500–503.

Fearon ER, Vogelstein B. A genetic model for colorectal tumorigenesis, *Cell* 1990;61:759–767.

Fidler IJ. Seed and soil revisited: contribution of the organ microenvironment to cancer metastasis, *Surg Oncol Clin N Am* 2001;10:257–269.

Fidler IJ, Hart IR. Biological diversity in metastatic neoplasms: origins and implications, *Science* 1982;217: 998–1003.

Folkman J. Tumor angiogenesis: a possible control point in tumor growth, *Ann Intern Med* 1975;82:96–100.

Folkman J. Angiogenesis. *Ann Rev Med* 2006;57:1–18.

Hanahan D, Weinberg RA. The hallmarks of cancer, *Cell* 2000;100:57–70.

Hicklin DJ, Ellis LM. Role of the vascular endothelial growth factor pathway in tumor growth and angiogenesis. *J Clin Oncol* 2006;23:1011–1027.

Hurwitz HL, Novotny W, Cartwright T, *et al.* Bevacizumab plus irinotecan, fleurouracil, and leucovorin for metastatic colorectal cancer, *N Engl J Med* 2004;350:2335–2342.

Jodele S, Blavier L, Yoon JM, DeClerck YA. Modifying the soil to affect the seed: role of stromal-derived matrix metalloproteinases in cancer progression. *Cancer Metastasis Rev* 2006;25:35–43.

Liotta LA, Steeg PS, Stetler-Stevenson WG. Cancer metastasis and angiogenesis: an imbalance of positive and negative regulation, *Cell* 1991;64:327–336.

Mocellin S, Provenzano M, Rossi CR, *et al.* DNA array-based gene profiling: from surgical specimen to molecular portrait of cancer. *Ann Surg* 2004;241:16–26.

Nowell PC. The clonal evolution of tumor cell populations, *Science* 1976;194:23–28.

Paget S. The distribution of secondary growths in cancer of the breast, *Lancet* 1889;1:571.

Pantel K, Brakenhoff RH. Dissecting the metastatic cascade, *Nat Rev Cancer* 2004;4:448–456

Schwartz GK, Shah MA. Targeting the cell cycle: a new approach to cancer therapy. *J Clin Oncol* 2005;23:9408–9421.

Stetler-Stevenson WG. Invasion and metastases. In: Devita VT, Hellman S, Rosenberg SA, editors: *Cancer: principles & practice of oncology,* ed 7, Philadelphia: Lippincott Williams and Wilkins, 2005.

3

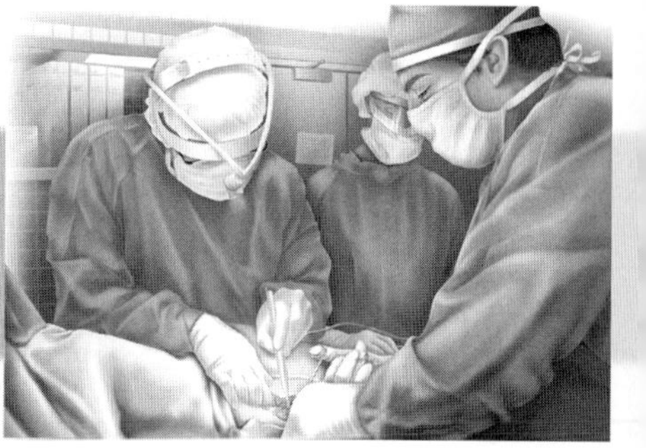

Basic Epidemiologic Methods for Cancer Investigations

Dana E. Rollison and Michael S. Sabel

Basic Epidemiologic Methods for Cancer Investigations: Key Points

- Distinguish between the three main types of epidemiologic studies.
- Define the terms *incidence, prevalence,* and *mortality*.
- Discuss the factors to consider in the various methods of sampling.
- Compare risk, relative risk, and attributable risk.
- Explain the principles governing patient selection for a clinical trial.
- Evaluate the various survival endpoints used in clinical trials.
- Analyze the concepts of error and statistical significance.
- Explain how bias influences an epidemiologic study.

As surgical oncologists, it is incumbent upon us to continuously evaluate the impact that our therapies are having and to search for new therapies that may improve patient outcomes or minimize morbidity. Surgical research can range from the basic science laboratory to the design of and participation in clinical trials to the retrospective review of one's own experience. Even those surgeons who do not directly participate in research must still possess an understanding of the principles of research so that they can interpret the literature and keep their practice current. This chapter will provide an overview of basic epidemiologic principles as they relate specifically to cancer research.

Types of Epidemiologic Studies

Descriptive Studies

Cancer epidemiology is the study of the distribution of cancer and its determinants among defined populations. Epidemiologic methods can be used to investigate cancer etiology; to evaluate the efficacy of interventions for cancer prevention, detection, or treatment; and to assess the burden of disease on society. There are many different types of epidemiologic studies, each with its advantages and disadvantages. Understanding the inherent limitations of studies is imperative for the interpretation of literature and the conducting of clinical research. The most basic types of epidemiologic studies are descriptive, in which rates of cancer incidence or mortality are described for specific populations over a certain period of time.

Incidence, Prevalence, and Mortality

The magnitude of cancer in a given population may be described using several different measures. Two simple measures are the **total number of new cancer cases** diagnosed within a given time period and the **total number of individuals living with cancer** during a given time period. Absolute numbers of cases may be useful for health care planning, because these are the numbers of patients who will require medical care. However, absolute numbers of cases do not take into account the size or the nature of the underlying population at risk. The larger the underlying population, the greater the number of expected cancer cases. Similarly, the age of the underlying population is crucial, because older age is the strongest overall cancer risk factor. **Total number of cancer deaths** is also determined in part by the size and age of the population at risk, in addition to other factors that may contribute to cancer survival (e.g., access to medical care).

The most commonly used population-based measures of cancer are incidence and mortality rates. These rates quantify the number of events in a specified population over a defined time period. Cancer **incidence** rates are defined as

BOX 3–1 MEASUREMENTS USED IN EPIDEMIOLOGY

$$\text{Incidence} = \frac{\text{Number of new cases diagnosed in a fixed time period}}{\text{Number of people at risk}}$$

$$\text{Prevalence} = \frac{\text{Number of people living with the disease}}{\text{Number of people at risk}}$$

$$\text{Mortality Rate} = \frac{\text{Number of cancer deaths in a fixed time period}}{\text{Number of people at risk}}$$

$$\text{Case Fatality Rate} = \frac{\text{Number of deaths from disease}}{\text{Number of people with the disease}}$$

$$\text{Proportional Mortality Ratio} = \frac{\text{Number of deaths from disease}}{\text{Total number of deaths}}$$

$$\text{Odds Ratio} = \frac{\text{Odds of exposure in cases}}{\text{Odds of exposure in controls}}$$

$$\text{Relative Risk} = \frac{\text{Incidence in exposed group}}{\text{Incidence in unexposed group}}$$

Attributable Risk among the exposed = Incidence in exposed group − Incidence in unexposed group the number of new cancer cases diagnosed during a fixed time period divided by the total population at risk. Cancer *mortality* rates are similarly defined as the number of cancer deaths during a fixed time period divided by the total population at risk. Population-based cancer incidence and mortality rates are typically expressed as the number of events per 100,000 individuals per year.

Although incident cancer cases include only those diagnosed during the specified time period, prevalent cases include all individuals living with cancer, regardless of when the cancer was diagnosed. Cancer *prevalence* can be described for a single point in time (i.e., "point prevalence") or for a defined time interval (i.e., "period prevalence"). *Point prevalence* may be expressed as the number of prevalent cases per number of individuals (e.g., per 100,000) or as a percentage or proportion, because time is not incorporated into the metric. *Period prevalence* is defined as the number of people with the disease divided by the total population during a defined period of time (typically 1 year). Although incidence is often used in studies of cancer etiology, prevalence is more relevant to the public health burden of cancer, because prevalent cases include all cases that involve accessing health care.

In parallel, the relationship between incidence and mortality rates depends on the fatality of the disease. Only when the disease is highly fatal and the interval between disease occurrence and death is short will mortality rates be similar to incidence rates. Cancers with which few people survive are said to have a high *case fatality rate,* which is equal to the number of deaths from a particular cancer divided by the total number of people diagnosed with that cancer. Case fatality rates are not technically rates, because they do not include time as a parameter and because they are frequently expressed as a proportion or percentage.

Age Adjustment

Incidence and mortality rates are often compared across different populations or over time to identify possible etiologies or to evaluate therapies. However, to maximize confidence that observed differences are indeed the result of a suspected etiologic factor or a therapy of interest, rate comparisons need to take into account other factors that may contribute to the observed differences. For example, age is the strongest risk factor for cancer overall. Therefore, a comparison of cancer incidence rates between two populations needs to consider the age distributions of the two populations. *Adjustment* (or *standardization*) is a method used to account for such differences between populations. Direct adjustment is one of two approaches that may be used to account for age and other factors.

Consider the following example. If one were to compare crude (i.e., unadjusted) cancer incidence rates between two different counties, A and B, located in state X and if the age distributions of residents within these two counties was known to differ greatly, then the following steps could be taken to account for age through direct adjustment. First, incidence rates would be calculated for each predefined age stratum in county A (i.e., ages 20–29, 30–39, 40–49, and so on) for a given year. These age-specific rates would then be applied to a standard population (i.e., the entire population of state X), and the rate would then by multiplied by the number of people in the given age stratum within the standard population. Cases are summed across age strata and divided by the total standard population to yield an age-adjusted incidence rate for county A; the same process would be conducted for county B. Comparing the age-adjusted cancer incidence rates for counties A and B ensures that any observed differences in rates are not the result of differences in age distributions across the two counties.

Age standardization may also be achieved through indirect adjustment whereby age-specific incidence rates from an external standard population are applied to the age-stratified population of interest to obtain the number of expected cancer cases. The observed number of cases is divided by the expected number of cases to yield a *standardized incidence ratio.* A standardized incidence ratio of greater than 1.0 indicates that there are more cancer cases in the population of interest than expected given the underlying age distribution. When cancer deaths are described instead of newly diagnosed cancer cases, the age-adjusted measure obtained is the *standardized mortality ratio.* Standardized mortality ratios are often used in epidemiologic studies of occupational exposures and cancer for comparing the observed number of cancer deaths in a given worker population with the number expected based on the general population. In addition to age, incidence and mortality rates are often adjusted for sex, race, or socioeconomic factors, all of which may affect cancer incidence or mortality rates.

Observational Studies

Although descriptive studies are an essential starting point for understanding the overall patterns of disease within a population, alternative study designs are needed for formal hypothesis testing. These studies include *experimental studies,* in which investigators deliver an intervention to one or more groups, and *observational studies,* in which investigators measure exposures and outcomes without intervening. Some types of studies may be relatively simple and inexpensive to conduct but challenging to interpret, whereas other, methodologically superior studies may be expensive, time-consuming, and, in some cases, unethical to conduct. For example, if one were interested in investigating whether exposure to asbestos was associated with a particular cancer, it would be unethical to expose some people to asbestos and then compare their cancer rates to a second experimental group of people who were not exposed. Therefore, observational studies are needed to investigate such etiologic questions. Although different study designs may be particularly useful for investigating different research questions, they all have some methodologic limitations, which must be considered when interpreting results.

Ecologic Studies

Ecologic studies investigate the correlation between an exposure and an outcome on the group level without including information about individuals. For example, an observed correlation between population-based national incidence rates of breast cancer and average dietary fat consumption for individual countries provides ecologic evidence for an association between dietary fat and breast cancer. Ecologic studies are relatively easy and inexpensive to conduct, because the data are usually readily available. However, ecologic studies do not incorporate data about individual exposures, and, thus, results should be interpreted with caution. The greater the variability in exposure levels within a given population, the less valid a population average will be as a surrogate for individual-level exposure. In the example, dietary fat consumption may vary greatly within a country, and it is not known whether women who had breast cancer also consumed diets high in fat. Additionally, average dietary fat consumption within a country may be associated with other socioeconomic factors, such as delayed childbearing, which may be more strongly related to breast cancer. When a factor is correlated with a disease in an ecologic study but the association is later disproved, the initial correlation is referred to as an *ecologic fallacy*. Although limited in design, ecologic studies may be particularly useful for generating hypotheses about the etiology of cancer, which may then be tested in studies of more sophisticated design.

Cross-Sectional Studies

Cross-sectional studies involve gathering information about a variety of factors at the individual level at a given point in time. In other words, they provide a "snapshot" view. As with ecologic studies, they are relatively simple to conduct, and they can be useful for generating new hypotheses. Because cross-sectional studies measure both the "exposure" and the "disease" at one point in time, these studies cannot establish the temporal sequence of these two factors. The relative timing of exposures is most important for those factors that may vary over time, such as diet, exercise, and medication history. For example, results from a cross-sectional survey of knee injuries and exercise might suggest that those who exercise regularly are less likely to have a knee injury. It is impossible to infer from these cross-sectional data whether exercise helps protect against injury or whether those with knee injuries were less likely to exercise as a result of pain caused by their injury.

One type of cross-sectional study is a population-based survey in which data are collected from a group of individuals and correlations between different factors are calculated. For example, data from the National Health Interview Survey (a population-based national survey that included questions about cancer screening use in 2000) was recently analyzed to assess factors associated with Papanicolaou (Pap) screening for cervical cancer. Women with low income and no health insurance coverage were less likely to have had a Pap test during the past 3 years. Inferences from these data are generalized to the entire U.S. population, although only 13,745 women were included in the survey. Clearly, it would have been impractical to study every woman in the United States, and, therefore, a representative *sample* of women was studied.

There are several techniques for selecting a subset of a population to study. *Probability sampling* refers to strategies used to choose that sample so that each individual has a predetermined probability of being selected. The simplest type of probability sampling is *random sampling,* with which each individual in the population has an equal chance of being chosen for the study. Random sampling maximizes the likelihood that the frequency distribution of a particular characteristic among the sample will be representative of the distribution among the underlying population. However, random sampling does not guarantee that the sample will be exactly equivalent to the underlying population; a particular subgroup may be oversampled or undersampled by chance alone. To minimize the probability that this will occur for a variable of importance, the researcher can identify key characteristics that may affect the final analysis (e.g., sex, age). Potential study participants are then divided into appropriate *strata* of these characteristics (i.e., "stratified") and randomly selected within these strata. *Stratified random sampling* helps ensure equal distributions of the stratified variables among the samples.

Although probability sampling helps to ensure that the sample is representative of the underlying population, it is not always employed in published studies. *Convenience sampling* is the process of selecting study participants from a group of individuals to which the researchers have easy access. For example, smaller medical studies will often incorporate blood samples from "healthy volunteers," sometimes including hospital or laboratory staff who may not represent the population as a whole (i.e., medical professionals may be more health conscious than the general population). Therefore, when evaluating published studies, it is important to critically assess the sampling strategy used, especially when the findings are generalized to the entire population.

Case-Control Studies

In the *case-control study* design, two groups of people are examined: one with the disease of interest ("cases") and one without the disease of interest ("controls"). Two common types of case-control studies of cancer are hospital-based studies and population-based studies, in which cancer cases may be identified through clinical centers or population-based cancer registries, respectively. Controls should be selected to be representative of the source population from which the cases arose (e.g., the controls would have been considered as study cases had they developed the disease). In hospital-based studies, possible sources of controls include spouses, friends, or visitors of the cases; patients with other types of cancer that would be unrelated to the exposure of interest; and patients of hospital departments other than oncology (e.g., orthopedics). Methods for identifying potential controls in population-based studies include random-digit dialing or driver's license records. Findings from population-based case-control studies may be generalized to all individuals in the underlying population, whereas hospital-based case-control studies are more prone to *selection bias.* Selection bias can result when cases and controls have different probabilities of selection into the study based on exposure status (see Bias and Confounding on page 36).

After cases and controls are selected, exposure data are obtained through a variety of methods, including questionnaires, interviews, and biomarker measurements. The prevalence of a given exposure is calculated separately for cases and controls, and the association between the exposure and cancer is estimated through calculation of an *odds ratio,* which is defined as the odds of exposure in the cases divided by the odds of exposure in the controls. An odds ratio of greater than 1 indicates that people with disease were more likely to have been exposed than people without disease, which suggests that there is an association between the exposure and the disease. Conversely, an odds ratio of less than 1 indicates that people with the disease were less likely to have been exposed, which suggests that the exposure may be protective against the disease. The odds ratio will approximate the *relative risk* when the disease or outcome is rare (see the description of relative risk in Cohort Studies below). This assumption holds true for most cancers.

The case-control design is ideal for studying rare diseases, including most cancers. Multiple exposures can be assessed with a case-control study, and multiple biospecimens are more easily obtained. Exposures are assessed retrospectively in case-control studies, and, therefore, temporality cannot be established. Additionally, retrospective exposure assessment entails problems of recall, whereby people have difficulty remembering exposures they may have encountered years before their cancer diagnosis. If case-control study participants know the study hypothesis before answering questions regarding exposures, *recall bias* may result; when this happens, the ability to recall exposures differs between cases and controls (see section on Bias and Confounding). However, because case-control studies are appropriate for the investigation of rare events, including most cancers, the case-control design is the most commonly used for epidemiologic investigations of cancer etiology.

Cohort Studies

A *cohort study* begins with the definition of two groups: one exposed to a factor of interest and the other unexposed to that factor. These two groups are then followed over time for cancer. Cohort studies can be either prospective, in which the investigator identifies the groups at the outset and follows them in real time, or retrospective, in which both baseline exposure and subsequent cancer incidence can be documented using historical records.

At the completion of a cohort study, the incidence of the disease in the exposed group is compared with that of the unexposed group. An association is estimated by a *relative risk,* which is the ratio of the cumulative incidence in the exposed group to the cumulative incidence of the unexposed group. (This could also be the mortality rate in the exposed group divided by the mortality rate in the unexposed group.) As was the case with the odds ratio, a relative risk of greater than 1 indicates that the exposed group had a higher risk of developing the disease than the unexposed group, whereas a risk ratio of less than 1 indicates that the exposure may be protective.

The *attributable risk* may also be calculated from a cohort study, and it represents the magnitude or proportion of disease that can be attributed to a particular exposure. The attributable risk for the exposed group is calculated by subtracting the incidence in the unexposed group from the incidence in the exposed group (see Text Box 3-1). The resulting incidence represents the extent of disease attributable to the exposure within the exposed group, taking into account the background risk of disease not associated with the exposure. Similarly, attributable risk may also be calculated for the total population by subtracting the incidence of disease in the unexposed group from the incidence of disease in the total population, where the incidence of disease in the total population is equal to the sum of the incidence of disease in the exposed and unexposed groups and weighted by the percentages of the population that are exposed or unexposed. Attributable risks may be expressed as a proportion for either the exposed group or the total population by dividing the attributable incidence by the total incidence in either the exposed group or the total population.

Because the magnitude of cancer associated with a given exposure in the general population is a function of both the strength of association between the exposure and cancer and the prevalence of that exposure, an exposure may be associated with a very high relative risk of cancer but a low attributable risk. For example, individuals belonging to families with Li–Fraumeni syndrome (a hereditary disorder associated with p53 dysfunction) are estimated to have 25 times the risk of developing central nervous system cancers by the age of 45 years as compared with the general population. However, only 4% of central nervous system cancers are attributed to Li–Fraumeni syndrome, because this disorder is extremely rare. Conversely, the relative risk of colon cancer associated with six main risk factors combined (obesity, physical inactivity, alcohol consumption, early adulthood cigarette smoking, red meat consumption, and low intake of folic acid from supplements) is only 2.0; however, together these factors account for an estimated 48% of colon cancer cases in the United States.

In addition to providing the data needed to calculate attributable risk, the cohort study design has several advantages. Cohort studies are ideal for investigating the natural history of a disease, because individuals may be followed forward prospectively, with the collection of certain measures repeated over time. In addition, multiple diseases or health outcomes may be compared between the exposed and unexposed groups (this cannot be done in case-control studies). The ability to establish temporality (the relative sequence of exposure and disease) is an important advantage of the cohort study. The establishment of the temporal relationship eliminates the potential misclassification of exposures as a result of recall.

Disadvantages of the cohort design include the inability to investigate exposures that were not ascertained at baseline, the limited ability to investigate rare diseases or health outcomes, and the relative expense required to follow large populations over long periods of time. These limitations are commonly encountered in studies of cancer etiology, because, unless the cohort under observation is a high-risk population, many subtypes of

BOX 3–2 EXAMPLE OF RELATIVE VS. ATTRIBUTABLE RISK

Assume that 2,000 women who took hormone replacement therapy (HRT) were followed for 10 years and that 40 developed breast cancer. An additional 1,500 women who did not take HRT were followed for the same amount of time, and 20 developed breast cancer.

The 10-year cumulative incidence of breast cancer for HRT users would be 40 out of 2,000, which equals 0.02, or 20 per 1,000.

The 10-year cumulative incidence of breast cancer for non-HRT users would be 20 out of 1,500, which equals 0.013, or 13 per 1,000

The *relative risk* of breast cancer among HRT users would be 40/2,000 ÷ 20/1,500, which equals 1.53.

This relative risk indicates that women who took HRT at baseline had a 53% increased risk of developing breast cancer over a 10-year period as compared with women who did not take HRT.

The *attributable risk* of breast cancer among HRT users would be 40/2,000 – 20/1,500, which equals 6.67 per 1,000.

This means that, over 10 years, for every 1,000 women who use HRT, 7 will develop breast cancer as a result of their use of HRT.

cancer are rarely diagnosed, and they are often associated with a long latency period. Another potential limitation of the cohort design is loss to follow up. Although losses will reduce sample size and statistical power, they may also introduce selection bias if those who are lost are different from those who are followed with respect to exposure status.

Nested Case-Control Studies

A commonly used design in cancer epidemiology is the *nested case-control study,* which incorporates features of both the cohort and the case-control study designs. The nested case-control design is particularly advantageous for studies of biologic precursors of cancer, because it reduces the number of biospecimens that need to be tested with a relatively minor loss in statistical efficiency. The investigator identifies cases of cancer diagnosed within an underlying cohort for which biospecimens (e.g., blood) have been previously banked. Controls are selected from cohort participants who did not develop cancer and who may be matched to the cases with regard to factors such as age and sex, usually at a ratio of one or two controls per case. For all cases and selected controls, the banked biospecimens are retrieved and tested in the laboratory for the biological precursor or "biomarker" of interest.

The following example of a nested case-control study describes an investigation of the association between circulating levels of antibodies to simian virus 40 (SV40) and the risk of developing non-Hodgkin lymphoma (NHL). Two cohorts were established in Washington County, MD, in 1974 and 1989, with blood specimens collected from more than 45,000 county residents. Cases of NHL diagnosed through 2003 were ascertained by linkage to the state cancer registry. If investigators had conducted a cohort study, then SV40 antibodies would have had to been measured in more than 45,000 blood samples, which is not cost-effective. Alternatively, the investigators selected a control group from the underlying cohort, matching two controls to each NHL case and measuring SV40 antibodies in the banked samples for the 170 cases and 340 controls. These antibody levels were then compared between the cases and controls to test the study hypothesis.

There are several advantages of the nested case-control study. For one, all cases and controls are from the same population. Because fewer study subjects exist than in full cohort studies and because much of the data are already gathered, the collection of data is less time-consuming and more cost-efficient. Finally, because exposures were assessed at baseline, a temporal relationship is established, and recall bias is eliminated.

Experimental Studies

In contrast with observational studies, experimental studies dictate that some aspect of the research is under the control of the researcher. The aim of the study is to determine how changes in the researcher's intervention (the independent variable) will affect some outcome (the dependent variable). Experimental or intervention studies in cancer can be conducted to evaluate the efficacy of cancer treatments, cancer screening tests, or dietary/behavioral/chemoprevention factors that may reduce the risk of cancer development (primary prevention), progression or recurrence (secondary prevention), or symptoms or treatment side effects (tertiary prevention).

TABLE 3-1 • *Clinical Trials*

Phase I	Evaluates safety
Phase II	Evaluates biologic response
Phase III	Evaluates efficacy
Phase IV	Evaluates the effectiveness of a drug in the general population after it has been approved

Types of Clinical Trials

A *phase I trial* is designed to evaluate the safety of the treatment (Table 3-1). In the case of a drug, it is often used to determine the dose that can be safely administered in the next set of trials. Phase I trials typically start with the administration of a low dose to a small group of patients (3 to 6). Participants in phase I trials are usually patients with advanced disease who have normal organ function. If no dose-limiting toxicity is seen, the dose is escalated for the next group of patients; this continues until the incidence of dose-limiting toxicity surpasses 33%. The recommended dose is then the highest dose for which the incidence of dose-limiting toxicity is less than 33%. Doses are usually escalated in steps, which are sometimes based on a modified Fibonacci sequence. Although this approach is designed to maximize patient safety, phase I trials may take a long time to complete, and large numbers of patients are often exposed to subtherapeutic doses. For this reason, other designs are being evaluated.

New treatments that are determined to be safe in phase I trials are evaluated for biologic response in *phase II trials*. Phase II trial participants are typically patients who have a likelihood of showing an effect but who have no other choices for effective therapy. These criteria translate to patients with good performance status and cancers that have not been exposed to many rounds of other therapies. As more effective therapies are developed and used clinically, the pool of patients that fits this description becomes increasingly limited.

The design of a phase II trial must include a clear definition of the response under investigation. To determine a response, the patient must have measurable disease, such as metastatic foci on a computed tomographic scan that can be objectively measured before and after treatment. A complete response (CR) is defined as the complete disappearance of disease. If the treatment is given to patients before surgical resection (e.g., such as is done with neoadjuvant trials), one must differentiate between a clinical complete response (cCR), which means disappearance on physical examination or imaging studies, and a pathologic complete response (pCR), which means no evidence of cancer is seen on the surgical specimen. A partial response (PR) reflects a lesion that decreases in size but does not completely disappear. PR is often defined by the percentage of change in the lesion, where a partial response may be defined by a decrease of more than 50% and a minor response defined by a decrease of less than 50%. *Stable disease* refers to lesions that did not change during therapy, whereas *progressive disease* refers to lesions that got larger.

The response rate (the percentage of patients who had a response to the therapy) can then be compared to a group of hisrtorical controls (previously recorded data from a reference group). If the response rate in the phase II trial is promising compared to historical controls, then further investigation is warranted. However, the treatment group may be critically different than the historical control group with respect to factors that change over time and are related to cancer survival, such as use of other medications and treatments. Therefore, phase II trials are useful in identifying treatments that should go on to phase III trials but do not provide satisfactory evidence to support clinical use.

Phase III trials of cancer are typically randomized trials designed to assess the efficacy of a new drug or intervention. In cancer treatment, the endpoints are more clinically relevant, and they include overall survival and symptom control. Overall survival and disease-free survival are often used in cancer screening trials, whereas cancer incidence is the ultimate endpoint in primary prevention trials. Regardless of the nature of the intervention and endpoints under investigation, a critical feature of the phase III trial design is participant selection and assignment to either the experimental group or a control group (either standard therapy or a placebo).

Patient Selection

For any particular trial, the eligibility criteria are established to determine which patients are suitable subjects for participation. Some eligibility criteria are necessary for safety (e.g., eliminating patients with renal disease from a trial involving a drug that requires renal clearance), whereas others are chosen to optimize the interpretation of the results. For example, some trials may restrict participants to patients who have a limited number of comorbid conditions so that treatment effects may be more easily distinguished from other underlying disease. The more narrow the eligibility criteria are, the more homogenous the study population will be, thus maximizing the ability to observe treatment effects. However, the narrower the eligibility criteria are, the less generalizable the results are to the general population. Once approved, new drugs may end up being wrongly used in subsets of patients who were not included in the the original trials. Also, narrow eligibility criteria makes it more difficult and expensive to enroll the required number of patients in the trial.

The method of assignment of eligible participants to a treatment or invention group in phase III trials has critical implications for the comparability of the two groups and the inferences that can be drawn from the observed results. Use of a nonrandom method of treatment assignment increases the probability that there may be important factors (other than the treatment) that differ between the two groups. For example, if patients with breast cancer were allowed to choose between two treatments (treatment A and treatment B), and treatment A required more time at the hospital, then working women may be more likely to select treatment B than nonworking women. If working women had different ethnic, socioeconomic, and/or physiologic profiles than nonworking women, and these factors were associated with prognosis, then any observed treatment effect would have to be adjusted for these confounding factors. Although confounders may be adjusted for in the statistical analysis of trials, not all confounders are measured or even known. Therefore, *randomization* is almost always used in phase III trials to achieve treatment and control groups that are comparable with respect to factors that may affect prognosis, including those that are unknown.

Random assignment to treatment groups is often conducted using random number tables (generated by computers) and assigning a number to each new subject. For example, if there are two groups, then all odd numbers could be allocated to one group, whereas all even numbers would be allocated to the other. Participants are usually allocated in blocks to avoid an imbalance in the number of participants between the two treatment groups if the study ends early. The randomization of subjects within successive blocks helps to ensure roughly equal-sized treatment and control groups, even with premature termination of the trial (Figure 3-1).

Because randomized treatment groups may be different by chance and because some factors are known to be strongly associated with the outcome a priori, *stratified randomization* may be conducted to ensure that confounding factors will be equally distributed between the two groups. To stratify samples, the researcher needs to identify characteristics that may affect the outcome if they are overrepresented in one group. For instance, if response is related to gender, the researcher may not want to take a chance that gender ends up not being equally distributed by chance, and so the subjects may be stratified by gender before randomization; this ensures an equal number of men and women in both groups. However, the more strata that are used, the larger the study population has to be, which may limit the practicality of the research.

The *masking* or *blinding* of study participants and/or investigators is essential for the minimization of bias in phase III trials. For example, sham procedures or placebo treatments may be used to mask treatment assignment, thus controlling for possible placebo effects. Ideally, investigators are also masked to the group assignment of each study participant to avoid potential bias in

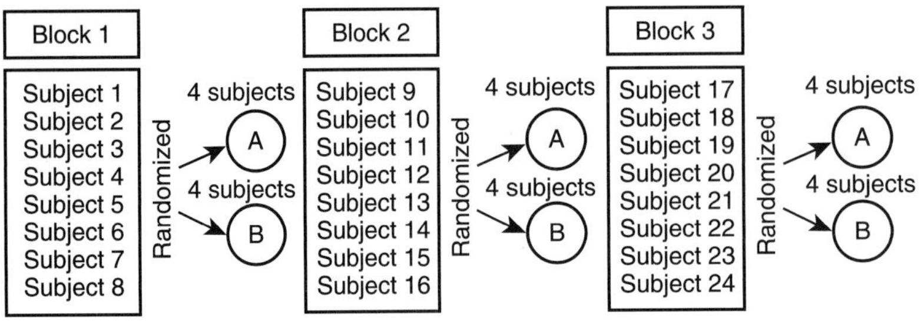

Figure 3–1. Block randomization of patients.

the assessment of clinical responses within participants. When both the investigators and the study participants are unaware of the group assignments, the study is considered ***double blind***.

Selection of Clinical Endpoints

The selection of a clinical endpoint in an experimental treatment trial has important implications for the inferences that will ultimately be drawn from the study results. In contrast with the indicators of biological response described for phase II trials above, clinical endpoints investigated in phase III treatment trials tend to be broader. The most global endpoint used in phase III cancer treatment trials is *overall survival,* which is defined as the proportion of people alive at a specified period after cancer diagnosis, regardless of cause of death. Five years has conventionally been used as the specified time period for cancer (i.e., the 5-year survival rate). Within any time period, a proportion of patients treated for cancer are going to die from their disease, and a proportion of patients are going to die from other diseases. In addition, some patients will have local-regional recurrences that are successfully treated, and others will develop distant recurrences but not die from them. To reflect these issues, survival rates are often qualified by the patient's disease status.

Disease-free survival refers to the proportion of people alive and without disease at a specified period after diagnosis. For example, a patient who is alive but who has liver metastases at the 5-year mark would be included in calculation of the overall survival rate but excluded from the disease-free survival rate. Overall survival and disease-free survival may provide different pictures of a new treatment. For example, an experimental treatment may increase disease-free survival but not overall survival, yet still could be important if overall quality of life is improved.

The definition of disease-free survival is important when interpreting results for overall survival, because some types of disease recurrence may not impact overall survival or be successfully treated. For example, in breast cancer, patients treated with breast conservation therapy may develop in-breast recurrences that can be treated by mastectomy without having a large impact on overall survival. In these situations, the researcher may be more interested in the proportion of patients who developed distant metastases, regardless of whether they had a local recurrence. *Distant disease–free survival* refers to the proportion of people alive and without distant metastases at a specified period after diagnosis, even if they had a local recurrence. The percentage of people who have survived a particular disease since diagnosis or treatment is known as disease-specific survival. Only deaths from the disease are counted; patients who died from some other cause are not counted. Cancer survival can be expressed in many ways, some of which may be appropriate for certain comparisons but inappropriate for others. Clinicians must understand the differences in the definitions of these measures to critically evaluate the appropriateness of the application of specific measures to different situations that commonly arise in the medical literature.

Survival Analysis

Survival curves are graphical tools that are commonly used to describe the survival experience of cancer patients in clinical treatment trials. In the case of a trial, a survival curve often represents the proportion of people alive (or alive without disease, in the case of disease-free survival), which is plotted on the y axis, as it corresponds with time, which is plotted on the x axis. The time metric can vary according to the objective of the analysis, and it may represent time since diagnosis or time since intervention. If the follow up of individuals is incomplete, then individuals must be "censored" at the time of loss to follow up or last observation if follow up is ongoing.

A common analytic tool used to calculate conditional survival probabilities while accounting for censored observations is the product limit method developed by Kaplan and Meier. Times of cancer deaths and censoring are ordered from least to greatest. At the time of the first cancer death, the number of patients alive is divided by the number of patients who were observed to survive up to the time of the event. The proportion of patients alive is calculated for all subsequent time points that correspond with patient deaths (e.g., the denominator at time point t does not include any individuals censored between time t-1 and time t). These probabilities are then plotted as a step function, which is commonly referred to as the *Kaplan–Meier curve* (Figure 3-2). A Kaplan–Meier curve is thus an estimate of the overall survival function. Importantly, the Kaplan–Meier analysis assumes that patients lost to follow up (censored observations) are similar to patients followed until the end of the study with respect to survival. One example of a violation of this assumption is if patients are lost to follow up because they fail to return to the clinic as a result of disease progression that renders them too sick to travel. In this scenario, the patients who are lost to follow up may have worse survival than patients who are followed throughout the study, and the analysis is then no longer valid.

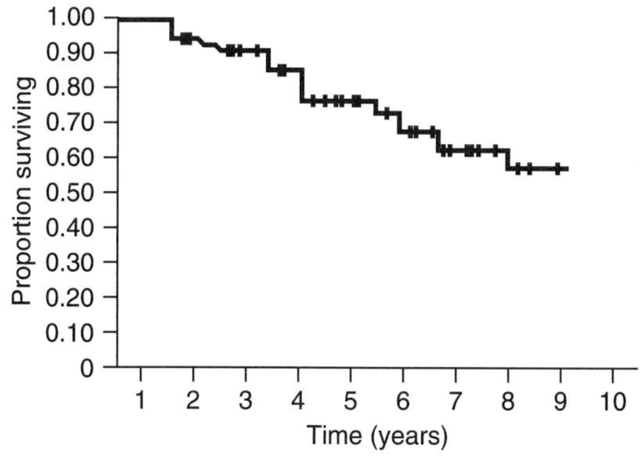

Figure 3-2. Kaplan–Meier survival curve. Intervals are defined by the survival times of the patients who have died. When graphed against time, the graph is a step function that starts at time 0 and ordinate 1.00. At each interval, the graph drops to the percentage of patients still alive. Tic marks are placed on the curve to represent the follow-up times of living patients.

Kaplan–Meier curves may be used to compare survival between two groups (e.g., experimental vs. standard therapy). After two curves are generated, the log-rank test (among others) may be used to determine the statistical significance of the observed difference between the two groups. If the two groups are thought to differ with respect to a factor that may influence survival (e.g., age), then other multivariable methods must be used to compare survival while adjusting for these factors (e.g., Cox proportional hazards). When applying statistical methods to evaluate the significance of observed differences in survival curves, it is essential to remember that these methods assume that the there is no interaction with time (i.e., the curves do not cross). For example, an intervention may be associated with improved survival immediately after the treatment but with worse survival overall. In this case, the survival curve for the intervention group would cross the curve for the control group. Analyzing the difference between these two curves would require careful consideration of this interaction with time.

Intention-to-Treat Analysis

One important principle when analyzing phase III trials is the *intention-to-treat* principle, which maintains patients in their original treatment assignment group for data analysis, regardless of crossover to another treatment group. If patients are excluded from the analysis for one reason or another, this can result in significant bias. For example, researchers studying a drug that needs to be taken every day for 6 months may wish to exclude patients in their analysis who did not take the drug for the full 6 months; they would argue that those patients are not valid because a poor outcome would be a result of a lack of compliance. However, it could be just the opposite; the patients with poorer outcomes ultimately stop taking the drug. Analyzing just the patients who finished the full 6 months of therapy would make the drug look effective when it truly was not. This is commonly seen in studies of neoadjuvant therapy before surgical resection. Consider an example in which patients with pancreatic cancer are randomized to a Whipple procedure followed by chemotherapy or to neoadjuvant chemotherapy followed by surgery. It is likely that the second group would have a repeat computed tomographic scan after chemotherapy and that some (the nonresponders) would have had progressive disease and would have not undergone the surgery. If comparisons are based solely on patients who had surgery, the results are biased in favor of neoadjuvant therapy by selecting out the worst patients (i.e., those who did not respond to the chemotherapy).

Interim Analyses and Stopping Rules

The decision to conduct an experimental study is a balanced consideration of the existing evidence in support of the intervention's efficacy and the degree of uncertainty surrounding this evidence. This balance is referred to as *clinical equipoise* and is a prerequisite for ethically conducting an experimental trial. If the evidence supporting the potential efficacy of an intervention is not compelling, then it is unethical to subject the participants to the unknown risks of the intervention. Conversely, if substantial evidence suggests that the intervention is efficacious, then it becomes unethical to withhold the intervention from the control group.

The balance of clinical equipoise may shift during the course of a trial as a result of preliminary observations from the study and/or the publication of results from other studies. Preliminary observations in a trial are formally assessed through *interim analyses,* which are planned at the outset of trial. For example, multicenter clinical trials are required to have a data-monitoring committee (independent from the researchers) that reviews results at designated time points during the trial. *Stopping rules* are predetermined guidelines for the level of evidence obtained from an interim analysis that would be required to terminate the trial prematurely. For example, the Women's Health Initiative, which was a randomized controlled trial of estrogen plus progestin for the prevention of coronary heart disease (along with other health endpoints), was stopped 3 years short of its 8.5-year design, in part as a result of an increased risk of breast cancer in the intervention group that was revealed by an interim analysis by the data-monitoring committee.

The Hawthorne Effect

Sometimes, the mere fact that you are closely examining a subject will have an impact on the outcome. This is classically called the *Hawthorne effect;* the term was originally used to describe the fact that worker productivity improved when factory illumination was increased and that it then improved again when illumination was decreased. It was not the illumination that increased worker productivity; rather, it was the fact that the workers were being watched more carefully. Similarly, participation in a clinical trial may affect how participants behave. If they know that they are being watched, people may avoid other unhealthy behaviors, or they may be quicker to contact a physician for a symptom than if they were not participating in a trial. Therefore, a treatment that is proven efficacious during a phase III trial may not be effective when introduced in practice. Factors that contribute to *effectiveness* include patient adherence to treatment, interactions with other medications, sociodemographic and lifestyle differences between the clinical trial participants and the general population, and long-term effects that were not observed in shorter-term trials. Post-marketing surveillance studies—sometimes referred to as *phase IV trials*—are observational studies that assess the effectiveness of a drug in the general population after it has been approved. Also, and more importantly, phase IV trials can detect late or rare adverse events that were not revealed in phase I, II, or III trials.

Sample Size and Statistical Significance

Type I and II Errors

Associations observed between two factors or differences observed between two groups may be true or spurious (i.e., the result of chance). To express the probability that an observed finding results from chance, a measure of statistical significance is calculated. The P value is one parameter used to convey statistical significance, and it represents the probability of obtaining the observed difference (or one more extreme) if the null hypothesis (no actual difference) is true. For example, if prostate-specific antigen (PSA) levels were compared between one group receiving an experimental treatment and another group receiving the standard of care, the null hypothesis would state that PSA levels do not differ between the two groups. The P value in this scenario would be interpreted as the probability of obtaining the observed difference in

PSA levels (or an even greater difference) if there truly was no difference between the two groups. Rejecting the null hypothesis when the null hypothesis is actually true is called a *type I error* (or α error), and a 5% probability for a type I error is conventionally considered to be acceptable in the literature. Thus, *P* values of less than .05 are deemed statistically significant. It is important to understand that the *P* value is a function of the magnitude of the difference between the two groups and the sample size of each group; thus, an association that is not statistically significant in a population of 20 may be statistically significant in a population of 100. However, the likelihood of the null hypothesis being falsely rejected is the same in both studies—namely 5%.

The conventional approach to testing the statistical significance of an observed risk ratio (i.e., odds ratio or relative risk) is to calculate the 95% confidence interval around the point estimate. In mathematical terms, the 95% confidence interval is the range in which one would expect the observed risk ratio to fall 95 times if the experiment was repeated 100 times. The null hypothesis states that the risk ratio equals 1.0, indicating that there is no difference between the two groups (in terms of the odds of exposure or the incidence of the endpoint). Therefore, if the confidence interval excludes 1.0, then the observed risk ratio is called *statistically significant*. If the confidence interval includes 1.0, then the observed association is not statistically significant, which means that the probability that the true risk ratio equals 1.0 is greater than 5%. Similar to the *P* value, the width of the confidence interval will decrease with increasing sample size.

Because measures of statistical significance are functions of sample size, investigators need to consider the sample size required to detect the expected difference between the two groups during the design phase of the study. When designing a phase III trial, the investigator estimates the magnitude of the expected difference in the outcome between the treatment and control groups and calculates the number of patients required to maximize the probability that this difference would be detected at a statistically significant level, assuming that the difference was real. This probability, which is also called *statistical power*, is equal to 1 minus the probability of committing a *type II error* (or β error), where the type II error is the probability of accepting the null hypothesis when the null hypothesis is untrue. Generally, one calculates sample size to achieve 80% or 90% power to detect a specified difference between the two groups at a significance level of 0.05. The difference between the groups is determined a priori, based on prior knowledge or, in a clinical trial, based on the smallest difference that is considered clinically important.

Superiority and Non-Inferiority Trials

A common error in research occurs when the failure of one treatment to prove itself superior to another is used to conclude that the two treatments are equivalent. Most trials are designed to show that one treatment is better than another, and the statistical design is such that the null hypothesis will be rejected; these are referred to as *superiority trials*. However, sometimes a researcher wants to show that an alternative treatment is not superior to the standard of care but rather that it is equal to it. Perhaps it is less morbid and the researcher wants to demonstrate that the same results can be obtained with fewer side effects, or maybe the researcher wants to demonstrate that the new treatment is better than no treatment but a no-treatment arm is not feasible. In these situations, investigators attempt to demonstrate therapeutic equivalence to an effective treatment.

Using a superiority trial to postulate therapeutic equivalence is a common error. Failure to reject the null hypotheses in a superiority trial may simply reflect an adequate sample size or an ineffectiveness of the standard treatment in this setting. When one wishes to conclude that a new treatment is equal to an old treatment, the trial must be designed as a *non-inferiority trial*. However these trials require large sample sizes to be meaningful, generally much larger than standard superiority trials.

Multiple Comparisons

Repeatedly performing statistical significance tests on multiple comparisons within a single study population increases the probability that one of these differences will test statistically significant by chance alone. For example, if a trial is designed to compare overall survival after 3 years for metastatic colon cancer patients treated with surgical resection versus chemotherapy alone, and overall survival is compared every 3 months over the course of trial, the probability that one of these comparisons will test statistically significant is greater than 0.05. If, based on these data, the authors conclude (and publish) that survival was significantly improved with surgical resection after 2 years, they have a greater chance of committing a type I error. Whenever published results do not represent a predesigned interim or final analysis, their statistical significance should be considered suspect.

Multiple comparisons can also be a limitation of analyses at the end of a study. For example, if 100 functional single nucleotide polymorphisms are measured in a single case-control study, five statistically significant associations may be observed as a result of chance alone. Some methods have been proposed to correct for multiple comparisons, including the Bonferroni method, whereby the α value is calculated as 0.05 divided by the number of comparisons. However, there is no one best method for correction.

Criteria for Assessing Causality

Because any study will have some probability of type I and II errors and because all studies have inherent methodologic limitations, the replication of findings across studies becomes an important tool for determining that an observed difference is true or that an observed association is causal. For this reason, the U.S. Food and Drug Administration will rarely approve a drug until at least two studies demonstrate a statistically significant benefit. Similarly, etiologic associations are not accepted as being causal until they are observed in multiple studies across different populations. Replication of findings, however, is only one of the criteria used to assess causality in epidemiology.

In 1964, the U.S. Department of Health issued a report about smoking and health that listed the criteria for causal inference; this was subsequently revised by Sir A. Bradford Hill in 1965 and by others in later years (Table 3-2). An association between an exposure and disease may be considered causal if the association is of strong magnitude and consistently observed across multiple study populations. Additionally, the exposure should be specifically associated with a particular disease, and higher levels of exposure should be associated with a greater risk of the disease (i.e., dose-response association). The association should be biologically plausible and coherent with existing knowledge about the natural history of the disease. Other explanations for the association should be considered and ruled out. Finally, the removal or elimination of the exposure should result in decreased risk of the disease. Although not all of these criteria will be applicable in every situation, they provide an important guide for an integrated review of existing evidence generated from a variety of scientific disciplines.

Evaluating Diagnostic Tests

A significant portion of oncology is diagnostic and involves trying to diagnose and stage cancer through serum assays, x-rays, and an

TABLE 3–2 • *Hill's Criteria of Causation*

The strength of the association	The stronger the association between cause and effect, the greater the chance of causation.
The consistency of the association	The association should be seen across numerous studies by different research teams.
The specificity of the association	The cause should lead to only one outcome, and the outcome should result from a single cause (however, this is rarely true in cancer epidemiology).
The temporal relationship	The cause must precede the outcome.
The biologic gradient (i.e., the dose-response relationship)	More exposure should lead to a higher incidence of the disease.
Biologic plausibility	The association should make sense from the perspective of biology.
Coherence (i.e., consistency with other knowledge)	The causal relationship should not conflict with what is known about the disease.
Consideration of alternate explanations	Alternate explanations for the observed association should be considered and ruled out.
Cessation of exposure	Eliminating the exposure should result in a decreased risk of disease.

increasing array of more advanced tests. Detecting cancer early through screening tests is also crucial to the secondary prevention of cancer. Therefore, evaluating the performance of these tests is critical to understanding both their uses and their limitations. Measures of a diagnostic test's validity are based on comparisons between true disease status and test results, as mapped in the 2-by-2 table in Figure 3-3. Observations in cell A represent the true positives (the patients who have the disease and who test positive for the disease). Cell B contains the false positives (those without disease who test positive for the disease). Observations in cell C are the false negatives (those patients who have the disease but who tested negative for the disease), and cell D includes the true negatives (those who the test accurately reported to not have the disease).

Sensitivity is the ability of a test to detect the disease when the disease is truly present (Table 3-3), and it is calculated by dividing the number of people with disease who test positive (true positives) by the total number of people with disease (true positives plus false negatives), or A/(A+C). *Specificity* is the ability of a test to correctly identify people who do not have the disease, and it is calculated by dividing the number of people without disease who test negative (true negatives) by the total number of people without disease (true negatives plus false positives), or D/(B+D). The false-positive rate is the percentage of people without the disease who have a positive test (B/[B+D]), whereas the false-negative rate is the percentage of people who have the disease who have a negative test (C/[A+C]).

Test result	True disease status: Patient has disease	True disease status: Patient does not have disease
Positive	A True positive	B False positive
Negative	C False negative	D True negative

Figure 3-3. Accuracy of diagnostic and screening tests.

Two additional measures of test performance include the positive and negative predictive values. The positive predictive value is the probability that a positive test result was obtained from a person who truly has the disease, and it is calculated by dividing the number of people who test positive and have the disease (true positives) by the total number of people who test positive (true positives plus false positives), or A/(A+B). Whereas the denominator for sensitivity was the total number of people who had the disease, the denominator for the positive predictive value is the total number of people who tested positive. The negative predictive value is the probability that a person with a negative test result truly does not have the disease. The negative predictive value is calculated by dividing the number of people without disease who test negative (true negatives) by the total number of people who test negative (true negatives plus false negatives), or D/(C+D).

TABLE 3–3 • *Measures of Diagnostic Validity and Accuracy*

True-positive rate (sensitivity)	$\frac{\text{People with positive test and disease}}{\text{All people with disease}}$	$\frac{A}{A+C}$
False-negative rate	$\frac{\text{People with negative test and disease}}{\text{All people with disease}}$	$\frac{C}{A+C}$
True-negative rate (specificity)	$\frac{\text{People with negative test and no disease}}{\text{All people without disease}}$	$\frac{D}{B+D}$
False-positive rate	$\frac{\text{People with positive test and no disease}}{\text{All people without disease}}$	$\frac{B}{B+D}$
Positive predictive value	$\frac{\text{People with positive test and disease}}{\text{All people with positive test}}$	$\frac{A}{A+B}$
Negative predictive value	$\frac{\text{People with negative test and no disease}}{\text{All people with negative test}}$	$\frac{D}{C+D}$
Accuracy	$\frac{\text{All true tests}}{\text{All tests}}$	$\frac{A+D}{A+B+C+D}$

Sensitivity and specificity are measures of diagnostic or screening test *validity*, and they are characteristic of the test, regardless of the setting in which it is used. Positive and negative predictive values vary with the prevalence of the disease in the population being tested. Specifically, the positive predictive value is positively correlated with disease prevalence, whereas the negative predictive value is inversely correlated with disease prevalence. A positive test result is more likely to be a true positive if the test is conducted in a population with a high prevalence of disease (see also Box 3-3). Finally, the *accuracy* of the test is defined as all of the true findings (A + D) divided by all of the findings (A + B + C + D).

Bias and Confounding

As stated throughout this chapter, methodologic limitations are inherent to epidemiologic studies, and they should be considered when interpreting study findings. When scrutinizing your own research or reading a journal article, it is important to keep these potential limitations in mind and to ask yourself how they may have affected the results. Some references to bias have been made earlier in the chapter and are further discussed here. Gordis defines *bias* as "any systematic error in the design, conduct or analysis of a study that results in a mistaken estimate of an exposure's effect on the risk of disease." Biases can generally be classified into selection biases and information biases, depending on whether the systematic error occurs with regard to participant selection or data collection and analysis. Many biases have been named, although most of these names are not consistently used across studies. Therefore, the clearest way to discuss potential biases in a given study is to describe how the bias may have occurred and the anticipated effect on the observed results.

Selection Bias

Selection bias results from a systematic error in the selection or follow up of study participants. For example, in a hospital-based study of smoking and bladder cancer, smoking status is compared between bladder-cancer cases and hospital-employee controls, and a strong association is observed between smoking and bladder cancer. Although smoking may be associated with bladder cancer in truth, the observed association may be overestimated, because hospital employees may be less likely to smoke than the general population. Selection bias can also occur in cohort studies if the participants who are lost to follow up over the course of the study are different from the participants who were followed for the whole study with respect to baseline exposures. In other words, if the people lost

BOX 3-3 CHANGE IN POSITIVE PREDICTIVE VALUE WITH CHANGE IN PREVALENCE TEST WITH A SENSITIVITY OF 99% AND A SPECIFICITY OF 95%

Illustrated below is an example of how positive predictive value (PPV) decreases with decreasing disease prevalence. Given a screening test with a sensitivity of 99% and a specificity of 95%, the PPV is calculated for two values of disease prevalence: 50% and 10%:

The disease of interest is very common (50% prevalence):

- Of 2,000 subjects, 1,000 will have disease.
- A total of 990 true positives and 10 false negatives are expected based on 99% sensitivity.
- Of 2,000 subjects, 1,000 will not have the disease.
- A total of 950 true negatives and 50 false positives are expected based on 95% specificity.
- The PPV is calculated as 990/(990+50), which equals 95%.

The disease of interest is less common (10% prevalence):

- Of 2,000 subjects, 200 will have disease.
- A total of 198 true positives and 2 false negatives are expected based on 99% sensitivity.
- Of 2,000 subjects, 1,800 will not have disease.
- A total of 1,710 true negatives and 90 false positives are expected based on 95% specificity.
- The PPV is calculated as 198/(198+90), which equals 69%.

to follow up were more likely to be exposed at baseline than people who were not lost to follow up, then the observed association between exposure and disease will be underestimated.

Incidence-prevalence bias (or Neyman bias) can occur in studies of prevalent disease. As discussed above, disease prevalence is a function of incidence and duration. If an exposure is more often reported among prevalent cases as compared with controls, investigators may conclude that the exposure could be involved in the etiology of the disease. However, if the exposure was associated with survival with that disease (and not incidence) then the inference made from the observed association is biased.

Information Bias

Information bias occurs through systematic errors in data collection or analysis. For example, in a case-control study of maternal illness during pregnancy and childhood cancer, mothers of cases may more consistently remember minor colds and illnesses during pregnancy than mothers of controls, perhaps because mothers of cases have spent more time thinking about pregnancy and possible causes of the child's cancer. In this situation, maternal illness would appear to be associated with childhood cancer, even if it was not truly involved in the etiology of disease. This phenomenon is commonly referred to as *recall bias*.

Generally speaking, humans do not remember exposures that occurred years—or sometimes decades—previously with great accuracy. Difficulty remembering will result in misclassification of exposure, and, when the degree of misclassification is equal for cases and controls, it is called *nondifferential. Nondifferential misclassification* will always result in a bias toward the null. Misclassification can also occur with exposures measured through laboratory tests; this is often referred to as *measurement error*. If the degree of measurement error is known from other validation studies, it can sometimes be accounted for during the data analysis.

More subtle examples of information bias include a *diagnostic suspicion bias* or a *surveillance bias*. If investigators are following cohort participants for the occurrence of disease and the investigators know the exposure status of the participants, they may be more likely to ascertain cases of disease in the exposed versus the unexposed by virtue of increased surveillance. For example, in a cohort study of water pollution and leukemia, physicians follow a group of exposed individuals and a group of unexposed individuals for incidence of leukemia. Exposed participants, knowing the potential dangers of their exposure, might seek medical care more often for nonspecific findings than will unexposed participants. The physicians, knowing that the group was exposed, may obtain more imaging studies or laboratory tests than will be obtained for the unexposed group. Therefore, more subjects may be diagnosed with leukemia within the follow-up period of the study (thus resulting in a higher risk ratio), even though the same number of patients in both groups would have developed the disease had the study period been extended.

Lead-Time Bias

Lead-time bias is a type of information bias specific to screening studies, and it is highlighted here because of its implications for cancer screening trials. Lead-time bias occurs when a disease is detected by a screening or surveillance test at an earlier time point than it would have been if it had been diagnosed by its clinical appearance; this time lag or "lead time" during which the disease is asymptomatic is not taken into account during the survival analysis (Figure 3-4). If survival time is measured from the time of cancer diagnosis, then the apparent increased survival time in the screened as compared with the control group will in truth be an artifactual difference. For example, assume that a randomized trial of spiral computed tomographic screening for the early detection of lung cancer in a high-risk group of smokers compares the survival time between the screened group and a control group. If survival time is calculated from the point that the lung cancer was detected, then the scanning would falsely appear to have resulted in improved survival, when in reality those patients lived the same amount of time after the point at which the disease would have been diagnosed by clinical symptoms.

Confounding

A *confounder* is a factor that is associated with both the exposure and the disease of interest. Confounding occurs when an observed association between an exposure and disease is due in part or in total to the third factor. For example, women who obtain a higher degree of educa-

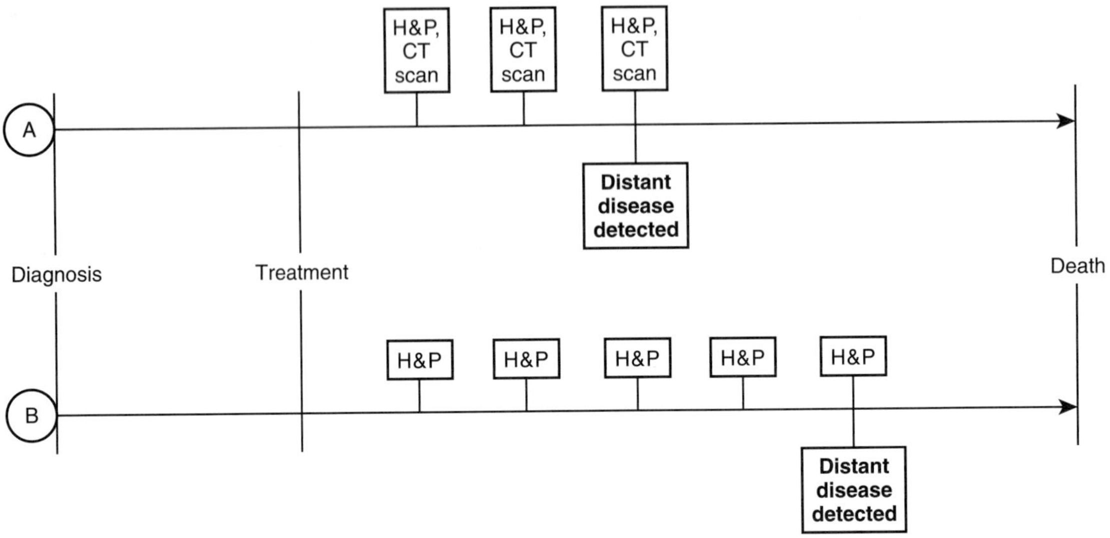

Figure 3–4. Lead-time bias for surveillance testing. If one measures survival from the time distant disease was detected, it would appear as though obtaining yearly CT scans did improve survival of stage IV cancer. However, if one appropriately measures survival from the time of treatment, it becomes apparent that yearly CT scans had no impact on survival.

tion have a higher incidence of breast cancer. Education itself is unlikely to be involved in the development of breast cancer; rather, it is more likely that there is a confounder, a third variable that is related to both breast cancer and the degree of education. One possibility might be the age at first full-term pregnancy. Women who have their first full-term pregnancy later in life (or who are nulliparous) have an increased risk of breast cancer as compared with women who have their first full-term pregnancy at younger ages. In addition, women with more education tend to postpone pregnancy until later in life. Therefore, the apparent association between education and breast cancer may be in part or entirely due to confounding by age at first full-term pregnancy.

Confounding may be addressed in several ways in both the design and analysis phases of a study. Cases may be matched to controls with regard to known confounders, thus eliminating the association between the confounder and disease status. Randomization in a clinical trial is another element of study design that may control for confounding by increasing the probability that both known and unknown confounders will be equally distributed between the intervention and control groups. Stratification is one way to adjust for confounding during the analysis phase. In the breast-cancer example, the subjects should be stratified on the basis of age of first full-term pregnancy; if this is done, odds ratios for education and breast cancer would be calculated separately for women with younger versus older ages at first pregnancy. If the observed association between education and breast cancer was attributed entirely to confounding by age at first full-term pregnancy, then the odds ratios for education and breast cancer would equal 1.0 in each strata. Multivariable regression models are analytic tools that are used to adjust for multiple confounders simultaneously.

Key Selected Reading

Adami H-O, Hunter DJ, Trichopoulos D, eds. *A textbook of cancer epidemiology,* New York: Oxford University Press, 2002.

Selected Readings

Black WC. Randomized clinical trials for cancer screening: rationale and design considerations for imaging tests. *J Clin Oncol* 2006;24:3252–3260.

Gordis L. *Epidemiology,* Philadelphia: WB Saunders, 2000.

Lee JJ, Feng L. Randomized phase II designs in cancer clinical trials: current status and future directions. *J Clin Oncol* 2005;23:4450–4457.

Meinert CL. *Clinical trials: design, conduct, and analysis,* New York: Oxford University Press, 1986.

Rothman KJ, Greenland S. *Modern epidemiology,* Philadelphia: Lippincott–Raven, 1998.

Sargent DJ, Conley BA, Allegra C, Collette L. Clinical trial designs for predictive marker validation in cancer treatment trials. *J Clin Oncol* 2005;23:2020–2027.

Schottenfeld D, Fraumeni JF, eds. *Cancer epidemiology and prevention,* New York: Oxford University Press, 1996.

4

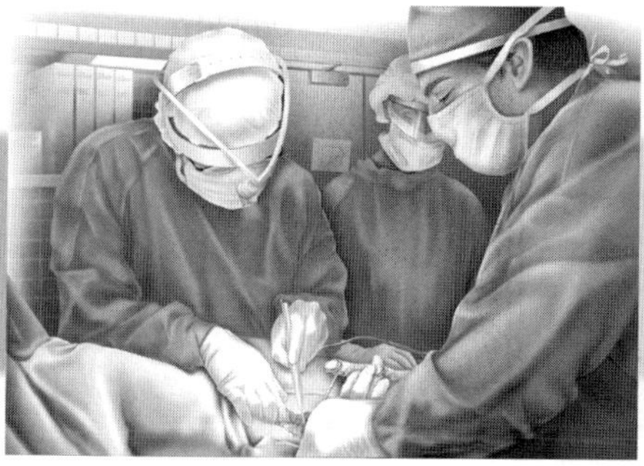

Principles of Surgical Therapy

Michael S. Sabel

Principles of Surgical Therapy: Key Points

- Identify the developments that shaped the field of surgical oncology.
- Compare the methods for the surgical collection of tissues.
- Explain the tumor classification systems used for staging tumors.
- Outline the factors to consider before surgery is performed.
- Detail the factors to consider when resecting a primary tumor.
- List the reasons for performing regional node dissection.
- Describe the circumstances in which metastatic disease resection is appropriate.
- List the prophylactic surgical procedures that can be undertaken.
- Discuss the role of palliative surgery.

The role of surgery in the treatment of cancer found its start with John Hunter (1728–1793), the "father of scientific surgery." He first described the concept that cancer could be a localized process amenable to surgical cure, and he also discussed the need for the removal of the regional lymphatic basin. As surgery itself became more feasible through a better understanding of anatomy and pathology, through the introduction of general anesthesia in 1842, and through the principles of antisepsis (first described by Lister in 1867), surgery became the cornerstone of cancer treatment, and it allowed the field to move beyond superficial tumors to the treatment of intra-abdominal malignancies. The description and implementation of major operations for cancer began to emerge over the next few decades, including total laryngectomy (Billroth in 1873), partial gastrectomy (Billroth in 1881), colectomy (Weir in 1885), radical mastectomy (Halsted in 1891), radical hysterectomy (Kelly in 1895), neck dissection (Crile in 1906), and abdominoperineal resection (Miles in 1908).

For the next several decades, surgery was the mainstay of cancer therapy, with the mortality and morbidity of surgery greatly outweighed by the potential for cure or palliation of symptoms. Cancer surgeons were in abundance, and they were the clinical leaders at major medical centers and the few dedicated cancer centers. During the mid-twentieth century came advances in cancer therapies outside of surgery, including the development of radiation treatments for superficial cancers, the discovery of the antitumor properties of the alkylating agent nitrogen mustard and the folic acid antagonists, and the concepts of hormonal alteration. As it became apparent that cancer could be treated using more than one modality, the field of oncology began to transform.

With these changes, the role of the surgical oncologist evolved as well, and it continues to do so as the management of cancer is altered by increased knowledge of genetics, molecular biology, and tumor immunology. Whereas previously surgery was almost always the first line of defense against a tumor, the escalating use of neoadjuvant therapies often shifts surgery to the second or third treatment employed. Surgery has expanded from a purely therapeutic role to include both palliation and prophylaxis. Because surgeons are the ones with direct access to tumors, they have cemented their role as physician-scientists, investigating novel molecular and immunologic therapies. As new discoveries continue to transform our approach to cancer, the field of surgical oncology will continue to evolve.

Goals of Cancer Surgery

With the expansion of the multidisciplinary approach to cancer, the role of the surgeon has changed significantly. In addition to the well-established curative role, surgeons are often asked to obtain tissue for diagnosis and staging, to debulk tumors as part of multimodality therapy, to palliate incurable patients, or to prevent cancer by the surgical removal of nonessential organs. In some cases, the surgical oncologist takes on the role of coordinator of care and oversees the various aspects of care and follow up of the cancer patient.

BOX 4–1 ROLE OF SURGERY IN THE MANAGEMENT OF CANCER

- Diagnosis of suspicious masses
- Staging established cancers
- Curative resection of primary cancers
- Prevention of cancer by prophylactic surgery
- Debulking cancer as part of multimodality therapy
- Palliation of incurable patients

Diagnosis and Staging

A surgical oncologist is often called upon to obtain tissue for diagnosing masses, for staging known cancers, or for monitoring a cancer's response to therapy. There are several methods by which tissue may be obtained.

Fine-Needle Aspiration

The fine-needle aspiration (FNA) involves obtaining cytological material from a mass using a fine-caliber hollow needle. This biopsy method is particularly useful for superficial, palpable masses such as thyroid nodules, lymph nodes, and breast masses. An FNA can be easily performed in the office using a 22-gauge needle on a syringe, preferably with a pistol-grip aspiration system (Figure 4-1). After preparing the skin with alcohol or Betadine, the mass is fixed between the physician's fingers, and the needle is passed several times through the tumor mass while constant suction is applied on the syringe. The aspirate can be immediately smeared on a slide, fixed in alcohol, and stained. Ultrasound or computed tomographic scanning can be used for guidance when an FNA is needed on a deeper mass.

The FNA biopsy has several advantages, including its ease of performance and the potentially fast turnover of cytology for obtaining a diagnosis. It is important to remember that the FNA obtains cytologic material and

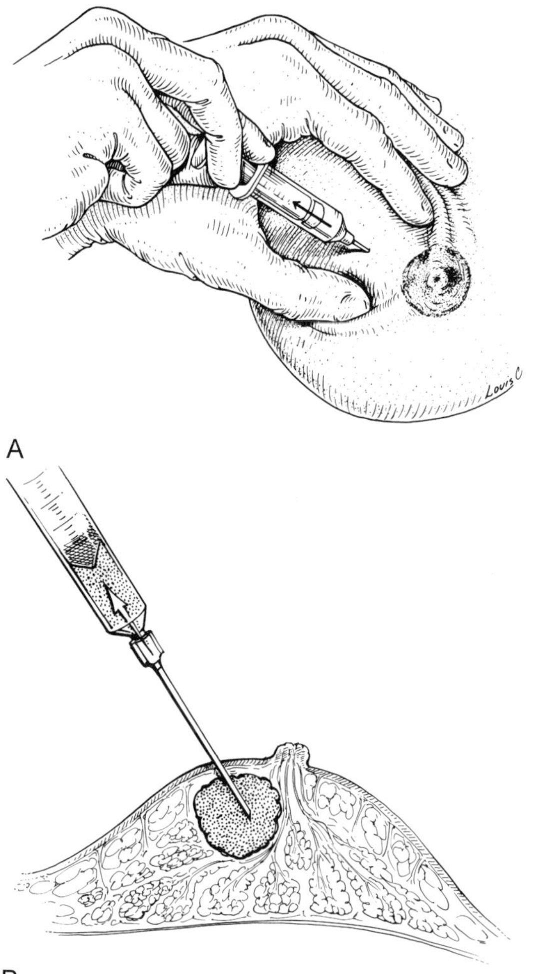

Figure 4–1. Fine-needle aspiration biopsy. (From Bland KI, Karakousis CP, Copeland EM. *Atlas of surgical oncology*, Philadelphia: WB Saunders, 1995, Figure 8-3.)

that it requires a cytopathologist for accurate interpretation. More importantly, an FNA shows cytology and not architecture. Both false-negative and false-positive results may occur. Given the possibility of a false-positive result, definitive therapy should not be undertaken without histologic confirmation (particularly a mastectomy for breast cancer). Either a core-needle biopsy can be performed preoperatively, or a frozen section can be obtained in the operating room. Given its limitations, FNA is more useful in specific situations, when the determination of atypical or malignant cells will help in diagnosis or treatment (e.g., before proceeding with a thyroid lobectomy). FNA is less useful for new, solid masses within the breast, where core-needle biopsy (see next page) can provide more definitive diagnosis and also allow for immunohistochemical staining. However, if a cyst is suspected, FNA can be both diagnostic and therapeutic. FNA is extremely useful for an abnormal lymph node and particularly for a cervical lymph node in which there is a concern of squamous cell cancer. If an excisional lymph node biopsy is done in this situation, the efficacy of the subsequent neck dissection may be compromised. Lymphoma is often in the differential diagnosis list for an enlarged lymph node, and it may be difficult to definitively diagnose using FNA alone, so excisional biopsy is usually required to make this diagnosis.

BOX 4–2 INDICATIONS FOR FINE-NEEDLE ASPIRATION BIOPSY

- Diagnosis of an enlarged lymph node
- Diagnosis of a thyroid nodule
- Diagnosis (and aspiration) of a suspected breast cyst
- Confirmation of recurrent or metastatic disease
- Proof of malignancy if it will affect subsequent treatment

BOX 4–3 PERFORMING A FINE-NEEDLE ASPIRATION BIOPSY

Use a 10- or 20-mL syringe with a small-gauge needle (21-23 gauge).

After cleansing the skin overlying the mass with alcohol, secure the mass between the thumb and forefinger.

Insert the needle into the mass, and apply suction by pulling back on the piston.

Advance the needle back and forth in four different directions under suction.

Before the needle is removed from the mass, the pull on the syringe piston is relaxed to avoid sucking the cells into the barrel of the syringe.

To fix the sample on a slide, disengage the needle and syringe, and attach them again after filling the syringe barrel with air to push the cells out onto a slide. A second clean slide can be placed directly over the sample (see Figure 4-1) to thin and disperse the cells. The two slides are then pulled apart within the plane of the slide surface, and they are immediately fixed and labeled.

Alternatively, the cells from the syringe needle can be irrigated into ThinPrep® solution and forwarded to a cytopathology laboratory that can process it accordingly.

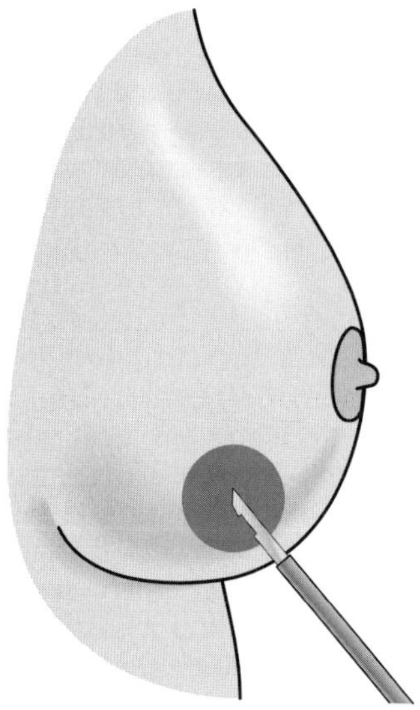

Figure 4–2. Core-needle biopsy.

Core-Needle Biopsy

When there is a palpable mass, it is often preferable to perform a core-needle biopsy under local anesthesia. Unlike FNA, which looks at cytology, core biopsy allows for the visualization of architecture and provides tissue for immunohistochemical staining. For lesions that are difficult to appreciate or that are only seen on imaging studies, image-guided core-needle biopsy may be performed. Although slightly more invasive than an FNA, there is minimal scarring and good patient tolerance of the procedure (Figure 4-2). Thus, it has become the procedure of choice for making a pathologic diagnosis in many areas of oncology. Core-needle biopsies often do not yield sufficient tissue for making a diagnosis of primary lymphoma or of a soft-tissue or bone sarcoma, particularly low-grade liposarcomas.

BOX 4–4 PERFORMING A CORE-NEEDLE BIOPSY

Outline the mass with a skin marker to indicate its location before administering local anesthesia.

Raise a small wheal of local anesthetic intradermally to the side of the lesion, where the initial incision will be made.

Make a small incision (2-4 mm) using a No. 11 scalpel blade. Take care to keep the entry point for the needle within the area of resection of the mass in the event that the result shows a malignancy.

Stabilize the mass with the nondominant hand.

Advance the central notched core into the lesion. Next, advance the outer sleeve over it, allowing for a small cylinder of tissue to be cut and sequestered within the notch (see Figure 4-3). A biopsy device with a trigger mechanism is less likely to push or indent the lesion, which can lead to sampling error.

Place the tissue in formalin solution. Take three to four samples to ensure adequate tissue representation and sufficient tissue for receptor studies.

Incisional Biopsy

Incisional biopsies are usually performed only when a core-needle biopsy is nondiagnostic and when it is not considered prudent to proceed with an excision of the mass or lesion. The most common indication is to biopsy a mass suspected to be a sarcoma so that a definitive resection or neoadjuvant therapy can be planned. Another common indication is when a mass is suspected to be lymphoma, and, therefore, the treatment would be chemotherapy rather than surgical resection. Advantages to incisional biopsy include the ability to obtain plenty of tissue for making a histologic diagnosis; however, the disadvantages to this approach are many, and it is only used under rare circumstances. Care should be taken when planning an incisional biopsy to keep the biopsy within the area of the definitive operation. Biopsies on the arm or leg should be done along the line of the long axis of the extremity. A poorly planned transverse incision can lead to an unnecessarily morbid procedure when the definitive resection must include margins around the area of previous dissection. Care should be taken to not violate tissue planes. Impeccable hemostasis should be obtained, because the complication of a postoperative hematoma can lead to the dissemination of tumor cells into tissues not previously exposed to the tumor.

Excisional Biopsy

Excisional biopsy involves the removal of the entire skin lesion or mass. Small, particularly superficial, mobile tumors can be difficult to isolate and biopsy with a needle. Small masses or skin lesions on the extremity or trunk that are potentially malignant are often best treated with an excisional biopsy, because it allows for definitive diagnosis without risking the violation of tissue planes. When performing an

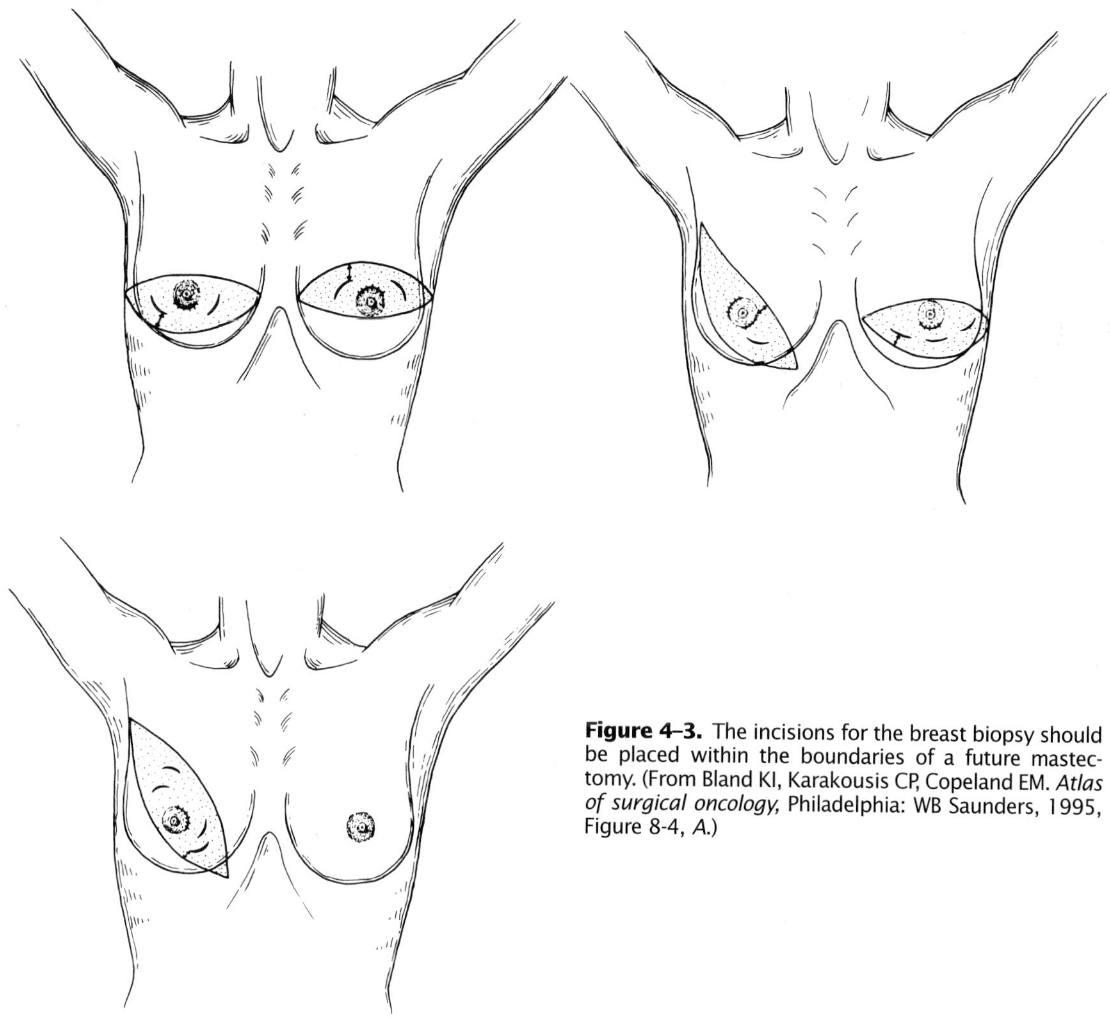

Figure 4–3. The incisions for the breast biopsy should be placed within the boundaries of a future mastectomy. (From Bland KI, Karakousis CP, Copeland EM. *Atlas of surgical oncology,* Philadelphia: WB Saunders, 1995, Figure 8-4, *A.*)

excisional biopsy, it is important to not interfere with a subsequent wider resection if the lesion is malignant. The specimen should be oriented in three dimensions for the pathologist to determine margins if surgical re-excision is needed. Incisions should be placed with the next operation in mind. For example, an incision on the breast should keep in mind a possible mastectomy (Figure 4-3), and incisions on the extremity should be done along the line of the long axis (Figure 4-4). Lymph node biopsies should be oriented so that the scar can be excised with the subsequent lymph node dissection, if needed.

Care should be taken when biopsying more than one lesion on a single patient. Separate instruments should be used for each biopsy in the event that not all of the lesions are malignant to avoid the cross contamination of malignant cells into a wound. Precise labeling of each biopsy is needed in case only one of the biopsied lesions is malignant to correctly

BOX 4–5 PRINCIPLES OF SURGICAL BIOPSIES

- Obtain sufficient tissue for diagnosis.
  - Consider a frozen section to assess adequacy.
- Handle tissue properly.
  - Orient tissue for accurate margins.
  - Send tissue in proper medium for special studies.
- The biopsy should not interfere with subsequent therapy.
  - Prevent hematomas that may distort the operative field.
  - Orient incisions with the next operation in mind.

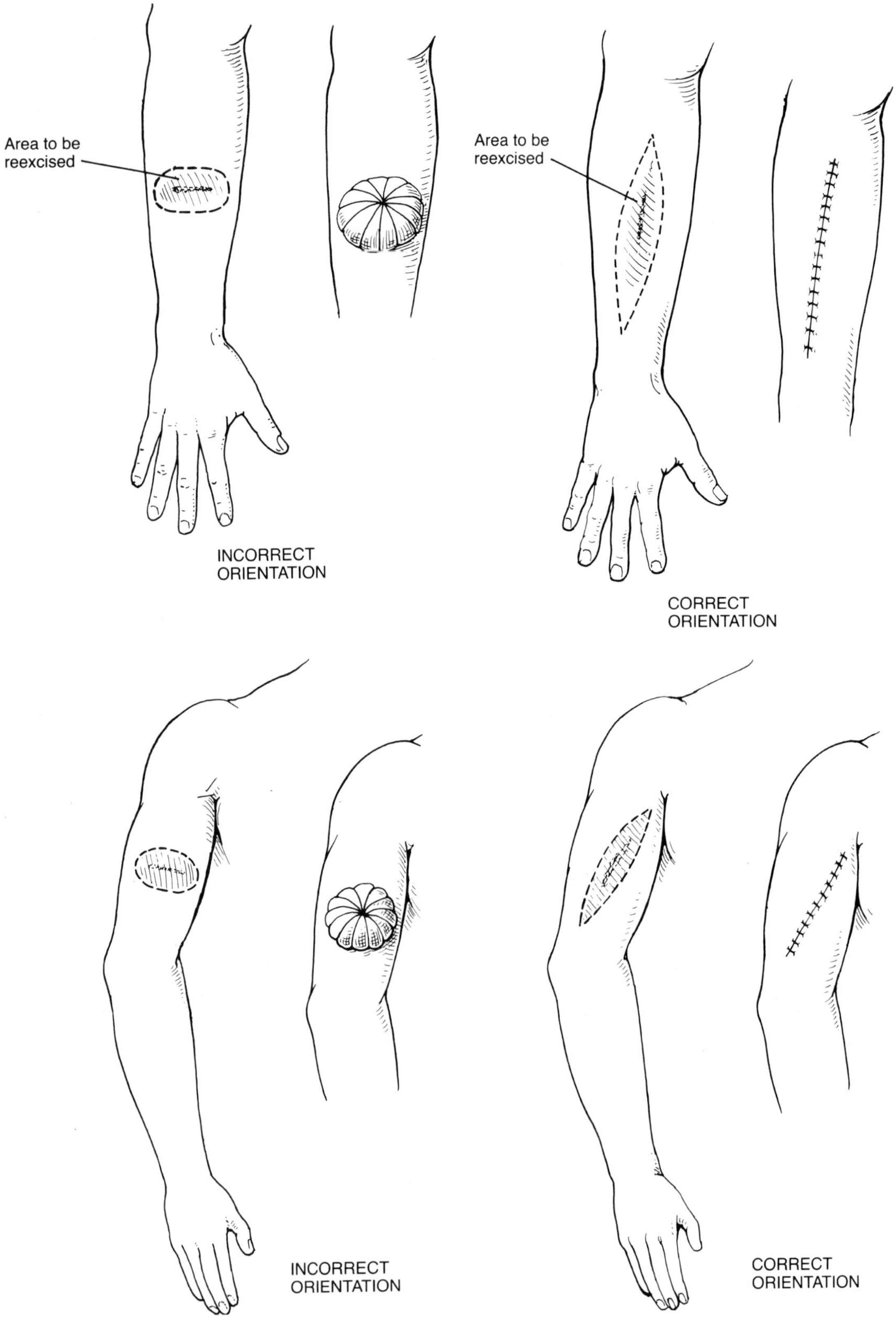

Figure 4–4. Excisional biopsy scar oriented correctly and incorrectly. (From Bland KI, Karakousis CP, Copeland EM. *Atlas of surgical oncology,* Philadelphia: WB Saunders, 1995, Figure 3-4.)

identify the area to be treated further. It is also important to ensure the proper handling of specimens. For example, lymph nodes for the potential workup of non-Hodgkin's lymphoma patients must be sent to the pathology department fresh to process part of the specimen for flow cytometry and/or gene rearrangement studies.

Tumor Staging

A crucial part of the surgical oncologist's role is staging the tumor. Tumor staging establishes the extent of disease, and it has important prognostic and therapeutic implications. Clinical staging is based on the results of a noninvasive evaluation, including physical examination and various imaging studies. Pathologic staging is based on findings in surgical tumor specimens and biopsies, and it allows for the evaluation of microscopic disease that is undetectable by imaging techniques. Pathologic staging may reveal more extensive tumor spread than the clinical evaluation suggests, or, in some instances, it may reveal less-extensive tumor spread, with falsely positive imaging studies detecting inflammatory changes. Pathologic staging, therefore, is much more reliable and prognostic. Clinicians must be careful when attempting to compare clinically and pathologically staged patients, because the two groups may have dramatically different outcomes.

The staging systems vary with different tumor types. Two major staging systems are currently in use. One was developed by the Union Internationale Contre le Cancer (UICC), and the other was developed by the American Joint Committee on Cancer (AJCC). The UICC system is based on the TNM classification. *T* refers to the primary tumor and is based on the size of the tumor and the invasion of surrounding structures. Tumors are characterized as T1 to T4 cancers, with the higher T stages for larger and more invasive tumors. *N* refers to regional lymph nodes, and classifications of N0 to N3 denote increasing degrees of lymph node involvement. Finally, *M* refers to distant metastatic disease, with M0 signifying no distant metastases and M1 and M2 indicating the presence of blood-borne metastatic disease. The AJCC system divides cancers into stages 0 to IV, with higher stages representing more widespread disease and a poorer prognosis. These two systems have been consolidated to conform to each other. It is important for the surgical oncologist to be familiar with these staging systems to plan surgery (including necessary staging tests, such as sentinel lymph node biopsy), to properly refer for adjuvant therapy, and to adequately counsel patients.

Surgery in the Oncologic Patient

Whenever surgery is being considered for patients with an underlying malignancy, the realistic benefits of surgery must be carefully weighed against the risks of the planned procedure. Many factors must be considered, such as the patient's underlying health status and expected long-term survival, the likelihood of either cure or successful palliation with surgery, and the potential risks of intervention. Both the Eastern Cooperative Oncology Group scale and the Karnofsky scale can be used to gauge the patient's performance status (Tables 4-1 and 4-2). Quality-of-life issues must be carefully considered.

When preparing for surgery on cancer patients, a thorough preoperative evaluation should focus on the anatomic and physiologic disturbances that can be associated with malignancy. Many patients with advanced cancer who are in need of surgery have evidence of malnutrition and cachexia. With advances in both parenteral and enteral nutrition in the 1980s, there was a push toward

TABLE 4–1 • *Eastern Cooperative Oncology Group (ECOG) Performance Status Criteria*

Grade	ECOG Status
0	Fully active, able to carry on all pre-disease performance without restriction.
1	Restricted in physically strenuous activity but ambulatory and able to carry out work of a light or sedentary nature (e.g., light housework, office work.)
2	Ambulatory and capable of all self-care but unable to carry out any work activities; up and about more than 50% of waking hours
3	Capable of only limited self-care; confined to bed or chair more than 50% of waking hours
4	Completely disabled; cannot carry on any self-care; totally confined to bed or chair
5	Dead

TABLE 4–2 • *Karnofsky Performance Status*

Grade	Karnofsky Scale
100	Normal, no complaints; no evidence of disease
90	Able to carry on normal activity; minor signs or symptoms of disease
80	Normal activity with effort; some signs or symptoms of disease
70	Cares for self but unable to carry on normal activity or to do active work
60	Requires occasional assistance but is able to care for most personal needs
50	Requires considerable assistance and frequent medical care
40	Disabled; requires special care and assistance
30	Severely disabled; hospitalization is indicted, although death is not imminent
20	Very ill; hospitalization and active supportive care are necessary
10	Moribund
0	Dead

BOX 4–6 FACTORS TO CONSIDER WHEN PLANNING SURGERY FOR CANCER PATIENTS

- Overall health of the patient and expected survival
  - Age
  - Performance status
  - Comorbidities
- Tumor type and stage
  - Long-term survival and potential benefits of surgery
  - Disturbances in anatomy and physiology caused by cancer
  - Elevated surgical risks as a result of cancer
- Technical complexity of the procedure
  - Potential surgical complications
  - Type of anesthesia needed
  - Quality-of-life issues
  - Experience of personnel

trying to maximize a patient's nutritional status before surgery. However, multiple randomized trials have failed to demonstrate an overall objective benefit of preoperative nutrition in patients with cancer. In certain situations, severely debilitated patients may benefit from preoperative alimentation. If enteral nutrition is feasible, this is preferred, because it is more physiologic, less costly, and associated with fewer infectious complications. Nutritional support should last at least 2 weeks if any true benefit is to be realized.

BOX 4–7 ADVANTAGES OF ENTERAL NUTRITION OVER PARENTERAL NUTRITION

- Cost
- Maintains gut mucosal mass and barrier function
- Supports gut immune function
- Maintains a balanced luminal microflora environment

Many tumors develop the ability to elaborate hormones or cytokines that can have deleterious physiologic consequences. These hormones may result in paraneoplastic syndromes that occur in approximately 10% of patients with advanced cancer. Another mechanism by which paraneoplastic syndromes may develop can be host antibodies to tumor antigens (Table 4-3). It is also important to remember that many cancers induce a hypercoagulable state that increases the risk of deep venous thrombosis and pulmonary embolism, so cancer patients should have appropriate deep venous thrombosis prophylaxis.

BOX 4–8 METABOLIC ABNORMALITIES IN PATIENTS WITH CACHEXIA

- Decreased energy balance and increased glucose consumption
- Increased fat breakdown and serum lipid levels
- Increased gluconeogenesis and hepatic glucose production
- Increased muscle proteolysis and amino acid release
- Increased hepatic protein synthesis and amino acid transport
- Decreased nitrogen balance and decreased muscle mass

More and more patients are being treated with neoadjuvant therapies, which can have profound effects on the patient and the subsequent surgery. Previous radiation therapy can be associated with delayed healing and wound complications; this may require the use of rotational or free tissue flaps to provide adequate

TABLE 4–3 • *Paraneoplastic Syndromes*

Syndrome	Associated Cancers	Suspected Mechanisms
Cushing's syndrome	Lung, pancreatic, adrenal, and neural tumors	ACTH or ACTH-like molecules
Syndrome of inappropriate ADH secretion	Lung and intracranial tumors	ADH secretion
Hypercalcemia	Lung, breast, parathyroid, renal, myeloma, prostate, and ovarian cancers	Osteolytic metastases or parathyroid-hormone–related peptide
Hypoglycemia	Sarcomas, islet cell tumors, and hepatocellular carcinoma	Insulin or insulin-like peptides
Myasthenia	Thymomas and lung cancer	Autoimmune
Encephalomyelitis	Lung, ovarian, and breast cancer	Autoimmune
Neuropathies	Myeloma, lung, breast, and ovarian cancer	Autoimmune
Cerebellar atrophy	Breast and ovarian cancer	Autoimmune
Acanthosis nigricans	Gastric, lung, and uterine cancer	Autoimmune
Dermatomyositis	Lung and breast cancer	Autoimmune
DIC	Pancreas, lung, stomach, and prostate cancer	Tumor products that activate and consume clotting factors

ACTH, Adrenocorticotropic hormone; *ADH,* antidiuretic hormone; *DIC,* disseminated intravascular coagulation.

coverage after resection. Chemotherapy can have physiologic effects that may increase surgical risks. Previous treatment with doxorubicin can be associated with cardiac dysfunction, and bleomycin can lead to decreased pulmonary function. Cancer patients treated with chemotherapy often have hematologic abnormalities as a side effect of either chemotherapy or the underlying disease. Neutropenia is a common side effect of many chemotherapeutic agents. Patients with severe neutropenia (absolute neutrophil count <500 per mm^3 [$0.5 \times 10^9/1$]) are at significant risk for perioperative infection. In many cases, an adequate amount of time can be scheduled between the final course of chemotherapy and the surgery to allow white blood cell counts to rise naturally or with the use of colony-stimulating factors. However, when the surgery is more urgent or patients have impaired hematopoiesis, the surgeon must be prepared to deal with the increased risks.

Curative Surgery

Resection of the Primary Tumor

The cornerstone of surgical oncology remains the en bloc resection of the primary cancer. The goal is to obtain complete local control wherein the entire tumor is removed with adequate margins of normal tissue so that it does not recur. For patients who have not yet developed distant micrometastases, this is curative. What constitutes an adequate margin varies from cancer to cancer and evolves with the results of well-designed, prospective clinical trials. Historically, cure was achieved with radical extirpative surgeries; the classic example is that of breast cancer. Before Halsted's description of the radical mastectomy, the surgical treatment of breast cancer resulted in a dismal local control rate of less than 30%. With a local control rate of greater than 90%, the radical mastectomy was adopted as the standard of care. However, it became apparent that, despite the lack of local recurrence, the overall survival of breast cancer patients was still poor. This was because of the large percentage of patients who had already developed distant disease by the time they came for evaluation. Since then, multiple large prospective trials have shown that a more limited resection is as effective as mastectomy for treating breast cancer, and this has become the preferred treatment. Other examples include randomized trials demonstrating no difference in survival with 2-cm versus 4-cm margins around malignant melanoma or 2-cm versus 5-cm distal margins for rectal cancer.

In some cases, a tumor will appear adherent or fixed to normal adjacent structures. In these cases, en bloc resection of the tumor is mandatory, and any attachment should be considered malignant in nature. Any violation of the cancer has the potential for tumor spillage and wound implantation. For example, the removal of a primary colon cancer requires an adequate margin of normal colon proximally and distally. In addition, if it involves an adjacent loop of small bowel or bladder, this will require the en bloc resection of the primary tumor along with removal of the involved segment of small bowel or bladder wall.

The emergence of multimodal therapy has dramatically affected the surgical approach to many primary cancers. This is especially the case when surgical resection of the tumor is combined with radiotherapy. Local control is significantly improved by using radiation after resection of breast, rectal, sarcoma, head, and neck squamous cell and pancreatic primary cancers. In fact, the addition of radiation therapy as an adjunctive therapy has allowed for less radical procedures to be performed with an improvement in the quality of life of patients. Classic examples include the use of lumpectomy and adjuvant radiation instead of mastectomy for breast cancer or limb-sparing surgery plus radiation instead of amputation for sarcoma. However, it should be stressed that, even with adjuvant radiation, local recurrence rates may still be unacceptably high if negative surgical margins are not obtained, and radiation should not be thought of as a substitute for adequate surgery.

In the cases of some malignancies, surgery has been replaced as the primary treatment modality. A prime example of this is the treatment of squamous cell carcinoma of the anus (see Chapter 20: Multimodality Therapy of Gastrointestinal Cancer). Although the primary treatment for this used to be an abdominoperineal resection, the discovery of an effective combination of chemotherapy and radiation has relegated surgery to a second-line treatment, and it is now reserved for those who relapse or who fail to respond to chemoradiation. This has spared the majority of patients the morbidity of an abdominoperineal resection. Other examples include the primary treatment of certain head and neck cancers with radiation alone or with chemoradiation.

In the case of other cancers, resection is still the mainstay of therapy, but it is performed after chemotherapy and/or radiation therapy has been administered. This preoperative use of chemotherapy or radiation is referred to as "neoadjuvant" therapy, and, in many cases, it has dramatically improved outcomes. One example is the treatment of childhood rhabdomyosarcomas. Before the 1980s, surgery was the primary therapy, but it had dismal results. The development of neoadjuvant chemoradiation followed by resection has resulted in the survival of more than 80% of patients with this cancer. The survival of women with locally advanced or inflammatory breast cancer has also dramatically improved with the use of neoadjuvant therapy. The use of neoadjuvant chemotherapy for breast cancer has been expanded to render many women who would have required mastectomy (because of large tumor size) appropriate for breast-sparing surgery. In cases in which neoadjuvant therapy is not needed, postoperative adjuvant chemotherapy and/or radiation therapy have become standard approaches for many solid tumors, and they have resulted in improved local control and overall survival.

Resection of Regional Lymph Nodes

The regional lymph nodes represent the most prevalent site of metastases for most solid tumors, and the presence of metastases in the lymph nodes represents an important prognostic factor in the staging of the cancer patient. For this reason, the regional lymph nodes are often removed at the time of resection of the primary cancer. In addition to providing crucial staging information, a lymphadenectomy provides regional control of the cancer, thereby preventing future recurrence in the draining basin and the subsequent and often more extensive dissection.

Somewhat less clear is the impact that regional node dissection has on survival. When the presence of cancer within the regional nodes is clinically evident and there is no evidence of distant metastases, the removal of the regional lymph nodes in addition to the primary tumor can result in a long-term survival benefit. In these cases, the removal of regional lymph nodes is clearly therapeutic. The timing of the procedure—as well as the extent—is more controversial. For some visceral solid tumors (e.g., gastric, pancreatic), the extent of lymphadenectomy at the time of primary tumor resection has been hypothesized to be important for optimizing local and regional control and to have an impact on overall survival. However, this has not been borne out in prospective randomized trials, and the more extended lymphadenectomy appears to result in more accurate staging but not improved survival in the majority of patients.

Another question is whether the "elective" removal of the regional lymph nodes in the hopes of removing micrometastatic disease before it recurs as clinically evident disease will improve survival. This approach hinges on whether a substantial portion of patients have microscopic disease in their lymph nodes (but not distant micrometastases at the time that their cancer is diagnosed) and, hence, would develop secondary metastases from the persistent tumor in the lymph nodes as it grows. Some would argue that this would be a very small subset (either because distant disease is already present or because it rarely metastasizes from the regional disease), and so they advocate a "watch and wait" approach. This involves performing a lymphadenectomy only when the patient relapses in a nodal basin, sparing the node-negative patients the morbidity of lymph node dissection. Despite retrospective data suggesting a survival benefit to elective lymph node dissection, prospective randomized trials of various tumor types have yet to demonstrate a survival advantage, but they have been largely underpowered to detect clinically significant effects. On the other hand, subset analysis suggests that a survival advantage may exist for certain populations of patients. With the development and implementation of the sentinel node biopsy, it is now possible to determine which patients have microscopic disease in their lymph nodes (Figure 4-5). This limits the complete dissection only to those patients with known microscopic disease. Although this clearly improves staging (see below), whether it has an impact on survival is a question that is being addressed by several ongoing prospective trials.

Resection of Metastatic Disease

Although the presence of metastatic disease has typically been considered outside the realm of surgical intervention, there are situations in which the resection of isolated metastases in patients with solid malignancies is a consideration. The selection of appropriate patients for the resection of metastases requires a thorough evaluation of the individual's disease status (including the original stage of disease, the disease-free interval, and the results of a complete staging workup); medical status; and assessment of the feasibility of resecting the metastatic site with a negative margin. This process identifies a small subset of patients that become surgical candidates. However, in the absence of prospective randomized trials (which are difficult to perform in this situation), it is not clear to what extent survival is improved because of the surgery itself rather than because of the selection of a subset of patients with an excellent prognosis. Nonetheless, there is a significant body of retrospective evidence indicating that this approach can result in significant long-term benefit.

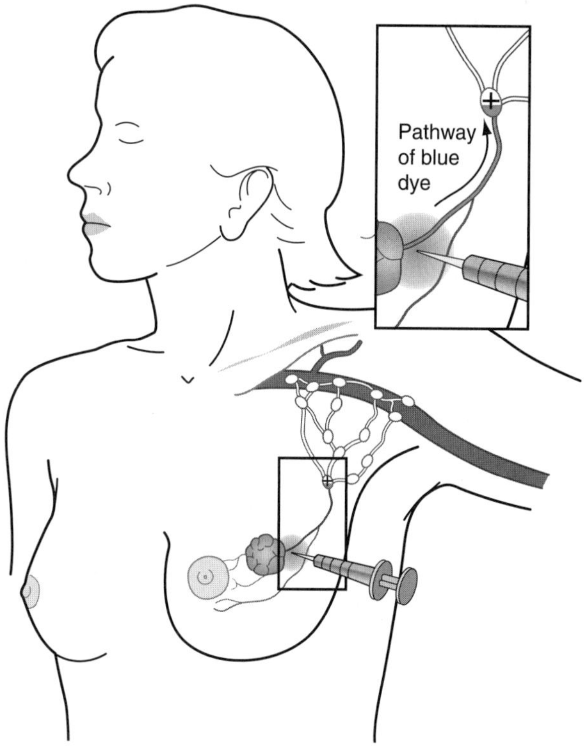

Figure 4-5. Sentinel lymph node biopsy. A tracer injected around the tumor maps to the first lymph node that receives drainage. This lymph node is the one most likely to harbor micrometastases if they exist.

There are several malignancies in which the resection of metastatic disease is often recommended. One such tumor is colorectal cancer, which often metastasizes to the liver. These cancers appear to have a pattern of spread that involves the liver as the initial visceral site. The resection of solitary or multiple colorectal liver metastases has resulted in a 25% to 40% overall 5-year survival rate, depending on the extent of liver involvement. The resection of lung metastases in patients with osteogenic or soft-tissue sarcomas has been established from numerous retrospective reports, because these cancers have a propensity to metastasize to the lung as the only site. Pulmonary metastasectomies for sarcoma result in approximately a 20% to 25% overall survival rate beyond 5 years. The resection of metastatic disease among patients with melanoma and breast cancer has also been advocated, and it can result in survival rates that appear much higher than the typical natural history of these diseases would dictate. One of the roles of the surgical oncologist is to judge when it is appropriate to offer this option.

Tumor Debulking

Finally, there is an occasional role for tumor debulking. Tumor debulking involves removing as much of the cancer as is feasible, even though it is known that a significant tumor burden remains. This is rarely recommended for most cancers, because it carries a high morbidity rate, and it rarely affects the natural history of the underlying cancer. However, there are situations in which this may be beneficial. Ovarian carcinomas often present with extensive intraperitoneal metastasis, thus making curative resections impossible. Cytoreductive surgery in this situation, followed by postoperative chemotherapy, appears to improve outcome, with median survival improving with decreasing amounts of residual disease (see Chapter 23: Gynecologic Cancers). The resection of functional neuroendocrine metastases to the liver, even if incomplete, can result not only in prolonged survival but also in palliation of the patient's symptoms. These tumors tend to be indolent in their growth rate; however, the symptoms associated with the metastatic disease can often be detrimental to the patient's quality of life.

Cancer Prevention

With the increasing understanding of inherited genetic mutations and the identification of patients who are predisposed to malignant transformation, surgery has now become an option for the prevention of cancer. With the ability to perform genetic screening for relevant mutations, cancer prevention can be implemented before the onset of symptoms or histologic changes. Although many interventions may ultimately be nonsurgical (e.g., tamoxifen for the chemoprevention of breast cancer), surgical therapy remains a primary option. It is for this reason that surgeons must be aware of those high-risk situations for which surgery may be considered to prevent subsequent malignant disease (Table 4-4).

BOX 4–9 FEATURES OF HEREDITARY CANCER SYNDROMES

- Early age of onset of disease
- Multiple family members with the same cancer on one side of the family tree
- Clustering of cancers known to be caused by a gene mutation
- Multiple primary cancers in one individual

TABLE 4–4 • *Possible Indications of Prophylactic Surgery*

Prophylactic Surgery	Potential Indications
Bilateral mastectomy	BRCA1 or BRCA2 mutation Familial breast cancer Atypical hyperplasia or lobular carcinoma in situ Unilateral breast cancer in a young patient (<40 years)
Bilateral oophorectomy	BRCA1 or BRCA2 mutation Familial ovarian cancer Hereditary nonpolyposis colorectal cancer At the time of hysterectomy for endometrial cancer At the time of colon resection for colon cancer
Thyroidectomy	RET oncogene mutation Multiple endocrine neoplasia (MEN) type 2A MEN type 2B Familial non-MEN medullary thyroid carcinoma
Total procto-colectomy	Familial adenomatous polyposis or APC mutation HNPCC germline mutation Ulcerative colitis

APC, Adenomatosis polyposis coli; *HNPCC*, hereditary nonpolyposis colorectal cancer.

Prophylactic Colectomy

One of the earliest examples of surgical prophylaxis is the recommendation for total proctocolectomy for some patients with ulcerative colitis (e.g., those who developed the disease at a young age, those who have a long duration of colitis), because these patients are at high risk of developing colorectal cancer. Familial adenomatous polyposis coli syndrome, which is defined by the diffuse involvement of the colon and rectum with adenomatous polyps, universally leads to colorectal cancer if the large intestine is left in place. With the identification of the adenomatous polyposis coli gene, which is responsible for familial adenomatous polyposis coli syndrome, the role of screening and prophylactic proctocolectomy changed dramatically. Today, children of families in which an adenomatous polyposis coli gene mutation has been identified can have genetic testing before polyps become evident. Carriers can be screened and then undergo resection after polyps appear, usually during their late teens or early twenties.

The potential role of prophylactic colectomy will expand as additional syndromes and genes that carry an increased risk of colorectal cancer are identified. Hereditary nonpolyposis colorectal carcinoma, or Lynch syndrome, is an autosomal dominant disorder that is estimated to be responsible for 5% to 10% of all colorectal cancers. Although some of the genes responsible for this syndrome have been identified, the mutations do not have a 100% penetrance, so cancer will not develop in all carriers. However, prophylactic surgery may be a consideration for some carriers, and the remainder should have aggressive screening.

Prophylactic Mastectomy

Another example of prophylactic surgery is bilateral mastectomies for women at high risk of developing breast cancer. Before the identification of the BRCA genes, prophylactic mastectomies were typically reserved as an option for women with lobular carcinoma in situ. However, with the identification of BRCA1 and BRCA2, the role of prophylactic mastectomies has been greatly expanded. Women with BRCA1 or BRCA2 mutations carry a high lifetime probability of breast cancer; however, bilateral mastectomy will result in a 90% to 95% risk reduction. Even a total mastectomy cannot remove all breast tissue; this reduction is not 100%. The potential benefits of prophylactic mastectomy must be weighed against quality-of-life issues and the morbidity of the surgery. In addition, other methods of prophylaxis (e.g., tamoxifen chemoprevention, bilateral oophorectomy) must be considered. Along with the increased risk of breast cancer with BRCA1 and BRCA2 mutations, the risk of ovarian cancer is also increased. Bilateral oophorectomy after childbearing is complete will not only reduce the risk of ovarian cancer, but it may also decrease the risk of breast cancer.

Prophylactic Thyroidectomy

Increased genetic knowledge has also changed our approach to thyroid cancer. Medullary thyroid cancer is a well-established component of multiple endocrine neoplasia syndrome type 2a (MEN 2a) or type 2b (MEN 2b). Previously, family members at risk for MEN 2 underwent annual screening for elevated calcitonin levels; however, this only detected medullary thyroid cancer after it developed. Mutations in the RET oncogene are present in almost all cases of MEN 2a and 2b. Now, family members of MEN patients can be screened for the presence of an RET mutation. Those without the mutation need not undergo additional screening, whereas those with the mutation should undergo total thyroidectomy at a young age.

Palliation

Surgical intervention is sometimes required in the face of unresectable advanced cancer to palliate the patient. Common indications for palliation include pain, bleeding, obstruction,

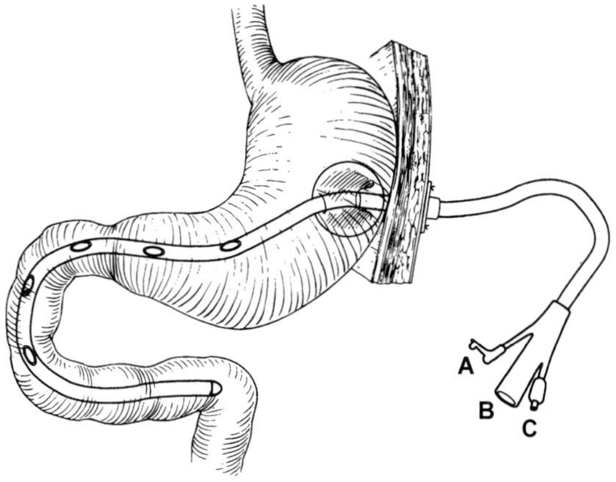

Figure 4-6. Gastrojejunostomy tube with feeding port. This is often placed to provide both decompression and nutrition. (From Bland KI, Karakousis CP, Copeland EM. *Atlas of surgical oncology*, Philadelphia: WB Saunders, 1995, Figure 28-2.)

BOX 4–10 EXAMPLES OF PALLIATIVE SURGERY FOR CANCER

- Resection of a primary tumor for pain or bleeding
- Bowel resection for bleeding or obstruction
- Placement of a gastrostomy tube for decompression
- Placement of a jejunostomy tube for enteral feedings or of a vascular access for hyperalimentation

malnutrition, or infection. The surgeon needs to consider several factors before operating on a patient in this situation, specifically whether the risks of surgery are outweighed by the potential improvement in the quality of life of the patient. Other factors to consider include the expected survival of the individual, the potential morbidity of the procedure, the likelihood that the procedure will successfully palliate the patient, and whether there are alternative nonsurgical methods of palliation available.

A common indication for palliative surgery is the obstruction of a hollow viscus, which can give rise to perforation. The hollow viscus could be the bowel, the biliary tree, the endobronchial tree, the ureter, or the bladder. Bleeding from a tumor is another frequent indication for intervention. The surgeon may also be involved when a metastatic lesion is causing pain by compressing on an organ or adjacent nerves. Malnutrition is often a problem in the patient with cancer, especially one with advanced, unresectable disease. Nutrition can be supplemented or replaced by intravenous hyperalimentation or enteral feedings via gastrostomy or jejunostomy tubes. Commonly, the surgeon is involved in the placement of vascular access and/or feeding tubes for enteral nutrition (Figure 4-6). The surgeon needs to assess the relative risk-to-benefit ratio for resecting a symptomatic mass knowing that it will not have an impact on the overall survival of the patient. If the quality of life of the individual can be improved at an acceptable operative risk, then the surgical intervention is warranted.

Clinical Trials

At the very heart of evidence-based medicine are clinical trials. Although the earliest cancer trials dealt primarily with nonsurgical issues, surgeons quickly became involved in significant roles in oncology trials. These trials continue to answer many important questions regarding the optimum surgical treatment and adjuvant therapy for cancer. As surgeons, we have an obligation not only to the patient we are presently treating but also those patients who will follow. The improved success and decreased morbidity of the treatments that we offer today are only possible because of the involvement of surgeons and their patients in the clinical trials of the past. Because the newest discoveries in all fields of oncology will have a direct impact on surgical therapy, it is imperative that surgeons continue to play prominent roles as both leaders and participants in multidisciplinary cooperative group trials. As such, they should incorporate clinical trials into their practice and encourage patient accrual.

Key Selected Reading

Chang AE, Ganz PA, Hayes DF, *et al. Oncology: An Evidence-Based Approach.* New York: Springer-Verlag, 2005.

Selected Readings

American Joint Committee on Cancer. *AJCC Cancer Staging Manual,* ed 6, New York: Springer Verlag, 2002.
Arnold SM, Lieberman FS, Foon KA. Paraneoplastic syndromes. In: Devita FT, Hellman S, Rosenberg SA, eds. *Cancer, principles & practice of oncology,* ed 7, Philadelphia: Lippincott Williams and Wilkins, 2005.
Barentsz J, Takahashi S, Oyen W, *et al.* Commonly used imaging techniques for diagnosis and staging. *J Clin Oncol* 2006;24:3234–3244.
Bertagnolli MM. Surgical prevention of cancer. *J Clin Oncol* 2005;23:324–332.
Birkmeyer JD, Stukel TA, Siewers AE, *et al.* Surgeon volume and operative mortality in the United States, *N Engl J Med* 2003;349:2117–2127.
Cotran CS, Kumar V, Robbins SL, eds. *Robbins pathologic basis of disease,* ed 6, Philadelphia: WB Saunders, 1999.
Edge SB, Cookfair DL, Watroba N. The role of the surgeon in quality cancer care. *Curr Probl Surg* 2003;40:511–590.
Ferrell BR. Palliative care: an essential aspect of quality cancer care. *Surg Oncol Clin N Am* 2004;13:401–411.
Garber JE, Offit K. Hereditary cancer predisposition syndromes. *J Clin Oncol* 2005;23:276–292.
Goldman L, Caldera DL, Nussbaum SR, *et al.* Multifactorial index of cardiac risk in noncardiac surgical procedures. *N Engl J Med* 1977;297:845–850.
Jemal A, Murray T, Ward E, *et al.* Cancer statistics, 2005, *CA Cancer J Clin* 2005;55:10-30.
McCahill LE, Krouse R, Chu D, *et al.* Indications and use of palliative surgery—results of Society of Surgical Oncology survey, *Ann Surg Oncol* 2002;9:104–112.
Miltenburg DM, Conklin L, Sastri S. The role of genetic screening and prophylactic surgery in surgical oncology, *J Am Coll Surg* 2000;190:619–628.

5

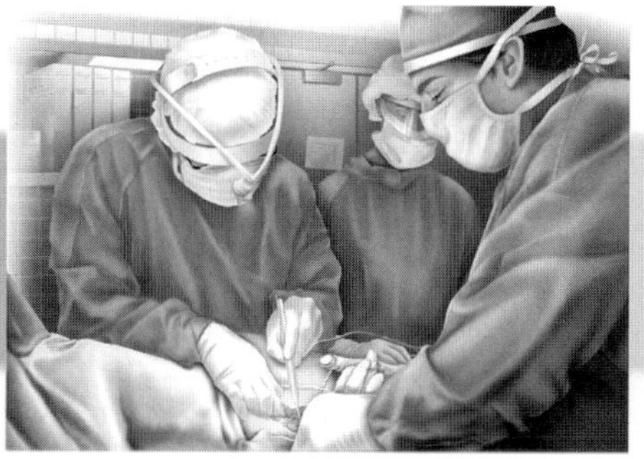

Principles of Chemotherapy

Elaina M. Gartner

CLASSES OF CHEMOTHERAPEUTIC AGENTS

PRINCIPLES OF CHEMOTHERAPY USE

TREATMENT OF CHEMOTHERAPY TOXICITY

Principles of Chemotherapy: Key Points

- Describe the mechanisms of action of alkylating agents, platinum analogues, antimicrotubule agents, topoisomerase inhibitors, antimetabolites, and antitumor antibiotics.
- Explain the principles supporting the use of combination chemotherapy.
- Discuss the benefits of using adjuvant chemotherapy.
- Outline the purposes, advantages, and disadvantages of neoadjuvant chemotherapy.
- List the treatments used for the symptoms of chemotherapy toxicity.

Treatment with chemotherapy is considered for cancer patients in a variety of situations, and it can be given with either curative or palliative intent. Chemotherapeutic agents inhibit cell growth and cause apoptosis through interference with normal cellular functions, primarily progression through the cell cycle. In general, tumors that are slowly growing are considered less sensitive to chemotherapy than tumors that are growing more rapidly; this is most likely because only a small proportion of cells in a slowly growing tumor are progressing through the cell cycle when chemotherapy is given. The converse is not necessarily true: rapidly growing, aggressive tumors often acquire resistance to chemotherapy. The mechanisms of action and resistance of the major classes of chemotherapeutic agents are discussed in this chapter. Specific chemotherapeutic agents commonly used to treat solid tumors, their side effects, and important precautions regarding their use are presented in the accompanying tables.

Chemotherapeutic agents may be used alone or in combination. In general, combination therapies are more effective, and they are more often used when chemotherapy is meant to be curative. When treating with curative intent, the dose intensity (i.e., the amount of chemotherapy administered within a certain period of time) is very important. The dose intensity achieved with standard therapy (as opposed to high-dose therapy, which requires stem cell rescue [i.e., bone marrow transplant]) is more likely to lead to cure than doses that are reduced as a result of toxicity. The uses of chemotherapy for curative and palliative purposes are outlined in this chapter.

Unfortunately, in addition to damaging cancer cells, normal tissues progressing through the cell cycle may be damaged during chemotherapy, and this may lead to significant toxicity. This is the reason for some of the most familiar side effects of chemotherapy. For example, damage to the gastric mucosa may contribute to nausea and vomiting; neutropenia, anemia, and thrombocytopenia may be caused by damage to the bone marrow (myelosuppression). This chapter will provide an overview of the common side effects of chemotherapy and their treatments.

Classes of Chemotherapeutic Agents

Alkylating Agents

A variety of chemotherapeutic agents, including the nitrogen mustards, first used during the 1940s, fall into this category. All alkylating agents contain an alkyl group ($-CH_2C$). This alkyl group is able to covalently bind DNA, thus causing DNA damage. Agents with single alkyl groups are thought to damage DNA bases or to cause single-stranded DNA breaks. Agents with two alkyl groups form DNA cross-links, which lead to interference with DNA synthesis and transcription as well as double-stranded DNA breaks.

Cancer cells may develop resistance to alkylating agents through decreasing cellular uptake of the drugs, increasing activity of DNA repair enzymes, or increasing levels of thiol-containing proteins (e.g., glutathione). Glutathione is thought to bind these drugs, thereby preventing their interaction with DNA.

Specific alkylating agents that are commonly used to treat solid tumors are listed in Table 5-1. Although they do not contain alkyl groups, dacarbazine and temozolomide are included, because they are thought to be metabolized into active forms that contain alkyl groups.

BOX 5–1 CHARACTERISTICS SHARED BY ALKYLATING AGENTS AND PLATINUM ANALOGUES

- They bind and damage DNA.
- Resistance develops by decreased cellular uptake, increased activity of DNA repair enzymes, or increased levels of thiol-containing proteins.

Platinum Analogues

The platinum analogues have a similar mechanism of action to the alkylating agents. They bind DNA to form interstrand and intrastrand cross-links, which lead to the inhibition of DNA synthesis and transcription.

The mechanisms of cancer-cell resistance are also similar to alkylating agents: decreased cellular uptake of the drugs, increased activity of DNA repair enzymes, and increased thiol-containing proteins. In addition, resistance to both cisplatin and carboplatin has been associated with a deficiency of mismatch repair genes (MMRs). It is thought that MMRs are involved in proapoptotic signaling and that their absence prevents cell death. It is not known why this mechanism of resistance appears to be specific to cisplatin and carboplatin, but the efficacy of the newest platinum analogue, oxaliplatin, is not affected by a deficiency of MMRs.

The platinum analogues are listed in Table 5-2.

Antimicrotubule Agents

During mitosis, the protein tubulin polymerizes to form microtubules, which are involved in the segregation of chromosomes. There are three mechanisms by which chemotherapeutic agents inhibit microtubules. The vinca alkaloids (vinblastine, vincristine, and vinorelbine) bind to tubulin and arrest further polymerization when incorporated into the microtubule. Estramustine also inhibits microtubule assembly by binding microtubule-associated proteins. The taxanes (paclitaxel and docetaxel) bind and stabilize microtubules, thus preventing their disassembly at the end of mitosis. A new class of drugs, called epothilones, have a similar mechanism of action to the taxanes and are currently being evaluated in clinical trials.

Cancer-cell resistance to the vinca alkaloids and taxanes is conferred by mutations in the tubule protein that alter drug-binding affinity and by expression of the multidrug resistance (MDR) gene. The MDR gene encodes a glyco-

TABLE 5-1 • *Alkylating Agents*

Agent	Active Tumors	Side Effects	Precautions
Cyclophosphamide	Breast Ovarian Sarcoma Neuroblastoma Wilms' tumor Germ cell tumors	Myelosuppression Nausea/vomiting Alopecia Infertility Hemorrhagic cystitis SIADH 2° malignancies	Encourage oral fluids (2-3 L/day) to prevent hemorrhagic cystitis May increase the effects of anticoagulation
Ifosfamide	Sarcoma Germ cell tumors Lung Bladder Head and neck Cervical	Myelosuppression Nausea/vomiting Alopecia Infertility Hemorrhagic cystitis CNS toxicity (lethargy → coma) SIADH	Administer IVF or bladder irrigation with intravenous/PO mesna to prevent hemorrhagic cystitis May increase the effects of anticoagulation
Streptozocin	Pancreatic Neuroendocrine tumors Carcinoid tumors	Renal failure Proteinuria Nausea/vomiting Hyperglycemia Myelosuppression Hepatotoxicity	
Thiotepa	Breast Ovarian Bladder	Myelosuppression Nausea/vomiting Mucositis Hypersensitivity Rash Hemorrhagic cystitis 2° malignancies	Have resuscitation supplies nearby during administration for hypersensitivity reactions
Carmustine	Glioblastoma multiforme Medulloblastoma Glioma Astrocytoma Ependymoma	Myelosuppression Nausea/vomiting Hepatotoxicity Infertility Pulmonary toxicity Renal failure 2° malignancies	Obtain baseline pulmonary function tests with DLCO and monitor Increased toxicity if given with valproic acid May decrease activity of phenytoin
Dacarbazine	Melanoma Sarcoma Neuroblastoma	Myelosuppression Nausea/vomiting Flu-like syndrome Photosensitivity	May decrease activity of phenytoin
Temozolomide	Melanoma Astrocytoma Brain metastases	Myelosuppression Nausea/vomiting Flu-like syndrome Photosensitivity Hepatotoxicity	

CNS, Central nervous system; *DLCO,* carbon monoxide diffusion in the lung; *IVF,* intravenous fluids; *PO,* by mouth; *SIADH,* syndrome of inappropriate secretion of antidiuretic hormone.

protein (P170) that actively pumps drugs out of the cell. The mechanisms of estramustine resistance are unknown.

Antimicrotubule agents commonly used to treat solid tumors are listed in Table 5-3.

Topoisomerase Inhibitors

The topoisomerases are required for proper chromosomal structure. Topoisomerase I cleaves and relegates a single strand of DNA to allow DNA unwinding. Topoisomerase II cleaves and relegates both strands of DNA to allow DNA untwisting. Cells are most sensitive to the topoisomerase inhibitors during DNA synthesis. Irinotecan and topotecan—also known as the *camptothecins*—are topoisomerase-I inhibitors, and they bind to the topoisomerase-I–DNA complex, thus preventing relegation and causing single-stranded DNA breaks. Etoposide is a topoisomerase-II inhibitor that causes double-stranded DNA breaks by a similar mechanism.

TABLE 5-2 • *Platinum Analogues*

Agent	Active Tumors	Side Effects	Precautions
Cisplatin	Germ cell tumors Ovarian Lung Bladder Head and neck Esophageal	Renal failure Nausea/vomiting Myelosuppression Neurotoxicity Alopecia Ototoxicity Optic neuritis SIADH Hypomagnesemia	Administer IVF before, during, and after treatment to prevent renal failure Consider baseline audiology examination to monitor ototoxicity Increased toxicity if given with valproic acid May decrease activity of phenytoin May decrease activity of valproic acid or carbamazepine
Carboplatin	Lung Ovarian Head and neck Bladder Endometrial Germ cell tumors Breast cancer	Myelosuppression Nausea/vomiting Neurotoxicity Renal failure	May decrease activity of phenytoin
Oxaliplatin	Colorectal Gastric	Neurotoxicity Nausea/vomiting Diarrhea Myelosuppression Hypersensitivity	Warn patients to avoid exposure to cold to prevent exacerbation of neurotoxicity

IVF, Intravenous fluids; *SIADH,* syndrome of inappropriate secretion of antidiuretic hormone.

Like the antimicrotubule agents, cancer resistance can develop through MDR gene expression and altered binding affinity of the target proteins: in this case, the topoisomerases. Additionally, decreased expression of the topoisomerases can lead to resistance. Irinotecan must be converted to its active metabolite, SN-38, and decreased conversion will result in resistance to this agent.

The topoisomerase inhibitors are listed in Table 5-4.

Antimetabolites

Antimetabolites are structural analogues to a variety of cellular substrates. There are three antimetabolites that are commonly used to treat solid tumors. These agents are discussed below, and they are listed in Table 5-5.

5-Fluorouracil (5-FU) is metabolized to FdUMP; FdUMP inhibits the enzyme thymidylate synthase, which is involved in thymidine synthesis. FdUMP and another metabolite, FdUTP, are misincorporated into DNA, thus inhibiting further DNA synthesis and transcription. The metabolite FUMP is misincorporated into RNA, which leads to aberrant RNA processing. Two agents related to 5-FU have important roles in cancer treatment. Capecitabine is an oral prodrug of 5-FU that is converted to 5-FU by the enzyme thymidine phosphorylase. FUDR is a form of 5-FU administered by intrahepatic arterial infusion. Given this way, almost all of the FUDR is removed by the liver through first-pass metabolism, with very little (<10%) passing into the systemic circulation.

Cells may become resistant to 5-FU through the increased expression of thymidylate synthase, the increased salvage of thymidine, the increased activity of DNA repair enzymes, or the increased expression of dihydropyrimidine dehydrogenase, which metabolizes and inactivates 5-FU.

Methotrexate is a folate analogue that binds to dihydrofolate reductase (DHFR) and that inhibits its ability to reduce folate. Reduced folate is required for the synthesis of thymidylate, purines, serine, and methionine. The increased expression of DHFR and altered DHFR, with lower binding affinity, are mechanisms of cancer-cell resistance.

Gemcitabine is a deoxycytidine analogue. The incorporation of its metabolite, dFdCTP, into DNA leads to the termination of DNA

TABLE 5-3 • Antimicrotubule Agents

Agent	Active Tumors	Side Effects	Precautions
Vinblastine	Germ cell tumors Melanoma Renal	Myelosuppression Mucositis Alopecia Neurotoxicity Autonomic dysfunction (hypertension) Constipation SIADH Hypersensitivity	Consider a prophylactic stool softener for constipation Activity reduced by phenytoin and carbamazepine May decrease activity of phenytoin
Vinorelbine	Breast Ovarian Lung (non-small cell)	Myelosuppression Nausea/vomiting Neurotoxicity Alopecia Constipation Diarrhea Mucositis SIADH Hypersensitivity Hepatotoxicity	Activity reduced by phenytoin and carbamazepine
Paclitaxel	Breast Lung Ovarian Head and neck Esophageal Prostate Bladder Germ cell tumors	Myelosuppression Hypersensitivity Neurotoxicity Alopecia Mucositis Diarrhea Cardiac arrhythmia Hepatotoxicity	Dexamethasone, antihistamines, and H_2 blockers should be administered before treatment to avoid hypersensitivity Resuscitation supplies should be available during administration Activity reduced by phenytoin and carbamazepine
Docetaxel	Breast Lung Ovarian Head and neck Esophageal Bladder Gastric	Myelosuppression Hypersensitivity Fluid retention Neurotoxicity Alopecia Arthralgias Myalgias Mucositis Diarrhea Rash	Administer dexamethasone prior to and after treatment to prevent hypersensitivity and fluid retention Resuscitation supplies should be available during administration Activity reduced by phenytoin and carbamazepine
Estramustine	Prostate	Nausea/vomiting Gynecomastia Diarrhea Rash Thromboembolism	

SIADH, Syndrome of inappropriate secretion of antidiuretic hormone.

synthesis. Its incorporation into RNA leads to faulty translation. Cancer-cell resistance develops with the increased expression of deoxycytidine synthase, which increases available deoxycytidine, or with the decreased expression of deoxycytidine kinase, which decreases the amount of gemcitabine metabolized to dFdCTP.

Antitumor Antibiotics

Most of the antitumor antibiotics have been derived from the *Streptomyces* species of fungus. All of the agents discussed in this section, except mitomycin-C, intercalate into DNA and inhibit its synthesis and transcription. In addition to this mechanism of action, mitoxantrone and doxorubicin inhibit topoisomerase II. Bleomycin and doxorubicin cause DNA breaks through the formation of free radicals. Mitomycin-C is metabolized to an alkylating agent, and it damages DNA through forming cross-links.

MDR gene expression contributes to cancer-cell resistance of doxorubicin, mitoxantrone, and mitomycin-C. Resistance to mitoxantrone and doxorubicin is also conferred by alterations in topoisomerase II (as with the

TABLE 5–4 • *Topoisomerase Inhibitors*

Agent	Active Tumors	Side Effects	Precautions
Irinotecan	Colorectal Lung Esophageal	Myelosuppression Diarrhea Alopecia Nausea/vomiting Hepatotoxicity Acute cholinergic effect (diarrhea, abdominal cramping, diaphoresis)	Treat acute cholinergic effect with atropine Treat diarrhea aggressively with loperamide Activity reduced by phenytoin
Topotecan	Ovarian Lung	Myelosuppression Nausea/vomiting Flu-like syndrome Alopecia Hepatotoxicity	Activity reduced by phenytoin
Etoposide	Lung Germ cell tumors Gastric	Myelosuppression Nausea/vomiting Alopecia Hypersensitivity 2° malignancies	Treat hypersensitivity with steroids, antihistamines, and H_2 blockers Increased toxicity if given with valproic acid May decrease activity of phenytoin

TABLE 5–5 • *Antimetabolites*

Agent	Active Tumors	Side Effects	Precautions
5-Fluorouracil	Colorectal Breast Anal Esophageal Gastric Pancreatic Hepatoma Head and neck Ovarian	Myelosuppression* Diarrhea* Mucositis* Hand-foot syndrome* Blepharitis Cardiac ischemia	Severe toxicity in patients with DHD deficiency May increase toxicity of anti-epileptic medications.
Capecitabine	Colorectal Breast	Mucositis Hand-foot syndrome Diarrhea Nausea/vomiting Hepatotoxicity Blepharitis Cardiac ischemia	Severe toxicity in patients with DHD deficiency May increase the effects of Coumadin
Flourodeoxyuridine (FUDR)	Colorectal or gastrointestinal adenocarcinoma metastases to the liver	Hepatotoxicity Diarrhea Myelosuppression Mucositis Hand-foot syndrome Blepharitis Cardiac ischemia Gastric ulcers	Severe toxicity in patients with DHD deficiency Acid blockers should be administered to prevent gastric ulceration Cholecystectomy is usually performed at the time of liver pump implantation to prevent drug-induced cholecystitis
Methotrexate	Breast Head and neck Sarcoma Bladder Gestational trophoblastic cancer Carcinomatous meningitis	Myelosuppression Mucositis Hepatotoxicity Renal failure Pneumonitis Arachnoiditis (when given intrathecally)	Accumulates in 3rd space fluid; should not be given to patients with ascites, pleural effusions, and the like May increase the effects of Coumadin Ineffective if given with folate Activity reduced by phenytoin and carbamazepine May decrease activity of phenytoin or valproic acid

TABLE 5-5 • *Antimetabolites*—Cont'd

Agent	Active Tumors	Side Effects	Precautions
Gemcitabine	Pancreatic Lung (non-small cell) Breast Bladder Sarcoma	Myelosuppression Nausea/vomiting Flu-like syndrome Hepatotoxicity Dyspnea Rash Hemolytic-uremic syndrome	Potent radiosensitizier

DHD, Dihydropyrimidine dehydrogenase.

*The side effects of 5-fluorouracil (5-FU) vary according to the schedule. Myelosuppression is more common when 5-FU is given on a weekly bolus schedule, whereas diarrhea is more common when 5-FU is given as daily boluses for 5 days. Mucositis and hand-foot syndrome are more likely to occur with continuous infusion schedules. The side effects of capecitabine are similar to those of continuous infusion 5-FU.

BOX 5–2 DIHYDROPYRIMIDINE DEHYDROGENASE

A small percentage of patients are deficient in dihydropyrimidine dehydrogenase (DHD), the enzyme that is responsible for 5-fluorouracil (5-FU) catabolism. DHD deficiency results in severe, often life-threatening, 5-FU toxicity, including diarrhea with hemodynamic collapse or neutropenia. Routine testing for DHD deficiency is not currently done, but it should be considered for patients with significant 5-FU toxicity. 5-FU must be discontinued in patients with DHD deficiency or severe 5-FU toxicity.

BOX 5–3 LEUCOVORIN

Leucovorin is a tetrahydrofolate that is often used with 5-fluorouracil (5-FU) or methotrexate for opposing reasons. Leucovorin potentiates the action of 5-FU by further inhibiting thymidylate synthase. Therefore, it is administered with 5-FU to achieve a greater antitumor effect. However, because leucovorin is already a reduced folate, it inhibits the antineoplastic action of methotrexate. Therefore, it is used after methotrexate to prevent or treat methotrexate toxicity.

topoisomerase inhibitors) and increased glutathione (as with the alkylating agents). Increased DNA repair enzymes contribute to bleomycin and mitomycin-C resistance.

The antitumor antibiotics are listed in Table 5-6.

Principles of Chemotherapy Use

Combination Chemotherapy

Chemotherapeutic agents are usually used in combination (rather than as single-agent therapy) to increase their efficacy. The most desirable combinations are those in which the agents used act synergistically. Chemotherapy combinations are more likely to produce this effect if their mechanisms of action and resistance are different. For example, the combination of bleomycin (intercalating agent), etoposide (topoisomerase-II inhibitor), and cisplatin (DNA cross-linking agent) is a highly effective regimen for testicular cancer. However, when combining chemotherapeutic agents, the potential overlapping toxicities must also be considered to avoid excessive toxicity. Doses may be adjusted to make a combination more tolerable, but dose reductions may interfere with the efficacy of the combination. Maintaining dose intensity is very important, especially when chemotherapy is given with curative intent.

Adjuvant Treatment

Adjuvant chemotherapy is given after surgery that has been performed with curative intent to improve the chance of cure. At the time of surgery, all visible tumor tissue is removed; however, microscopic tumor deposits may still be present locally or at distant locations. Because chemotherapy is most effective against very

TABLE 5–6 • *Antitumor Antibiotics*

Agent	Active Tumors	Side Effects	Precautions
Doxorubicin	Breast Ovarian Lung Bladder Thyroid Hepatoma Gastric Wilms' tumor Neuroblastoma	Myelosuppression Nausea/vomiting Cardiotoxicity Alopecia Mucositis Diarrhea Rash (radiation recall)	Infuse through a central venous catheter due to vesicant properties Obtain baseline LVEF and monitor for cardiotoxicity May decrease activity of valproic acid or carbamazepine
Mitoxantrone	Prostate	Myelosuppression Nausea/vomiting Cardiotoxicity Alopecia Hepatotoxicity 2° malignancy	Obtain baseline LVEF and monitor for cardiotoxicity
Bleomycin	Germ cell tumors	Skin reactions Alopecia Pulmonary toxicity Fever	Obtain baseline PFTs with DLCO and monitor Obtain baseline chest x-ray and monitor Avoid $FiO_2 > 50\%$, which may worsen pulmonary toxicity May decrease activity of phenytoin
Mitomycin-C	Anal Cervical Bladder Pancreatic Lung (non-small cell) Breast	Myelosuppression Nausea/vomiting Mucositis Pulmonary toxicity/ARDS Renal failure Hemolytic-uremic syndrome Cystitis (intravesicular treatment)	Avoid $FiO_2 > 50\%$, which may worsen pulmonary toxicity

ARDS, Acute respiratory distress syndrome; *DLCO,* carbon monoxide diffusion in the lung; *FiO_2,* fractional concentration of oxygen in inspired gas; *LVEF,* left ventricular ejection fraction; *PFTs,* pulmonary function tests.

small tumors, microscopic tumor deposits may be killed by chemotherapy. Therefore, chemotherapy is given with curative intent, and maintaining dose intensity throughout treatment is very important to ensure maximum antitumor effects.

The benefit gained from adjuvant chemotherapy can be thought of in terms of absolute benefit or relative benefit. For example, treatment with adjuvant 5-FU/leucovorin is the standard of care for colon cancer after it is found in regional lymph nodes. In that circumstance, the chance of cure after surgery is approximately 50%, but it can be increased to approximately 70% by adjuvant treatment with 5-FU/leucovorin. This translates into a 20% absolute benefit and a 40% relative benefit (i.e., 40% more patients are cured with chemotherapy than without chemotherapy). Although the improvement in cure rate seems impressive, it is important to understand the meaning of these statistics on an individual-patient basis. With a 20% absolute benefit, 80% of patients experience the inconvenience and side effects of chemotherapy without gaining any survival improvement themselves (Figure 5-1). Unfortunately, it is currently impossible to determine which patients will benefit and which will not before they are treated.

BOX 5–4 COMBINATION CHEMOTHERAPY

- It increases efficacy.
- Most desirable are those regimens in which agents act synergistically.
- Potential overlaps in toxicity must be considered.
- It is important to maintain dose intensity, especially when treatment is given with curative intent.

Whether or not a patient receives adjuvant chemotherapy is determined by a balance

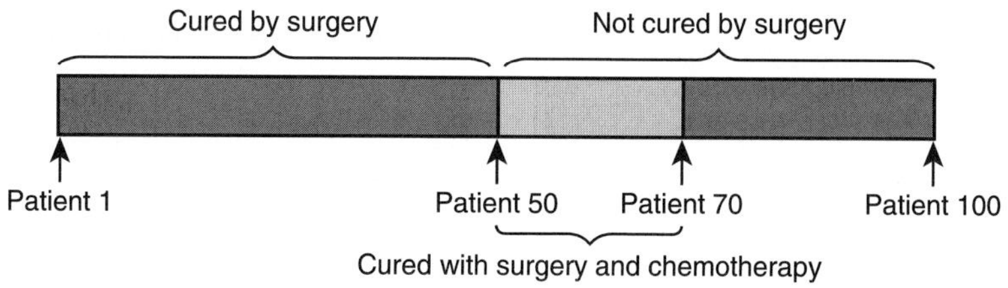

Figure 5-1. Schematic of the survival of adjuvant chemotherapy among patients with TX N1 colon cancer. Only patients in the yellow range will be cured by the addition of adjuvant chemotherapy, although all patients will receive it. Patients 1 through 50 would have been cured with surgery alone; Patients 71 through 100 are not cured with surgery or chemotherapy.

among the expected benefit of treatment, the patient's comorbid conditions and general health, and the patient's wishes. Patients in poor health may be no more likely to experience toxicity from treatment, but it is often much more difficult for them to recover from such side effects. These issues should be discussed in detail by the patient and an oncologist before treatment.

Adjuvant chemotherapy is usually not started within 4 weeks of surgery to prevent problems with wound healing. However, it should ideally be started within 6 to 10 weeks of surgery, because adjuvant treatments in most clinical trials were started during this timeframe; it is not known whether the same benefit can be expected if the treatment is delayed beyond this time. Typical adjuvant regimens for common malignancies and their approximate benefits are listed in Table 5-7.

Neoadjuvant Treatment

Neoadjuvant chemotherapy is usually given to reduce the size of a tumor before surgery, thereby making complete resection more likely or allowing for tissue or organ preservation. In a few studies, neoadjuvant treatment has been shown to prolong survival. Additionally, response to neoadjuvant chemotherapy appears to be an important predictor of survival.

TABLE 5-7 • *Adjuvant Chemotherapy Regimens*

Tumor	Stage	Regimen	Relapse-Free Survival* (percentage; no. of years)	Absolute Benefit†	Concurrent Radiation?
Gastric	IB-IV (M0)	5-Fluorouracil/leucovorin	45–50%; 3	15–20%	Yes
Breast	I-IIIA (N1)	Doxorubicin/cyclophosphamide or cyclophosphamide/methotrexate/5-fluorouracil	50–80%; 3	2–10%	No
	IIA-IIIA (N1)	Paclitaxel or docetaxel§	70%; 5	5%§	No
Colon	III	5-Fluorouracil/leucovorin	60–75%; 5	20–30%	No
Rectal	II-III	5-Fluorouracil/leucovorin	60–65%	15–20%	Yes
Colorectal	IV (liver)	5-Fluorouracil/leucovorin and intrahepatic fluorodeoxyuridine	55–60%; 2	30–35%	No
Lung (non-small cell)	T1-3/N0-1	Cisplatin/etoposide or vinca alkaloid	35–40%; 5	5%	No

*Relapse-free survival of patients treated with surgery and adjuvant chemotherapy (with or without radiation, as indicated in the last column).

†Absolute benefit represents percentage of relapse-free survival above surgery alone.

§Given after doxorubicin/cyclophosphamide; here, absolute benefit represents percentage of relapse-free survival above doxorubicin/cyclophosphamide only as adjuvant therapy.

The disadvantage of such treatment is that staging is based on clinical findings, and the true pathologic stage may not be determined at the time of surgery if there has been a good response to chemotherapy. In certain circumstances, this may have an impact on adjuvant therapy or prognosis estimates. For example, a borderline-large breast mass without palpable lymph nodes may be treated with neoadjuvant chemotherapy to make breast conservation surgery more likely to be successful with negative margins. If there is a good response to treatment in the primary tumor, it is also likely that there will be a good response in any affected lymph nodes. If previously positive lymph nodes are negative at the time of surgery, this may change whether further adjuvant chemotherapy is offered. However, residual disease in lymph nodes after neoadjuvant treatment is also prognostic. Breast cancer patients with a pathological complete remission have a much better prognosis than those with residual disease at the time of surgery.

Surgical treatment should be delayed until patients have recovered from the most significant toxicities of chemotherapy, such as neutropenia. Neoadjuvant regimens and their purposes for specific tumor types are listed in Table 5-8. Neoadjuvant treatments for many other tumor types, such as for unresectable pancreatic cancer, are currently being evaluated in clinical trials, but they are not yet proven to be beneficial. Although neoadjuvant chemotherapy can be considered for a variety of patients with locally advanced disease, it is preferable that these patients receive treatment as part of an appropriate clinical trial.

Chemotherapy Without Surgery

In general, nonhematologic malignancies are cured by surgery rather than chemotherapy, but there are a few exceptions. Anal cancer is cured in approximately 80% of patients with combined chemoradiation using 5-FU/mitomycin-C as the first-line treatment. Testicular cancer, even when widely metastatic, is curable with bleomycin/etoposide/cisplatin in approximately 85% of patients.

However, the majority of patients for whom treatment with chemotherapy alone is appropriate have metastatic disease that is not curable. For these patients, treatment with chemotherapy is intended to prolong survival and/or improve quality of life. Response rates range from 20% to 75%, depending on the tumor type and the chemotherapy regimen. However, even a complete remission is rarely durable. Most partial or complete remissions last only months.

As with adjuvant chemotherapy, the patient's general health must be considered when deciding which chemotherapy regimen, if any, to recommend. Because the disease is not curable, treatments with single agents, which are less toxic than combination chemotherapy, are often considered. A patient's wishes must also be followed; some patients are more willing than others to tolerate the side effects of chemotherapy. As noted previously, decreased dose intensity is associated with decreased efficacy. Although this principle remains important when treatment is given for metastatic disease, there is more willingness to reduce doses for toxicity because the disease is not curable.

TABLE 5–8 • *Neoadjuvant Chemotherapy Regimens*

Tumor	Regimen	Purpose	Concurrent Radiation?
Rectal	5-Fluorouracil/leucovorin	Sphincter sparing	Yes
Head and neck	Cisplatin/5-fluorouracil	Convert to resectable disease Improved delivery of chemotherapy Larynx sparing	Maybe
Breast	Doxorubicin/cyclophosphamide	Breast conservation Convert to resectable disease	No
Thymoma	Cisplatin/doxorubicin containing	Convert to resectable disease	No
Esophageal	Platinum/5-fluorouracil containing	Improved survival?	Maybe
Bladder	Methotrexate/vinblastine/ Doxorubicin/cisplatin	Bladder-sparing surgery possible Improved survival (57% vs. 43% with surgery only at 5 years)	No

Treatment of Chemotherapy Toxicity

When chemotherapy toxicity develops, medical intervention may or may not be necessary, depending on the toxicity and its severity. There are no adequate treatments for some toxicities, such as neuropathy and pulmonary toxicity. If these develop to a significant extent, treatment must be discontinued. Cardiotoxicity resulting from doxorubicin is predictable for cumulative doses above 550 mg/m^2. If doses approaching this level are required, dexrazoxane may be administered to prevent cardiotoxicity, but patients must be carefully monitored. Although alopecia only resolves after chemotherapy is stopped, it is not considered a significant enough side effect to cause therapy to be discontinued. Nausea, vomiting, diarrhea, flu-like symptoms, and myelosuppression are treatable side effects, and they can usually be controlled when dose intensity is an issue.

BOX 5–5 TREATABLE CHEMOTHERAPY SIDE EFFECTS AND THERAPIES

- Nausea and vomiting: lorazepam, metoclopramide or prochlorperazine, omeprazole or cimetidine, serotonin 5-HT3 receptor blockers (e.g., Ondansetron)
- Diarrhea: loperamide
- Flu-like symptoms: acetaminophen or ibuprofen
- Myelosuppression: antibiotics, growth factor support (e.g., Darbepoietan, granulocyte-colony–stimulation factor), transfusion

Nausea and Vomiting

Nausea and vomiting are mainly caused by serotonin release from the gastrointestinal mucosa, which leads to stimulation of the emesis center of the medulla. Therefore, prophylactic antiemetic medications containing 5-HT$_3$ serotonin antagonists (e.g., ondansetron), are used with the more emetogenic chemotherapy regimens. Dexamethasone may improve the response to 5-HT$_3$ serotonin antagonists. The benzodiazepine lorazepam is useful for anxious patients. Metoclopramide or prochlorperazine are useful for nausea occurring several days after treatment and for chemotherapy regimens of lower emetogenic potential. Finally, gastric mucosal damage can contribute to nausea; in these cases, an acid blocker such as omeprazole or cimetidine may be beneficial.

Flu-like Symptoms and Diarrhea

Fever, arthralgias, and myalgias may occur and are usually controlled with acetaminophen or ibuprofen. Patients receiving treatments associated with diarrhea should be instructed about the use of loperamide (usually two tablets after each loose stool) to prevent severe diarrhea.

Myelosuppression

Myelosuppression is a very common side effect of many chemotherapy regimens, and it may manifest as neutropenia, anemia, or thrombocytopenia. It usually occurs within 5 to 15 days of treatment. Mild neutropenia, which is an absolute neutrophil count of >1000/mm^3, does not require any action, although doses of chemotherapy may be reduced. Patients with more significant neutropenia should be instructed to report fevers, because they are at increased risk of infection. Antibiotics are required to treat neutropenic fever, even if a source is not found. Granulocyte colony-stimulation factor should be considered for patients in whom a prolonged neutrophil recovery is expected, such as patients with impaired bone marrow function before treatment. After a neutropenic fever, patients should receive prophylactic granulocyte-colony–stimulation factor during subsequent cycles of chemotherapy. Pegfilgrastim, which is longer acting and requires only one dose, may also be given.

Anemia is treated with erythropoietin or blood transfusion if the patient is symptomatic. Patients who feel fatigued and who have a hemoglobin level of <10 gm/dL are likely to benefit from erythropoietin. Darbepoetin, which is a longer-acting version of erythropoietin, may also be used. There is currently no effective treatment for thrombocytopenia other than platelet transfusion.

Conclusion

Although chemotherapeutic agents have different mechanisms of action, they all interfere with normal cellular processes. In addition to causing tumor cell death, this interference affects normal dividing cells, thus leading to significant side effects. Side effects should be treated to improve patient quality of life during treatment and also to maintain dose intensity. This is especially important for treatment given for curative intent, such as in the adjuvant and neoadjuvant settings. Chemotherapy given for palliative purposes (i.e., that given for most metastatic disease) also loses benefit with decreased dose intensity; however, this must be balanced against quality-of-life issues.

Key Reading

Chu E, DeVita VT. *Physicians' cancer chemotherapy drug manual,* Sudbury, Mass: Jones and Bartlett Publishers, Inc., 2003.

Selected Readings

Bosl GJ, Motzer RJ. Testicular germ-cell cancer, *N Engl J Med* 1997;337:242–253.

Chau I, Chan S, Cunningham D. Overview of preoperative and postoperative therapy for colorectal cancer: the European and United States perspectives, *Clin Colorectal Cancer* 2003;3:19–33.

Coleman RE. Current and future status of adjuvant therapy for breast cancer, *Cancer* 2003;97(3 Suppl): 880–886.

Crown J, Dieras V, Kaufmann M, *et al.* Chemotherapy for metastatic breast cancer—report of a European expert panel, Lancet Oncol 2002;3:719–726.

Floyd JD, Nguyen DT, Lobins RL, *et al.* Cardiotoxicity of cancer therapy. *J Clin Oncol* 2005;23:7685–7696.

Forastiere AA, Goepfert H, Maor M, *et al.* Concurrent chemotherapy and radiotherapy for organ preservation in advanced laryngeal cancer, *N Engl J Med* 2003;349:2091–2098.

Grossman HB, Natale RB, Tangen CM, *et al.* Neoadjuvant chemotherapy plus cystectomy compared with cystectomy alone for locally advanced bladder cancer, *N Engl J Med* 2003;349:859–866.

International Multicentre Pooled Analysis of Colon Cancer Trials (IMPACT) Investigators. Efficacy of adjuvant fluorouracil and folinic acid in colon cancer, *Lancet* 1995;345:939–944.

Kaufmann M, von Minkwitz G, Thuss-Patience PC, *et al.* International expert panel on the use of primary (preoperative) systemic treatment of operable breast cancer: review and recommendations, *J Clin Oncol* 2003;13:2600–2608.

Kemeny N, Huang Y, Cohen AM, *et al.* Hepatic arterial infusion of chemotherapy after resection of hepatic metastases from colorectal cancer, *N Engl J Med* 1999;41:2039–2048.

Martel CL, Gumerlock PH, Meyers FJ, Lara PN. Current strategies in management of hormone refractory prostate cancer, *Cancer Treat Rev* 2003;29:171–187.

O'Connell MJ, Martenson JA, Wieand HS, *et al.* Improving adjuvant therapy for rectal cancer by combining protracted-infusion fluorouracil with radiation therapy after curative surgery, *N Engl J Med* 1994;331:502–507.

Rizzo JD, Lichtin AE, Woolf SH, *et al.* American Society of Clinical Oncology; American Society of Hematology: Use of epoetin in patients with cancer: evidence-based clinical practice guidelines of the American Society of Clinical Oncology and the American Society of Hematology, *J Clin Oncol* 2002;20:4083–4107.

Rubenstein EB. Colony stimulating factors in patients with fever and neutropenia, *Int J Antimicrob Agents* 2000;16:117–121.

Ryan DP, Compton CC, Mayer RJ. Carcinoma of the anal canal, *N Engl J Med* 2000;342:792–800.

Schuchter LM, Hensley ML, Meropol NJ, Winer EP. American Society of Clinical Oncology Chemotherapy and Radiotherapy Expert Panel: 2002 Update of recommendations for the use of chemotherapy and radiotherapy protectants: clinical practice guidelines of the American Society of Clinical Oncology, *J Clin Oncol* 2002;20:2895–2903.

Urschel JD, Vasan H. A meta-analysis of randomized controlled trials that compared neoadjuvant chemoradiation and surgery to surgery alone for resectable esophageal cancer, *Am J Surg* 2003;185: 538–543.

Verstappen CC, Heimans JJ, Hoekman K, Postma TJ. Neurotoxic complications of chemotherapy in patients with cancer: clinical signs and optimal management, *Drugs* 2003;63:1549–1563.

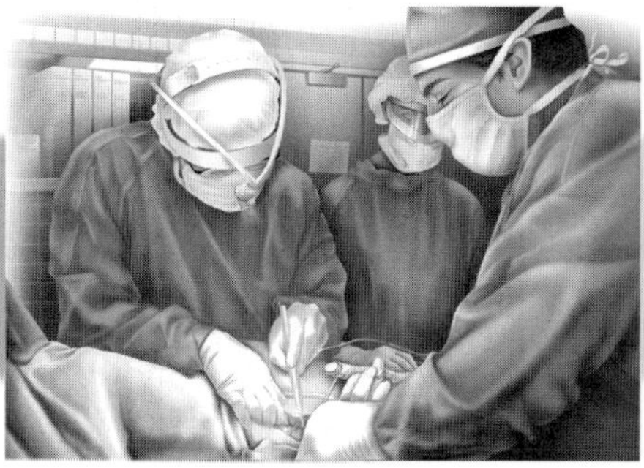

6

Principles of Radiation Therapy

Michael E. Ray and Michael S. Sabel

- DEFINING IONIZING RADIATION
- HOW RADIATION KILLS CELLS
- RADIATION DELIVERY
- RADIATION TREATMENT PLANNING
- ADVERSE EFFECTS OF RADIATION
- IMPROVING THE EFFECTS OF RADIATION
- CLINICAL APPLICATIONS OF RADIATION THERAPY

Principles of Radiation Therapy: Key Points

- Describe the three methods by which photons transfer energy to tissue.
- Explain the ways of measuring the interaction between energy and tissue.
- Outline the processes that contribute to sublethal damage repair.
- List the "four Rs" of radiobiology.
- Differentiate teletherapy from brachytherapy.
- List the steps to follow when planning radiation treatment.
- Describe the major acute and late radiation adverse effects.
- Explain altered fractionation and intensity-modulated radiation therapy.
- Name the main clinical uses of radiation treatment.

Shortly after x-rays were discovered in 1895 by Wilhelm Roentgen, their effects on biologic tissues were realized. In 1898, Henri Becquerel accidentally left 200 mg of radium in his pocket, which caused erythema and skin ulceration that took weeks to heal. Subsequent experiments demonstrated that radiation had different effects on different tissues and that these effects could be manipulated to kill malignant cells while sparing normal ones. Hence, the field of radiation oncology was born, and further advances in the delivery of higher energy radiation beams for the deeper penetration of tissues with less damage to the skin greatly expanded its versatility for the treatment of cancer.

Ionizing radiation is defined as energy with sufficient strength to cause the ejection of an orbital electron from an atom when the radiation is absorbed. When this occurs in biologic tissue, the ejected electrons can damage molecules that are crucial to the survival of the cell, thereby resulting in cell death. Radiation oncology is a specialty that combines the fields of radiation physics, cell and tumor biology, and clinical oncology (Figure 6-1). In this chapter, we will review how ionizing radiation interacts with tissue, both physically and biologically, and we will then focus on how to apply these concepts to the treatment of cancer patients.

Ionizing Radiation

Ionizing radiation can take either an electromagnetic form, such as high-energy photons, or particulate forms, such as electrons, protons, neutrons, alpha particles, or other particles. Most radiation oncology departments treat patients with either photons or electrons. Electrons interact directly with tissue to cause ionization; this is in contrast with photons, which affect tissues by the electrons that they eject. Electron beams deliver a high skin dose and exhibit a rapid fall-off after only a few centimeters. Electron absorption in human tissue is also affected when the beam passes through low-density air cavities (increased dose) or high-density bone (decreased dose). In modern clinical practice, electron beams are commonly used to treat superficial targets (e.g., skin cancers, lymph nodes) that are within a few centimeters of the surface of the body, because electrons are unable to penetrate into deeper tissues.

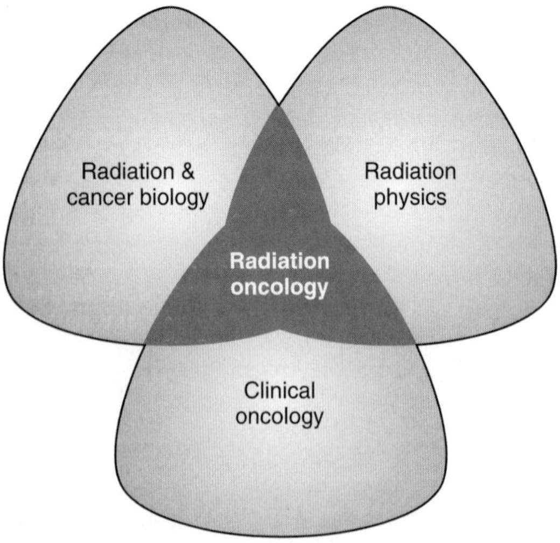

Figure 6–1. The field of radiation oncology represents the overlap of multiple disciplines, including radiation and cancer biology, radiation physics, and clinical oncology.

More commonly, electromagnetic radiation (high-energy photons) is used to treat cancer; this consists of either gamma rays (photons created from the decay of radioactive nuclei) or x-rays (photons created by the interaction of accelerated electrons with the electrons and nuclei of atoms in an x-ray tube). Photons transfer energy to tissue in three ways: via the photoelectric effect, via the Compton effect, and via pair production. With the *photoelectric effect,* the incoming photon undergoes a collision with a tightly bound electron. In doing so, all of the energy

BOX 6–1 TRANSFER OF ENERGY TO TISSUE

Photoelectric Effect

- Incoming photon collides with a tightly bound electron so that all energy is transferred to the electron
- Dominant interaction at photon energies of 10–25 keV

Compton Effect

- Most important interaction
- Photon collides with free electron and transfers some energy, thus scattering photon and electron
- Additional interactions of lower energy are possible while the electron begins to ionize with the transferred energy
- Dominant interaction at photon energies of 60 keV to 20 MeV

Pair Production

- Photon interacts with nucleus of atom, which absorbs energy
- Pair of electrons results: one positively charged (positron) and one negatively charged
- Positron ionizes until it combines with a free electron, after which the resulting two photons scatter
- Dominant interaction at photon energies of ≥25 MeV

of the photon is transferred to the electron. The photon ceases to exist, whereas the electron departs and begins to directly ionize surrounding molecules.

The *Compton effect* is the most important interaction between photons and tissue at the typical photon energies used in radiation therapy. As opposed to colliding with a tightly bound electron, in this case, the photon collides with a "free electron," which is one that is not tightly bound to the atom relative to the incident photon energy. As a result of the collision, the photon transfers some of its energy to the electron, thereby scattering both the photon and the electron in various directions. The photon can then undergo additional interactions (with a subsequently lower energy), whereas the electron begins to ionize with the energy it gained from the photon.

Finally, *pair production* refers to the interaction between the photon and the nucleus of an atom (as opposed to an electron). When the nucleus absorbs the photon's energy, a pair of electrons is formed: one positively charged and one negatively charged. The positively charged electron (a positron) ionizes until it combines with a free electron, thus forming two photons that scatter in opposite directions.

Which effect takes places depends on the energy of the photon and the tissue being treated. The basic unit of energy used in radiation oncology is the electron volt (eV); 10^3 eV is equal to 1 keV, and 10^6 eV is equal to 1 MeV. The likelihood of a photoelectric interaction is directly proportional to the atomic number (Z) of the absorbing material taken to the third power, and it is inversely proportional to the energy (E) of the photon taken to the third power. Photoelectric effects tend to occur at photon energies in the 10 to 25 keV range. The photoelectric effect is the basis for the excellent contrast between bone (high Z) and soft tissues (low Z) using relatively low-energy diagnostic x-rays, and it is why lead is such a good shielding agent for low-energy photons. The probability of a Compton interaction is not dependent on the atomic number, but it is inversely proportional to the energy of the incoming photon. Compton interactions predominate in the 60 keV to 20 MeV photon energy range, which includes the typical energy range used in radiation therapy. The probability of pair production is proportional to the logarithm of the energy of the incoming photon, and, like the photoelectric effect, it is dependent on the atomic number of the tissue. The energy range in which pair production dominates is 25 MeV or greater, although it does occur at low frequencies at energies used in clinical radiation therapy.

To quantify the interaction of this energy with tissue, one must first measure the ionization produced in air by the beam of radiation. This quantity is known as *exposure*, and it is measured in Roentgens (R). One can then correct for the presence of soft tissue and calculate the *absorbed dose*; this is the amount of energy absorbed per unit of mass. This was previously measured in rads, but today it is typically measured as joules per kilogram, or Gray (Gy); 100 rad is equal to 1 Gy, which is equal to 100 centiGy. The dose absorbed by tissues as a result of these interactions can then be measured and plotted to form a percentage depth dose curve (Figure 6-2). As photons enter tissue, the dose increases at first, as photons collide with electrons triggering ionization events; it then begins to fall off as a result of attenuation of the photon beam by tissue and the fact that radiation falls off with the square of the distance from the source (this is the result of a law of physics known as

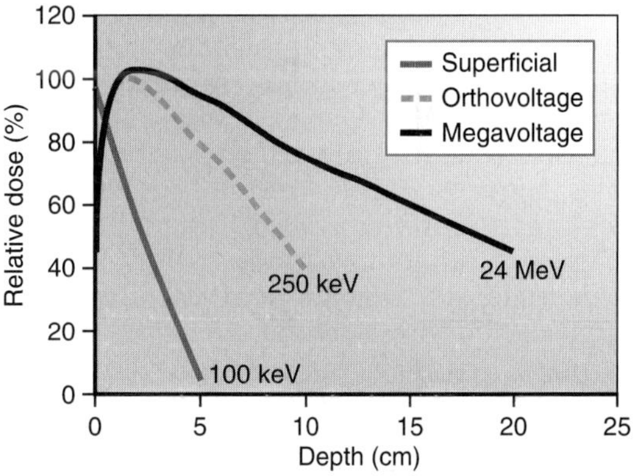

Figure 6-2. A depth-dose plot displays the relative percentage of the deposition of dose as a beam of ionizing radiation penetrates to various depths of biologic tissue. In general, the relative dose decreases as the radiation penetrates more deeply into tissue as a result of attenuation of the beam and increased distance from the radiation source. Higher-energy radiation beams penetrate more deeply into tissue, whereas low-energy beams fall off rapidly at depth. High-energy beams have a superficial "buildup" of a few centimeters in which electrons are mobilized to deposit the full dose at a depth specific to the beam energy. Because of this, modern megavoltage radiation therapy is much more skin-sparing than historical treatment delivery using lower energy sources, such as cobalt-60.

the *inverse square law,* which is discussed further below). As energy increases, attenuation by tissue decreases, and the dose depth penetration increases, bringing a larger dose to deep tissues while relatively sparing the skin surface.

There are different ranges of electromagnetic radiation used in clinical practice, although megavoltage equipment predominates in modern clinical practice. *Superficial radiation* uses low-energy photons from 10 to 125 keV. Uncommonly used, this has very little penetration, and it can only be used to treat very superficial tumors. *Orthovoltage radiation* uses photon energies from 125 to 400 keV. This can treat slightly deeper structures, and it is occasionally used for skin cancers in modern practice. Photon energies above 400 keV are referred to as *supervoltage radiation,* and those of more than 1 MeV are referred to as *megavoltage radiation.* At these energies, Compton interactions predominate, and the maximum dose is not reached at the skin but at some depth below the surface that is a function of the beam energy.

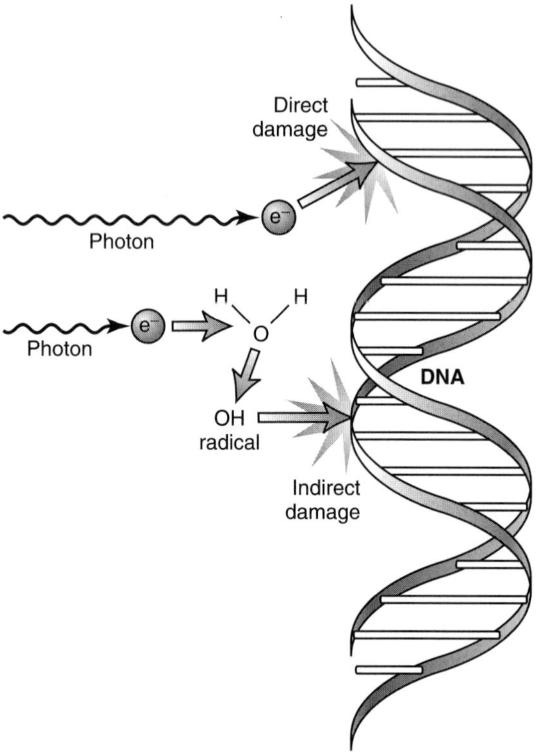

Figure 6–3. Radiation may cause ionization of a high-energy electron that directly causes a DNA strand break (direct damage). Alternatively, radiation may cause ionization of a high-energy electron that then interacts with a water molecule, thereby forming free-radical molecules, such as hydroxyl radicals. These highly reactive species rapidly interact with neighboring molecules such as DNA (indirect damage), again resulting in DNA strand breaks.

How Radiation Kills Cells

When ionizing radiation encounters biological tissues, ejected electrons either interact directly with the target molecules within the cell, or they interact indirectly with water to produce free radicals (e.g., hydroxyl radicals) that subsequently interact with target molecules (Figure 6-3). During their brief life span, electrons and free radicals interact with molecules in a random fashion. If they interact with molecules that are not crucial to cell survival, the effect of the radiation will be harmless. If they react with biologically important molecules, the effect will be detrimental. Molecular oxygen prolongs the life of reactive radicals, thereby increasing the likelihood that it will have a detrimental effect. This is why tumor hypoxia tends to increase resistance to radiation. Sulfhydryl compounds and other antioxidants reduce the life span of free radicals by combining with them, thereby also increasing cellular resistance to radiation.

Although ionizing radiation may damage many molecules within the cell, the most critical injury with respect to cell death appears to be DNA damage in the form of single- or double-strand breaks (Figure 6-4). Cells have relatively efficient repair mechanisms for single-strand breaks in DNA, because there is an intact template on which to replicate a repair patch. However, repair errors may occur and result in mutations, and this ultimately lead to the increased incidence of secondary malignancies.

Double-strand breaks in DNA are much more difficult for cells to repair, because the integrity of the molecule is compromised with the creation of two free ends that separate from one another in space, leaving no template upon which to repair the break. Cellular mechanisms for double-strand break repair do exist; however, their efficiency is variable, and repair may not be sufficient before cells trigger pathways that lead to programmed cell death (apoptosis) or before they enter into mitosis with damaged DNA, thereby leading to mitotic catastrophe and cell death. Therefore, the ability of ionizing radiation to kill cells depends not only on the generation of enough

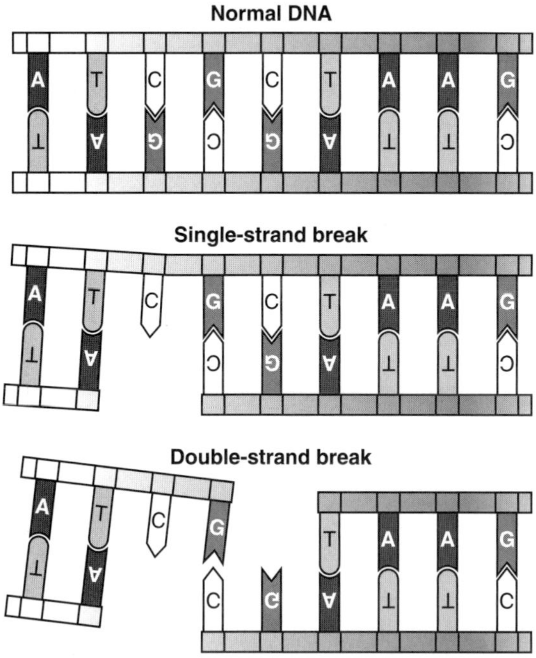

Figure 6–4. Radiation exerts its biological effects by damaging biological molecules within the cell, mainly DNA. DNA damage occurs when the double-helix "backbone" of the molecule is broken. Single-strand breaks are damaging to the cell; however, the integrity of the molecule can be relatively easily restored by DNA repair mechanisms within the cell. When DNA suffers a double-strand break, the broken ends of the DNA molecule can physically separate in space. These lesions are much more damaging because of the infidelity and inefficiency of cellular mechanisms to reapproximate and repair double-strand breaks.

DNA double-strand breaks to overwhelm repair pathways but also on the time the cell has to repair those breaks before the next mitotic cell division.

This explains the phenomenon known as *sublethal damage repair,* during which increased cell survival is observed if a dose of radiation is divided into two fractions separated by a time interval. As the time interval between the fractions increases, the surviving fraction of the cells also increases as the cells are able to repair double-strand DNA breaks. Furthermore, if the time interval is sufficiently long, the cells will once again begin to proliferate via a process known as *repopulation.*

Radiation cell killing is highly dependent on the phase of the cell cycle of the injured cell. The most sensitive phase of the cell cycle is M phase, which occurs just as a cell is about to undergo mitosis, with another sensitive phase occurring during the early part of G1. Cells in S phase and late G1 are relatively more resistant to the lethal effects of radiation. In a population of cells within a tumor or a normal tissue, there will typically be a distribution of cells within various phases of the cell cycle. Those cells in sensitive phases will likely be killed, whereas those in more resistant phases will more likely survive, which leads to a temporary phase synchronization in the cell population until the cells can reassort back into the sensitive cell cycle phases.

Of course, in clinical radiation therapy, the goal is to kill the cancer cells but spare the normal cells. Delivering a single large dose of radiation will have a high rate of tumor cell killing, but the concordant killing of the normal tissue cells may limit the clinical utility. This has led to the development of the multi-fraction regimens commonly used today, which typically deliver daily fractions of 1.8 to 2.5 Gy. The advantages of fractionated courses of radiation therapy are explained by the *four Rs* of radiobiology: repair (of sublethal damage); repopulation (of cells within tumor or tissue); reassortment (of cells within the cell cycle); and reoxygenation (of hypoxic tumor tissue).

BOX 6–2 THE "FOUR Rs" OF RADIOBIOLOGY

1. Repair (of sublethal damage)
2. Repopulation (of cells within tumor or tissue)
3. Reassortment (of cells within the cell cycle)
4. Reoxygenation (of hypoxic tumor tissue)

Fractionation of a radiation dose spares normal tissues because of their greater ability to repair sublethal damage between dose fractions and to repopulate with cells if the overall time is sufficiently long. Although tumors may also repair sublethal damage and repopulate, there is increased damage to the tumor, because dividing a dose into a number of fractions allows for the reoxygenation of hypoxic regions within the tumor and the reassortment of tumor cells into radiosensitive phases of the cell cycle between dose fractions. Actively cycling cell populations, such as those within tumors, reassort themselves to a greater degree than cells within slowly proliferating tissues that are not actively cycling. Furthermore, tumors frequently have hypoxic regions that are radioresistant, and the interval between fractions again allows for reoxygenation before the subsequent fraction.

Radiation Delivery

Teletherapy

Radiation is administered by two methods: either by an external machine (teletherapy) or by the implantation of radioactive sources in or around the tumor (brachytherapy). In the past, teletherapy radiation was delivered using cobalt-60, a radioisotope produced in nuclear reactors. Although cobalt machines are very reliable, their usefulness is limited by a relatively low energy output (about 1.2 MeV). Because of this, cobalt therapy is unable to penetrate to deep tumors without significant skin toxicity. Furthermore, because of the significant size of the cobalt source, geometric factors create difficulty for achieving sharp beam edges, which are necessary to limit the dose to normal tissues. Today, external radiation is most often administered using a linear accelerator, which is capable of producing higher-energy photons without the geometric disadvantages associated with cobalt-60 units.

No matter the source, the beam of radiation needs to be modified to get optimal delivery of the desired dose to the tumor while minimizing the dose to the normal tissues. Typically, the beam of radiation is rectangular, with a relatively flat depth-dose curve in the center, with fall-off on the sides (Figure 6-5, *A*). The "edges" of the beam are defined as a point at which the dose is 50% of that at a central reference point. Collimators are thick shielding devices made from materials with a high atomic number such as lead. Primary collimators at the head of the machine create a rectangular beam, and additional devices, such as wedges, compensators, blocks, or multileaf collimators, are used to further modify the beam to desired specifications. Wedges allow for a higher fluence through on one side of the beam with less on the opposite side, thereby altering the angle seen on depth-dose charts at varying angles from 15° to 60° (Figure 6-5, *B*). Wedges or compensators can also optimize the dose distribution if the treatment surface is curved or irregular. The beam can also be shaped using individually fashioned blocks that are custom made for each patient's anatomy and for their tumor size and shape. In modern linear accelerators, multileaf collimators have replaced handmade blocks, and these allow for automated and precise field shaping without the use of cumbersome handmade blocks.

The patient is positioned on a table, known as a *couch*. Modern treatment units use isocentric techniques in which the entire room is engineered around a central point. In three dimensions, the couch, treatment gantry, and collimator all rotate around the three axes at the *isocenter*. After the patient is lined up using external marks in reference to the isocenter of the room, treatment can be delivered precisely and accurately to the target identified during the treatment planning process.

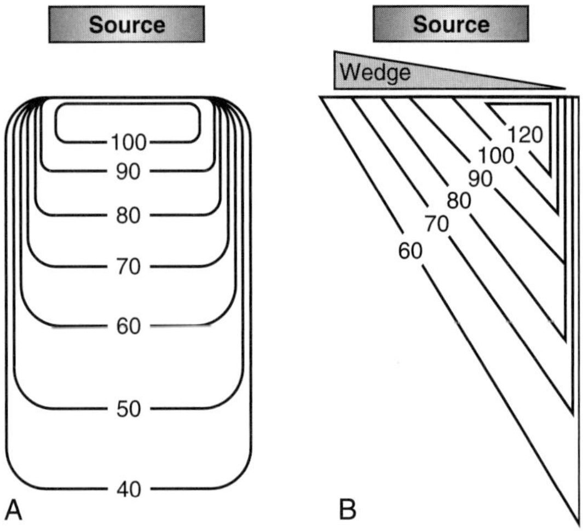

Figure 6–5. One of the simplest methods of changing the shape of a radiation beam's dose distribution in tissue is to use beam modifiers like wedges. An unmodified radiation beam penetrating tissue is shown in cross section in **A. B,** A wedge-shaped piece of metal has been placed in the path of the radiation beam. Radiation passing through the thicker metal on the "heel" side of the wedge is relatively more attenuated, and it will subsequently penetrate less deeply into tissue. Radiation passing through the thinner metal on the "toe" side of the wedge will be less attenuated, and it will penetrate more deeply into tissue. This produces a triangular-shaped depth-dose distribution when viewed in cross section.

Brachytherapy

Brachytherapy (*brachy* comes from the Greek for "short distance") involves the placement of sealed radioactive sources into or next to the target tissue. It takes advantage of the inverse square law, which states that the intensity of electromagnetic radiation dissipates as the inverse square of the distance from the source. Thus, if radioactive sources can be placed so that the tumor is within a centimeter of the sources, the dose received by normal tissues just 2 cm distant from the source and 1 cm distant from the tumor would be one fourth of the dose received by the tumor (Figure 6-6). This can allow for the delivery of a high dose to the tumor with only a modest dose to normal tissue (Figure 6-6).

Implantation techniques are as diverse as the applications for brachytherapy. The surgical approach to the target volume may be interstitial (e.g., prostate seed implantation), intracavitary (e.g., gynecologic applicators), transluminal (e.g., endoscopic applications), or surface mold techniques (e.g., eye plaques for ocular melanoma). The implants may be permanent or temporary, and the dose may be delivered using low (0.02-4 Gy/hr), medium, or high (>12 Gy/hr) dose rates. Many modern applications use afterloading techniques that place treatment applicators and load radioactive sources afterward to reduce radiation exposure for therapy personnel. Modern remote afterloading equipment uses pneumatically or motor-driven source transport mechanisms to robotically transfer radioactive sources between a shielded safe and the treatment applicator while personnel are safely outside of the treatment room.

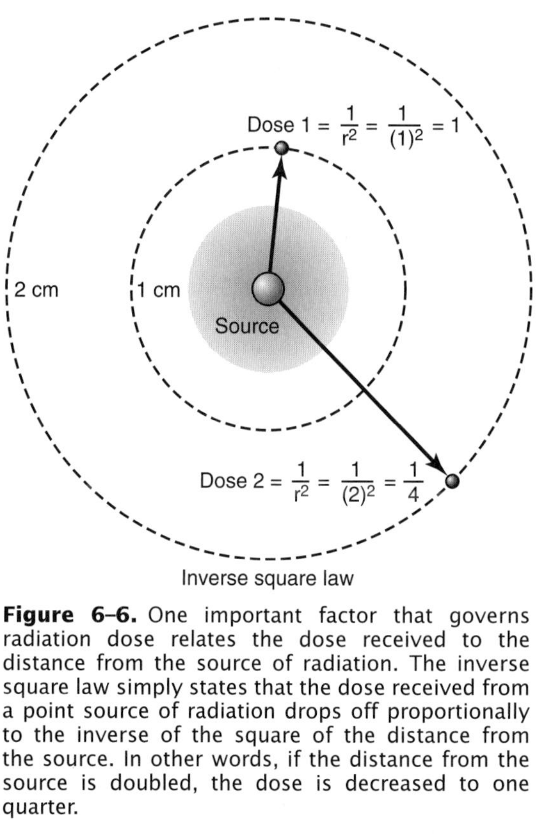

Figure 6–6. One important factor that governs radiation dose relates the dose received to the distance from the source of radiation. The inverse square law simply states that the dose received from a point source of radiation drops off proportionally to the inverse of the square of the distance from the source. In other words, if the distance from the source is doubled, the dose is decreased to one quarter.

As mentioned in the introduction, Dr. Becquerel discovered the power of brachytherapy more than 100 years ago. It was first applied therapeutically during the early 1900s, and interest has again surged during the last few decades. Historically, early radiotherapists used radium sources for intracavitary and interstitial applications. Alternative isotopes have now been developed that offer improved safety and physical properties that make them suited for various applications (Table 6-1). Among the most commonly used isotopes are cesium-137 for low-dose rate procedures (e.g., temporary tandem and colpostat insertions for cervical cancer), iridium-192 for temporary low- and high-dose rate interstitial and intracavitary procedures, and iodine-125 or palladium-103 for permanent interstitial prostate seed implants.

Radiation Treatment Planning

After a patient has been evaluated and a course of radiation deemed to be of use, planning is initiated. This process involves five steps:

1) *Determining the region that requires treatment:* This is done by a combination of physical examination; plain x-rays; computed tomographic scanning, magnetic resonance imaging, and positron emission tomography scanning; and

TABLE 6–1 • *Common Brachytherapy Sources and Applications*

Isotope	Half-Life	Energy	Application
Radium-226	1,600 years	0.83 MeV	Historical interstitial and surface molds
Cobalt-60	5.26 years	1.17–1.33 MeV	Teletherapy and brachytherapy
Cesium-137	30.0 years	0.662 MeV	LDR intracavitary gynecologic implants
Iridium-192	74.2 days	0.38 MeV	HDR applications; interstitial LDR
Gold-198	2.7 days	0.412 MeV	Eye plaques; permanent interstitial
Iodine-125	60.2 days	0.028 MeV	Permanent interstitial
Palladium-103	17.0 days	0.021 MeV	Permanent interstitial

HDR, High-dose rate; *LDR,* low-dose rate.

knowledge of the clinicopathologic characteristics of the disease, including patterns of spread and failure patterns.

2) *Localizing the patient and the involved region in three-dimensional space (in a manner that can be referenced to the linear accelerator):* Initially, the optimal patient position is determined to allow for a combination of beams to treat the target while minimizing the normal-tissue dose. Immobilization devices, such as custom-made foam cradles or mesh-plastic masks, are constructed to allow for comfortable and reproducible patient positioning for daily treatment. The conventional x-ray simulator is a device that is a geometric mock-up of a clinical linear accelerator with the same isocentric design described earlier. Instead of a high-energy beam source powered by a linear accelerator, a fluoroscopic unit consisting of a diagnostic quality x-ray tube and detector are mounted on the device. This allows the patient to be positioned and manipulated using adjustments of the couch, gantry, and collimator angles under fluoroscopic guidance exactly as the patient would be set up on the treatment machine. After a satisfactory beam arrangement is determined, plain x-ray films document the proper setup, and this setup can be translated to the treatment unit. Blocks are drawn by hand on the simulation x-rays, and they are then fabricated and fixed to a tray that can be mounted on the linear accelerator during treatment. More recently, the computed tomography simulator has been introduced. This device performs precisely the same functions, but the accuracy of localization is greatly increased by soft-tissue information. A three-dimensional representation of the patient is generated by computer from the computed tomography data. All of the manipulation of the couch, gantry, and collimator—as well as the functions of block design—can be performed in virtual space on a computer workstation instead of requiring the patient to remain immobilized for prolonged periods during simulation. At the end of this session, reference marks are placed on the patient (tattoos), which will be used in reference to the isocenter to facilitate accurate and precise daily setup.

3) *Determining beam arrangement:* The complexity of this step varies tremendously depending on the clinical setting. In some cases (e.g., a proposed treatment of a bone metastasis to the upper thoracic spine), a single posterior field may be sufficient to treat the tumor. In other cases, such as when an effort is being made to treat the tumor but spare the parotid glands (e.g., head and neck cancer), it may be necessary to use 6 to 10 distinct treatment apertures (fields), each of which may be subdivided into segments to vary the intensity of radiation across the field (this is called *intensity modulated radiation therapy*, or IMRT). In traditional (forward) radiation planning, a beam arrangement is constructed inside the planning system; the expected dose distribution produced by this arrangement is calculated, and the physician decides whether the goals of planning have been achieved. If not, another beam arrangement is attempted. Plans can be displayed using isodose lines or three-dimensional surfaces that indicate the region that is receiving more than a particular dose (Figure 6-7). Treatment planning tools, such as dose-volume histograms, yield additional information to help evaluate potential plans. An exciting area of research is that of *automated-dose optimization* (also called *inverse planning*), in which the physician defines a set of objectives that are to be met when treating the tumor and avoiding normal tissue; a computer then determines the beam arrangement that would produce a satisfactory dose distribution.

4) *Verification of beam arrangement:* After an acceptable plan is determined, the patient is aligned to reference markers on the linear accelerator couch, and the beam arrangement is evaluated. Diagnostic images (and/or portal images, which are analogous to fluoroscopy images for the treatment unit) are obtained to verify that the planned beams treat the regions predicted by the treatment planning process.

5) *Treatment:* Radiation is typically delivered in daily fractions, from as few as 1 to more than 40. Traditionally the radiation therapist manually aligns the patient and manipulates the machine position and configuration to administer therapy. More recently, this process has been computer controlled, thus permitting complex, multifield plans to be delivered accurately and efficiently. Each treatment

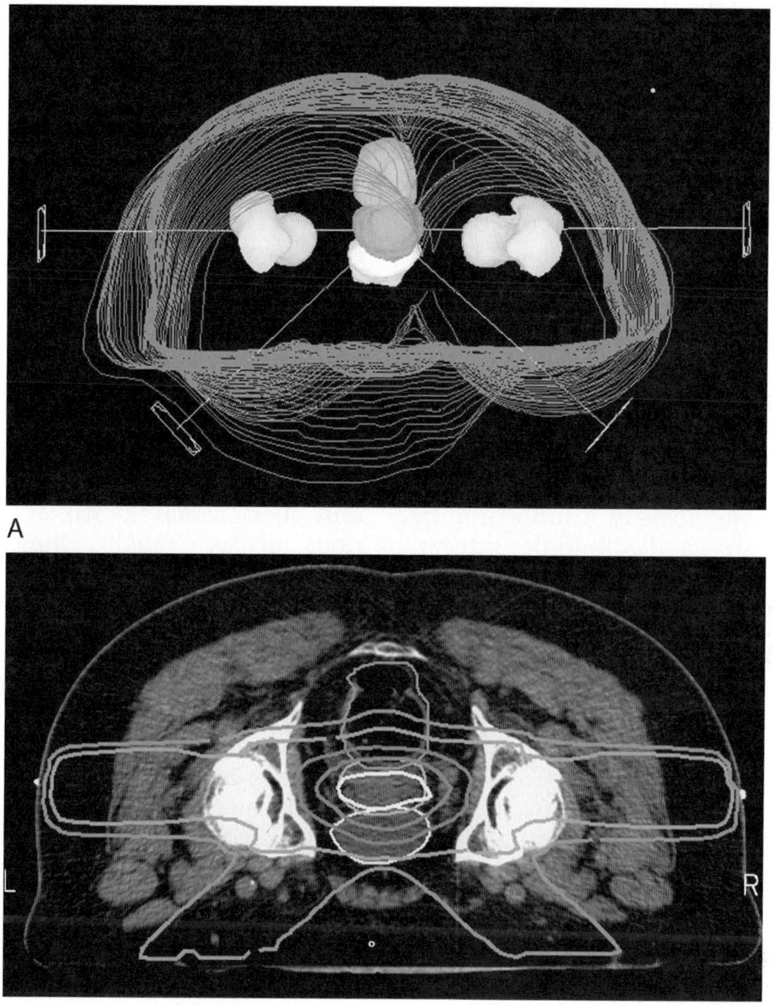

Figure 6–7. Three-dimensional conformal treatment planning involves choosing combinations of radiation beams with appropriate angles, shapes, energies, and other modifications in an effort to maximize conformation of the radiation dose to the target while minimizing the radiation dose to normal structures. **A,** A configuration of radiation beams to treat the prostate gland while sparing the rectum and bladder. **B,** The relative doses received by various tissues are displayed with isodose lines overlaid on a CT scan.

typically takes less than 15 minutes. Most of this time is spent aligning the patient and the machine; the radiation beam is on for only a minute or two. Treatment is similar to undergoing a diagnostic x-ray, and the patient will not feel the beam when it is on.

BOX 6–3 ADVERSE EFFECTS OF RADIATION

- Acute radiation effects
- Late radiation effects
  - Immunosuppression
  - Secondary malignancies

Adverse Effects of Radiation

Acute Radiation Effects

Acute radiation effects are those toxicities that occur within a few weeks to months of radiation therapy. They occur mainly in classic self-renewing tissues that are characterized by constant mitosis within a stem cell compartment, thus producing progeny that "turn over" the tissue cell population every few days to weeks. This includes bone marrow, skin and its appendages, and mucosal surfaces of the oropharynx, esophagus, stomach, intestines, rectum, bladder, and vagina. Actively proliferating stem cells produce progeny that divide and differentiate into mature functioning cells. Radiation mainly kills actively dividing cells within the stem cell compartment while having minimal effect on the mitotically inactive mature-functioning cells. After the normal life span of the mature cells expires, the normal turnover and replacement with new cells does not occur because of radiation killing of the dividing stem cells. Therefore, the timing of maximum acute effects is determined by the normal life span of mature cells within the affected tissue, which ranges from a few days for intestinal epithelium to a few weeks for skin, mucosal surfaces, and hematopoietic tissues.

Similar to tumors, normal tissue effects are influenced by the four Rs of radiobiology. Acute normal tissue toxicity is influenced by both fraction size and the time interval between fractions. The more rapidly a given dose is delivered during the overall treatment period, the more severe the acute effects will be. This is relevant for the strategies that modify dose and fractionation, as discussed below. A decrease in fraction size or prolongation of the interval between fractions allows the cell populations to repair and repopulate, thereby decreasing the severity of acute toxicity.

The acute toxicities observed during clinical radiation therapy obviously depend on the anatomic site being treated. Head and neck irradiation are among the most toxic during the acute period because of significant mucositis of the oral cavity, oropharynx, larynx, and cervical esophagus. Skin and the salivary glands are also affected. Mucositis, yeast superinfection, desquamation, pain, xerostomia, odynophagia, dysphagia, dehydration, and malnutrition are all common clinical scenarios that radiation oncologists manage when delivering head and neck radiotherapy, and concomitant chemotherapy can further add to acute toxicity. Other common acute effects observed during radiation therapy directed at other anatomic sites include dysphagia and cough from thoracic radiation; nausea, vomiting, and diarrhea from abdominal radiation; and dysuria, proctitis, pain, and perineal desquamation from pelvic radiation.

Self-renewing tissues have tremendous reserve and are able to rapidly repopulate as long as the stem cell population is not completely sterilized. With modern clinical radiation therapy, most acute effects are temporary, and complete recovery is typical within a few weeks to months after the completion of treatment. Acute effects to non–self-renewing tissues are exceptions, such as xerostomia, which is a permanent side effect of head and neck radiotherapy that encompasses the salivary glands.

Late Radiation Effects

Late effects are those toxicities that occur months to years after radiotherapy and that are more commonly permanent. Mitotically inactive tissues without the capacity for self-renewal are commonly involved. The mechanisms that cause late effects may include direct damage to the parenchymal cells within an organ or indirect effects as a result of microvascular damage. Each organ is characterized by a *tolerance dose,* which is a radiation dose above which the risk of organ complications increases rapidly. These normal tissue tolerances are the true dose-limiting factors in clinical radiation therapy, because late complications can be permanent and, in some cases, life threatening.

An important fact is that the risk of late complications is increased by using a large fraction size; this again relates to the repair capacities of normal tissues. This is relevant for strategies that alter dose and fractionation, as discussed later. In addition to dose, the risk of complications is also influenced by the volume of the organ tissue irradiated. In general, increasing the dose and the volume irradiated leads to the increased risk of organ complications.

The types of late complications induced by radiation can vary. For the brain, late toxicity may mean necrosis of the brain tissue, whereas in the kidney it may mean nephrotic syndrome and organ failure (Table 6-2). The tolerance doses for different organs vary over a large range, from a few Gray causing sterility after testicular irradiation to more than 100 Gy causing necrosis or perforation of the uterus. Late complications may include fibrosis, necrosis, ulceration and bleeding, chronic edema, telangiectasias and pigmentation changes, cataract formation, nerve damage, lung pneumonitis and fibrosis, pericarditis, myocardial damage, bone fracture, liver or kidney failure, sterility, intestinal obstruction, and fistula and stricture formation.

Immunosuppression

The hematopoietic system is acutely sensitive to ionizing radiation, because it is a classic self-renewing tissue. Similar to the effects of

TABLE 6–2 • *Tolerance Doses of Normal Organs Resulting in Approximately 5% Risk of Complications Within 5 Years After Radiation*

Organ	Tolerance Dose (5% at 5 years)	Complication
Testes	1 Gy	Sterilization
Ovaries (age dependent)	2-10 Gy	Sterilization
Bone marrow	2.5 Gy	Aplasia
Lens	10 Gy	Cataract
Kidney	20 Gy	Kidney failure
Salivary gland	30 Gy	Permanent xerostomia
Spinal cord	50 Gy	Infarction (paralysis)
Intestine	50 Gy	Obstruction, ulcer, perforation
Skin (100 cm^2)	55 Gy	Dermatitis, telangiectasia
Oral mucosa	60 Gy	Ulceration, mucositis
Brain	60 Gy	Necrosis
Peripheral nerve	60 Gy	Neuritis
Uterus	100 Gy	Necrosis/perforation

systemic chemotherapy, the irradiation of stem cells within the bone marrow depletes the renewal of mature blood cells, thus leading to nadirs in white blood cell and platelet counts 2 to 3 weeks after exposure. Furthermore, the irradiation of lymphocytes triggers rapid apoptosis, so the irradiation of a large field can cause a rapid lymphopenia. A single whole body exposure of 2 to 8 Gy may be lethal as a result of immunosuppressive effects; this is known as the *hematopoietic syndrome*. Although whole-body irradiation is only used clinically as part of preparative regimens for bone marrow transplants, even local radiation can have immunosuppressive effects if large areas of bone marrow are irradiated. Furthermore, direct damage to lymphocytes as they pass through the area being targeted or by the radiation-induced release of immunosuppressive cytokines may contribute to immunosuppressive effects. The clinical consequence of most radiation therapy regimens on the immune system appears to be small; however, it is unclear how this might affect the combination of radiation therapy and immunotherapy.

Secondary Malignancies

The most serious of late effects from radiation may be the induction of second malignancies. Radiation-associated second malignancies generally arise as solid tumors that are distinct from the original tumor but that originate within the irradiated area. New malignancies at distant sites outside of the radiation fields are unlikely to be related to previous radiation. Second malignancies arise as a consequence of somatic mutations induced by DNA damage inflicted by radiation but that are incompletely repaired by the cell. A latency period of 8 or 10 or even 20 or 30 years is not uncommon before additional genetic or environmental factors combine with radiation-induced mutations to result in a clinically detectable second malignancy. The influence of dose and volume on secondary malignancy risk has been difficult to quantify; however, the age and developmental status of the

BOX 6–4 CHARACTERISTICS OF RADIATION-INDUCED SECONDARY MALIGNANCIES

- Usually arise as solid tumors that are distinct from the original tumor but within the irradiated area
- Caused by somatic mutations induced by radiation damage to DNA that is incompletely repaired
- Latency periods of 20 to 30 years not uncommon, with a minimum of 4 to 7 years
- Age and developmental status of patient important determining factors
  - Pediatric and adolescent patients at increased risk
- Older patients at low risk

patient appear to be critical. In particular, pediatric and adolescent patients have a substantial risk of second malignancy after therapeutic radiation, whereas older adults have quite a low risk. This likely relates to the vastly different life expectancies between pediatric and adult patients and the long latency period associated with secondary malignancies. In addition, pediatric and adolescent patients are in developmental stages when various tissues are still undergoing active division and differentiation (e.g., breast development in the adolescent female). This most likely explains the high risk (35% to 40%) of secondary breast cancer among female patients treated for Hodgkin's disease with thoracic radiation therapy during their teenage years. Various sarcomas are other tumor types that may be induced by radiation, and these include angiosarcomas that may arise in areas of chronic lymphedema caused by axillary surgery and radiation for breast cancer.

Improving the Effects of Radiation

Dose, Time, and Fractionation

Standard fractionation for radiation therapy in current clinical practice within the United States is the delivery of one treatment of 1.8 to 2.0 Gy per day, Monday through Friday, to total doses felt to be potentially curative for the tumor (usually 60 to 70 Gy) within tolerance of the normal tissues within the treated volume. This approach produces a fairly well understood chance of tumor control and risk of normal tissue damage (as a function of volume). By altering the fractionation schemes, one may be able to improve the outcome for patients undergoing curative treatment or to simplify the treatment for patients receiving palliative therapy. Two forms of altered fractionation have been tested for patients undergoing curative treatment: *hyperfractionation* and *accelerated fractionation* (Table 6-3).

With hyperfractionation, the dose per fraction is significantly decreased, whereas the number of dose fractions is increased (usually delivered twice daily). The total dose is usually slightly increased, and the overall treatment time is unchanged. With accelerated fractionation, the overall treatment time is significantly decreased, whereas the number of dose fractions, the total dose, and the fraction size are unchanged or slightly decreased. Accelerated hyperfractionation incorporates the concepts of both of these strategies.

The rationale for altering fractionation is based on radiobiologic considerations of the four Rs and observations from clinical practice. Late effects are more sensitive to changes in the size of the dose per fraction, whereas acute reactions and tumor response are more sensitive to changes in the overall rate of dose delivery. Depending on whether the dose is limited by acute reactions (e.g., severe mucositis during head and neck irradiation) or late effects (e.g., severe fibrosis, fistula formation), alterations to fraction size and schedule can be made to improve the therapeutic ratio. Hyperfractionation uses smaller fraction sizes, thereby decreasing the risk for late effects while delivering a similar overall dose at a similar rate and not compromising tumor control. Accelerated fractionation decreases the overall treatment time, thereby increasing the likelihood of tumor control as well as acute toxicity while using similar fraction size, total dose, and number of fractions in an attempt to not increase the risk of late effects. Accelerated fractionation attempts to address the issue of accelerated repopulation, during which tumors may increase their rate of proliferation during a course of fractionated radiation.

TABLE 6–3 • *Comparison of Hyperfractionation and Accelerated Fractionation*

Hyperfractionation	Accelerated Fractionation
Dose per fraction decreased	Fraction size unchanged or decreased slightly
Number of dose fractions increased	Number of dose fractions unchanged or decreased slightly
Total dose slightly increased	Total dose unchanged or decreased slightly
Treatment time unchanged	Overall treatment time significantly decreased
No alteration of tumor control	Improved likelihood of tumor control
Lower risk for late effects	Greater acute toxicity

Altered fractionation has been found to improve local control rates in multiple clinical trials, particularly among patients with head and neck cancer, and it may represent the standard of care for selected malignancies. Most altered-fractionation protocols attempt to incorporate some degree of both hyperfractionation and acceleration, trading some increase in temporary acute reactions for the promise of improved tumor control without significantly increasing risks of late effects.

Radiosensitization and the Halogenated Pyrimidines

Radiosensitizers are drugs or chemical compounds that enhance the lethal effects of radiation. Importantly, a good radiosensitizer must have a favorable *therapeutic ratio*. In other words, it must have a differential effect between tumors and normal tissues to be clinically useful. The best examples and the most clinically used category of radiosensitizers in modern clinical practice are the halogenated pyrimidines, including 5-fluorouracil (5-FU). The precise mechanism by which 5-FU and other nucleoside analogues radiosensitize cells remains unclear; however, halogenated nucleoside analogues are incorporated into the DNA of cycling tumor cells, and the intracellular pools of deoxyribonucleotides are depleted. Intravenous 5-FU remains the most commonly used agent clinically; however, the oral agent capecitabine (a prodrug that is converted to 5-FU within the body) is being actively investigated for use in combination with radiation therapy. Gemcitabine is another commonly used chemotherapeutic agent with powerful radiosensitizing properties, even when used at very low doses. Although early trials showed significant toxicity from combining gemcitabine and radiation, ongoing studies seek to optimize this powerful combination by limiting the gemcitabine dose and/or radiation doses and field sizes.

Targeting Tumor Hypoxia as a Mechanism of Radioresistance

The presence of hypoxia decreases the likelihood that radiation will be effective, and it may be a component of tumor radiation resistance in the clinic. Therefore, there has been considerable interest in measuring and improving tumor oxygenation. Early attempts centered around hyperbaric oxygen. Some reports suggested increased cure rates for head and neck and cervical cancers when hyperbaric oxygen was combined with radiation as compared with conventional daily fractionation. However, the cost and cumbersomeness of the technique and the difficulty for the patient has led most radiotherapy centers to abandon the technique. Simple interventions to improve tumor oxygenation (e.g., giving blood transfusions to anemic patients) have been shown to be associated with improved local control in patients with uterine cervix cancer.

Radiosensitizers that are selectively targeted against hypoxic tumor cells may represent another technique to combat the effect of hypoxia. These molecules mimic oxygen in their effect of increasing the life span of free radicals, and, in addition, they may be directly cytotoxic to hypoxic cells, or they may sensitize cells to chemotherapeutic agents. Misonidazole and its related nitroimidazole compounds have been shown to significantly improve radiosensitivity in hypoxic cells in culture, but they have shown disappointing results when tested in clinical trials. Tirapazamine is a hypoxic cell cytotoxin that appears to be highly selective in tissue culture studies; however, the few clinical experiences with the compound have been hampered by toxicity concerns.

Improved Delivery

Three-dimensional conformal radiation therapy is a geometric shaping of the radiation beam so that the fields conform closely to the shape of the tumor. Radiation beams can be delivered from any angle in three dimensions. Combining multiple shaped beams from multiple angles allows an increased dose to the tumor and possibly better control while relatively sparing the surrounding normal tissues. This has been one of the most important fundamental advances in radiation therapy over the past couple of decades.

Similar three-dimensional techniques are employed in various types of radiosurgery, where a small target volume can be treated with a high dose of radiation therapy using multiple beams. Radiosurgery is typically performed for small lesions in the brain, with a rigid immobilization frame bolted to the patient's skull. Radiosurgery can be delivered using conventional linear accelerators or a sophisticated cobalt-60 teletherapy unit called a *gamma knife*.

With the improved capabilities of the computed tomography scan-simulator, modern radiation therapy is not only more precise, but it allows for the shaping of the intensity of the radiation beam as well; this is referred to as IMRT. Modern IMRT planning systems use inverse planning computer algorithms that optimize the shapes and fluence patterns of all of the treatment beams with the goal of making the treatment as conformal as possible. In this way, a more uniform dose distribution is delivered around the tumor, with minimal dose received by the surrounding normal tissues.

Brachytherapy, as discussed previously, represents another method for improving dose delivery simply by virtue of the inverse square law. By placing radioactive sources within the target volume, the target will receive a relatively high dose, whereas the rapid fall-off in dose will provide a relative sparing of the adjacent normal tissues.

Other forms of teletherapy may offer improved delivery as well. Proton-beam radiotherapy offers specific physical advantages over electron and photon beam therapy. Because protons deposit an enormous amount of energy just before stopping, proton-beam therapy is capable of achieving steep dose gradients to conform high-dose radiation to a target, even when the target is adjacent to critical normal structures that must be spared. Because of the cost, only a handful of proton-beam facilities exist in the world.

Clinical Applications of Radiation Therapy

Radiation Therapy as Definitive Local Treatment

Although radiation therapy is typically used in combination with other treatments, radiation can also be used as monotherapy with curative intent. Many malignancies can be cured with this therapy, with high rates of success. Examples of tumors with high control rates when treated with radiation alone include basal and squamous skin cancers, benign brain tumors, ocular melanomas, head and neck cancers (particularly small laryngeal cancers), certain lymphomas, and prostate cancer. Some tumor types are better treated using combined treatment; however, cancers of the esophagus, lung, and anal canal, as well as other lymphomas, can be treated with curative intent using radiation alone.

Radiation therapy can also be used as definitive local treatment in combination with systemic therapies (e.g., chemotherapy, hormonal therapy). Examples of this treatment approach include sequential or concurrent chemotherapy and radiation for limited stage small-cell or stage III non–small-cell lung carcinoma and combined androgen deprivation and radiation therapy for clinically localized prostate cancer.

Organ Preservation Strategies

An important related treatment concept concerns the use of radiation (with or without chemotherapy) for organ preservation. For example, combined chemotherapy and radiation therapy can replace radical surgery for the treatment of advanced head and neck cancers, achieving comparable local control and survival while preserving critical organs, such as the larynx. This strategy of organ conservation permits voice preservation in approximately two thirds of patients with advanced larynx cancer. The use of chemotherapy and radiotherapy to treat anal cancer can also be viewed in this light, with chemoradiotherapy producing organ conservation and cure rates superior to those of the radical surgery used decades ago.

The treatment of early-stage breast cancer provides an example where conservative surgery may be combined with radiation therapy to achieve results that are comparable with those of more radical surgery. No fewer than seven randomized trials have demonstrated that lumpectomy plus radiation produces survival equal to that of modified radical mastectomy while allowing for the preservation of the breast. Another important example is in the treatment of soft-tissue sarcoma, in which limb-sparing surgery plus radiation produces equivalent survival and comparable local control to that resulting from amputation. Finally, investigations of bladder-preserving therapy using maximal transurethral resection followed by concurrent chemotherapy and radiation therapy have shown survival rates comparable with radical cystectomy series.

Combining Radiation Therapy and Surgery

Radiation therapy also plays a crucial role in adjuvant therapy after surgery, because the two modalities are often complementary. Surgery removes gross disease, whereas radiation therapy is most effective for sterilizing residual microscopic disease. Several organ-preserving strategies already discussed use the two treatment modalities in this way. The benefit of adjuvant radiation therapy depends on the risk of local recurrence. Furthermore, the acute and late toxicities of radiation therapy must be weighed against the local control benefit. If the risk of local recurrence is small, or if a local recurrence can be easily dealt with by a second surgical resection, the benefits of adjuvant radiation therapy may not outweigh the risk of acute and late effects. On the other hand, when complete resection of the tumor still carries a high risk of residual occult disease and local recurrence creates excessive morbidity, adjuvant radiotherapy is often recommended. In some cases, the prevention of local recurrence not only increases local control, but it also improves the disease-free and overall survival. Indeed, there is accumulating evidence that radiation therapy in the postmastectomy setting for high-risk breast cancer not only improves local control, but it may also improve overall survival. It is important to note, however, that radiation will not compensate for inadequate surgery. If gross disease or positive margins remain, higher doses to larger volumes may be required, which may be poorly tolerated and less successful.

Radiation therapy may be delivered after surgery in the adjuvant setting or before surgery in the neoadjuvant setting. Advantages of postoperative radiation therapy include complete anatomic and pathologic information, often allowing for more accurate treatment portals based on the known residual tumor burden. Surgical clips delineating the tumor bed or areas of residual tumor or positive margins are very useful for the treating radiation oncologist, and they indicate the importance of multidisciplinary patient management. Ideally, the radiation oncologist may attend the surgical procedure to view the anatomy of the tumor bed and the placement of surgical clips that will aid subsequent radiation treatment planning. The tumor can be assessed pathologically without the effects of the radiation. In addition, tissue healing after surgery is better in nonirradiated tissues.

However, in some cases, it is preferable to deliver preoperative radiation. Radiation can shrink the tumor, thus diminishing the extent of the resection or making an unresectable tumor resectable. Preoperative radiation therapy for rectal cancer may enable consideration of a low anterior resection as opposed to abdominoperineal resection. Preoperative treatment of abdominal masses (e.g., a large retroperitoneal sarcoma) enables the radiation oncologist to conform the radiation more accurately to the tumor and to limit normal tissue radiation. In the postoperative setting, the radiation fields would treat large areas of normal bowel and other tissues that fall back into place after tumor removal and that may become fixed in place by adhesions, thus increasing the risks of normal tissue toxicity. In addition, oxygenation may be better in the preoperative setting before resection disrupts the native vasculature.

Palliative Radiation

Radiation is also important for the palliation of symptoms produced by cancers, even when cure is not possible. Treatment is highly effective for relieving the pain that results from bony metastases. The combination of systemic treatment with narcotics and adjuvant medications (e.g., antidepressants, antiepileptics, antiinflammatories) with localized radiation to sites of severe pain can relieve pain in the great majority of patients. Radiation therapy may also be used for the palliation of tumors that may obstruct the respiratory, gastrointestinal, or genitourinary tracts.

A special category that does not fit neatly into the foregoing discussion concerns the role of radiation during oncologic emergencies. These include superior vena cava syndrome resulting from tumor occlusion of the superior vena cava (typically resulting from either lymphoma or lung cancer) and spinal cord compression. In both of these cases, the prompt initiation of radiation therapy (usually in combination with steroids) may reverse life-threatening or neurologically devastating situations.

Key Selected Reading

Chao K, Perez C, Brady L. *Radiation oncology: management decisions,* ed 2. Philadelphia: Lippincott Williams & Wilkins, 2002.

Selected Readings

Elshaikh M, Ljungman M, Ten Haken R, Lichter AS. Advances in radiation oncology. *Ann Rev Med* 2006; 57:19–31.

Kahn F. *The physics of radiation therapy,* ed 3. Philadelphia: Lippincott Williams & Wilkins, 2003.

Leibel S, Phillips T. *Textbook of radiation oncology,* ed 2. Philadelphia: Saunders; 2004.

Mittal B, Purdy J, Ang KK. *Advances in radiation therapy.* Boston: Kluwer Academic Publishers; 1998.

Purdy J. *3-D conformal and intensity modulated radiation therapy: physics and clinical applications.* Madison, Wis.: Advanced Medical Publishing, 2001.

7

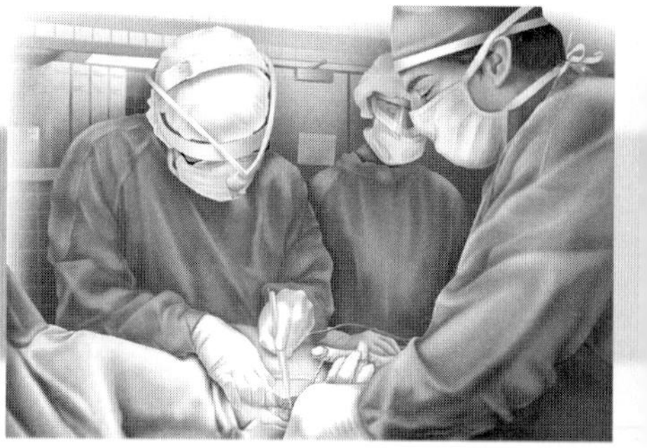

Principles of Immunotherapy

Michael S. Sabel and Alisha Arora

Principles of Immunotherapy: Key Points

- Describe and compare the two types of tumor-specific immune responses.
- Discuss the various types of antigens that can serve as targets for immunotherapy.
- Explain the mechanisms of passive immunotherapy.
- Describe the approaches to nonspecific active immunotherapy.
- Discuss the principles of cancer vaccines and the various types of vaccines used.

The concept of activating the immune system to reject tumors dates back at least several millennia. The treatment of tumors by the injection of infected purulent materials has been documented in both Eastern and Western ancient medical writings. In 1893, William Coley, a surgeon at Memorial Hospital in New York, reported that injecting a sarcoma with streptococcal broth cultures resulted in tumor regression. When the injections were stopped, tumor growth resumed. Injection of a new streptococcal culture elicited a life-threatening attack of erysipelas, but the tumor regressed significantly, and the patient lived for 8 more years. On the basis of these results, Coley began treating inoperable patients with "Coley's toxin," which consisted of either viable or killed bacteria. At the time, William Coley had little knowledge of the mechanisms involved in the generation of an immune response. As knowledge of the components of the immune system has grown, interest in harnessing its power as a therapy against cancer has also grown.

Principles of Antitumor Immune Responses

Understanding the methods by which the immune system may recognize and destroy tumor cells is essential to understanding approaches to immunotherapy. There are two broad types of tumor-specific immune responses (Table 7-1). The first is the humoral arm, which involves antibody production by B cells. The humoral response is triggered by the interaction between the variable region of an antibody with specific epitopes on cell-surface molecules. The other response happens via the cellular arm, which is mediated by cytotoxic (CD8+) T cells. This response involves the recognition of antigens by T cell receptors when they are presented by the cell in conjunction with the major histocompatibility complex (MHC) molecules. Antibodies are not capable of detecting the small processed peptides on MHC molecules located on the cell surface, and so the nature of the antigens recognized by the humoral and cellular arm are quite different. However, the humoral and cell-mediated immune responses overlap in that the activation of a B cell response usually requires the presence of helper T cells. Which immune response is more important in generating antitumor immunity is subject to debate; interestingly, cancer patients who exhibit both responses appear to fare better than those who demonstrate only one type of response or no response.

Tumor Antigens

The key to the specificity of immunotherapy is the presence of cancer-specific antigens to which either a humoral or cellular response can be initiated. The immune system's ability to differentiate between "self" and "nonself" is frequently referred to, so it may seem intuitive that, because cancer cells originate from "self," they would have few if any unique antigens. This is not true, however, and there are several types of antigens that can serve as targets for immunotherapy (Table 7-2). One category includes antigens that are encoded by the genetic alterations responsible for the malignancy. The aberrant proteins that result from genetic mutations not only deprive the cell of the wild-type functions (resulting in malignant transformation), but also they can lead to new "nonself" proteins exhibiting increased immunogenicity. Point mutations of the p53 oncogene, for example, have resulted in proteins that the immune system is capable of recognizing as foreign.

The next category is that of antigens present on germ-line cells but not on normal cells. These antigens, which are exemplified by the cancer-testis antigens, are sometimes expressed on cancer cells as a result of changes in transcriptional regulation. Because

TABLE 7–1 • *Humoral vs. Cellular Immune Response*

	Humoral Response	Cellular Response
Principal cell	B lymphocyte	T lymphocyte
Recognizing molecule	Immunoglobulin	T cell receptor
Types of antigens recognized	Proteins, polysaccharides, nucleic acids, others	Proteins
State of antigens	Free or cell-surface	Processed
Methods of cellular death	Antibody-dependent cell-mediated cytotoxicity Complement-dependent cytotoxicity Opsonization	Granulocyte exocytosis Triggering of target cell receptors

TABLE 7–2 • *Examples of Tumor Antigens*

Mutated oncoproteins	ras, p53
Cancer-testis antigens	MAGE-1, MAGE-3, BAGE, GAGE-1, GAGE-2, NY-ESO-1
Differentiation proteins	Tyrosinase, Gp100, Mart-1/Melen-A, Gp75/TRP-1, PSA, PSMA
Overexpressed self proteins	CEA, HER-2/neu, PSA
Viral proteins	E6, E7 (human papilloma virus), EBV, HCV

germ-line cells do not express MHC molecules, these antigens are normally silent; when expressed on cancer cells, however, they are capable of eliciting an immune response. The MAGE family of antigens, (MAGE-1 was the first human gene product identified in a patient with cancer that was recognized by CD8+ T cells), along with the related GAGE and BAGE families, are the classic examples.

Differentiation antigens are shared by both cancer cells and normal cells, but they are massively overexpressed in cancerous tissue. It is possible that an immune response to these antigens could also stimulate an autoimmune destruction of the normal tissues that express them. The clinical significance of this, however, may be trivial. In the treatment of melanoma, for example, destruction of normal melanocytes would result in vitiligo, which, although not aesthetically desirable, is well tolerated physiologically. In fact, vitiligo has been described as a side effect of immunotherapy, and it has been associated with an improved prognosis.

Viral antigens, which are gene products of oncogenic viruses that can elicit immune responses, comprise the fourth category. Examples include the E6 and E7 proteins from human papilloma virus type 16 (which causes cervical cancer) that have been shown to induce T-cell responses.

Antigen Presentation

The key to the generation of an immune response through either arm of the immune system is the ability of antigen-presenting cells (APCs) to process and present tumor-related peptide antigens. Monocytes, macrophages, and B cells can all function as APCs, but the most powerful APC is the dendritic cell (Figure 7-1). Proteins are phagocytosed by dendritic cells and partially digested into smaller polypeptides. These small peptide antigens are then bound to MHC molecules in the endoplasmic reticulum and transported onto the cell surface (Figure 7-2). These unique antigen:MHC complexes can then be recognized by naïve T lymphocytes through the T cell receptor. When a naïve helper (CD4+) T cell recognizes the antigen being expressed on the MHC class II molecule and also recognizes co-stimulatory molecules present on the APC, it becomes activated. That co-stimulation signal—when CD28 on the T cell recognizes B7 on the dendritic cell—is crucial for activation to take place. Activation results in proliferation and differentiation. The activated helper T cell can then promote either a cellular T helper 1 response or a humoral T helper 2 response. If a naïve T cell recognizes the antigen:MHC complex in the absence of co-stimulation (as frequently happens when a naïve T cell comes in direct contact with a tumor cell), the T cell becomes tolerant. This is one way the body

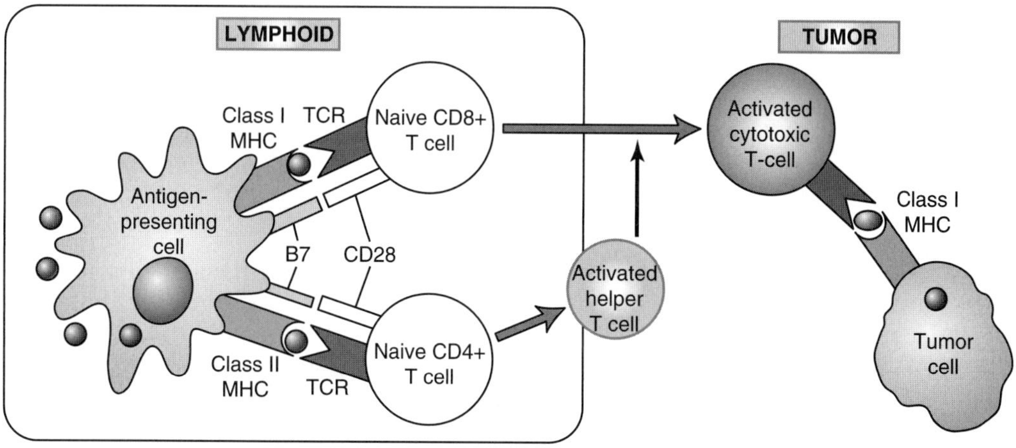

Figure 7-1. A naïve T cell that recognizes antigen on the surface of an antigen-presenting cell becomes activated when it receives two signals: one through the T cell receptor and major histocompatibility complex and one through the co-stimulatory signal through B7 on the antigen-presenting cell and CD28 on the T cell. The T cell becomes activated and both secretes and responds to interleukin-2, which drives expansion and differentiation. The cytotoxic T cells are then released into the periphery, and, when they encounter the specific antigen (in this case, on a tumor cell), this triggers their effector actions.

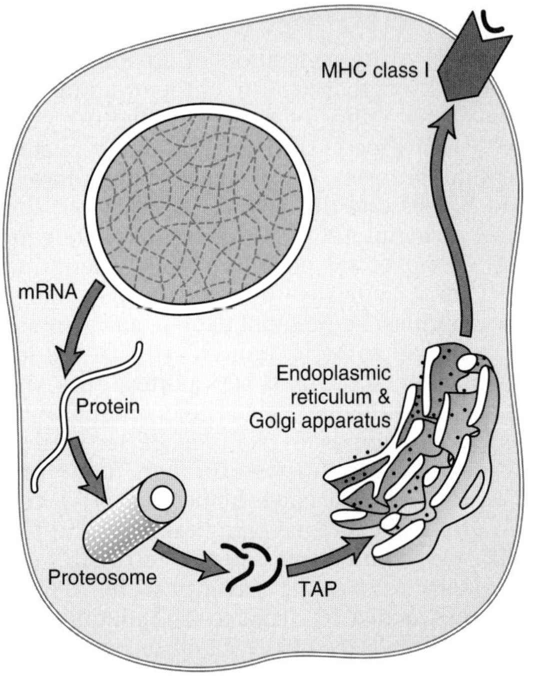

Figure 7–2. Proteosomes degrade proteins into peptide fragments, which are transported into the lumen of the endoplasmic reticulum by the peptide transporter TAP. Newly synthesized major histocompatibility complex class I α chains assemble in the endoplasmic reticulum and are bound to β2 microglobulin and TAP. When the peptide fragments delivered by TAP are bound to the major histocompatibility complex class I molecule, it is released, and it is transported through the Golgi apparatus to the cell surface.

prevents autoimmune disease, but it also results in tolerance by the immune system of the cancer.

Immune Responses

A cellular response occurs when a naïve cytotoxic T cell recognizes antigen being presented on the surface of an APC (Figure 7-1). The T cell receptor on cytotoxic T cells recognizes antigen presented not on MHC class II molecules but rather on MHC class I molecules. MHC class I molecules are present on both immune and nonimmune cells, and they collect peptides derived from proteins in the cytosol for expression on the cell surface (Figure 7-2). As with the helper T cell, a second co-stimulatory signal is necessary for the cytotoxic T cell to become activated.

There are two types of helper T cells, and the type of response that develops depends on which type of helper T cell is activated. For a cellular response to occur, a type 1 helper T cell (Th1) is necessary. When a Th1 is activated, it releases cytokines that promote the proliferation and differentiation of cytotoxic T cells, such as interleukin-2 (IL-2), interferon-gamma (IFN-γ), tumor necrosis factor-alpha (TNF-α), and granulocyte-macrophage colony-stimulating factor (GM-CSF). Between the recognition of the antigen by the T cell receptor, the co-stimulation through CD28 and B7, and the presence of these type 1 cytokines, a naïve cytotoxic T cell will activate, proliferate, and travel out to the periphery. Once there, activated cytotoxic T cells destroy tumor cells via the T cell receptor recognition of tumor-specific antigen presented on MHC class I molecules at the tumor cell surface. Activated T cells do not require any second or co-stimulatory signal. After the antigen-specific T cells bind to the MHC I receptor-tumor antigen complex, they can destroy the tumor cell via the release of granules that contain granzyme B and perforin and also via the induction of the FAS/FAS ligand apoptosis.

If instead of a Th1 a type 2 helper T cell (Th2) is activated, the response will be geared toward a humoral response rather than a cellular response. Type 2 helper T cells produce B cells, and they produce B cell stimulatory cytokines, including IL-4, IL-5, and IL-10. This leads to B cell proliferation and differentiation into plasma cells, which then produce antigen-specific antibodies. Unlike cellular responses, which are directed toward antigens presented on class I MHC receptors, antibody-dependent mechanisms rely on the recognition of cell-surface antigens. When antibodies recognize antigen expressed on the surface of the tumor cell, the cell can be killed by a variety of methods (Figure 7-3).

Antibody-dependent cell-mediated cytotoxicity involves the attachment of tumor-specific antibodies to tumor cells and the subsequent destruction of the tumor cell by immunocompetent cells, most commonly the natural killer cell. Fc receptors on immunocompetent cells recognize the Fc portion of antibodies adhering to surface tumor antigens. After recognition and attachment via its Fc receptors, the natural killer cell can destroy the target tumor cell through the release of granules containing

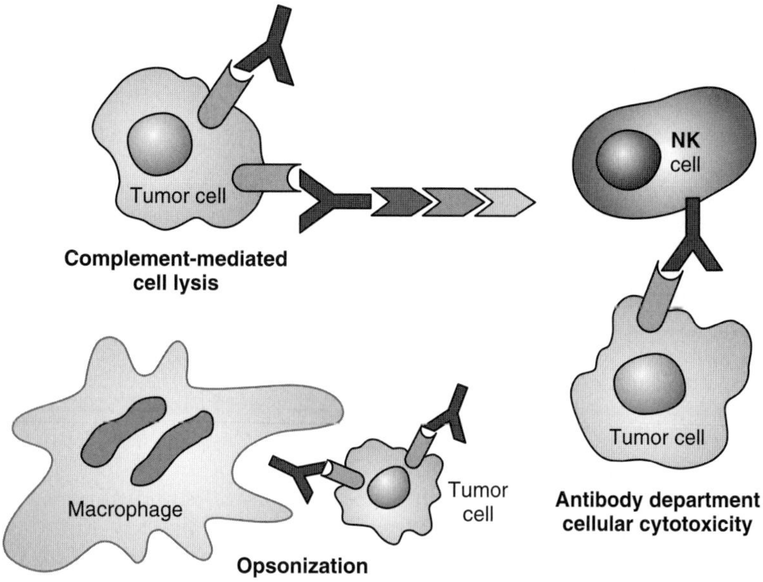

Figure 7–3. Antibodies can lead to tumor cell death by three mechanisms. Bound antibodies form a receptor for the first protein of the complement system, which leads to a protein complex on the surface of the cell that can kill the cell directly (complement-mediated cell lysis). Antibodies coating a tumor cell render it recognizable by macrophages, which then ingest and destroy it (opsonization). Natural killer cells recognize and rapidly kill cells coated with immunoglobulin G antibody (antibody-dependent cellular cytotoxicity).

perforin and granzyme B and/or through the activation of the FAS pathway apoptosis system in the target cell. Perforin molecules make holes or pores in the cell membrane, thereby disrupting the osmotic barrier and killing the cell via osmotic lysis.

Similarly, complement-dependent cell-mediated cytotoxicity involves the recognition and attachment of complement-fixing antibodies to tumor-specific surface antigens, followed by complement activation. Sequential activation of the components of the complement system ultimately leads to the formation of the membrane attack complex, which forms transmembrane pores that disrupt the osmotic barrier of the membrane and lead to osmotic lysis.

A third mechanism of tumor destruction through the humoral arm is opsonization. During this process, tumor-specific antibodies attach to their target antigens on tumor cell surfaces, thus marking them for engulfment by macrophages. This can also lead to processing and presentation of new tumor-specific antigens by the macrophage in addition to direct destruction of the tumor cells.

TYPES OF IMMUNOTHERAPY

There are several methods by which the immune system may be incorporated into cancer therapy. Immunotherapy can be categorized as either active or passive. With passive immunotherapy, the host need not mount an immune response; rather, the therapeutic agent will directly or indirectly mediate tumor killing. Examples of passive immunotherapy include the use of monoclonal antibodies or adoptive immunotherapy. Adoptive immunotherapy typically denotes passive immunotherapy with cells (e.g., lymphocytes, macrophages). Active immunotherapy, on the other hand, refers to the delivery of materials designed to elicit an immune response by the host. This can further be broken down into nonspecific and specific active immunotherapies.

BOX 7–2 TYPES OF IMMUNOTHERAPIES

- Passive immunotherapy
  - Monoclonal antibodies
  - Adoptive immunotherapy
- Active nonspecific immunotherapy
  - Immunostimulants
  - Cytokines
- Active specific immunotherapy
  - Peptide and ganglioside vaccines
  - Nucleic acid vaccines
  - Anti-idiotype vaccines
  - Allogeneic cellular vaccines
  - Autologous cellular vaccines
  - Dendritic cell vaccines

Nonspecific agents are those that stimulate the immune system globally but that do not selectively stimulate tumor-specific effector cells. These agents include immunostimulants and cytokines. Specific active immunotherapy is designed to elicit an immune response to one or more tumor antigens. The prime example of this approach is the use of tumor vaccines.

Passive Immunotherapy

Monoclonal Antibodies

The development of monoclonal antibodies with unique specificity to tumor antigens has allowed for multiple attempts to use them as a mode of cancer therapy (Table 7-3). They may either be used alone to mediate complement-dependent or antibody-dependent cellular cytotoxicity, or they may be linked to therapeutic drugs or toxins so that the conjugate may be targeted specifically to cancer cells. In addition to their relative selectivity and minimal toxicity, they are easily mass produced for widespread application. Their success is unfortunately limited by the relatively low amount of antibody that reaches the tumor and by their limited ability to destroy tumor tissue. Murine monoclonal antibodies are often inactivated by the development of human anti-mouse antibodies, although recombinant chimeric antibodies that combine the constant region of human antibodies with the variable region of mouse antibodies can help overcome this.

BOX 7–3 IMMUNOCONJUGATES

- Immunotoxins
  - Antibodies conjugated to toxins from plants (ricin) or microorganisms *(Pseudomonas)*
- Immunodrug conjugates
  - Antibodies directly conjugated to drugs (doxorubicin) or antibodies used to target liposome-encapsulated drugs (liposomal doxorubicin, antisense RNA, radionuclides)
- Radioimmunoconjugates
  - Antibodies conjugated to radionuclides (^{90}Y, ^{131}I)

BOX 7–4 DRAWBACKS TO CANCER THERAPY WITH MONOCLONAL ANTIBODIES

- Antigenic modulation by tumor cells
- Impaired delivery of antibodies to tumor sites
- Low tumor specificity of target antigens
- Shed or internalized targets
- Human anti-mouse antibody responses

Rituximab (Rituxan) is an anti-CD20 monoclonal antibody that is approved for the treatment of relapsed or refractory low grade or follicular non-Hodgkin's lymphoma. Rituximab can directly induce cell death by mediating complement or antibody-dependent cellular cytotoxicity or by directly inducing apoptosis. It is well tolerated with only minor infusion-related symptoms, such as fever, chills, and aches.

Trastuzumab (Herceptin) is the first monoclonal antibody to be effective against solid tumors. Trastuzumab binds to HER-2/neu, a transmembrane glycoprotein receptor with intrinsic tyrosine kinase activity that is overexpressed in 25% to 30% of human breast cancers. Although it is a monoclonal antibody, trastuzumab more likely exerts its effects through internalization and interruption of the tyrosine kinase pathway than as a

TABLE 7–3 • *Monoclonal Antibodies Used In Cancer Treatment*

Monoclonal Antibody	Targeted Antigen	Clinical Use
Rituximab (Rituxan)	CD20	Lymphoma
Alemtuzumab (Campath)	CD52	Chronic lymphocytic leukemia
Trastuzumab (Herceptin)	HER-2/neu	Breast cancer
Edrecolomab (17-1A)	EpCAM	Colon cancer (in trials)
Bevacizumab (Avastin)	VEGF	Colon cancer
Cetuximab (Erbitux)	EGFR	Colon cancer

true immunotherapy (i.e., killing cancer cells through antibody-dependent cytotoxicity).

Edrecolomab is a monoclonal antibody directed to 17-1A/EpCAM, a tumor-associated antigen that is commonly expressed on colorectal carcinomas. Early studies of this antibody in the adjuvant setting for stage III colorectal cancer were promising, and randomized trials are ongoing. Antibodies directed against carcinoembryonic antigen (CEA) are also being evaluated as an adjuvant therapy for colorectal cancer.

Adoptive T Cell Immunotherapy

A cellular immune response to cancer appears to be more effective than an antibody response, but attempts to stimulate a cellular response through the use of immunostimulants or vaccines have had limited success. For this reason, the passive administration of cells with pre-existing antitumor activity to the tumor-bearing host has generated significant interest. Early attempts were limited by the ability to generate large enough numbers of tumor-specific cells for transfer; however, several new approaches have been developed to augment this. At present, the cost, complexity, and variability of these strategies still limit their use to investigational studies.

Tumor-infiltrating lymphocytes infiltrate growing tumors, and they can be isolated by producing single-cell suspensions from the tumor in the presence of IL-2. They have been isolated from virtually all types of tumors, and they are capable of recognizing tumor-associated antigens. Researchers have also looked at harvesting lymphocytes from lymph nodes that drain the site of the tumor or that drain the site of a vaccine and using these T cells for adoptive immunotherapy.

Another cell for adoptive immunotherapy that has generated interest is the lymphokine-activated killer (LAK) cell. LAK cells can be obtained by growing human peripheral blood lymphocytes in the presence of high doses of IL-2. The resultant cells represent a lytic population that has properties similar to both natural killer cells and cytotoxic T lymphocytes. They appear capable of lysing tumor cells but not normal cells, although the exact cell-surface determinants recognized by LAK cells remain a mystery. How these cells may be used to fight cancer is the subject of ongoing research.

Nonspecific Active Immunotherapy

Immunostimulants

Before the mechanisms by which the immune system can eradicate tumor cells were understood, early attempts at immunotherapy involved nonspecific stimulation of the immune system. The premise was that any increase in immune reactivity would be associated with a concomitant increase in the antitumor immune response. Coley's toxins are the classic example, and several other nonspecific immunostimulants have been explored as methods to stimulate a systemic immune response against cancer.

Probably the most widely embraced immunostimulant investigated has been the bacille Calmette–Guérin (BCG), a modified form of the tubercle bacillus. BCG is a nonspecific immune stimulant that has generated interest as an immunotherapy for melanoma for more than 30 years, ever since it was demonstrated that intralesional injection of viable BCG organisms could lead to the regression of intradermal metastases of melanoma. The observation that response was occasionally seen in noninjected nodules suggested that BCG could induce a systemic immune response of potential therapeutic benefit. Instillation of BCG in the bladder eliminates superficial bladder cancers and prevents tumor recurrences; it is one of several standard therapies for patients with bladder cancer.

Corynebacterium parvum is another microbe that can stimulate the human immune system. As compared with BCG, it holds the clinical advantage of being heat-killed and thus does not require viable organisms for efficacy. Systemic injection of *C parvum* enhances antibody responses and activates circulating and noncirculating macrophages. Despite early promising results, however, randomized trials failed to show a significant benefit, and *C parvum* has never been widely adopted as a therapeutic agent for melanoma or any other malignancy. Multiple other immunostimulants (e.g., transfer factor, Isoprinosine, thymostimuline) have been studied, but they have failed to make a clinical impact. A newer agent—a streptococcal preparation called OK-432 (Picibanil)—is presently being studied as a nonspecific immunostimulant for the adjuvant treatment of gastric cancer.

Cytokines

Cytokines are naturally occurring soluble proteins produced by mononuclear cells of the immune system that can affect the growth and function of cells through interaction with specific cell-surface receptors. Cytokines were originally identified by the function they exhibited in in vitro assays, a fact that led to confusion when the same molecules were described by different investigators based on multiple functions. After molecular biologic techniques became available to clone the genes for these cytokines, to express them in bacteria, and to purify and produce them in large amounts, researchers were not only able to study them but also to use them as therapeutics. There have been more than 50 cytokines isolated to date (Table 7-4). Several cytokines have subsequently been approved by the U.S. Food and Drug Administration for clinical use, and others are being investigated (Table 7-5).

Interferons

The interferons were originally described as proteins produced by virally infected cells that serve to protect against further viral infection through a variety of effects. These include increased antigen presentation via the increased expression of MHC and antigens, the enhancement of natural killer cell function, and the enhancement of antibody-dependent cellular cytotoxicity. In addition, the interferons exert direct anti-angiogenic, cytotoxic, and cytostatic effects. There are several subtypes of interferons, including interferon-alpha (IFN-α), interferon-beta (IFN-β), and IFN-γ. Although the anticancer effects of IFN-β and IFN-γ have been disappointing, several hematologic and solid tumors have proved responsive to IFN-α. Chronic myelogenous leukemia is characterized by the proliferation and accumulation of

TABLE 7–4 • *Cytokines*

Cytokine	Principle Cell Source	Biologic Effects
IL-1α and β	Monocytes/macrophages, dendritic cells, B cells, T cells, fibroblasts, endothelial and epithelial cells	Induces IL-2 production and IL-2 receptor expression; co-stimulates T cells; induces inflammation and nonspecific immune responses
IL-2	T cells	Induces T cell proliferation and differentiation; chemotactic for T cells
IL-4	T cells, mast cells	Induces antigen expression by B cells and monocytes; growth factor for B cells; increases antibody secretion
IL-6	T cells, monocytes/macrophages, fibroblasts	Co-stimulates T cells; induces IL-2 production; enhances MHC class I expression; enhances B cell differentiation and immunoglobulin secretion
IL-10	T cells, B cells	Inhibits cytokine synthesis by Th1 T cells; inhibits macrophage activity; inhibits natural killer cell production of IFN-γ
IL-12	Monocytes/macrophages, dendritic cells	Stimulates activated T cells; promotes a Th1 response; synergizes with IL-2; enhances natural killer activity
IFN-α	Leukocytes	Enhances antigen expression; augments natural killer activity, inhibits suppressor T cells; activates CTL
IFN-γ	T cells, natural killer cells, monocytes/ macrophages	Enhances antigen expression; activates macrophages; augments natural killer activity; regulates differentiation
TNF-α	Monocytes/macrophages, T cells	Stimulates T cell proliferation; enhances natural killer activity; induces acute phase responses; stimulates production of cytokines; mediates septic shock and inflammation
GM-CSF	Fibroblasts, stromal cells, endothelial cells	Stimulates growth of granulocyte and monocyte progenitors; enhances ADCC

ADCC, Antibody-dependent cell-mediated cytotoxicity; *CTL,* cytotoxic lymphocytes; *GM-CSF,* granulocyte-macrophage colony-stimulating factor; *IFN,* interferon; *IL,* interleukin; *MHC,* major histocompatibility complex; *Th1,* type 1 helper T cell; *TNF,* tumor necrosis factor.

TABLE 7-5 • *Cytokines Used In Cancer Treatment*

Cytokine	Cancer
IL-2	Renal cell carcinoma, melanoma
GM-CSF	Supportive therapy, melanoma
Interferon-α	Melanoma, chronic myelogenous leukemia (CML), cutaneous T-cell lymphoma, hairy cell leukemia, Kaposi's sarcoma
TNF-α	Regional therapy of melanoma and sarcoma

BOX 7-5 EFFECTS OF INTERFERONS

Immunologic Effects

- Increases proliferation and cytolytic activity of natural killer cells
- Increases differentiation and major histocompatibility complex class II expression on antigen-presenting cells
- Promotes Th1 response; increases cytolytic activity of T cells
- Increases immunoglobulin G production by B cells

Nonimmunologic Effects

- Antiangiogenesis
- Directly cytostatic and cytotoxic to tumor cells
- Antimetastatic

mature myeloid cells and their progenitors with the marker Philadelphia chromosome. Chronic myelogenous leukemia, cutaneous T cell lymphoma, and hairy cell leukemia all respond to IFN-α. Several phase III trials have confirmed the benefit of adjuvant IFN-α after the surgical resection of cutaneous melanoma. Kaposi's sarcoma is a common clinical manifestation of human immunodeficiency virus infection, and it can also be responsive to IFN-α, although the high doses required and subsequent side effects often limit its usefulness. It is unclear whether the predominant antitumor effect of interferon is its direct antiproliferative activity or its immunologic actions.

BOX 7-6 CLINICAL USES OF INTERFERONS

- Chronic myelogenous leukemia
- Hairy cell leukemia
- Non-Hodgkin's lymphoma
- Kaposi's sarcoma
- Malignant melanoma
- Renal cell carcinoma
- Intravesical therapy of bladder cancer

BOX 7-7 POSSIBLE TOXICITIES OF INTERFERONS

- Fever and chills
- Tachyphylaxis
- Muscle pain, joint pain, headache
- Fatigue
- Nausea and vomiting, anorexia, weight loss
- Anemia, neutropenia, thrombocytopenia
- Supraventricular tachydysrhythmias
- Hepatic dysfunction
- Depression, adult respiratory distress syndrome, and prerenal azotemia

Interleukin-2

IL-2 was originally described as the "T cell growth factor," because it is required for the differentiation and proliferation of activated T cells. In addition to increasing the cytotoxicity of killer T cells, it can enhance the secretion of immunoglobulins by B cells and the secretion of other cytokines, such as IL-1, TNF-α, and IFN-γ. As such, it seems like an ideal choice for immunotherapy. The major drawback of IL-2 is the significant dose-related toxicity. IL-2 leads to significant interstitial edema, vascular depletion, and lymphoid infiltration into vital organs. This can lead to severe hypotension and resultant ischemic damage to the heart, liver, kidneys, and bowel. Thus, the use of IL-2 is limited to patients with excellent performance status, normal pulmonary and cardiac function, and no active infections. Despite these limitations, IL-2 has proven to be an effective therapy for selected patients with metastatic melanoma and metastatic renal cell carcinoma.

BOX 7–8 POSSIBLE TOXICITIES OF INTERLEUKIN-2

- Fever and chills
- Fatigue, lethargy, confusion
- Nausea, diarrhea
- Anemia, thrombocytopenia, eosinophilia
- Neutrophil chemotactic defect
  - Predisposition to infection and sepsis
- Hepatic dysfunction
- Myocarditis
- Capillary leak syndrome
  - Fluid retention, hypotension

Tumor Necrosis Factor-α

Tumor necrosis factor earned its name when it was discovered that it induced a hemorrhagic necrosis of tumors in mice. This comes from both direct cytotoxic effects as well as the induction of other cytokines. Unfortunately, systemic TNF-α is associated with extremely severe systemic toxicity, including coagulopathy, pulmonary failure, pancytopenia, and shock. Although it has no role as a systemic therapy, it is possible to use TNF-α in a locoregional fashion. Isolated limb perfusion allows for the restriction of toxic therapeutics to an extremity while minimizing systemic uptake. In combination with melphalan (Alkeran), TNF-α produced high response rates in extremity sarcomas and melanomas. TNF-α is currently approved in Europe for the regional treatment of extremity soft-tissue sarcomas. Recent investigations of TNF-α in the United States, in combination with melphalan for hyperthermic limb perfusion for patients with melanoma, have not been as encouraging.

Active Specific Immunotherapy: Vaccines

The goal of nonspecific immunotherapy is to stimulate the immune system globally. It rests on the assumption that the immune system has at least a minimal capacity to recognize and ablate tumor cells; this global augmentation aims to improve that baseline antitumor response to clinically relevant levels. Active specific immunotherapy, on the other hand, assumes that the host has no significant recognition of the tumor. Therefore, the goal is to generate a host immune response to known or unknown tumor-associated antigens. These are generally referred to as *cancer vaccines,* although this term can be somewhat misleading. We are used to referring to vaccines as protective against infectious agents; that is, they are meant to stimulate the immune system against antigens to which it has not yet been exposed. By contrast, cancer vaccines are designed to stimulate an immune response against antigens on cells to which the immune system has already been exposed (and failed to eradicate).

Many different vaccine strategies are under investigation, each with advantages and disadvantages with regard to clinical feasibility and cost, the number of antigens available, and the mechanism of response (cellular, humoral or both) (Table 7-6). Some vaccine strategies use specific peptide antigens. These are highly purified, and therefore they are less likely to contain potentially irrelevant material. This has important implications regarding standardization and quality control. Several other

TABLE 7–6 • *Relative Advantages and Disadvantages of Various Vaccine Approaches*

Vaccine	Advantages	Disadvantages
Peptide or protein vaccine	Easy to produce Safe	Requires known antigens Must match patient's HLA status Weakly immunogenic
Allogeneic cellular vaccine	Relatively easy to produce Presents multiple antigens	Efficacy may be related to patient's HLA status Contains many irrelevant antigens
Autologous cellular vaccine	Highly patient specific Strongly immunogenic	Individualized cell processing needed Costly Requires harvestable tumor
Dendritic cell vaccine	Highly patient specific Strongly immunogenic	Individualized cell processing needed Costly and technically difficult May require accessible tumor

approaches use whole cells, which contain many antigens. These cells can be either allogeneic or autologous, and they can be used either intact or lysed. These vaccines are generally less focused, and they are more difficult to standardize and analyze; however, this approach theoretically has the greatest potential for eliciting an immune response that is directed against multiple antigenic targets.

Peptide Vaccines

If a tumor-specific protein is known to be immunogenic, it is possible to use that protein as a vaccine. The entire protein can be used, which allows the patient's own immune system to cleave and bind peptides, or only selected immunogenic peptides (one or multiple) can be used. Simply immunizing the patient with the protein would not typically be sufficient, because the majority of tumor antigens are weakly immunogenic. To improve the immunogenicity, proteins or peptides are often delivered to the patient, along with an immune adjuvant meant to induce inflammation and to push the immune process to move toward immunity rather than tolerance. Alum, BCG, and DETOX (detoxified Freund's adjuvant, which is composed of monophosphoryl lipid A and a purified mycobacterial cell-wall skeleton) are examples of adjuvants meant to cause a generalized or nonspecific inflammatory response that will increase the likelihood of the immune system recognizing the vaccinating antigens. Cytokines—including IL-2, IL-12, IFN-α, IFN-γ, TNF, and GM-CSF—have also been given simultaneously with the vaccines to further stimulate the immune response.

Unfortunately, peptide vaccines have several drawbacks that limit their potential clinical benefit. For example, the cancer can escape immune recognition rather simply through antigenic modulation. In the same way that chemotherapy will not be curative if a small population of tumor cells develops resistance to the chemotherapeutic agent, if a subpopulation no longer expresses that antigen, then it is no longer susceptible to that immunotherapy. Peptide vaccines are limited by the fact that, even if a peptide vaccine is immunogenic, it may not be the right peptide for many patients. Even commonly expressed tumor antigens are not present on all patients' tumors, or they may be present in varying degrees. In addition, the T cell's recognition of an antigen depends on the presentation of that antigen on a specific MHC molecule. Only certain human lymphocyte antigen (HLA) phenotypes can present any given peptide to induce an immune response, so peptides will only be immunogenic in a limited subset of patients. A classic example is that of the MART-1/Melan-A antigen in melanoma. The antigen is expressed by 80% of melanomas, but the peptide only binds to HLA-A2. Approximately 45% of Caucasians have HLA-A2, so only 36% (80% of 45%) of all melanoma patients given a MART-1/Melen-A vaccine would have the potential to generate a therapeutic antitumor immune response.

Ganglioside Vaccines

Gangliosides are a group of related acidic glycosphingolipids that contain a ceramide chain, which is incorporated into the lipid bilayer of the plasma membrane. The carbohydrate moieties are present on the cell surface, and they are available for antibody recognition. Gangliosides are present on neoplastic cells and on some nonneoplastic cells (particularly neural tissues). The various gangliosides differ in their expression on cancers and normal tissues and in their intrinsic immunogenicity.

Gangliosides can be targets for both passive and active immunotherapy, although their use as targets for passive immunotherapy have not demonstrated consistent laboratory or clinical responses. Because gangliosides are not proteins being degraded and expressed in the context of MHC but, rather, they are cell-surface molecules, active specific immunotherapy should stimulate a humoral response. The most well-studied ganglioside vaccine is the GM2 vaccine in melanoma. Ganglioside GM2 is expressed on a large percentage of melanoma specimens, but it is rarely detected on normal tissues, and about 5% of melanoma patients have naturally occurring anti-GM2 antibodies. To further increase humoral response to GM2 vaccination, the ganglioside was conjugated to the xenogeneic protein keyhole limpet hemocyanin, and the vaccine was delivered with the saponin-derived adjuvant QS-21. This resulted in high levels of anti-GM2 antibodies in a very high percentage of patients. Although this vaccine was not as good as interferon for stage III melanoma, studies in earlier-stage melanoma are ongoing.

Autologous Cellular Vaccines

Peptide vaccines are only applicable if one has a target antigen in mind. For many cancers, only a few tumor-associated antigens have been defined, and these may not be present in a significant percentage of patients or be sufficiently immunogenic. Presumably, any patient's cancer may have multiple antigens to which an immune response may be directed. Using the patient's cancer as the vaccine precludes the need to identify these antigens specifically. This approach theoretically ensures that all biologically relevant antigens are presented to the immune system. Autologous tumor cells are harvested from the patient, irradiated, and returned to the patient to stimulate a tumor-specific immune response. Early attempts to use irradiated autologous tumor cells as vaccines had little success as a result of the poor immunogenicity of native tumor cells themselves; however, the immunogenicity could be increased through the use of adjuvants.

There are several drawbacks to autologous cellular vaccines. First and foremost, the approach is limited to individuals with sufficient tumor to prepare a vaccine. This has restricted trials to patients with bulky nodal or accessible distant metastatic disease. Such patients have a poor overall prognosis, and they are likely to have significant residual tumor burden, thus making them less-than-ideal candidates for any immunotherapeutic approach. Second, even when it is available, in most cases only enough tumor is obtained to provide for a limited number of vaccinations. Third, the technical complexities inherent in procuring tumor and preparing a vaccine have, to date, largely precluded the widespread conducting of multi-institutional trials to formally test the efficacy of these vaccines.

Allogeneic Tumor Cell Vaccines

Many tumor-associated antigens are shared among a large number of patients. Therefore, it is reasonable to expect that one could create a vaccine from cultured cell lines that would stimulate an antitumor immune response in any patient who shared some of those antigens. This is the principle behind allogeneic tumor cell vaccines. This approach offers several advantages over autologous vaccines: allogeneic vaccines are readily available, even for patients who lack sufficient tumor to produce an autologous tumor cell vaccine, and they can be standardized, preserved, and distributed in a manner akin to any other therapeutic agent. Because of this, they are more readily available for evaluation in large, prospective, randomized trials. Several allogeneic tumor cell vaccines are currently being studied.

Canvaxin is an allogeneic melanoma vaccine composed of three viable irradiated melanoma cell lines, which were specifically chosen for their high content of immunogenic melanoma-associated antigens. In a phase II study of patients with metastatic melanoma, Canvaxin plus BCG significantly improved the median survival of treated patients as compared with historical controls, particularly patients who underwent the resection of clinically detectable disease before vaccination. Case-control studies of Canvaxin among both stage IV melanoma patients after the complete resection of metastases and among stage III patients have demonstrated promising results as compared with historical controls. However, a multicenter, randomized controlled trial comparing Canvaxin plus BCG with placebo plus BCG failed to demonstrate any benefit in either stage III- or stage IV-resected melanoma patients.

As opposed to using whole cells, Melacine consists of a lysate of two homogenized melanoma cell lines that are combined with the adjuvant DETOX. On the basis of early promising results, a phase III trial compared Melacine with combination chemotherapy (dacarbazine, cisplatin, Carmustine [BCNU], and tamoxifen) among patients with metastatic melanoma. Although this trial demonstrated no statistical difference in median survival, Melacine had much less toxicity. On the basis of these results, Melacine was approved in Canada in May 2000 for the treatment of advanced melanoma.

A large study of Melacine as an adjuvant therapy for patients with intermediate-thickness, node-negative melanoma failed to demonstrate an overall improvement in relapse-free or overall survival, but prospective subset analysis was suggestive of significant antitumor activity. A major secondary aim of the trial was to determine if the effectiveness of the vaccine varied based on the patient's HLA class I allele expression. It had previously been reported that there was a strong association between patient HLA phenotype and evidence of clinical benefit from Melacine. Indeed, the trial did demonstrate that patients expressing either HLA-A2 or HLA-C3 who received the vaccine had a significantly improved disease-free survival as compared with controls and with patients who received the vaccine but who were not A2 or C3 positive.

There are other methods under investigation to increase the immunogenicity of cellular vaccines beyond immunologic adjuvants such as BCG or DETOX. Advances in the ability to genetically modify cells ex vivo presents one such method. One approach is to introduce genes for cytokines into tumor cells. Much of the difficulty with using cytokine therapy is that high levels must be achieved in the serum to induce a local therapeutic benefit. The introduction of the genes for cytokines into tumor cells results in a sustained release of those cytokines at the site of the vaccine. Locally secreted cytokines can recruit APCs at the vaccine site and enhance in vivo lymphocyte activation and expansion, thereby augmenting the immune response. Cytokine-gene–modified cellular vaccines have been formulated from both autologous and allogeneic tumor cells engineered to secrete IL-2, IL-4, IL-7, IL-12, IFN-γ, or GM-CSF.

Dendritic Cell Vaccines

Most of the aforementioned vaccine therapies depend on dendritic cells (DCs) to take up tumor-associated antigens and to present them to T cells to generate an immune response. DCs are a unique system of cells that induce, sustain, and regulate immune responses. DCs express a variety of molecules at various stages of maturation, thereby allowing them to capture antigens, process them, and then present them to naïve T cells. This is why GM-CSF, with its DC-maturing properties, is a popular adjuvant for vaccine therapies. An alternate approach is to bypass the need for DC to take up and process antigen by delivering to the patient DCs that are already expressing tumor antigens.

After DCs are obtained from the patient through leukapheresis, there are several ways that DC vaccines may be created. One method is to load exogenous peptides onto the empty MHC class I molecules of mature DCs. This approach is limited, however, to known tumor antigens and to patients of a given HLA type. Another approach is to expose immature DCs to tumor lysates. This allows for both MHC class I and class II epitopes to be processed and for the diversification of immune responses.

BOX 7–9 METHODS FOR LOADING ANTIGEN ONTO DENDRITIC CELLS

- Presenting tumor lysates to be taken up by immature dendritic cells
- Ex vivo antigen loading onto mature dendritic cells
- Transduction of dendritic cells with purified tumor RNA
- Transfecting dendritic cells with the genes of antigens
- Fusing dendritic cells with tumor cells

This approach is attractive in that immune responses can be generated without the need for the characterization of tumor-specific antigens. However, like autologous cellular vaccines, it is only applicable to patients from whom enough tumor may be procured. Alternative approaches have used the transfection of tumor cells with tumor RNA; the transduction of DCs with retroviruses, poxviruses, or adenoviruses encoding specific antigens; or the fusion of tumor cells with DCs.

OBSTACLES TO IMMUNOTHERAPY

Much of the emphasis in immunotherapy has centered on the creation of an immune response to tumor-specific antigens, but this is only half of the story. A clinically relevant immune response has two tiers. The first tier is the generation of antibodies or cytotoxic T cells that can recognize tumor-specific antigens. The second tier is the ability of those antibodies or T cells to not just recognize cells expressing those antigens but to kill the malignant cells. Tumor cells are not passive bystanders to the immune response (Figure 7-4). Instead, they develop mechanisms to evade immune recognition. Cancers can escape immune recognition rather simply through antigenic modulation. Patients with progressive disease after immunotherapy often exhibit "antigen loss." In the case of T cell–based therapies, tumor cells that lose the ability to bind antigen to MHC or that do not express the antigen:MHC complex on the cell surface also escape immune recognition. Tumor cells can produce immunosuppressive cytokines, such as IL-10 or TGF-β, which inhibits DC

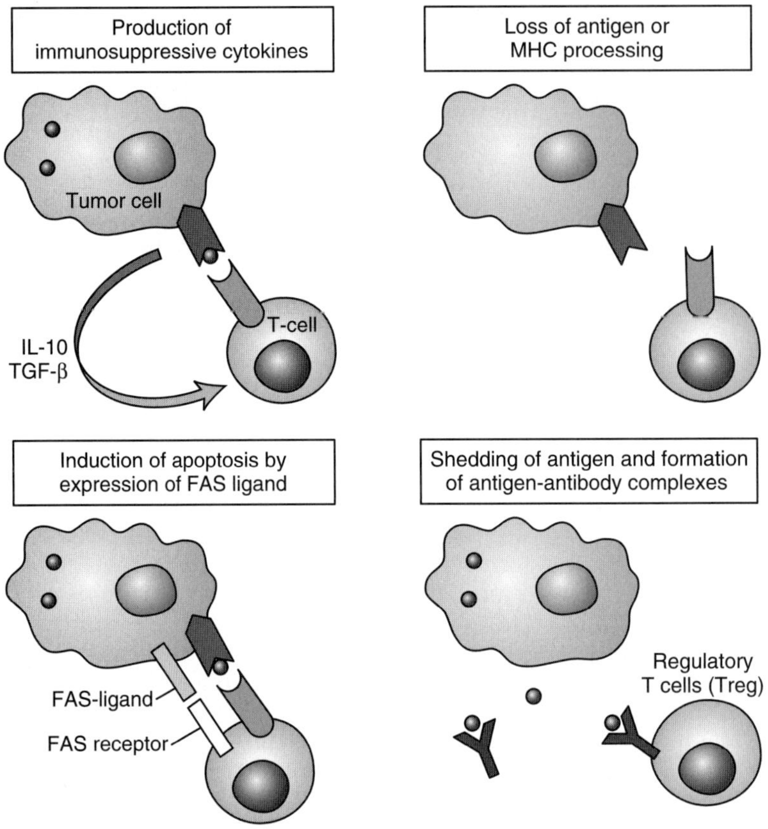

Figure 7–4. Methods by which a tumor may escape immune recognition.

migration and antigen presentation. The expression of FAS ligand molecules on tumor cells can interact with FAS receptors on T cells, thus leading to T cell death by apoptosis. Tumor cells can shed antigen, and this antigen alone—or in complex with antibodies—can induce regulatory (or suppressor) T cells, which can suppress the immune response.

Conclusion

With its innate ability to recognize unique cell-associated antigens, to target specific cells for death, and to maintain a memory for these antigens, the immune system seems ideal for eradicating cancer. However, by the time they become clinically apparent, cancer cells have developed several mechanisms by which they can escape immune recognition. The study of immunotherapy centers on methods to augment the immune recognition and ablation of cancer cells and to help tilt this clinical balance back in the favor of the patient. The use of antibodies to target specific receptors or to deliver agents directly to cancer cells and the systemic administration of cytokines as biologic agents represent successful translations of immunotherapy into clinical practice. Other immunotherapeutic approaches, such as adoptive immunotherapy, seem promising for select patients. The most enthusiasm exists for cancer vaccines, given their potential to prevent disease recurrence with minimal toxicity. Despite considerable research, however, there has yet to be a cancer vaccine that demonstrates an increased overall survival in a prospective, randomized trial. Many questions still need to be answered regarding the best method of vaccination, how to increase the ability of effector cells to kill the cancer, and methods to negate tumor escape mechanisms before the routine use of cancer vaccines in clinical practice will be seen.

Key Reading

Ribas A, Butterfield LH, Glaspy JA, Economo JS. Current developments in cancer vaccines and cellular immunotherapy. *J Clin Oncol* 2003;21:2415–2432.

Selected Readings

Allen TM. Ligand-targeted therapeutics in anticancer therapy, *Nat Rev Cancer* 2002;2:750.

Allen TM, Lotze MT, Dutcher JP, *et al.* High-dose recombinant interleukin-2 therapy for patients with metastatic melanoma: analysis of 270 patients treated between 1985 and 1993, *J Clin Oncol* 1999; 17:2105.

Dermine S, Armstrong A, Hawkins RE, Stern PL. Cancer vaccines and immunotherapy, *Br Med Bull* 2002;62: 149–162.

Faries MB. Evaluation of immunotherapy in the treatment of melanoma. *Surg Oncol Clin N Am* 2006;15:399–418.

Fyfe G, Fisher RI, Rosenberg SA, et al. Results of treatment of 255 patients with metastatic renal cell carcinoma who received high-dose recombinant interleukin-2 therapy, *J Clin Oncol* 1995;13: 688–696.

Janeway CA, Travers P, Walport W, Capra JD, eds. *Immunobiology: the immune system in health and disease.* New York: Garland Publishing, 2001.

Jonasch E, Haluska FG. Interferon in oncologic practice: review of interferon biology, clinical applications and toxicities, *Oncologist* 2002;6:34.

Mapara MY, Sykes M. Tolerance and cancer: mechanisms of tumor evasion and strategies for breaking tolerance. *J Clin Oncol* 2004;22:1136–1151.

Mocellin S, Rossi CR, Lise M, Marincola FM. Adjuvant immunotherapy for solid tumors: from promise to clinical application, *Cancer Immunol Immunother* 2002; 51:583–595.

Pardoll DM. Spinning molecular immunology into successful immunotherapy, *Nat Rev Immunol* 2002; 2:227–238.

Rosenberg SA. Shedding light on immunotherapy for cancer. *N Engl J Med* 2004;350:1461–1463.

Sabel MS, Nehs MA. Immunologic approaches to breast cancer treatment. *Surg Oncol Clin N Am* 2005; 14:1–31.

Trinchieri G. Interleukin-12: a proinflammatory cytokine with immunoregulatory functions that bridge innate resistance and antigen-specific adaptive immunity, *Annu Rev Immunol* 1995;13:251–276.

Webster WS, Small EJ, Rini BI, Kwon ED. Prostate cancer immunology: biology, therapeutics, and challenges. *J Clin Oncol* 2005;23:8262–8269.

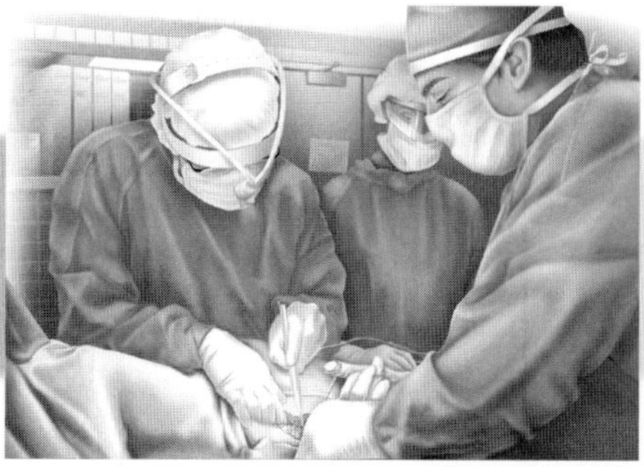

8

Noninvasive Breast Cancer

Erika A. Newman and Michael S. Sabel

Noninvasive Breast Cancer: Key Points

- Describe ductal carcinoma in situ lesions and risk factors.
- List the elements emphasized in a histopathologic analysis of ductal carcinoma in situ.
- Differentiate the various presentations of ductal carcinoma in situ lesions.
- Identify the primary treatment options for ductal carcinoma in situ.
- Differentiate lobular carcinoma in situ from ductal carcinoma in situ.
- Detail the three management options for lobular carcinoma in situ.

Ductal Carcinoma In Situ

Ductal carcinoma in situ (DCIS) and *intraductal carcinoma* are terms that are used interchangeably for a clinical entity that is limited to the confines of the basement membrane. DCIS typically starts in the small- to medium-sized ducts, with exaggerated ductal cellular proliferation. Frequently diagnosed on screening mammography, this lesion is a precursor to invasive ductal carcinoma. Although it is thought of as innocuous, DCIS encompasses a variable group of lesions with a wide spectrum of histologic and pathologic features, diverse malignant potential, and multiple treatment options.

Incidence

The widespread use of screening mammography has resulted in an unprecedented increase in the detection of noninvasive breast cancer. Before this era, DCIS was an altogether different disease entity. Before widespread mammographic screening, DCIS presented as either a palpable mass, nipple discharge, or Paget's disease, and it represented a small fraction of breast cancer cases (1% to 3%). As a result of a lack of clinical data regarding DCIS, treatment recommendations ranged from simple observation to modified radical mastectomy. Between 1983 and 1989, as screening mammography became widespread, incidence rates increased dramatically. The incidence of DCIS continues

BOX 8–1 TYPES OF DUCTAL CARCINOMA IN SITU LESIONS

- *Multifocal ductal carcinoma in situ (DCIS):* An entity in which multiple, apparently separate foci of disease occur within the same quadrant of the breast. Upon closer evaluation using three-dimensional reconstructions of the cross-sectional segments, 99% of these seemingly disconnected areas are in essence unifocal, harboring disease that arises from convolutions of the same duct system.
- *Multicentric DCIS:* A type of disease in which the foci of disease present in different quadrants of the breast, arising simultaneously in different, disconnected duct systems. On average, 30% cases of DCIS are believed to be multicentric.
- *Microinvasive DCIS:* Defined by the American Joint Committee on Cancer as the extension of cancer cells beyond the basement membrane and into adjacent tissues, with no focus more than 1 mm in its greatest dimension. Lesions fulfilling this criterion are staged as T1mic, which is a subset of T1 breast cancer. Only the focus with the largest dimension is used to classify the lesion, and the sizes of individual foci are not added together.
- *Extensive intraductal component:* A particular morphology of invasive carcinoma with associated DCIS comprising more than 25% of the tumor volume, along with an additional extratumoral focus of DCIS.
- *Paget's disease of the breast:* Clinically defined by finding eczematous, scaly skin at the nipple and areolar complex. It is associated with underlying breast cancer (invasive and/or in situ) in 97% of cases. A less-common presentation of breast cancer, Paget's disease should be considered in any patient with a persistent nipple and areolar complex abnormality.

to increase exponentially, with more than 62,000 cases expected in 2006. Today, DCIS accounts for more than 20% of all new cancer diagnoses and approximately 42% of all mammographically detected malignancies. It remains unresolved how much of this increase is attributable to more rampant screening and how much is a true increased occurrence of the disease. The risk factors for DCIS and invasive cancer are similar and include a personal history of breast cancer, family history, nulliparity, or older age at first birth.

Pathology

Although the concept of a localized preinvasive form of breast cancer dates back to 1906, the actual term in situ was not coined until 1932. Basically, DCIS is thought to be an exaggerated multiplication of cells in the ductal system with a propensity toward longitudinal rather than radial growth; these cells remain within the confines of the basement membranes. A constellation of subtypes have been recognized, each with their own individual architectural characteristics, invasive potential, and prognostic significance.

Historically, DCIS has been classified into five subtypes based on architectural pattern: micropapillary, papillary, cribriform, solid, and comedo. These types are postulated to represent steps in evolution and worsening malignant potential (Table 8-1; Figures 8-1, 8-2, 8-3, and 8-4). More recently, the emphasis has been on the presence of necrosis and nuclear grade. This is based on the fact that these factors have the most significant association with microinvasive disease and the propensity for recurrence. DCIS is not associated with a high risk of regional or distant recurrence, so the focus centers on local control, particularly on preventing an invasive recurrence. This is particularly true as more women opt for breast conservation. Hence, the current recommendation is for each histopathologic result to individually comment on morphology, nuclear grade, and necrosis. Several systems exist for classifying DCIS by these features (Table 8-2).

Natural History of DCIS

Ductal carcinoma in situ is generally thought to be a precursor lesion to invasive carcinoma: a step in the transition from normal cells of the duct to frankly invasive cancer. It is important to keep in mind, however, that the progression from cellular proliferation to atypical hyperplasia to noninvasive cancer and ultimately to invasive cancer has been hypothesized yet never proven. Evidence from past studies of patients with DCIS left untreated as

TABLE 8–1 • *Traditional Architectural Classification of Ductal Carcinoma In Situ*

Architectural Pattern	Cytologic Features	Calcifications	Cell Necrosis
Micropapillary	Intraluminal projection of cells, club shaped, lack fibrovascular cores	Minimal, small	Limited to single cells
Papillary	Intraluminal projection of tumor cells, fibrovascular cores	Minimal, small	Variable
Cribriform	Small cells, small hypochromatic nuclei, back-to-back glands	Minimal, small	Limited to single cells
Solid	Not as well defined, tumor cells fill and distend involved space	Variable	Not significant
Comedo	Large cells, nuclear pleomorphism, mitotic activity, often associated with microinvasion	Linear, branching	Prominent

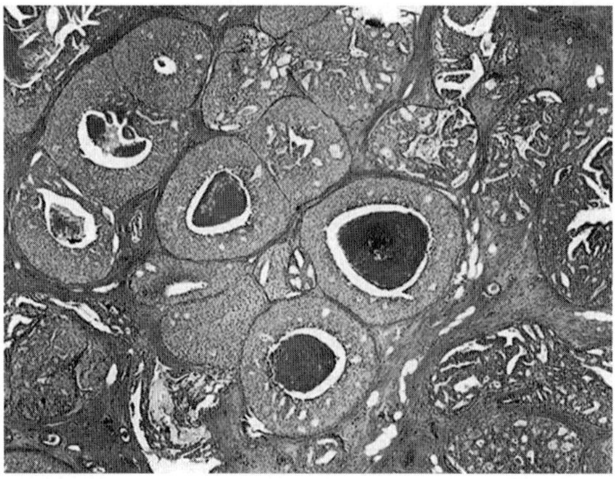

Figure 8–1. Ductal carcinoma in situ. Comedo variant showing large cells with pleomorphic nuclei. (Courtesy of Celina Kleer, MD, Department of Pathology, University of Michigan.)

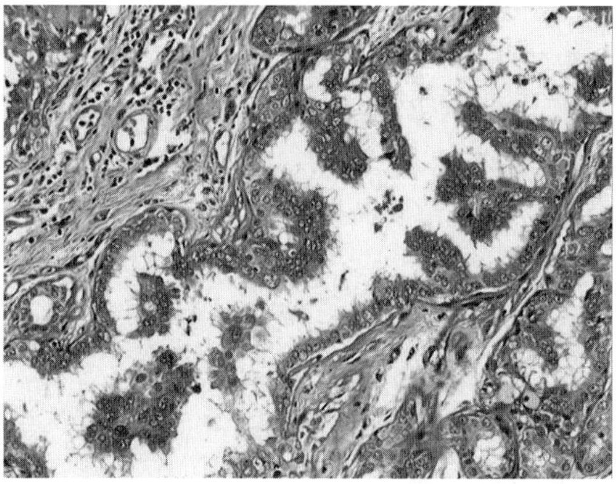

Figure 8–3. Micropapillary variant of ductal carcinoma in situ. (Courtesy of Celina Kleer, MD, Department of Pathology, University of Michigan.)

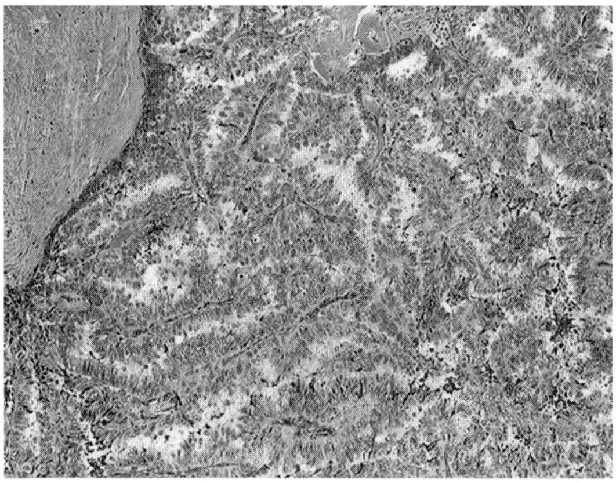

Figure 8–2. Papillary variant of ductal carcinoma in situ. (Courtesy of Celina Kleer, MD, Department of Pathology, University of Michigan.)

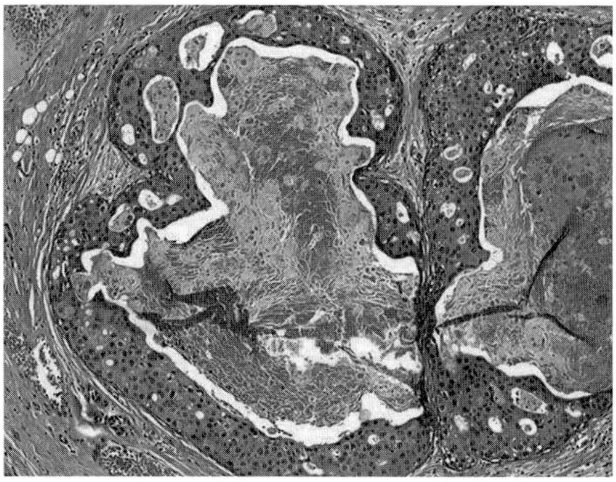

Figure 8–4. High-grade ductal carcinoma in situ. (Courtesy of Celina Kleer, MD, Department of Pathology, University of Michigan.)

TABLE 8-2 • *Histopathologic Classification of Ductal Carcinoma In Situ*

European	Van Nuys	Lagios
Well differentiated	Non high grade, no necrosis	Low grade
Moderately differentiated	Non high grade, with necrosis	Intermediate grade
Poorly differentiated	High grade	High grade

a result of missed diagnoses provides valuable insights. Aftcr 30 years of follow up, approximately two thirds of these patients progressed to invasive disease. This clearly demonstrates that most DCIS lesions will evolve into invasive cancers; however, a significant proportion do not. The disease-free subset most likely represents low-grade disease with small residual tumor burden or even lesions that were incidentally completely excised during biopsy.

Studies suggest that DCIS most commonly originates from a single site, with longitudinal extension along the ductal systems. Cross-sectional proliferation and progression to invasion occurs concurrently; thus, the larger the area of DCIS, the more likely it is that there are microinvasive foci. There is a much higher prevalence of invasive disease in cases of diffuse DCIS.

By definition, unless microinvasive disease is present, DCIS does not invade through the basement membrane and, therefore, cannot spread to the regional lymph nodes or distally. A review of modified radical mastectomy specimens performed for DCIS more than two decades ago showed concurrent axillary disease in only 2% to 3% of patients. Similar proportions were seen to develop distant metastasis, despite adequate local treatment. This most likely represents missed foci of microinvasion, although the possibility of an inherently aggressive form of DCIS cannot be ruled out.

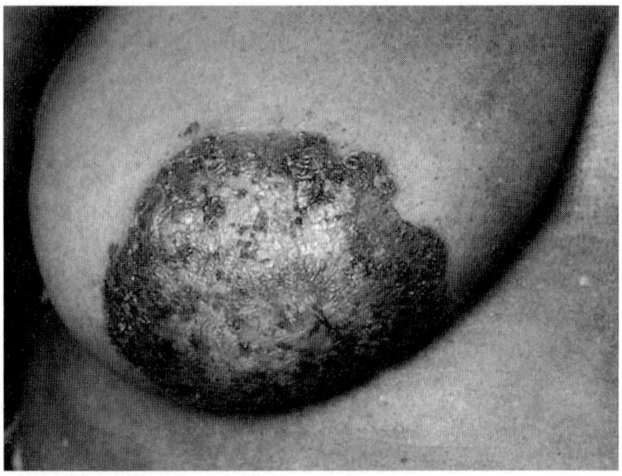

Figure 8-5. Paget's disease of the breast. Classical scaly, eczematous, nipple-areolar complex. (Courtesy of Celina Kleer, MD, Department of Pathology, University of Michigan.)

Presentation

Although today most DCIS patients present with an abnormality on routine screening mammogram, approximately 9% of patients still present with a palpable mass, nipple discharge, or Paget's disease of the breast (a chronic, eczematous, scaly rash at the nipple and areolar complex) (Figure 8-5). Any patient presenting with these findings should undergo mammographic imaging.

Because more than 90% of DCIS lesions diagnosed today are clinically occult, dependence on imaging modalities has become obligatory. Mammography has emerged as the primary imaging tool for the detection and diagnosis of DCIS. Microcalcifications are the most common mammographic characteristic of DCIS, and they are observed in more than 90% of cases (Figure 8-6). Less frequently, mammographic findings may include prominent ducts, mass, or architectural changes.

There is evidence to suggest correlation between the histopathologic subtype of DCIS and features of associated mammographic calcifications. The most characteristic feature of comedo DCIS is casting-type calcifications: linear branching patterns that depict alignment in a ductal distribution. Conversely, noncomedo DCIS is more often associated with fine punctuate calcifications that usually present as a cluster or as a noncalcific mass. Up to 94% of comedo DCIS have mammographic calcifications, 87% of which are linear. Alternatively, only 53% of noncomedo DCIS had calcifications. In addition, the mammographic estimation of lesion size for comedo DCIS was more accurate than for the other subtypes.

Other available imaging techniques—including ultrasonography, magnetic resonance imaging (MRI), scintimammography, and computerized thermography—are relatively insensitive in the absence of invasion.

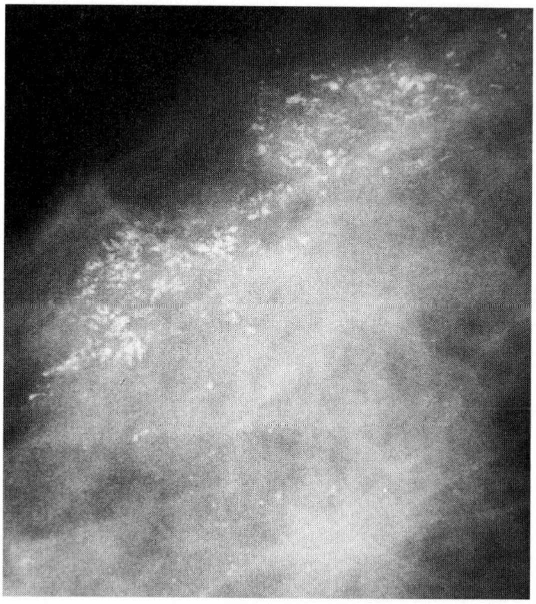

Figure 8–6. Mammographic findings of ductal carcinoma in situ with microcalcifications.

Sonographic features of DCIS include a higher proportion of oval- or lobulated-shaped areas, with uniform isoechoic texture and bilateral edge shadowing. Calcifications may be detected by a high frequency probe in up to 60% of lesions, usually the comedo subtype. Ultrasound's sensitivity is estimated as 62% for comedo DCIS as compared with only 30% for noncomedo lesions. Breast MRI is the most recent adjunct to breast imaging. The use of MRI for evaluating invasive breast cancer is still evolving, and recent data suggest a possible role of MRI for accurately assessing the extent of disease as well as for detecting multicentricity or residual disease after resection. Although estimating the extent of disease in DCIS is equally as important, the ability of MRI to do this accurately is still under investigation, and the role of MRI for DCIS remains experimental.

An abnormality detected on mammography obligates histopathologic evaluation. The various available options include fine-needle aspiration (FNA); percutaneous core needle biopsy under stereotactic, sonographic, or tactile guidance (when palpable); and surgical biopsy with or without wire localization. The absolute sensitivity of FNA for the diagnosis of DCIS is only in the range of 51% to 55%, with more than 35% of indeterminate cytology lesions later confirmed as DCIS. Cytology cannot differentiate in situ versus invasive cancer, and, therefore, FNA is inadequate for the diagnosis of DCIS. On the other hand, stereotactically guided core biopsy with specimen imaging to confirm the retrieval of microcalcifications has a sensitivity up to 91% to 94%. Ultrasound-guided biopsy techniques have similar results. Wire localization of microcalcifications with surgical excision is used for diagnosis if the above-mentioned procedures cannot be performed as a result of technical or patient-related factors, a situation which is becoming increasingly rare.

It is important to remember that image-guided core biopsy techniques may understage malignant microcalcifications. Studies indicate that approximately 10% to 15% of 14-gauge (G) core biopsy specimens revealing atypical hyperplasia, which is a benign condition, get upgraded to DCIS. Similarly, DCIS diagnosed by a core biopsy may get upgraded to DCIS with microinvasion or frankly invasive cancer. This rate of upstaging may be reduced by using larger 11-G or 8-G core samples. It is recommended that atypical ductal hyperplasia diagnosed by a core biopsy be completely excised via wire-localization excision to rule out any residual DCIS or invasive cancer.

Treatment

With the evolution of current knowledge of the disease process and its pattern of behavior, treatment options have evolved accordingly. Today, a variety of treatment options ranging from excision alone (lumpectomy or breast-conserving therapy) to mastectomy, with or without radiation therapy (XRT), have been proposed for DCIS. When treating invasive breast cancer, local control efforts may be tempered by the likelihood of distant recurrences and overall survival. For noninvasive breast cancer, there is an extremely low likelihood of distant disease, and the overall survival should approach 99% to 100%. Therefore, the goal of therapy centers squarely on local control. Approximately half of all recurrences will be invasive, with the associated risk of metastases and decreased survival.

After DCIS has been established with tissue biopsy, the treatment is directed at the complete resection of all disease and the prevention of recurrence. Treatment must be individualized to each patient to accomplish these goals. The extent of disease, the size of the lesion, any prior history of breast cancer and/or XRT, occult invasive cancer coexisting with the in situ lesion, and multicentricity are important factors for determining the best treatment for disease control. Patients should be counseled and involved in the decision-making process.

Mastectomy

Historically, mastectomy was the treatment of choice for DCIS, with cure rates approaching 98% to 99% (Table 8-3). Reported failure rates after mastectomy are in the range of 1% to 3%, and almost all of these are invasive carcinomas presenting as chest wall, axillary, or distant recurrence. This may be explained by the fact that high-grade comedo DCIS may contain areas of invasion or microinvasion that remain undiagnosed with standard histopathologic evaluation protocols.

Although mastectomy has the lowest reported failure rate and is considered the gold standard for the management of DCIS, it may be more aggressive than is necessary for most women with DCIS. With the advent of breast-conservation therapy options for invasive cancer, its application was successfully extended to DCIS. However, mastectomy is still the treatment of choice for several specific situations. Multicentric DCIS is one indication for mastectomy. Some patients will have diffuse microcalcifications throughout the breast on mammography. This often represents diffuse disease, and, even in those cases in which these calcifications are associated with benign disease, they hamper the ability to detect recurrence on surveillance mammography. When DCIS is not multicentric but rather is limited to one area within the breast, the size of this region relative to the size of the breast is an important consideration for whether mastectomy is indicated. This is obviously relative and must be individually considered for each patient, but a large area of disease that cannot be excised with a cosmetically acceptable result should be a relative indication for mastectomy. Likewise, the inability to obtain histologically negative margins after multiple attempts is another indication to proceed with mastectomy. In addition, contraindications to radiation, which plays a significant role in breast conservation, must be considered. These include women in the first or second trimester of pregnancy; women with connective-tissue disorders such as scleroderma, who have unusually high complications from radiation; and women who have had previous radiation to the area.

BOX 8–2 INDICATIONS FOR MASTECTOMY IN DUCTAL CARCINOMA IN SITU CASES

- Multicentric disease
- Diffuse microcalcifications on mammography
- Large tumor size with predictably bad cosmetic outcome
- Contraindication to radiation
  - Pregnancy
  - Connective-tissue disorder (scleroderma)
  - Previous radiation therapy
- Patient preference

Breast-Conservation Therapy

During the mid-1980s to the 1990s there were various authors who reported their experiences with breast-conservation therapy (BCT) for DCIS, employing lumpectomy as the primary treatment modality, with or without XRT (Tables 8-4 and 8-5). These studies provided compelling evidence in favor of BCT. A strong argument for the use of adjuvant radiation came unintentionally

TABLE 8–3 • *Results of Ductal Carcinoma In Situ Treated with Mastectomy*

Report	Patients	Median Follow Up (Years)	Local Recurrence Rate (%)
Jha et al (2001)	176	7.3	0
Kinne et al (1989)	82	11.5	1.2
Sunshine et al (1985)	70	10	3
Silverstein et al (1995)	167	7.6	1.2
Ward et al (1992)	123	10	1
Cutuli et al (2001)	145	91	2.1

TABLE 8–4 • *Trials of Lumpectomy with and without Radiation for Ductal Carcinoma In Situ*

	National Surgical Adjuvant Breast and Bowel Project Protocol B-17	European Organization for Research and Treatment 10853	UK DCIS
No. of patients	813	1,002	1,030
Follow up (in years)	12	4	4.4
Recurrence rate, excision alone	32%	16%	14%
Percentage invasive	50%	50%	40%
Recurrence rate, excision plus radiation therapy	12%	9%	6%
Percentage invasive	30%	40%	50%

TABLE 8–5 • *Retrospective Recurrence Rates after Lumpectomy and Radiation Therapy for Ductal Carcinoma In Situ*

Report	No. of Patients	Median Follow Up (Years)	5-Year Local Recurrence (%)
Hiramatsu et al (1995)	54	6.2	2
Kestin et al (2000)	146	7.2	8
Mirza et al (2000)	87	11	13
Nakamura et al (2002)	260	8.8	18
Silverstein et al (1995)	133	7.8	7
Fowble et al (1996)	110	5.3	1
Kuske et al (1993)	44	4.0	7

from the National Surgical Adjuvant Breast and Bowel Project (NSABP) protocol B-06. Designed to evaluate invasive breast cancers, the protocol recruited a small group of women (78 patients) who were confirmed to have DCIS upon histopathologic reevaluation. Recurrence rates were in the range of 43% for lumpectomy alone, but they were only 9% for the lumpectomy plus XRT arm.

This prompted the NSABP to launch protocol B-17, a prospective randomized trial comparing lumpectomy alone to lumpectomy plus XRT (50 Gy) for the treatment of DCIS. More than 800 patients were recruited in total for both arms of the study, which has a mean follow up of 90 months. Local failure rate for the group treated with lumpectomy alone was approximately twice that of the lumpectomy plus XRT group: 26.8% as compared with 12.1%, with half of the recurrent tumors being invasive in the former and one third being invasive in the latter. Pathologic findings from protocol B-17 showed that the two biggest predictors of ipsilateral recurrence were comedo necrosis and the presence of involved specimen margins.

A similar trial was simultaneously launched in Europe by the European Organization for Research and Treatment. After a median follow-up time of 51 months, a recurrence rate of 16% was observed in the group treated with lumpectomy alone; 50% of these were invasive cancers. Patients treated with lumpectomy with subsequent XRT revealed a recurrence rate of 9%; 40% of these were invasive cancers.

BOX 8–3 RADIATION THERAPY AFTER LUMPECTOMY FOR DUCTAL CARCINOMA IN SITU

- This treatment reduces ipsilateral breast tumor recurrence by 50–60%.
- It also reduces ipsilateral invasive breast tumor recurrence by 50–60%.
- After radiation therapy, the annual rate of an invasive recurrence is 0.5–1% per year.
- Radiation therapy does not improve survival.

Although there have been no prospective, randomized trials comparing mastectomy to BCT for the treatment of DCIS, the large treatment registries have suggested that, although local recurrence rates may be lower after mastectomy than after BCT, there are no differences in overall survival. The reported cause-specific mortality from DCIS treated with either mastectomy or lumpectomy plus XRT is similar (in the range of 1% to 2%). For DCIS, there is little risk of metastasis; however, the potential of an invasive recurrence remains. It is imperative that the basis of all treatment options for DCIS be the minimization of the potential risk of an invasive recurrence. At the present time, most patients are candidates for BCT. The initial attempt should be to widely excise the entire area, with acceptable margins. Careful preoperative planning is paramount, because the initial operation is the best chance to achieve complete excision and to offer good cosmetic results.

As with all lumpectomies, the surgical specimen should be accurately oriented and, if appropriate, imaged to confirm complete excision of the radiographic abnormality. If the lesion is seen to abut a specific margin, an additional surgical margin should be obtained in the corresponding quadrant. Orienting the specimen correctly and inking it with a six-color system allows the pathologist to inform the surgeon if a margin is either involved or close, thereby allowing for a more directed re-excision. This provides a better cosmetic outcome as compared with having to re-excise the entire lumpectomy cavity. Surgical clips left along all six biopsy cavity boundaries are instrumental for delineating the site for the accurate planning of an adjuvant radiation therapy boost dose or partial breast irradiation.

The accurate pathologic assessment of margin status is imperative. There is no consensus to date on what comprises the ideal negative margin for DCIS. Most institutions strive for at least 3 mm of circumferential disease-free tissue. Inadequate margins necessitate re-excision (hence the importance of orienting and labeling the specimen at the time of lumpectomy to guide subsequent surgery). Noninvasive cancers presenting with calcifications require postoperative mammography to ascertain complete excision. Residual suspicious calcifications require localization and re-excision.

It is clear that postoperative radiation as a component of BCT offers excellent local control (see Table 8-5). However, radiation is not without its side effects and costs. Whole-breast irradiation is time consuming and can cause cardiac or pulmonary side effects; there is also the risk of second malignancies. Given the fact that many cases of DCIS treated by excision alone do not recur, it seems likely that there is a subset of patients who may be treated by lumpectomy alone. With careful attention to grade, size, and margin width, there may be a subset of patients who could be treated by lumpectomy alone. This may be appropriate treatment for patients with extremely low risk: mammographically detected DCIS exhibiting favorable histopathologic features (low grade, no necrosis) when resected with an adequate negative margin. However, the definition of "adequate margins of excision" varies among institutions and has not been clearly defined. Ongoing prospective studies in both Europe and the United States are attempting to answer these questions. Until then, for most patients qualifying for BCT, lumpectomy plus postsurgical XRT is the treatment of choice to minimize the risk of local recurrence.

Management of the Axilla

The standard of care for the treatment of noninvasive breast cancer does not include regional lymph node excision. Historically, the analyses of data from studies of mastectomy and lymphadenectomy performed for the treatment of DCIS revealed axillary metastasis in 2% of cases. These were commonly attributable to possible foci of invasive disease that may have been present in the specimen and that remained undetected.

The advent of lymphatic mapping for breast cancer a few years ago opened up new vistas for the detection of axillary disease via minimally invasive modalities. When applied to noninvasive breast cancer, early results have shown wide variability, with some series describing 3% to 6% of patients with pure DCIS having a

BOX 8–4 INDICATIONS FOR SENTINEL LYMPH NODE BIOPSY FOR DUCTAL CARCINOMA IN SITU

- Microinvasion
- Having mastectomy for diffuse disease
- High suspicion of harboring invasive disease
    - Extensive high-grade disease or necrosis on core biopsy
    - Imaging studies suggestive of invasion

positive sentinel lymph node (SLN). The prognostic significance of these rates was questioned widely, and the exclusion of the SLN detected by immunohistochemistry (for which the prognostic implications are not known) resulted in a significant decrease in the positivity rates.

Therefore, neither lymph-node dissection nor lymphatic mapping and SLN biopsy should play a role in the routine management of pure DCIS, with two notable exceptions. The first is when there is a high likelihood of finding invasive disease. This would include cases in which core biopsy demonstrated extensive high-grade disease or in which there is a suspicion of invasion on imaging studies. In these cases, it is reasonable to perform an SLN biopsy in conjunction with lumpectomy; however, for patients being treated with BCT, axillary staging can be deferred until the diagnosis of invasion is confirmed. Any patients with documented microinvasion should undergo axillary evaluation by SLN biopsy. The second indication for lymphatic mapping in the management of DCIS is for the patient undergoing mastectomy for diffuse DCIS, particularly if it is high grade. In this case, should microinvasive disease be discovered during pathologic examination, it would not be possible to then stage the patient by SLN biopsy, and an axillary lymph-node dissection might be necessary.

Hormonal Therapy for DCIS

Tamoxifen, which is a competitive inhibitor of estrogen, has been shown to reduce the risk of both invasive and noninvasive breast cancer among high-risk women. The NSABP protocol B-24 studied the use of tamoxifen among women with DCIS undergoing BCT and XRT. There was an overall risk reduction of 37% for patients receiving tamoxifen, irrespective of resection margin, tumor size, or grade. There was also a decrease in the risk of contralateral invasive and noninvasive cancer of 52% (Table 8-6). Alternatively, a trial from the United Kingdom, Australia, and New Zealand failed to demonstrate a significant benefit of tamoxifen for preventing either ipsilateral or contralateral events. The trial was a smaller study with a design that allowed for some patient choice, so the results must be interpreted with care.

However, these results suggest that a selective approach must be used when deciding which women with DCIS should receive adjuvant tamoxifen. The potential benefits of tamoxifen for reducing both recurrence and second breast malignancies must be weighed against the potential side effects, which include venous thromboembolism and uterine cancer. The baseline risk of recurrence, the age of the patient, and the relative risk of side effects must be considered. In addition, the estrogen receptor (ER) status should be considered. In a study derived from the NSABP protocol B-24 drug arm comparing the response of ER-positive versus ER-negative patients to tamoxifen, recurrence rates were 10% for the ER-positive group as compared with 23% for the ER-negative group. Therefore, many institutions have begun routinely evaluating DCIS for ER status by immunohistochemistry.

Recently, the aromatase inhibitor anastrazole has received growing attention. Results of the Anastrazole and Tamoxifen: Alone or in Combination trial, which randomized 9,000 patients with early-stage breast cancer to receive anastrozole versus tamoxifen versus the combination revealed a statistically significant risk reduction of new breast cancers in the anastrozole arm ($P = .007$). However, there is no data about the use of aromatase inhibitors in patients with DCIS. There are presently two ongoing trials that address this issue (NSABP protocol B-35 in the United States and IBIS-II in Great Britain).

Lobular Carcinoma in Situ

Lobular carcinoma in situ (LCIS) is a relatively uncommon disease that arises from the

TABLE 8–6 • *Results of National Surgical Adjuvant Breast and Bowel Project Protocol B-24: Tamoxifen Versus Placebo after Lumpectomy Plus Radiation Therapy*

Study Arms	No. of Patients	Local Recurrence	Invasive Recurrence	Survival
Lumpectomy plus radiation therapy plus placebo	902	87 (9.6%)	40/87 (46%)	97%
Lumpectomy plus radiation therapy plus tamoxifen	902	63 (7%)	23/63 (37%)	97%

lobules and terminal ducts of the breast. It is rarely suspected before biopsy, because it does not form a palpable mass, nor can it be routinely detected by mammography. Rather, it is usually an incidental microscopic finding. What makes LCIS confusing is that, as opposed to DCIS, LCIS is not a premalignant lesion, but rather it is considered an indicator of increased risk of subsequent invasive cancer (Table 8-7). The subsequent cancer could be either ductal or lobular, and it may be in either the ipsilateral or the contralateral breast.

Diagnosis

LCIS does not form a mass or calcifications; therefore, it has none of the clinical features associated with DCIS. It is usually discovered during biopsy for either a palpable mass or suspicious calcifications found on mammogram and found incidentally adjacent to the area in question during the pathological review. Before 1980, LCIS was found in only 0.6% of all breast biopsies. Since the advent of screening mammography as well as the increase in breast biopsies, LCIS is now found in 1.1% of all biopsies, and it comprises approximately 5% of all breast carcinomas. The true incidence of LCIS in the population is unknown.

LCIS is recognized by intraepithelial proliferation of the terminal lobular-ductal unit with expanded and filled acini. The lobular architecture remains undisturbed, and the basement membrane is never penetrated (Figure 8-7). In contrast with DCIS, the cells of LCIS have a rather homogeneous morphology and are without evidence of necrosis or calcification.

Numerous reports have confirmed that LCIS is multicentric as well as multifocal, and it is found in other areas of the breast in up to 80% of cases. It is also found in the contralateral breast in 50% to 90% of cases. It is for these reasons that LCIS discovered at one site should serve as an indicator of possible pathology at any site in both breasts.

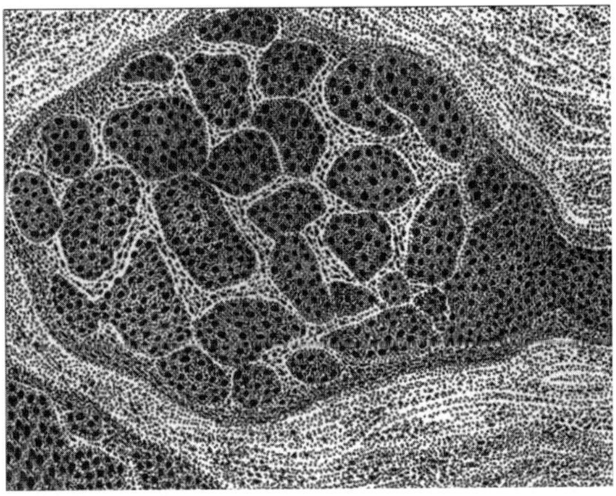

Figure 8–7. Typical pathologic findings of lobular carcinoma in situ with intraepithelial proliferation of the terminal lobular-ductal unit and distended acini. (Courtesy of Celina Kleer, MD, Department of Pathology, University of Michigan.)

Natural History of LCIS

It appears unlikely that LCIS directly progresses to invasive disease in the same way that DCIS appears to progress to invasive ductal carcinoma. The molecular characteristics are consistent with a relatively benign biologic behavior, and the invasive tumors that do develop are more often invasive ductal rather than invasive lobular (although women with LCIS have a higher incidence of invasive lobular cancer than the general population). Whereas lobular carcinoma typically represents 5% to 10% of breast cancers, among women with LCIS, it accounts for 25% of subsequent cancers. The subsequent cancer is almost as likely to be in the contralateral breast as it is to be in the ipsilateral.

For this reason, LCIS is not treated as a premalignant lesion (with an attempt to resect to

TABLE 8–7 • *Lobular Carcinoma In Situ Versus Ductal Carcinoma In Situ*

	Lobular Carcinoma In Situ	Ductal Carcinoma In Situ
Presentation	Incidental on biopsy	Mammographic (90%), palpable mass, nipple discharge, Paget's disease (10%)
Findings on mammogram	None	Microcalcifications
Subsequent invasive cancer	Lobular or ductal, either breast	Ductal, site of diagnosis
Treatment choices	Observation, tamoxifen, bilateral prophylactic mastectomy	Breast-conservation therapy, mastectomy

negative margins) but rather as a marker of increased risk. Patients who have LCIS diagnosed during core needle biopsy should undergo a wire-localized biopsy, because there is a chance of missing an adjacent invasive lobular carcinoma (Table 8-8). However, patients who have positive margins of LCIS on an excisional biopsy do not require re-excision. Instead, these patients should be thought of as high-risk patients, and they should be counseled about preventative options. The absolute risk of developing invasive cancer after a biopsy demonstrating LCIS is approximately 7 to 18 times higher than it is among the general population.

Management Options

Observation

As knowledge of the biology of LCIS has developed and its natural history clarified, treatment has likewise evolved (Table 8–9). LCIS is now viewed in much the same way as any other risk factors for breast cancer (family or personal history, atypical hyperplasia), and, as with any high-risk patient, careful observation with *lifelong* surveillance is one option. There is no indication for wide local excision (to clear margins), radiation therapy, or ipsilateral mastectomy given the bilaterality, multifocality, and multicentricity of LCIS. Furthermore, these operations have not been shown to decrease the risk of subsequent invasive cancer over observation alone. Historically, an attempt was made at performing unilateral mastectomy with blind contralateral mirror-image biopsies. This is no longer advocated, because the chances of finding a lesion requiring treatment are low, and women with a negative contralateral biopsy had the same incidence of subsequent cancers as those with positive biopsies. Most centers recommend examinations every 4 to 6

TABLE 8–8 • *Risk of Finding Cancer on Excisional Biopsy after Core Biopsy Demonstrating Lobular Carcinoma In Situ*

Report	Cases of Lobular Carcinoma In Situ on Core Biopsy	No. of Excisional Biopsies after Core Biopsy	Cases Upgraded on Excisional Biopsy
Liberman (1999)	14	14	2/14 (14%)
Georgian-Smith (2001)	7	7	2/7 (28%)
Berg (2001)	10	8	0/8 (0%)
Renshaw (2002)	36	9	0/9 (0%)
Yeh (2003)	3	3	0/3 (0%)
Middleton (2003)	14	9	2/9 (22%)
Crisi (2003)	9	9	2/9 (22%)
Foster (2004)	15	12	4/12 (33)
Total	108	71	12 (17%)

TABLE 8–9 • *Management Options for Lobular Carcinoma In Situ*

Management Option	Advantages	Disadvantages
Observation	No side effects of therapy, no negative	Subsequent risk of invasive breast cancer that may not cosmetic effects be detected by screening examinations
Tamoxifen, 20 mg by mouth daily every day for 5 years	Reduces risk of invasive cancer by more than 50%, no negative cosmetic effects	Hot flashes, risk of venous thromboembolism or endometrial cancer, risk of invasive breast cancer still present
Bilateral mastectomy with or without immediate reconstruction	Reduces risk of invasive cancer by more than 95%	Major surgery with potential complications and psychological implications

months, with annual diagnostic mammograms occurring for the patient's lifetime. Recently, the utility of MRI as a screening test has been investigated. Although MRI has been reported to detect more cancers than mammography among high-risk women, it also has significantly more false positives. More studies are necessary to determine what role MRI might have in the surveillance of women with LCIS.

Bilateral Mastectomy

If the patient is deemed extremely high risk (women having a strong family history in addition to LCIS) or does not feel comfortable with observation or chemoprevention, then bilateral mastectomy is a rational and appropriate therapy for LCIS. This treatment addresses the bilateral nature of the disease, and it has the clear benefit of risk reduction. There is no risk of regional or distant metastasis, so axillary dissection is not required. Patients should be offered immediate reconstruction after bilateral mastectomy.

Tamoxifen

A third option—for women who want to reduce their risk yet who are not willing to undergo bilateral mastectomy—is chemoprevention. The NSABP protocol 1 trial prospectively studied the effect of tamoxifen on the prevention of breast cancer, and it included women who had been diagnosed with LCIS. The study randomized nearly 13,200 women with various risk factors for breast cancer to receive tamoxifen or placebo. There was a 55% risk reduction among women with LCIS who were treated with tamoxifen as compared with placebo. Tamoxifen has now emerged as a major element in the management of LCIS, and recent trends show fewer women with LCIS undergoing prophylactic mastectomies. Most patients will benefit from chemoprevention with tamoxifen, but there are adverse effects that many women will perceive as outweighing the benefit. These include hot flashes, fibroids, polyps, cataracts, and venous thromboembolism. Postmenopausal women carry the additional serious risk of endometrial cancer. Patients receiving tamoxifen should be followed closely for adverse effects. The current dosing recommendations are 20 mg per day for 5 years.

Key Selected Reading

Silverstein, MJ. *Ductal carcinoma in situ of the breast,* 2nd ed. Philadelphia: Lippincott Williams & Wilkins, 2002.

Selected Readings

Bao T, Prowell T, Stearns V. Chemoprevention of breast cancer: tamoxifen, raloxifene, and beyond. *Am J Ther* 2006;13:337–348.

Bodian CA, Perzin KH, Lattes R. Lobular neoplasia: long term risk of breast cancer and relation to other factors, *Cancer* 1996;78:1024–1034.

Burstein HJ, Polyak K, Wong JS, *et al.* Ductal carcinoma in situ of the breast. *N Engl J Med* 2004;350: 1430–1441.

Dupont W, Parl F, Hartmann W, *et al.* Breast cancer risk associated with proliferative breast disease and atypical hyperplasia, *Cancer* 1993;71:1258–1265.

Fisher B, Costantino JP, Wickerhan L, *et al.* Tamoxifen for prevention of breast cancer: report of the National Surgical Adjuvant Breast and Bowel Project P-1 study, *J Natl Cancer Inst* 1998;90:1371–1388.

Fisher B, Dignam J, Wolmark N, *et al.* Lumpectomy and radiation therapy for the treatment of intraductal breast cancer: findings from the National Surgical Adjuvant Breast and Bowel Project B-17, *J Clin Oncol* 1998;16:441–452.

Fisher B, Dignam J, Wolmark N, *et al.* National Surgical Adjuvant Breast and Bowel Project B24 randomized controlled trial, *Lancet* 1999;353:1993.

Fisher B, Dignam J, Wolmark N, *et al.* Tamoxifen in treatment of intraductal breast cancer: National Surgical Adjuvant Breast and Bowel Project B-24 randomised controlled trial, *Lancet* 1999;353:1310–1319.

Fisher ER, Costantino J, Fisher B, *et al.* Pathological findings from the National Surgical Adjuvant Breast and Bowel Project Protocol B-17, *Cancer* 1995; 75:1310–1390.

Frykberg ER. Lobular carcinoma in situ of the breast, *Breast J* 1999;5:296–303.

Haagensen CD, Bodian, D, Haagensen DE. *Lobular neoplasia (lobular carcinoma in situ) breast carcinoma: risk and detection.* Philadelphia: WB Saunders, 1981, p. 238.

Houghton J, George WD, Cuzick J. UK Coordinating Committee on Cancer Research (UKCCCR). Radiotherapy and tamoxifen in women with completely excised ductal carcinoma in situ of the breast in the UK, Australia and New Zealand. *Lancet* 2003; 362(9378):95–102.

Julien JP, Bijker N, Fentiman IS, *et al.* Radiotherapy in breast conserving treatment for ductal carcinoma in situ: first results of the EORTC randomized phase III trial 10853, *Lancet* 2001;355:528–535.

Julien JP, Bijker N, Fentiman IS, *et al.* Radiotherapy in breast-conserving treatment for ductal carcinoma in situ: first results of the EORTC randomized phase III trial 10853. EORTC Breast Cancer Cooperative

Group and EORTC Radiotherapy Group, *Lancet* 2000;355;528–533.

Mizra NQ, Vlastos G, Meric F, *et al.* Ductal carcinoma in situ: long term results of breast conserving therapy, *Ann Surg Oncol* 2000;7:656–664.

Morrow M, Schnitt SJ. Treatment selection in ductal carcinoma in situ, *JAMA* 2000;283:453–455.

Orel SG, Mendonca MH, Reynolds C, *et al.* MR imaging of ductal carcinoma in situ, *Radiology* 1997; 202:413–420.

Page DL, Kidd TE, Depont WD, *et al.* Lobular neoplasia of the breast: higher risk for subsequent invasive cancer predicted by more extensive disease, *Hum Pathol* 1991;22:1232–1239.

Romero L, Klein L, Ye W, *et al.* Outcome after invasive recurrence in patients with ductal carcinoma in situ of the breast, *Am J Surg* 2004;188:371–376.

Silverstein MJ, *et al.* A prognostic index for ductal carcinoma in situ of the breast, *Cancer* 1996; 77:2267–2274.

Tsikitis VL, Chung MA. Biology of ductal carcinoma in situ classification based on biologic potential. *Am J Clin Oncol* 2006;29:305–310.

Winchester DP, Jeske JM, Goldschmidt RA. The diagnosis and management of ductal carcinoma in-situ of the breast, *CA Cancer J Clin* 2000;50:184–200.

9

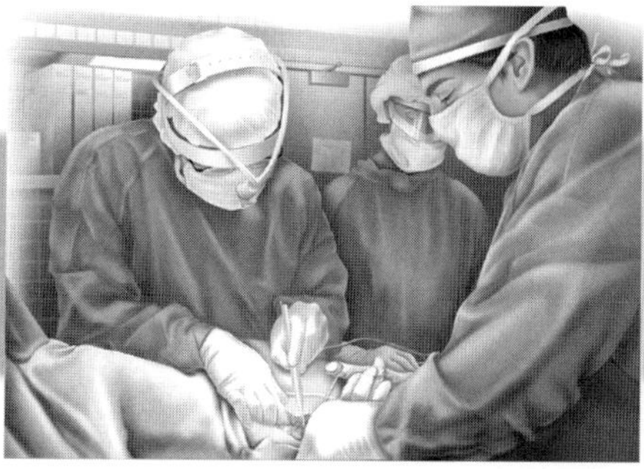

Invasive Breast Cancer

Elizabeth A. Shaughnessy

- ASSESSMENT AND DIAGNOSTICS
- CLINICAL STAGING
- TREATMENT OPTIONS
- SURGICAL THERAPY
- PATHOLOGY REPORT
- SYSTEMIC THERAPY
- RADIATION THERAPY
- SURGICAL AND OTHER COMPLICATIONS
- SPECIAL CONSIDERATIONS

Invasive Breast Cancer: Key Points

- Describe the steps taken in breast cancer assessment and diagnosis.
- Contrast the various biopsy techniques.
- List the components considered during the clinical staging of breast carcinomas.
- Explain the guidelines for choosing breast-conservation surgery.
- Describe the principles of axillary assessment and sentinel node biopsy.
- Outline the technique for mastectomy.
- List the steps taken in axillary lymph node dissection.
- List the steps taken in sentinel lymph node biopsy.
- Review the content of the pathology report.
- Compare the benefits and drawbacks of hormonal therapy and chemotherapy.
- Discuss the role of radiation therapy.
- List the complications associated with breast cancer management.

Historically, the successful treatment of breast cancer began with the work of Halsted and the radical mastectomy. As care has advanced in the context of clinical trials, surgical management still addresses the same two key concepts: management of the breast and management of the axilla. However, over the past century, the treatment of breast cancer has evolved into a multimodality approach, frequently including systemic therapies and radiotherapy and often offering more than one option for those who present with early-stage disease.

The incidence rate of breast cancer was increasing during the 1980s, but it leveled off during the 1990s. In 2006, it is estimated that there will be more than 214,000 cases in the United States. The good news is that the mortality rate is falling. This trend in declining mortality was first identified in 1995, and it is reflected in the cancer statistics of multiple industrialized countries. Whether this reflects the impact of breast cancer screening, the emergence of many effective options for systemic treatment, or both is difficult to dissect. The observation of an actual decrease in cancer mortality after the initiation of screening methods may take decades, as demonstrated by the delayed reduction of cervical cancer mortality with Papanicolaou's staining of cervical smears. It is likely that both screening and treatment play a role, because newly diagnosed patients with metastatic disease are beginning to live for 6 years or longer given the many options for systemic therapies.

No single cause has been identified for breast cancer initiation; it is probable that several pathways are possible from a molecular standpoint. For those with hereditary concerns, BRCA1 and BRCA2 gene mutations carry the greatest influence, but other cancer syndromes may predispose the individual as well. These include the Lynch II syndrome of hereditary colon cancer, Li-Fraumeni syndrome with p53 mutations, ataxia-telangiectasia syndrome, Cowden's syndrome, and others. Given a low incidence of breast cancers among men (1 in 100-200 cases), these are more likely to reflect a hereditary influence, especially that of the BRCA2 mutation. However, hereditary breast cancer constitutes less than 15% of all cases of newly diagnosed cases among women.

BOX 9–1 GENETIC SYNDROMES THAT INCLUDE BREAST CANCER

- Breast-ovarian syndrome (BRCA1 or BRCA2 mutation)
- Lynch II syndrome of hereditary colon cancer (microsatellite instability)
- Li–Fraumeni syndrome (p53 mutations)
- Ataxia-telangiectasia syndrome
- Cowden's syndrome (possibly PTEN mutation)

Risk factors extend beyond just hereditary influence. Younger age at menarche, older age at menopause, the number of pregnancies, and an older age at first pregnancy presumably reflect the degree of hormonal influence on the cycling breast cells. Extensions of these influences can also be seen in the higher rate of breast cancer among women with polycystic ovarian syndrome. Traditionally, the Gail Model of breast cancer risk includes some of these, and newer versions (http://bcra.nci.nih.gov/brc/) take racial differences in breast cancer incidence into account, as influenced by the observations within the context of the Breast Cancer Prevention Trial of the National Surgical Breast and Bowel Project (NSABP). In general, black women have a lower incidence of breast cancer, but they generally present at a younger average age and usually with a slightly more advanced stage as compared with the white population.

Assessment and Diagnostics

Patients generally seek consultation with a surgeon who is familiar with breast management either because of breast symptoms (e.g., breast pain, nipple discharge, a palpable mass) or an abnormality on screening mammography. The initial history should include a description of the problem, its duration, and its associated symptoms. The history should also encompass aspects of breast cancer risk, which include the gynecologic history, exogenous hormone use, and a family history of breast and ovarian cancers. The previous history of a breast biopsy also constitutes increased risk; the presence of atypical ductal or lobular hyperplasia or lobular carcinoma in situ in such biopsies places the patient at increased risk for breast cancer development.

Beyond the initial history, a focused physical examination should be incorporated to address any concerns. After inspection, the breast should be palpated. The texture of the breast should be appreciated, because masses, areas of thickening, or induration should be distinct from the overall texture. With a complaint of pain, attention should be paid to the area in question; it should first be palpated softly, and then with greater pressure. A distinction needs to be made between actual breast pain and pain of the chest wall muscle; examination can then be facilitated by having the woman lie more on her side so that the breast falls away from the lateral chest wall. When dealing with breast discharge, it should be noted whether the discharge is spontaneous or expressed, unilateral or bilateral, or if it has blood in it (Figure 9-1). The pathologic discharge is generally spontaneous and unilateral; the etiologies of bilateral discharge tend to be systemic, such as medication or hormonal perturbations (e.g., hyperthyroidism, prolactinemia). A thick, cheesy, or pasty discharge, often bilateral and not spontaneous, is usually a reflection of duct ectasia.

Further investigation should proceed with breast imaging (usually diagnostic mammography), except perhaps mass lesions identified in young women or girls. In this situation, ultrasound is a reasonable modality. Ultrasound is usually employed to discern whether a mass lesion (on examination or by mammogram) constitutes a cystic or a solid mass. Use of breast magnetic resonance imaging (MRI) is gaining momentum in the patient with dense breast tissue, especially in the context of a family history of breast cancer. However, this technique, although sensitive, is not considered the standard of care for the management of most breast complaints.

Simple cysts can be aspirated or followed; complex cysts associated with a solid mass or that are septated are usually excised, because they are associated with a small chance of an adjacent malignancy. Similarly, recurrent cysts should be excised after two aspirations with recurrence as a result of a higher rate of associated malignancy in this context. Solid lesions should be assessed with regard to their characteristics; obscured or indistinct margins and margins that are lobulated or spiculated are suspicious for malignancy. Although in certain situations it may be acceptable to clinically follow a benign-appearing solid mass with serial clinical examinations and ultrasounds, most solid masses require some type of tissue biopsy.

Biopsy Techniques

When approaching a mass, several biopsy approaches are available if the mass is palpable. Fine-needle aspiration (FNA) can be performed in the clinical setting with a minimum of equipment. If the mass is cystic, the fluid contents may be removed in their near entirety. It should be noted whether the mass completely resolves with aspiration, because a

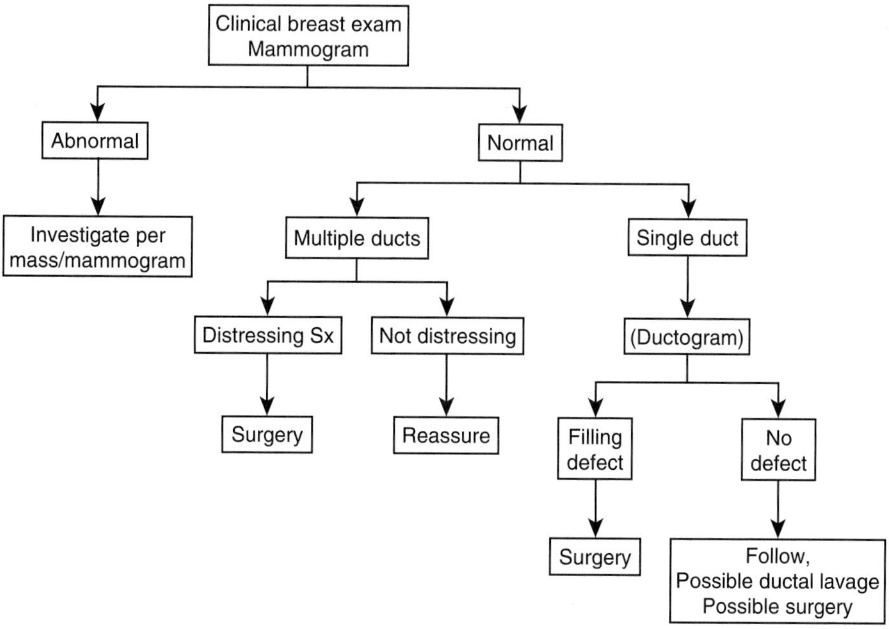

Figure 9–1. Algorithm for the management of breast discharge.

residual mass makes this clinically suspicious for a complex cyst and requires excision. Should the fluid context contain blood, it should be forwarded for cytologic evaluation. The incidence of cancer associated with a nonbloody aspirate is less than 1 in 1,000, and nonbloody fluid is generally not forwarded for further evaluation. If the mass is solid, loose cells can be pulled into the hub of the needle after multiple passes in at least four different directions for an accurate sampling. These cells can then be placed on slides and fixed, or they can be released in fixative fluid and prepared per ThinPrep technology. In this context, with a competent cytologist, the sensitivity of FNA for malignant cells is approximately 92%. The definitive diagnosis of benign conditions may or may not be possible. However, if there is triple concordance between the examination, imaging, and FNA results, the diagnostic accuracy ranges from 93% to 99%. In the context of triple concordance, it is reasonable to follow a patient as long as the patient is counseled and understands the risks of a potentially small delay in diagnosis. Should the mass enlarge, sampling error is assumed, and excisional biopsy is recommended. If the triple results are discordant, the biopsy should probably be excised because of the possibility of sampling error with the aspiration technique.

In the context of a palpable mass of sufficient size, a percutaneous core biopsy could be performed under local anesthesia. Unlike FNA, with which only loose cells are evaluated, core biopsy allows for assessment of architecture, which may discern between intraductal and invasive cells, if malignant. This too can be performed in the outpatient clinical setting; deep masses, which may be missed with a percutaneous approach, or masses seen only on imaging may benefit by image-guided core biopsy for tissue assessment. This includes stereotactic core biopsy as well as ultrasound guidance. In general, this technique reflects 96% sensitivity for detecting malignancy. This technique is a sampling type of biopsy, and thus there is a risk of sampling error. The results should always be interpreted in light of the physical examination and breast imaging findings. However, the finding of atypical cells on FNA or on core biopsy must prompt excision of the abnormality; noninvasive or invasive carcinoma has been found adjacent to the biopsy site in 10% to 40% of cases, depending on the literature cited.

Excisional biopsy can also be performed, and it is considered the gold standard, because it yields 100% sensitivity for palpable lesions and 98% sensitivity if performed with needle localization. Local anesthesia is generally used, with or without intravenous sedation, but general anesthesia is used in some settings. Usually, the mass is outlined on the skin with a sterile skin marker before proceeding; the local anesthetic can obscure palpation of the mass after it is injected. Lesions that are more centrally located are usually approached with a periareolar incision around a limited segment of the border; most others use Langer's skin lines, because they overlie the mass for incision and provide a better cosmetic result (Figure 9-2). Alternatively, a radial incision may also be used in the inferior aspect of the breast with a minimum of contour distortion. After the initial skin incision, the excision for a suspicious mass is approached with an attempt to excise the mass in its entirety, with a 1-cm margin of nor-

BOX 9–2 APPROXIMATE SENSITIVITIES OF BIOPSY TECHNIQUES

Fine-needle aspiration	94%
Core biopsy	96%
Excisional biopsy	100%
Wire-localized excisional biopsy	98%

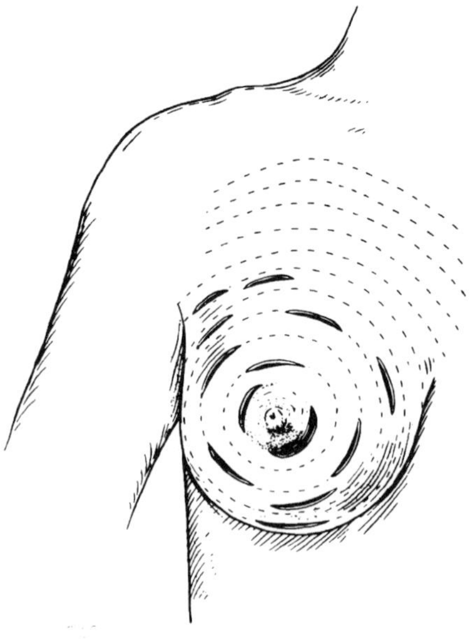

Figure 9–2. Curvilinear incisions made parallel to Langer's skin lines heal with less distortion. (From Bland KI, Copeland EM III, eds. *The breast: comprehensive management of benign and malignant masses*, ed 3. Philadelphia: WB Saunders, 2004, p. 797, with permission.)

mal tissue circumferentially. This biopsy may constitute a lumpectomy should the lesion prove to be a breast cancer. As with all excisions, hemostasis is maintained. Electrocautery may be used in the excision; most laboratories have moved beyond the assessment of estrogen and progesterone receptors by functional assay to immunohistochemical staining. After the mass is ready to be completely excised, a short suture is placed on the superior aspect, and a long suture is placed on the lateral aspect, per usual convention, to orient the specimen. This should be mentioned on the pathology submission sheet for use by the pathologist. Preferably, the specimen has been removed en bloc rather than piecemeal to ensure accuracy of the margins should it prove to be a cancer. In general, frozen section is not performed intraoperatively for definitive diagnosis, because the technique is only 80% accurate, and adipose tissue resists freezing. After the lesion has been submitted for evaluation by pathology and hemostasis has been assured, the wound is then checked for any other palpable lesions. If none is found, the wound is closed, usually without reapproximating the deep breast tissue. A two-layer closure suffices for the subcutaneous tissue and skin.

Image guidance is essential for addressing nonpalpable lesions. In the case of cysts identified by ultrasound, ultrasound guidance is used to aspirate, when indicated. Masses may be approached by mammography (stereotactic biopsy) or ultrasound guidance for core biopsy, assuming that the method used adequately identified the lesion. For example, microcalcifications seen only mammographically would need stereotactic core biopsy for sampling. In all of these cases, the procedure would necessitate performance by a person sufficiently trained in these radiologic techniques; usually this would require referral, except for those surgeons who have pursued specialized training in stereotactic biopsy or breast ultrasound. Not all patients are candidates for these techniques. Stereotactic biopsy has a weight restriction of 300 lb for the table. Furthermore, lesions located close to the chest wall, immediately deep to the skin, or in the tail of Spence would be difficult or impossible to access given the physical restrictions of the instrumentation. As with any sampling technique, the pathology result should be examined in light of the imaging result (obviously, not the physical examination, because it is not palpable). Should there not be concordance, excision should be sought.

It is worth mentioning that the identification of atypical cells, atypical ductal or lobular hyperplasia, or papillary lesions on stereotactic core biopsy prompts further excision of breast tissue using wire localization. These lesions may be associated with a significant chance (up to 10%) of finding further adjacent malignancy that was not adequately sampled as a consequence of sampling error. This possibility should be discussed with the patient initially so that she understands that further surgery may be warranted with this approach.

For nonpalpable lesions, the biopsy method of choice may be excision with wire localization. This technique involves the placement of a wire, possibly with the needle, before the planned surgery. During the placement of the guidewire, the radiologist places a needle within the breast near the lesion and then passes a wire through the needle with a curve or hook at its tip to stabilize the wire within the breast tissue (Figures 9-3 and 9-4). In most cases, the radiologist places the tip of the wire or needle near the lesion in question using the imaging modality that identified the lesion. Localization mammograms should be checked before performance of the biopsy; some radiologists will localize the lesion halfway along the wire or needle, whereas others place it near the tip. Often a dia-

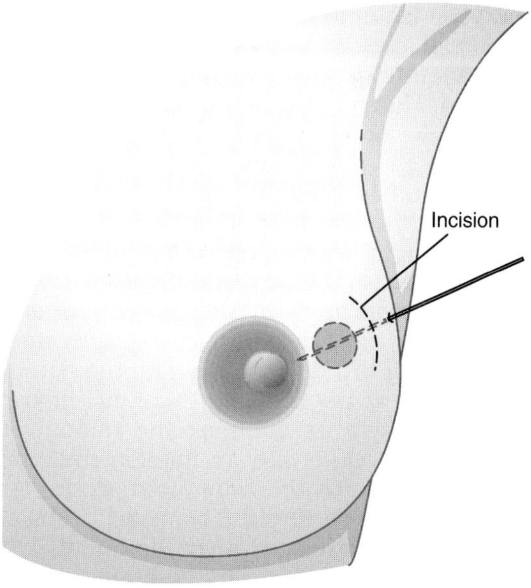

Figure 9-3. When localizing the lesion, the needle may be placed through the lesion, usually near the tip. The surgeon may plan the incision through the needle insertion site or closer to the needle tip. If the incision is made between the needle insertion site and the lesion, the distal wire is delivered into the wound. (From Kinne DW, ed. *Multidisciplinary atlas of breast surgery*. Philadelphia: Lippincott-Raven, 1998, p. 29, with permission.)

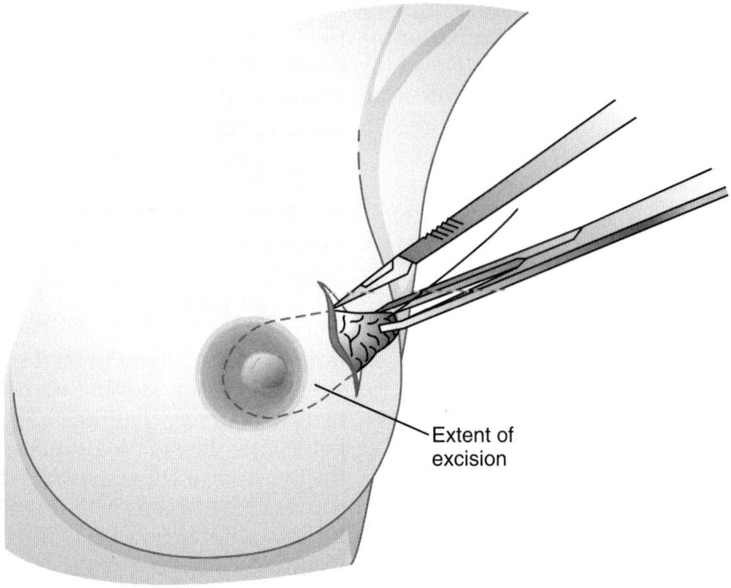

Figure 9–4. Excision is performed with stabilization of the tissue and wire with an Allis clamp. A cylinder of tissue with a radius of 1 to 2 cm is excised from the adjacent tissues until past the tip. (From Kinne DW, ed. *Multidisciplinary atlas of breast surgery*. Philadelphia: Lippincott-Raven, 1998, p. 29, with permission.)

gram depicting the relationship of the wire and the target lesion in multiple views is helpful.

Most of these biopsies are performed under local anesthesia, with or without intravenous sedation. The entry site of the wire is frequently the superior or lateral aspect of the breast. It is the site of the wire and its relation to the tip of the needle that determine the optimal surgical approach in most cases. After the patient has been brought to the operating room, her affected breast is prepared and draped with the needle and wire in place, having been prepared along with the breast. An incision is then planned near this tip and drawn on the skin in the manner as described for excisional biopsy above; this helps to minimize the amount of tissue incised. Otherwise, an incision could be made to encompass the wire insertion site. As with an excisional biopsy for a palpable mass, skin flaps are developed after the initial skin incision. Should the incision be separate from the needle insertion site, dissection is performed back to the wire insertion and the wire pulled into the biopsy site. The breast tissue is then excised at a radial distance of 1 to 2 cm from the needle and/or wire until it is past the tip or lesion, as appropriate. Before complete excision of the specimen from the breast, sutures are placed to orient the tissue by usual convention. To be assured that the abnormality has been excised, the specimen should undergo specimen radiography, if mammography was used for wire placement, to confirm the excision of the lesion in question. This has been shown to reduce the incidence of missed lesions to less than 2%, given that the needle or wire may be potentially dislodged or displaced.

Clinical Staging

After tissue confirmation has been made for breast carcinoma, clinical staging is then pursued (Table 9-1). The size of the tumor is approximated by palpation and imaging. The axillary nodes should be assessed in a similar manner, although most patients with axillary metastases will have normal exams. During the assessment for possible symptoms consistent with metastatic disease, questions pertain to the main four organ systems of involvement: bone, liver, lungs, and brain. The lungs are usually asymptomatic, unless significant amounts of lung are involved or there is lymphadenopathy at the carina. The liver, too, is rarely symptomatic. Patient complaints with liver metastases include a feeling of upper abdominal tightness and pain, sometimes accompanied by persistent nausea. Bone pain is far more predictive; symptoms correlate 95% of the time with

TABLE 9–1 • *Breast Cancer Stage Grouping*

Primary Tumor (T)			
TX	Primary tumor cannot be assessed		
T0	No evidence of primary tumor		
Tis	Carcinoma in situ		
T1	Tumor 2 cm or less in greatest dimension		
T2	Tumor more than 2 cm but less than 5 cm in greatest dimension		
T3	Tumor morc than 5 cm in greatest dimension		
T4	Tumor of any size with direct extension to chest wall or skin or inflammatory carcinoma		
Regional Lymph Nodes (N)			
pNX	Regional lymph nodes cannot be assessed		
pN0	No regional lymph node metastasis		
pN0(i–)	No regional lymph node metastasis, negative IHC		
pN0(i+)	Positive IHC, no IHC cluster greater than 0.2 mm		
pN1	Metastasis in 1 to 3 axillary lymph nodes and/or internal mammary nodes with microscopic disease detected by sentinel lymph node biopsy		
pN2	Metastasis in 4 to 9 axillary lymph nodes or in clinically apparent internal mammary lymph nodes in the absence of axillary lymph nodes		
pN3	Metastasis in 10 or more axillary lymph nodes, in infraclavicular lymph nodes, or in clinically apparent internal mammary lymph nodes in the presence of 1 or more positive axillary lymph nodes; internal mammary nodes with microscopic disease detected by sentinel lymph node biopsy in the presence of 3 or more positive axillary lymph nodes		
Distant Metastases (M)			
MX	Distant metastasis cannot be assessed		
M0	No distant metastasis		
M1	Distant metastasis		
Clinical Stage Grouping			
Stage	T	N	M
0	Tis	N0	M0
I	T1	N0	M0
IIA	T0	N1	M0
	T1	N1	M0
	T2	N0	M0
IIB	T2	N1	M0
	T3	N0	M0
IIIA	T0	N2	M0
	T1	N2	M0
	T2	N2	M0
	T3	N1	M0
	T3	N2	M0
IIIB	T4	N0	M0
	T4	N1	M0
	T4	N2	M0
IIIC	Any T	N3	M0
IV	Any T	Any N	M1

IHC, Immunohistochemistry.

skeletal involvement. Brain metastases are usually a late event, but assessment should be pursued if neurologic symptoms as reported.

For those tumors that are less than 2 cm and that do not involve palpable lymphadenopathy, there is less than a 3% chance of disease being metastatic to a distant organ. In light of this information, cost-effective practices would speak against testing the asymptomatic patient to detect metastatic spread if the patient has a T1 lesion. However, palpable lymphadenopathy or symptoms suggestive of possible bone or liver involvement should prompt further investigation. To assess the extent of disease, a bone scan is usually employed for a general survey. Because it is highly sensitive to those processes that involve bone, it will detect common diseases, such as arthritis, bursitis, and old fractures, as well as bone islands. Because is it impractical to do a total body bone radiologic survey, the bone scan provides a venue for identifying an area of abnormality that needs additional radiologic attention. Thus, further studies such as radiographs, computed tomographic (CT) scans, or MRIs may be indicated, depending on the finding and its location. When assessing the lung, chest x-ray or CT scanning of the chest can be done. In areas that are endemic for molds, small granulomatous disease may be sufficiently prevalent that the greater sensitivity of CT leads to a needless pursuit of tissue to confirm or refute the presence of metastases or repeated evaluation of lesions to check for persistence or growth of these small lesions. Alternatively, a chest CT with extension below the diaphragm may visualize the liver sufficiently such that an abdominal CT is not needed for liver assessment. In most locales, CT of the abdomen is a necessary separate component of the assessment to fully visualize the liver if there is any question of metastases. Serum tests of liver function generally lack sensitivity and are seldom elevated until significant amounts of liver have been replaced by tumor. Still, these serum tests will be need to be performed to verify function should chemotherapy or antihormonal therapy be considered.

Treatment Options

For the majority of patients diagnosed with breast cancer, the initial discussion of therapeutic options usually falls to the surgeon in the context of discussion of the biopsy results. The complexity of treatments available for patients can sometimes be overwhelming for the patients in the context of their newly diagnosed breast cancer. Consider discussion in two settings. The basic options available to an individual are provided during the first visit, keeping the issues very simple so as not to confuse the patient. Pamphlets and brochures prepared by reputable agencies are provided to the patient for further education, and a list of reputable Web sites should be provided for the patient's education. At the return visit, which is established for the purpose of decision making, it is helpful to review the past information in discussion and to go into greater detail about the fine points of both decision making and potential complications. Encourage all patients to bring a family member or friend to both visits; there is so much information provided that it is difficult to remember it all, and this other person may be able to provide a more objective opinion and perspective. The involvement of the patient in the decisions regarding her care helps to return some sense of control to her life, and it appears to lead to greater compliance with the treatment plan.

An understanding of the surgical options is expected of the surgeon in the context of treatment discussions. A basic understanding of the role for the adjuvant treatment modalities of systemic therapy and radiotherapy is also needed by the surgeon to communicate this to the newly diagnosed breast cancer patient and to provide her with some foundation of knowledge on which to base an informed decision regarding care.

Surgical Therapy

The more radical surgical options of the past were based on the Halstedian perspective in which breast cancer was felt to spread in a systematic, orderly fashion, first to the lymphatics and lymph nodes and then beyond. However, this understanding of tumor biology did not necessarily explain those patients who developed distant metastatic spread despite more radical procedures. This opened the door to multimodality therapy and studies that addressed the possibility of breast conservation. Multiple prospective randomized trials compared mastectomy with breast conservation with radiotherapy, with no survival advantage for either treatment. Consequently, either is an acceptable option for the appropriate patient.

The basic guidelines for breast conservation in a patient with breast cancer would include the patient's desire to have such a procedure. Beyond that, the patient necessarily has to be reliable and able to follow through with her therapy of radiation and long-term surveillance (Table 9-2). The inclusion of radiotherapy for local control may not be possible for the patient who is pregnant or who has had prior radiation to the field (e.g., a patient with a history of Hodgkin's disease who received mantle radiation). Patients with active collagen vascular disease, especially systemic lupus erythematosus and scleroderma, may have an extreme scarring response to the radiation as well as necrosis, yielding a cosmetic result that may not be acceptable to the patient. The trials that examined survival with breast conservation as compared with treatment with mastectomy restricted its use to a single primary tumor; multicentric disease was treated with mastectomy. Above all, the focus is to obtain negative margins, which may not be possible in some patients with lumpectomy. Those patients who present with diffuse suspicious or indeterminate microcalcifications may reflect extensive carcinoma or in situ carcinoma. These may be very difficult to deal with when following the patient postoperatively; the suspicious nature of the calcifications may prompt repeated biopsy given the patient's history of malignancy. However, this would not be the case with calcifications that are felt to be benign.

In studies that examined the use of breast conservation, surgery was restricted to those patients with a tumor size of 4 cm or less. Breast conservation may not be practical or cosmetically acceptable in a patient with a small breast, whereas a woman with a very large breast may be able to sustain an excellent cosmetic outcome from breast conservation, even if the mass was much larger. What is important is that there does not appear to be an absolute tumor size beyond which the surgery cannot be performed with an acceptable outcome; however, there does seem to be a restriction based on the relative size relationship of the tumor to the breast volume. Contraindications include extensive disease precluding acceptable cosmesis (large extent of disease relative to breast size, multicentric disease, extensive multifocal disease) or a contraindication to radiation (prior breast/chest radiation, first/second trimester of pregnancy, collagen vascular disease). Trials that examined the use of neoadjuvant (preoperative) chemotherapy have demonstrated that larger tumors may be reduced sufficiently in size as to allow breast conservation in approximately one third of patients.

For patients not deemed to be appropriate for breast conservation, mastectomy is recommended. This procedure is an option for any patient diagnosed with breast cancer. As a method of local control, it generally is not coupled with radiotherapy of the chest wall, unless the tumor is greater than 5 cm or there are four or more lymph nodes involved with metastatic breast cancer. In these latter two instances, there is an increased risk of chest-wall recurrence. For cancers that are not regarded as high risk for local recurrence (specifically stage I or II cancers), the resection can be performed using skin-sparing incisions if immediate reconstruction is performed as well (see later). This has been shown to be oncologically sound, because the local tumor recurrence is no greater in this setting than with standard mastectomy and delayed recon-

TABLE 9-2 • *Breast Conservation Guidelines*

Relative/Absolute Contraindication	No Contraindication
Prior breast radiation	Contralateral breast cancer
First or second trimester of pregnancy	Family history of breast cancer
Negative margin excision not possible	Clinically palpable lymph nodes, not fixed
Multicentric disease	Tumor histology
Collagen vascular disease	Age
Diffuse microcalcifications on mammography	Tumor location within breast

(Modified from Baker RJ, Fischer JE, eds. *Mastery of surgery,* ed 4. Philadelphia: Lippincott Williams and Wilkins, 2001, with permission.)

struction. Furthermore, the local recurrences are nearly always subcutaneous (i.e., deep to the native skin flap rather than against the chest wall).

For those persons who present with early breast cancer, the approach to a surgical discussion regarding management revolves around two concepts: the management of the breast and the management of the ipsilateral axilla. Assuming that the patient has undergone the appropriate testing and history to check for metastatic disease, if indicated, most patients with stage I or II disease proceed with surgery first. Those patients with breast cancer who are candidates for breast conservation should be made aware that they have more than one option; it is up to the surgeon to summarize these options, their advantages and disadvantages, and their benefits and risks. Optimally, this could be done within the setting of a multidisciplinary clinical setting. However, that is not always possible, thus placing the responsibility of a brief discussion of the roles of radiotherapy and systemic therapy on the shoulders of the surgeon as well.

Most would agree that assessment of the axilla is necessary for the proper staging and consequent management of the patient with breast cancer. The paradigm for management of the axilla has recently shifted. Because an axillary dissection carries with it the risks of significant morbidity (which includes nerve or vascular injury, seroma formation, and chromic ipsilateral upper extremity lymphedema), it is preferable to be more selective when performing axillary dissection in an effort to reduce these morbid outcomes. Hence, the technique of sentinel lymph node biopsy was developed for use among patients with breast cancer to help identify those persons who may be at risk for axillary metastases. Surveillance Epidemiology and End Results data indicate that 20% of those women with a T1 tumor have axillary metastases. For them, it would behoove the surgeon to identify that individual and complete the axillary node dissection.

As defined, a sentinel lymph node (or nodes) is the node that is most likely to drain the interstitial fluids from a tissue region containing the tumor. The rationale is that these nodes then would be most likely to reveal a nodal metastasis if it is present within the axilla. This technique has been validated by studies of sentinel lymph node biopsy within the context of a full axillary lymph node dissection. Sentinel lymph nodes can be identified in more than 95% of patients using a combination of both isosulfan blue and Tc99 technetium sulfur colloid injection. Furthermore, the status of the sentinel lymph node accurately reflected the status of the axilla as a whole, with a 5% to 10% false-negative rate.

The sentinel lymph node biopsy is a diagnostic test to identify patients with nodal metastasis who may benefit from selective axillary lymph node dissection. Patients with palpable enlarged lymph nodes do not require a sentinel node biopsy but rather should undergo FNA to document regional disease and then undergo a completion axillary lymph node dissection. The use of sentinel lymph node biopsy can be minimized by performing axillary ultrasound on patients with documented invasive breast cancers, with FNA of any suspicious-appearing lymph nodes.

Technical Aspects

Breast Conservation

The partial mastectomy (i.e., lumpectomy, segmentectomy) is approached in a manner similar to that of excisional biopsy (see above), using needle localization, if necessary. Preoperative evaluation of the mammographic studies, should they reflect the presence of the cancer, may help guide the surgeon in gauging the extent of disease present and the volume of breast tissue/tumor to be resected. Assuming that diagnosis made preoperatively by either a sampling method of biopsy or by excisional biopsy with positive margins, frozen section could be employed if there is concern for a positive margin intraoperatively. Breast tissue does not freeze well because it contains a significant amount of fat; thus, intraoperative identification of ductal carcinoma in situ by frozen section can seldom be performed accurately. It may be the case that an excisional biopsy, previously performed with negative margins, constitutes the lumpectomy. Care should be taken to orient the margins so that the pathologist may guide the surgeon should additional resection be necessary. Before closing, the adjacent tissues should be checked for additional residual masses and titanium clips placed at the margins of the lumpectomy site to guide the postoperative radiation therapy boost to the cancer site. Should a final pathology evaluation reveal a positive margin, reexcision is still an option, and it does not affect overall survival.

In conjunction with management of the breast, axillary management should be addressed. If using sentinel lymph node biopsy as a decision-making tool, the sentinel lymph node biopsy should be performed first. In that manner, the sentinel lymph node(s) could be analyzed by touch prep or frozen section while the breast resection is taking place. Consequently, after completing the breast resection, the surgeon could proceed with completion of the axillary lymph node dissection, if indicated, or close. See the sections about technical aspects of sentinel lymph node biopsy and axillary lymph node dissection below.

Mastectomy

When preparing for a mastectomy with immediate reconstruction, coordinated operative arrangements are, obviously, made with the plastic and reconstructive surgical teams in advance. Should sentinel lymph node biopsy be used in conjunction with mastectomy for decisions regarding whether to complete the axillary lymph node dissection, it is performed first as was described in the context of breast conservation. However, the incision for the sentinel lymph node biopsy must be considered in the context of the surgical incision. For those persons having the more classical ellipse with inclusion of the nipple-areolar complex, these incision lines should be drawn on the skin; following identification of the axillary hot spot, a portion of the incision closest to the hot spot could be used for performance of the sentinel lymph node biopsy. For a description of sentinel lymph node biopsy, see below. Many different variations of ellipses can be considered to include prior biopsy incisions, with the nipple-areolar complex within the ellipse (Figure 9-5). A skin-sparing incision can be used if the patient's cancer is not close to the skin (Figure 9-6). A small counter-incision within the axilla can also be employed for access to perform the sentinel lymph node biopsy (approximately 3 to 4 cm in length) within a preexisting skin fold just below the hair-bearing area of the axilla. This has not been shown to place the skin flap in jeopardy for the development of necrosis.

When approaching removal of the breast with a (potential) axillary lymph node dissection, the patient is placed in the supine position, with the ipsilateral upper extremity on an armboard orthogonal to the chest. The breast, ipsilateral chest, lateral thorax, and upper extremity are then prepared into the field. In all cases, the nipple-areolar complex is included in the excised specimen. Often, use of a headlamp by the surgeon can obviate difficulties with shadows created when using a skin-sparing incision. Should a skin-sparing incision be used, as with an ellipse, the skin flaps are raised circumferentially, dissecting between the investing adipose of the skin and the adipose of the breast. The superior flap is raised nearly to the clavicle, and the inferior flap is raised to the inframammary fold. The latter may lie inferior to the insertion of the pectoralis major muscle. This flap is raised medially to the edge of the sternal border and laterally to the lateral border of the latissimus dorsi muscle. The skin flaps include a layer of subcutaneous adipose that is approximately 4 to 5 mm in depth. The breast is dissected off the chest wall, and this includes the investing fascia of the pectoralis major with the specimen. Use of electrocautery in dissection reduces blood loss during the extirpation from the muscle surface. However, despite the apparent electrocautery stimulation of muscle, it can also be used to safely and easily excise the breast from the pectoralis major muscle if this dissection is performed in a superior to inferior (or inferior to superior) direction. By maintaining a continuous electric stimulus with contact of the cautery pen in parallel with the muscle fibers, the continuous stimulation produces tetany and minimal fiber contraction. Furthermore, the use of cautery in this context lends itself to less muscle damage, thereby reducing muscle loss, blood loss, and postoperative pain. Special attention must be given to dissection along the sternal border, where perforating vessels from the internal mammary artery and veins are expected. The breast tissue is slowly delivered through the skin opening as it is dissected off the chest wall, offering increasingly larger exposure. Given the size of the breast removed from this envelope, the opening can shift significantly toward or over the axilla if this is a skin-sparing incision.

In the context of the classical ellipse incision, removal of the breast is generally not performed if a full axillary lymph node dissection is to be completed as well; the resection is done en bloc. However, the limited access of a skin-sparing incision precludes adequate access to the axilla with the breast attached. Thus, with the latter incision, the breast is usually removed separately and oriented with

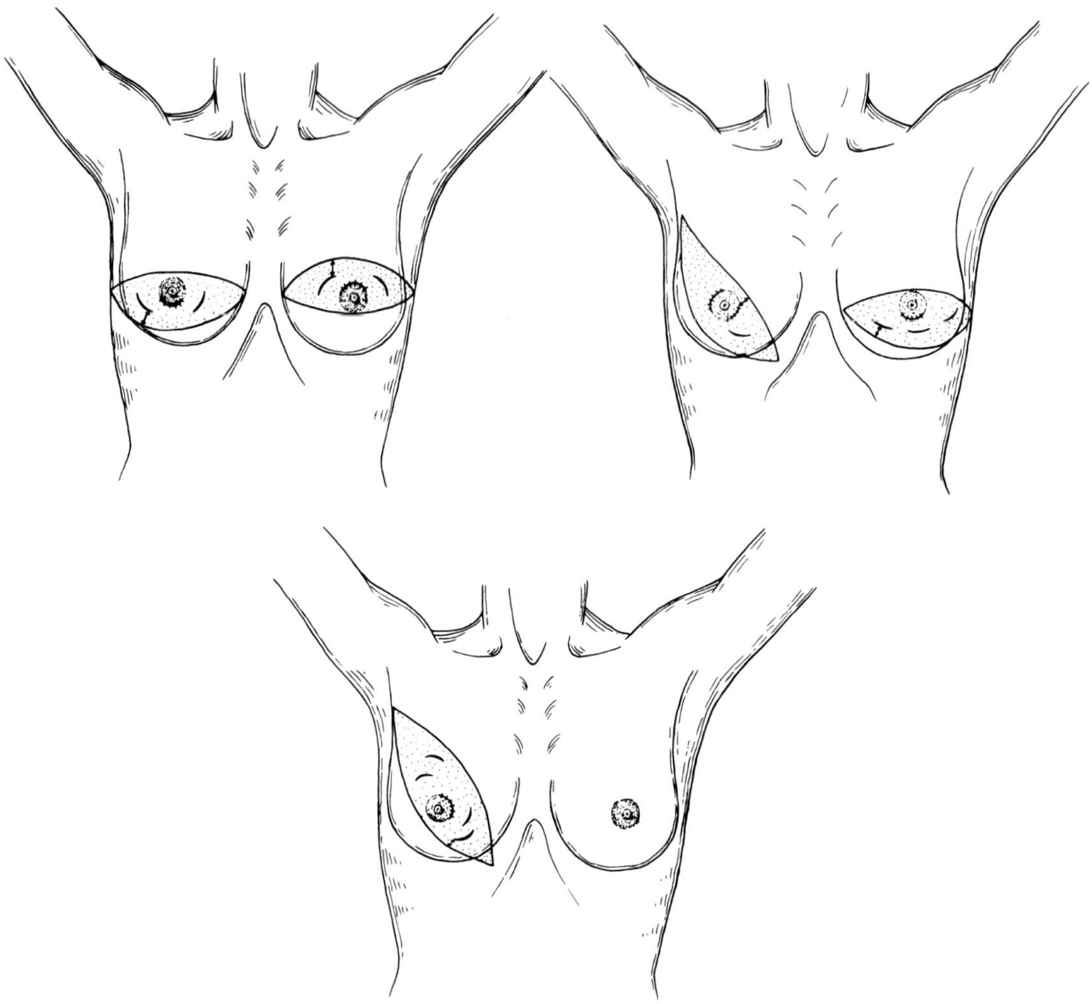

Figure 9–5. An elliptical incision for mastectomy is planned to include the nipple-areolar complex and the skin overlying the tumor. If there is an incision from the diagnostic biopsy, this is included within the ellipse as well. (From Bland KI, Copeland EM III, eds. *The breast: comprehensive management of benign and malignant diseases*. Philadelphia: WB Saunders, 1991, p. 798, with permission.)

sutures before it is passed off the field and before proceeding with axillary management. The extent of dissection laterally toward the axilla in the extirpation of the breast as the tail of Spence is not easy to discern. Pay careful attention to the contour of the breast as it extends into the axilla; a few lymph nodes may be attached, and they may be intraparenchymal. It is reasonable to include them in the resection. If only the breast is removed, full dissection and identification of the long thoracic nerve or the thoracodorsal neurovascular bundle is usually not necessary, because the dissection has not taken place as posteriorly as these structures. However, in the thin individual, there may a minimum of axillary tissue present deep to the breast. Care should be taken to avoid these structures.

Axillary Lymph Node Dissection

If an axillary lymph node dissection is to be completed—either as the procedure planned in the context of a modified radical mastectomy or as a consequence of a sentinel lymph node with evidence of metastatic breast cancer—the usual procedure includes the removal of axillary levels I and II. There is a very low rate of nodal metastases to level III lymph nodes, and these are usually not dissected unless there is palpable nodal disease at level II. In many cases, after the breast has been removed using a skin-sparing incision, the envelope is sufficiently loose and the opening sufficiently large that an axillary dissection can be performed through it when the skin is shifted laterally. This is not a concern

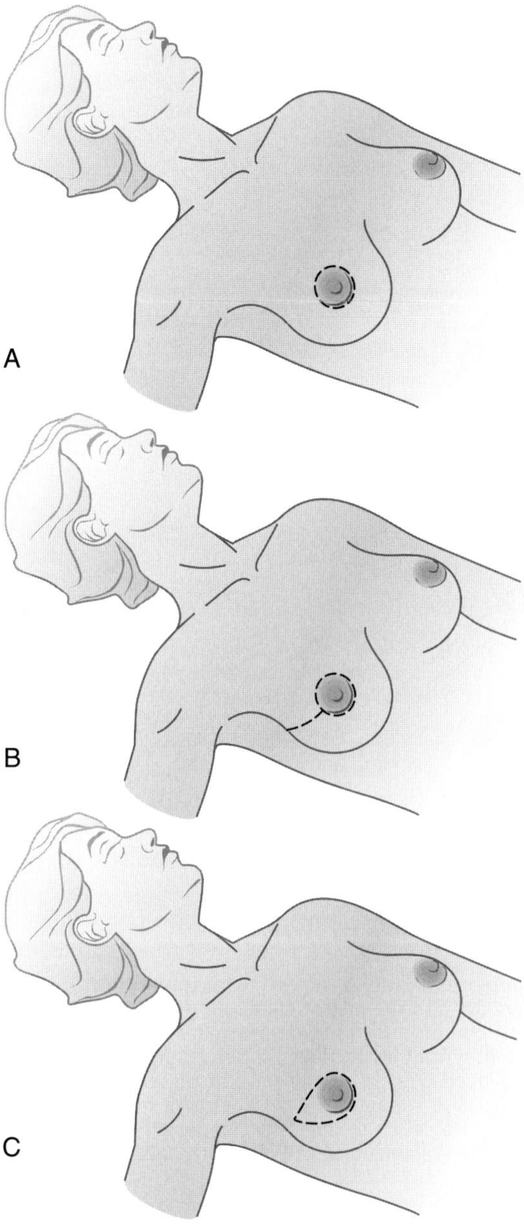

Figure 9–6. Skin-sparing incisions that are commonly used are **(A)** periareolar, **(B)** tennis racket, and **(C)** teardrop. The latter two allow for greater access to the axilla after the breast is excised if the patient has a small breast. (From Baker RJ, Fischer JE, eds. *Mastery of surgery,* ed 4. Philadelphia: Lippincott Williams and Wilkins, 2001, p. 606, with permission.)

with the breast left in situ for resection en bloc and incised with the classical ellipse. Should a skin-sparing incision limit access to the axillary contents in conjunction with a small breast envelope, a separate counter-incision made below the hair-bearing area (preferably within a skin fold or as an extension of the sentinel lymph node biopsy incision) may be used. This would be the same incision used for axillary dissection in the context of breast conservation, and it would extend at most to the anterior and posterior axillary folds (Figure 9-7). Alternatively, a lateral extension to a periareolar incision can be made to increase exposure of that area, approximating a tennis racket incision (Figure 9-6, *B*). Inclusion of the ipsilateral upper extremity in the skin preparation of the operative field permits the extremity to be maneuvered into a position at a right angle to the table, if necessary, thus opening up the space under the pectoralis muscles for a full level II access by release of their tension (Figure 9-8).

Initially, skin flaps are raised superiorly up to the axillary fold, anteriorly to the lateral edge of the pectoralis major muscle, posteriorly to the lateral border of the latissimus dorsi muscle, and inferiorly to the projection of the inferior mammary fold as it wraps laterally around the thorax (Figure 9-9). This can be done with electrocautery or with the scalpel, depending on the technique with which the surgeon is most comfortable. As with the breast, the adipose investing the skin should be left in continuity with the skin so as to not devascularize the tissue. After these flaps are raised, the fascia along the lateral border of the pectoralis major muscle is

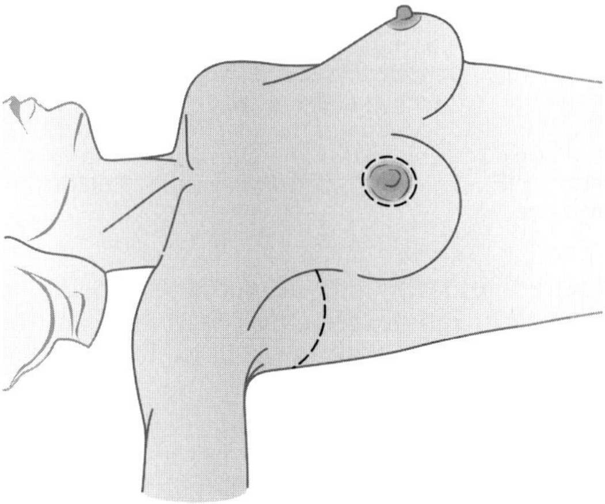

Figure 9–7. An additional incision within the axilla to complete the axillary dissection is rarely needed, except in very small–breasted individuals. A curvilinear incision *(dashed lines)* is made between the anterior and posterior axillary folds, just below the hair-bearing area, preferably within an existing skin fold. (From Baker RJ, Fischer JE, eds. *Mastery of surgery,* ed 4. Philadelphia: Lippincott Williams and Wilkins, 2001, p. 608, with permission.)

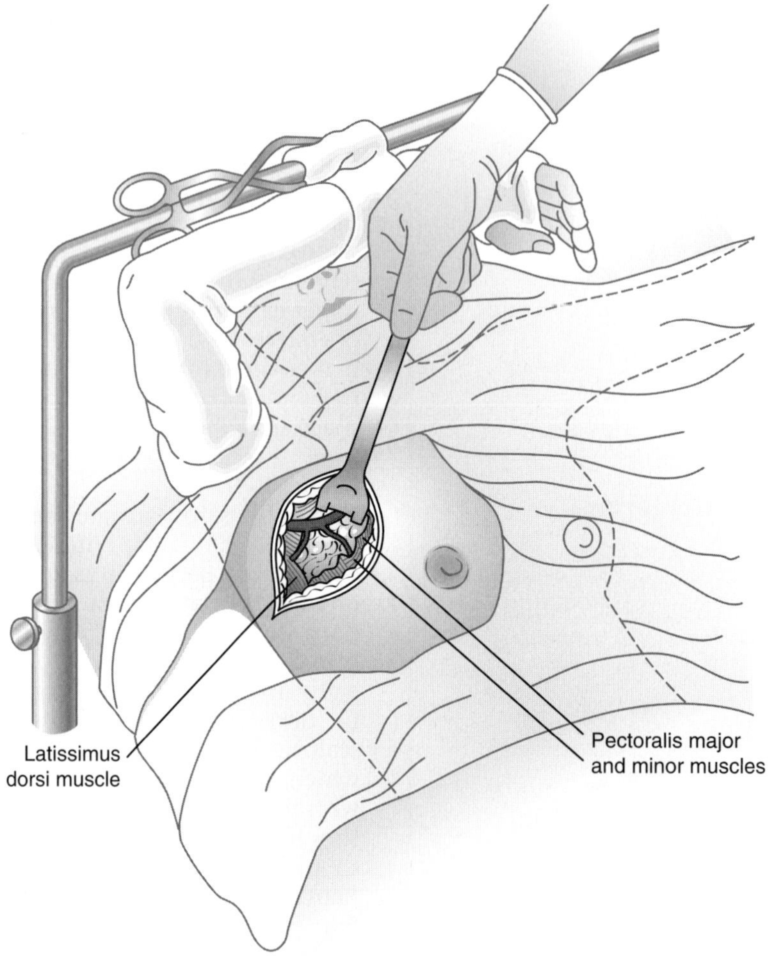

Figure 9–8. Intraoperative positioning of the ipsilateral upper extremity anteriorly with the arm orthogonal to the table can provide greater ease of access to the tissues deep to the pectoralis minor muscle. Usually the pectoralis minor muscle can be spared (no division) without compromise in the performance of a level I or II axillary lymph node dissection. To assist with this positioning, a rigid ether screen is set up at the start of the case, approximately at the level of the nose, with drapes placed over it. At the time of dissection, a sterile towel is wrapped around the wrist of the patient, which is used to suspend the patient's arm from the bar of the ether screen. A large, nonpiercing clamp is applied to the towel to secure it to the bar. (From Baker RJ, Fischer JE, eds. *Mastery of surgery*, ed 4. Philadelphia: Lippincott Williams and Wilkins, 2001, p. 609, with permission.)

incised and the muscle retracted medially, exposing the underlying pectoralis minor muscle. At this point, an interpectoral dissection could be performed by incision of the interpectoral tissue medially over the pectoralis minor muscle and by mobilizing it medially using traction and a light touch with dissection on the medial edge, keeping the tissue in continuity with the axillary contents. The fascia along the lateral border of the pectoralis minor muscle is then incised, with care taken to avoid the medial pectoral neurovascular bundle; the pectoralis minor muscle is then retracted medially with a Richardson retractor. This helps to expose the clavipectoral fascia within the axilla. This latter fascia is then carefully incised approximately at the level at which the axillary vein is expected. Tension on the axillary contents can help to reveal a small flash of "blue" vein from deep beneath the adipose.

The dissection then proceeds immediately inferior to this vein along the anterior aspect for its length within levels I and II. No major branches will be found anterior for this length. Tension is placed on the adventitial tissues below the vein in level II, and the tissue is carefully dissected and mobilized laterally, again preserving the medial pectoral neurovascular bundle and keeping the level II

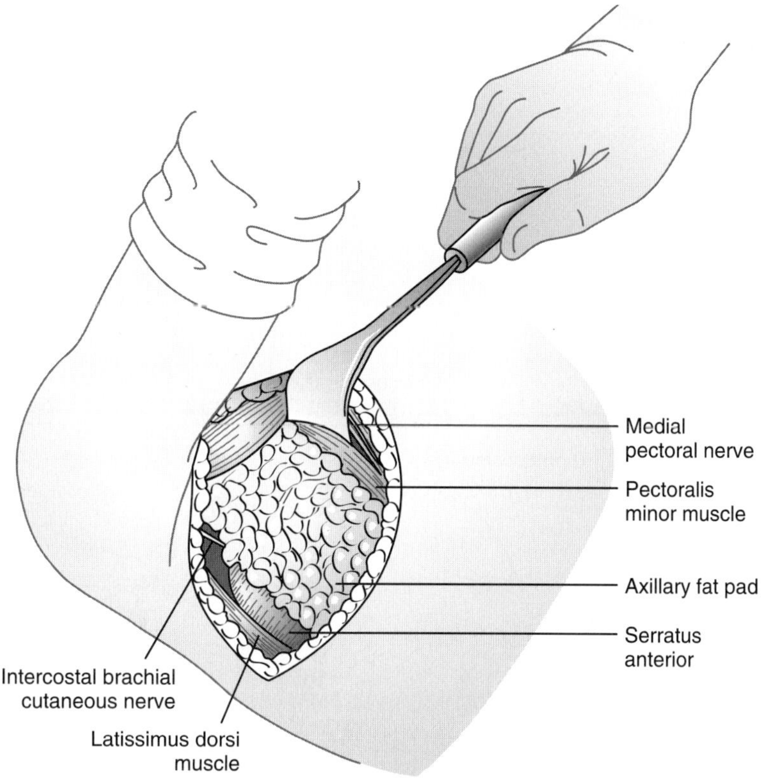

Figure 9-9. After identification and dissection along the lateral borders of the pectoralis major and latissimus dorsi muscles, the pectoralis major muscle is retracted medially to assist with the identification of the axillary vein and in the level II dissection. (From Kinne DW, ed. *Multidisciplinary atlas of breast surgery*. Philadelphia: Lippincott-Raven, 1998, p. 101, with permission.)

contents in continuity with the axilla. With tension on the more inferior axillary contents, the parallel intercostobrachial nerve can then usually be identified interiorly and thus preserved. On occasion, this nerve may have branched into multiple small branches upon reaching the axilla. In this context, it is quite difficult to identify and preserve these. The patient should be made aware that this may be the case during the preoperative risk discussion. When identifying the venous tributaries to the axillary vein, the thoracodorsal vein will be found coursing posteriorly, often deep to a more anterior venous branch to the axilla (Figure 9-10). Anatomic variants include the thoracodorsal vein branching closer to the chest wall than the lateral border of the latissimus dorsi muscle, the thoracodorsal vein branching from that more anterior branch and not from the axillary vein directly, a bifid axillary vein, and, rarely, a trifid vein. On occasion, a small strip of pectoralis muscle will reach across the axilla anteriorly and insert into the superior humerus. This strip of muscle can be divided for adequate access. After the thoracodorsal vein is identified, the vascular bundle is carefully dissected inferiorly, with care taken to dissect only anteriorly and to not touch the bundle. The nerve will join the bundle medially; it may join superiorly at the level of the vein, or it may gradually angle in from the chest wall. After this is definitively identified and the bundle freed laterally from the axilla and the lateral border of the latissimus dorsi, the larger and more anterior venous branch to the axillary contents is ligated and divided. Attention can then turn to identification of the long thoracic nerve.

At a distance of about 1 to 1.5 cm from the thoracic cage, near the beginning of the superior curvature of the thorax below the axillary vein, a plane of blunt dissection is developed using two fingers. After this is deepened to approximately the midaxillary line, a finger is inserted and stroked against the thoracic cage to identify the long thoracic nerve. If not felt, extend the dissection slightly more posteriorly. If there is still no success, it is likely that the nerve is just outside of the blunt dissection, away from the wall. The tissue that is then lateral to that plane should be developed to identify the nerve. After the nerve is identified, that plane is extended inferiorly for the

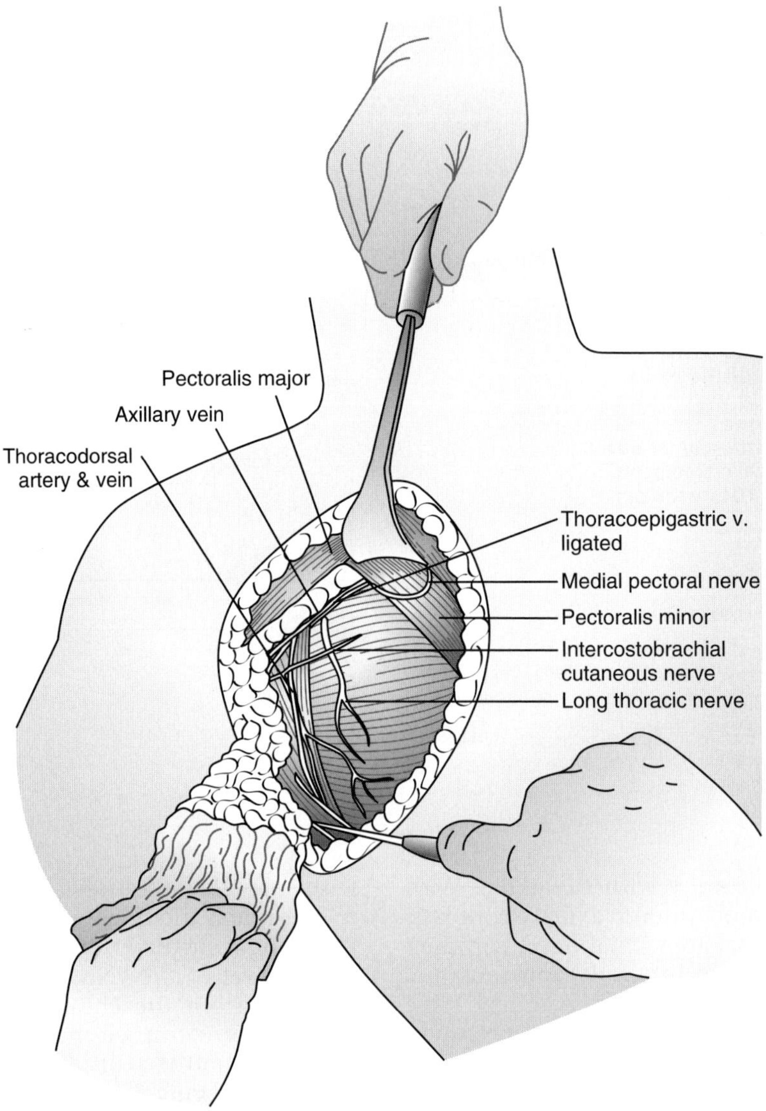

Figure 9–10. Axillary dissection proceeds with preservation of the long thoracic nerve and the thoracodorsal neurovascular bundle, the medial pectoral nerve, and, preferably, the intercostobrachial nerve. (From Kinne DW, ed. *Multidisciplinary atlas of breast surgery*. Philadelphia: Lippincott-Raven, 1998, p. 104, with permission.)

length of the operative field. Dissection between the long thoracic nerve and the chest wall should be avoided, because the vascular supply to the nerve can sometimes be tenuous.

The axillary contents between the thoracodorsal neurovascular bundle and the long thoracic nerve can then be divided sharply. The former nerve can be protected by the side of the hand while visualizing the long thoracic nerve and wielding the cautery over the finger away from the bundle. Alternatively, a clamp could be placed on this tissue, free of both nerves, divided, and then tied.

After irrigating the operative field and ensuring hemostasis, the patient can then be turned over to the reconstructive surgical team if immediate reconstruction is to be performed. Otherwise, a drain such as a flat Jackson-Pratt is placed dependently under the inferior chest wall flap, with a second drain in the axilla. Both are brought out through the low lateral axilla through separate stab wounds and secured externally with suture. The chest incision is then closed in two layers: a deep dermal layer of 3-0 dissolvable suture and a running subcuticular layer of a 4-0 dissolvable suture.

Sentinel Lymph Node Biopsy

The incidence of women presenting at stages 0 or I has shifted from 15% in the 1960s to more than 50% today. Because this defines a subset of patients in whom lymph node involvement should theoretically be absent, the question arose as to whether more harm than good was being caused by performing a full axillary lymph node dissection. The modern technique of sentinel lymph node biopsy was recently repopularized for melanoma, and it has now been applied successfully to breast cancer. The intent was to identify those persons in whom a complete lymph node dissection could possibly be avoided.

One specific prospective, randomized study set up by the NSABP, the B-32 trial, was designed as an equivalency trial to determine whether decisions regarding axillary management based on sentinel lymph node results are equivalent to those of full axillary lymph node dissection in terms of survival. Secondary endpoints will look at the incidence of surgical complications, such as neurologic deficit, lymphedema of the ipsilateral upper extremity, and ipsilateral shoulder range of motion. However, because survival is an endpoint, data will necessarily have to mature 10 years before a definitive answer will be obtained. In the meantime, a recent trial from Italy looking at the predictive power of the sentinel lymph node noted that, among 516 women randomized to axillary lymph node dissection based on sentinel lymph node results as compared with full axillary lymph node dissection, the number of recurrences between the two groups over a median 42-month follow-up was not statistically different. The women had no evidence of axillary recurrences, and the incidence of paresthesias, decreased arm mobility, or arm swelling was less among those who received the sentinel lymph node biopsy. It should be noted, however, that this study only evaluated tumors that were less than 2 cm in size. Until the definitive randomized trial results mature, retrospective evidence of the accuracy of sentinel node biopsy has led to its general acceptance as a reasonable alternative to formal axillary dissection for regional staging.

The technique itself can use either a radiocolloid for a tracer, which is commonly Tc99 technetium sulfur colloid in the United States, with or without blue dye, which is usually in the form of isosulfan blue. Recently, some have turned to use of methylene blue dye; however, it is a vital dye (it stains living cells), and it may remain in the patient longer than isosulfan blue. Furthermore, should one have a mishap when handling the methylene blue, the blue will remain in the affected skin until it is sloughed. The injection of radiocolloid can be performed 1 to 4 hours before surgery, with 1 mCi of unfiltered radiopharmaceutical Tc99 technetium sulfur colloid, although others have studied injection the night before surgery. For a small, 2-cm tumor, a volume of 8 mL is used, and it is delivered in equal volumes around the existing tumor or tissue surrounding the biopsy cavity; neither the tumor itself nor the seroma cavity created by biopsy is injected. Larger volumes (same radioactivity) would be used with larger tumors or cavities to generate sufficient tissue turgor leading to lymphatic filling. Injection into the residual seroma after biopsy will likely fail to lead to the identification of a sentinel node, because the cavity can seal with time. Alternate sites that have proved to be as effective include injection of the dermis overlying the mass, because the skin lymphatics parallel those of the breast, or the periareolar location within the dermis, taking the shortest radial distance to the areolar border for injection. The latter rationale is based on the communication of breast and skin lymphatics via Sappey's plexus. It should be noted that skin lymphatics do not drain to the internal mammary chain. Thus, if the plan is to pursue these as well, an intraparenchymal injection should be used. The advantage of a periareolar injection is that it separates the high-intensity primary site signal away from the axilla, thereby allowing for the better detection of sentinel node hot spots.

To enhance lymphatic uptake and propagation, the patient massages her breast after injection. Lymphoscintigraphy could be performed in the interim, before the sentinel lymph node biopsy; it can provide the surgeon with a visual indication of where to expect the location of the sentinel lymph node hot spot(s). However, this is not absolutely necessary, given the use of the gamma probe intraoperatively (Figure 9-11).

The combined techniques are often used, because they maximize the ability to identify a sentinel lymph node. The use of either technique alone seems to hold a sensitivity of approximately 90% to 95%, whereas the combined use is at least 95% sensitive. This may not identify a node in a patient with prior breast surgery, where lymphatics may have

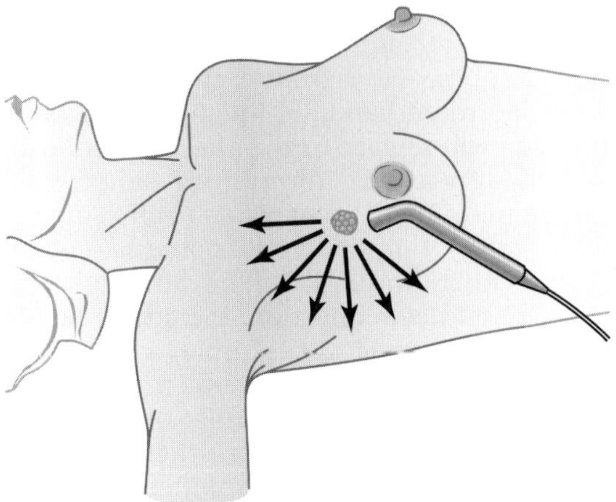

Figure 9–11. A gamma probe assists in the localization of radioisotope uptake in sentinel lymph nodes. When using the probe to trace radially from the tumor or biopsy cavity *(arrows)*, one can detect increased uptake at hot spots, which signifies the location of a sentinel node or nodes. (From Baker RJ, Fischer JE, eds. *Mastery of surgery*, ed 4. Philadelphia: Lippincott Williams and Wilkins, 2001, p. 599, with permission.)

been interrupted. Sentinel lymph nodes are most commonly identified in the ipsilateral axilla. However, occasionally, they have been identified in the supraclavicular fossa, the neck, the internal mammary chain, or the epigastrium. These areas should be surveyed by the gamma probe to be certain that the sentinel lymph node(s) are addressed. Should no hot spot be identifiable at the time of anesthesia, one problem with the patient who has been without eating or drinking since midnight the night before is that she is dehydrated. Uptake of the compound by the lymphatics is dependent on tissue turgor. After injection of the blue dye (see later), an additional 20 mL of injectable sterile saline can be administered similarly to increase tissue turgor and to enhance the flow through the lymphatics. In all cases, the area should be vigorously massaged to assist with this propagation.

The isosulfan blue dye is injected at the time of the surgery. After the patient has been administered general anesthesia and is positioned appropriately, 5 mL of sterile isosulfan blue dye is injected into the parenchyma in a similar manner to minimize skin "tattooing." Again, this is followed by breast massage, usually for at least 5 minutes, for the dye to propagate passively through the lymphatics.

Placement of the skin incision for the sentinel lymph node biopsy has been covered in the sections above, and it is pertinent with regard to whether breast conservation or mastectomy is planned. The gamma probe helps to guide incision placement. A survey of the lymphatic chains is performed before making any incision, and all hot spots are identified and marked on the skin for guidance. The probe is passed radially away from the tumor toward the axilla or toward the sternum if one plans to excise internal mammary nodes should they prove hot. Sometimes retraction of the breast medially can help to reduce the radioactive intensity of the signal from the injections around the tumor itself. Again, by marking the patient's skin with the location of the hot spot(s), the incisions can then be better planned, with the potential of extension should a full axillary lymph node dissection be warranted.

The sentinel lymph node biopsy should be performed promptly at the start of a case, because the dye and the radiocolloid will pass with time to secondary-echelon lymph nodes or beyond. This could lead to an excessive number of sentinel lymph nodes being identified, thus negating the intent of restricting the extent of operation, if possible. In the axilla, the dissection should begin along the edge of the lymphatic basin if relying on blue dye only, along the lateral edge of the pectoralis major muscle. This helps to avoid the misidentification of a secondary lymph node by direct approach. This also allows the surgeon to find and follow the blue dye contained within the lymphatic vessels and, with the use of careful sharp and blunt dissection, to follow the blue dye to the sentinel lymph node(s). If the blue dye did not reach the axilla or if radiocolloid is used, the gamma probe can be used to focus directly on the dissection toward the lymph node(s). The lymph node is dissected free from the adjacent tissues, and usually an ex vivo count is taken to quantify the amount of radioactivity. Intraoperative touch preparation of the resected nodes may positively identify the presence of carcinoma metastatic to the node. If consent has been obtained to do so, the axillary lymph node dissection could then be completed. However, permanent sectioning can possibly lead to the identification of such metastatic carcinoma postoperatively where none was seen previously. This then may precipitate a return to the operating theater at a future date for the completion of the dissection.

The technique of sentinel lymph node biopsy appears to lead to a lesser incidence of the same risks inherent to the full axillary lymph node dissection, specifically nerve or vascular injury, paresthesias, ipsilateral upper extremity lymphedema, and restricted shoulder range of motion. It also carries with it the potential for an allergic reaction to the blue dye or the sulfur colloid. The sulfur colloid appears to have less than a 0.5% chance of allergic reaction, whereas the incidence of isosulfan blue dye may have a 1.5% incidence of reaction, including anaphylaxis. The rashes associated with the blue dye include not only one which is red but also one which is blue. Because allergic reactions require previous exposure for sensitization, only recently has data suggested that a preexisting allergy to cosmetics may play a role. Certainly the incidence of these allergic reactions appear to be higher in allergy-prone individuals. In these cases, the allergies have been managed medically, with no ill effect sustained by the patient.

Operating room personnel, on the other hand, have been concerned about the potential harm that exposure to the radioisotope may carry. As studied in the worst-case analysis, the exposure to personnel within a case does not exceed natural background radiation, and, therefore, no additional precautions are necessary. As for pathology personnel, the tissue can be processed immediately and not first set aside to decay.

Pathology Report

The pathology report has become increasingly complex, in part in response to what is needed to stage the individual diagnosed with breast cancer and in part in response to the American College of Surgeons' guidelines with regard to content reporting. The pathology report should include the tumor size and its histology, but it should also include grade, histologic variants, presence and extent of ductal carcinoma in situ or other abnormal histology, and presence or absence of lymphatic or vascular invasion. Margin status should be addressed, specifically whether the margins are clear of cancer and also what the closest distance is to the margin.

The pathologist needs to address receptor status, specifically the presence of estrogen and progesterone steroid receptors as detected within the cancer and HER-2/neu receptor overexpression on the cell surface. These are included for two main reasons: (1) all have an impact on prognosis; and (2) there are therapeutic modalities that exploit the presence of these receptors on the tumor. The presence of estrogen or progesterone receptors is associated with a 15% overall survival advantage to the patient whose tumor expresses as compared with the patient whose tumor does not express. Those who have this expression have also been shown to respond to those therapies that target and block the estrogen receptor signal pathway. For example, tamoxifen is a compound that binds to the estrogen receptor; it competes with estradiol for the receptor binding site, consequently blocking the action of estrogen-mediated receptor-directed transcription. Similar-acting drugs include toremifene. Other sites of targeted interruption of the estradiol-receptor signal transduction pathway include drugs that target estradiol synthesis in the postmenopausal woman. The enzyme aromatase catalyzes the reaction to form estradiol in adrenal and adipose tissues. Aromatase inhibitors have been developed, such as anastrozole, letrozole, and exemestane, which lower circulating estradiol and improve survival for those taking the drug. Furthermore, the drug fulvestrant binds irreversibly to the estrogen receptor, thereby leading to its degradation.

The HER-2/neu receptor is an "orphan" receptor in that it does not have a specific known ligand that it binds on the cell surface. HER-2 can combine with the receptor for epidermal growth factor, HER-3, to form a functional dimer. Consequently, overexpression of HER-2 in the presence of epidermal growth factor can lead to mitotic stimulation of the cell, which is a bad prognostic factor for a patient with breast cancer. The synthetic monoclonal antibody trastuzumab, or Herceptin, can bind the HER-2 molecular on the cell surface. Use of trastuzumab in the context of metastatic breast cancer and as adjuvant therapy for node-positive breast cancer improves both disease-free and overall survival.

Systemic Therapy

Systemic therapy refers to agents with varying mechanisms of action targeted to kill actively dividing cells. The administration of these are sometimes a delicate balance between sufficient toxicity to the malignancy without substantial toxicity to the body's own actively dividing cells of the bone marrow or gut lumen. Today, systemic therapy for breast cancer typically involves hormonal therapy and chemotherapy. However, new systemic therapies, such as immunotherapies and targeted therapies, are on the horizon.

Hormonal Therapy

For many years, the selective estrogen receptor modulator tamoxifen has been the primary hormonal therapy used in the adjuvant setting. Today, tamoxifen still remains a highly effective agent in the therapy of all patients with breast cancers that express the estrogen receptor (ER). Tamoxifen acts at the level of the receptor, blocking the estrogen-signal pathway. However, tamoxifen can act as a weak estrogen in some tissues, depending on the distribution of alpha and beta subunits and transcription cofactors. Consequently, it is known to increase the risk of thromboembolic events and the risk of uterine cancer. It is prescribed for 5 years, because, after that point, there does not seem to be any further benefit to be gained in terms of local-regional tumor recurrence or in distant recurrence; however, the incidence of uterine cancer rises after that point.

Newer drugs, such as the aromatase inhibitors, may provide an equally potent effect in the treatment of these ER-positive cancers, without the threat of these serious events. Aromatase is the enzyme that controls the final step in estrogen steroidogenesis in the postmenopausal woman, unlike that seen in women who still have ovulatory cycles. In blocking this enzyme, circulating estrogen levels drop, thereby leading to a lack of estrogen to interact with cells that may possess the estrogen receptor. In the ATAC trial, which compared recurrence among patients taking anastrozole, an aromatase inhibitor, with tamoxifen use, the use of anastrozole was associated with fewer recurrences over a 5-year period. However, analysis of long-term survival benefit is still pending. Exemestane, which another aromatase inhibitor, and letrozole have been studied in the context of following tamoxifen therapy among women with previous ER-positive breast cancer. In both instances, the addition of the aromatase inhibitor after tamoxifen therapy appears to reduce the incidence of local recurrence by 50%. However, considering that chance is only 4% to 6% to begin with, the absolute value of that medication is on the order of a 2% to 3% reduction in cancer recurrence.

BOX 9-3 HORMONALLY TARGETED THERAPIES

• Selective estrogen receptor modulator	Tamoxifen Toremifene
• Aromatase inhibitor	Anastrozole Letrozole Exemestane
• Downregulator of estrogen receptor	Fulvestrant

Chemotherapy

Chemotherapy has been shown to provide significant survival benefit among women with node-negative cancers of 1 cm in size and larger, in addition to those with node-positive cancer. The more common chemotherapeutic regimens include cyclophosphamide (Cytoxan), methotrexate, and 5-fluorouracil, as well as cyclophosphamide with doxorubicin (Adriamycin). The former regimen is usually delivered at 3-week intervals (cycles) over 6 months, whereas the latter is delivered at 3-week intervals over 2 to 3 months. Both have equal efficacy in terms of survival benefit. Doxorubicin possesses potential cardiotoxicity at total doses of more than 400 mg/m^2; thus, its use is generally restricted to those women who have good cardiac function as evidenced by multiple gated acquisition scan and/or echocardiogram. Epirubicin, which is a drug that is related to doxorubicin but with less associated cardiotoxicity, is beginning to appear in experimental protocols in the United States; it is currently used in Europe. Hair loss is also most frequently associated with the use of doxorubicin, although cyclophosphamide can thin the hair significantly (Table 9-3).

The taxanes—paclitaxel (Taxol) and docetaxel (Taxotere)—also have activity when used to treat breast cancer. Docetaxel appears to have greater efficacy in the context of breast cancer. These drugs are seldom used as a single agent; rather, they have been used in combination with other regimens, usually cyclophosphamide with doxorubicin. However, the combined therapy shows no greater benefit than that with serial therapy, with the taxanes administered after one of the standard regimens.

Doxorubicin, cyclophosphamide, and tamoxifen can affect a woman's future ability to conceive. Premenopausal women receiving doxorubicin or cyclophosphamide usually stop menstruating, at least for the duration of their chemotherapy, and possibly beyond. If the menstrual cycle has not returned within 2 years after the completion of chemotherapy, it is unlikely to return. Tamoxifen is given to

TABLE 9-3 • *Chemotherapeutic Agents for Breast Cancer*

Agent	Side Effect/Toxicity
Cyclophosphamide	Alopecia, immunosuppression, hemorrhagic cystitis
Methotrexate	Immunosuppression, bone marrow suppression, intestinal tract epithelial sloughing, teratogen
5-Fluorouracil	Bone marrow suppression, intestinal tract epithelial sloughing
Doxorubicin	Alopecia, cardiomyopathy, myelosuppression, stomatitis, gastrointestinal disturbance
Paclitaxel/ Docetaxel	Numbness, hand-foot syndrome, nail discoloration, pericardial effusion

premenopausal women, and it variably affects the menstrual cycle. Women are cautioned to use barrier methods of birth control to reduce their chance of pregnancy while taking tamoxifen, because the drug may be teratogenic. However, after the completion of the recommended 5 years of therapy, a woman's fertility is reported to be reduced by approximately 50%.

Chemotherapy is generally administered postoperatively in the adjuvant setting, beginning 4 to 6 weeks after the definitive procedure. Neoadjuvant (preoperative) chemotherapy is the standard of care for patients who have locally advanced or inflammatory breast cancer. However, it is now being applied to those patients with large cancers who are not felt to be candidates for breast conservation upon initial presentation because of the large size of the cancer. Chemotherapy preoperatively allows for potential concentric shrinkage of the tumor, thus enabling approximately one third of patients to undergo breast conservation when mastectomy had previously been the only rational choice. Therapy delivered in this setting also allows the medical oncologist to observe which agents are truly effective against the malignancy; a response should be evident after two cycles if a response is to be seen at all. Should the cancer prove to be resistant to the agents, protocols that include other agents should be tried. In the NSABP B-27 trial of neoadjuvant therapy, one third of the patients experienced sufficient tumor shrinkage as to allow for breast conservation; however, there was no difference in overall survival benefit as compared with those who underwent postoperative therapy.

Trastuzumab (Herceptin) is a monoclonal antibody directed against the HER-2/neu receptor, which has shown a benefit in overall and disease-free survival among patients with metastatic disease and overexpression of HER-2. Early results from clinical trials also suggest a benefit to its use in the adjuvant setting in cancers that overexpress HER-2.

Radiation Therapy

Radiotherapy plays a role with lumpectomy (partial mastectomy, segmentectomy, tylectomy) in that the breast is radiated to consolidate local therapy. Radiation of the axilla is not typically included. The combination of radiation of the axilla with axillary lymph node dissection, in past studies, led to lymphedema in 30% of the patients treated in that manner when studied in the context of mastectomy as well.

Radiation of the chest wall with mastectomy is uncommon. Local chest wall recurrence is increased when the tumor is greater than 5 cm in its greatest diameter or when there are four or more lymph nodes harboring metastatic breast cancer. For circumstances of high risk for local/regional recurrence, such as muscle or skin invasion, gross extracapsular nodal tumor extension, positive margins, and, more controversially, those with lymph nodes greater than 2 cm in diameter or matted lymph nodes, radiation is often administered. Radiation works best after tumor debulking, which can include surgical and systemic treatments. Because radiation is generally delivered in doses based on normal tissue tolerance and volume of disease, those patients who undergo radiation are generally not felt to be candidates for repeat radiation to the same field in the context of recurrent disease in the future.

Radiation is delivered in divided doses for better tolerance by normal tissues. For the chest or the whole breast, the total dose is usually 50 Gy over 5 weeks following lumpectomy, and most centers deliver an additional 5 Gy as a "boost" to the operative site. More recently, attention has been given to partial breast radiation, with trials developing or ongoing to examine the feasibility of partial breast radiation, using CT guidance to design fields, brachytherapy using continuous temporary radioactive seeds in removable catheters, or MammoSite® balloon with interchangeable seed insertion for an outpatient. Furthermore, attention to the possibility of radiation after a 10-year interim is undergoing scrutiny in the context of a Radiation Therapy Oncology Group protocol examining the feasibility of brachytherapy seeds for radiotherapy in the ipsilateral breasts of patients with a second primary breast cancer.

Surgical and Other Complications

Complications can arise with any surgical procedure. Fat necrosis can occur with a loss of blood supply after surgery. This can form a hard, firm nodule, or it develop into an oil cyst. In the patient with a history of breast cancer, these hard nodules tend to be biopsied frequently out of concern for possible local recurrence. Obviously, bleeding and infection can be found in any surgical venue. The positioning of the patient is important to avoid neurapraxias. Usually the ipsilateral upper extremity is placed on an arm board perpendicular to the body and table at the same level as the table. A roll under the lateral thorax should be avoided. When raising skin flaps, the flap can be too thin to support skin viability; this can happen if the dissection of the flap is only as deep as the dermis. In the appropriate plane of dissection for the skin flaps, there will be a minimum of blood loss, because the vasculature between the breast and skin is not extensively shared.

During the performance of the axillary dissection, a loss of sensation will result, with the division of the intercostobrachial nerve or its branches affecting the medial arm, the axilla, or regions of the proximal back. Approximately 80% of women in whom this is divided regain some degree of sensation in the affected areas after 1 to 2 years. Injury could occur to one of the two main motor nerves. If transected, the loss of the long thoracic nerve can result in a wing scapula deformity. Division of the thoracodorsal nerve to the latissimus dorsi muscle will result in difficulties with climbing, swimming, and other activities that require movement of the shoulder girdle downward, such as tennis. Maintenance of this nerve is essential to its use in the latissimus dorsi rotational flap for reconstruction.

The medial and lateral pectoral neurovascular bundles can and should be preserved. The medial bundle is found along the lateral aspect of the pectoralis minor and major muscles. The lateral pectoral neurovascular bundle is found near the insertion of the pectoralis minor muscle on the coracoid process. If the pectoralis minor muscle is divided in an effort to perform a level III dissection, this may be sacrificed. However, there are few indications for this maneuver, and raised placement of the ipsilateral arm at a right angle to the table helps to open this space, thereby allowing sufficient access so that the muscle need not be divided. Injury to the axillary vein can occur, especially if care is not taken when exposing the lateral border of the latissimus dorsi muscle and it is extended too superiorly before exposure of the axillary vein.

Shoulder and arm motion can be limited if the patient is allowed to restrict the use of that arm during the immediate postoperative period. Active range-of-motion exercises are encouraged to begin within the first week to help maintain function. These exercises should be maintained intermittently for the first year, during the healing and remodeling of the area.

Lymphedema is the most feared chronic complication of the surgery, and it is found more frequently with the full axillary lymph node dissection. There are a select few who develop a very transitory slight edema, perhaps as a result of blockage of the lymphatics secondary to postoperative swelling at the axilla, which resolves with restoration of arm movement within the first few weeks. However, about 10% will develop a more chronic lymphedema over time, which can be greatly exacerbated with radiation therapy.

Excessive ipsilateral arm use can overload the draining lymphatics as a consequence of increased lymph flow and lead to temporary lymphedema in the occasional patient. The lymphedema can occur much later, after the patient has enjoyed no evidence of swelling, should she get lymphangitis with subsequent scarring of the lymphatics as a consequence of increased risk for the development of infection. Thus, all patients who have undergone a full axillary lymph node dissection are encouraged to avoid needle punctures for phlebotomy and blood-pressure cuff placement, and they are also cautioned to wear protective clothing, such as long sleeves and gloves for gardening, to reduce the incidence of skin injury and infection.

Lymphangiosarcoma of the arm from chronic lymphedema classically occurs 10 to 20 years after the development of the lymphedema. This goes by the eponym *Stewart-Treves syndrome* when applied to the lymphedema that results from axillary lymph node dissection; this sarcoma is rare (about 1 in 20,000 cases of lymphedema), but it is particularly aggressive. Nearly all of these patients have had radiation at the time of initial treatment, which raises the question of radiation as an additional causative agent. Patients who undergo radiation of the breast after breast conservation are also at risk of sarcoma development within the breast, again within a timeframe of 10 to 20 years after treatment.

Ionizing radiation can lead to vascular changes that are easily seen in the skin, such as telangiectasias. Vessels thicken as a consequence of subintimal hyaline sclerosis and endothelial proliferation, thus narrowing their lumen and potentially decreasing the perfusion to the tissue that has been irradiated. This leads to diminished capillary proliferation and eventual ectasia of the vessels that remain. Scarring occurs in the local tissues, contracting the radiated breast and leading to various degrees of increased density, fibrosis, and edema of the breast. Rarely is there osteonecrosis of the ribs with pain. As mentioned above, there is the rare incidence of malignancy (usually sarcoma) 10 to 20 years after therapy.

The complications of chemotherapy are usually a direct effect of their delivery as a controlled toxin, and they are acute (see adjuvant therapies above). However, numbness of the hands and feet experienced as a side effect of the taxanes can persist after treatment, and they seem to be found with a greater incidence among black women. For most patients who suffer hair loss, this is temporary. For some, cyclophosphamide can be associated with the rare development of leukemia or, for others, myelodysplastic syndrome, in which the bone marrow ceases to form sufficient blood elements. Both of these latter complications are life-threatening and difficult to manage. Doxorubicin (Adriamycin) can be associated with cardiotoxicity; the combination with trastuzumab (Herceptin) appears to heighten the cardiotoxicity and should be avoided in concomitant dosing.

Special Considerations

Breast Cancer and Pregnancy

The diagnosis of breast cancer during pregnancy presents challenges with regard to the concurrent treatment of the cancer while optimizing fetal outcome. The overall incidence of this phenomenon is low, but it may be possibly increasing because of the number of women who have delayed childbearing. Previously, 2.2 pregnancies out of 10,000 were complicated by breast cancer; that estimate is now 1 in 1,000. Fortunately, given the many options for women, therapy can usually be accomplished with minimal fetal risk.

Therapeutic abortion does not appear to improve survival for the mother, but it may be an option if maternal health is jeopardized or if fetal anomalies are suspected or confirmed. Stage per stage, survival is the same as it is for nonpregnant women with breast cancer. It may be the case that women are not diagnosed as promptly during pregnancy and thus present with more advanced stages. Therefore, they may do more poorly overall, but the prognosis for advanced-stage breast cancer is worse by virtue of its staging. Most patients with breast cancer present with a palpable mass during pregnancy. However, with the increasing size and density of the breast, these are more difficult to discern. A study from Memorial Sloan-Kettering would support this; 31% of pregnant women with breast cancer presented with smaller T1 tumors as compared with 50% of nonpregnant women.

With regard to available treatment options, chemotherapy is generally avoided during the first trimester. Chemotherapy during the first trimester is associated with an increased risk of spontaneous abortion, organ malformation, and fetal death, especially with methotrexate and 5-fluorouracil. Cyclophosphamide has also been associated with malformations. Chemotherapy can cross the placenta; thus, there is the potential for bone marrow toxicity as well as other organ damage. Fetal myocardial necrosis has been associated with the third-trimester administration of an anthracyclines. It does appear that the delivery of chemotherapy during the second or third trimester can generally be done safely with the combination of cyclophosphamide, doxorubicin, and 5-fluorouracil. Adjuvant tamoxifen therapy is not used in women during pregnancy; safety has not been demonstrated. However, the rare patient with metastatic disease will be faced with difficult decisions.

Usually, women undergo surgery first, delaying the use of chemotherapy for 4 to 6 weeks. Because radiation therapy during pregnancy is contraindicated, women who choose breast conservation or who need adjuvant radiation will need to wait until after parturition to receive this component of their therapy. This is of some concern for local recurrence if this delay is 3 to 8 months; however, because these women are usually candidates for systemic therapy, adjuvant chemotherapy is then delivered in the interim. Breast conservation or mastectomy can be safely performed during pregnancy. The surgeon should be aware that the breast of a pregnant woman has a greater blood supply than the breast of a nonpregnant woman. The surgical performance of a partial mastectomy will also have a greater risk of the formation of a mammary fistula. Mastectomy is often employed as a surgical option, and it eliminates the concern for the timing of radiation for most women. Reconstruction using a transverse rectus abdominal muscle flap is contraindicated given the pressure on the abdominal wall from pregnancy.

Male Breast Cancer

Breast cancer in males makes up 0.5% to 1% of all cases of breast carcinoma. There is a greater familial history, with approximate 25% to 30% of these men having a family history of female breast or ovarian carcinomas. Although germline mutations of BRCA2 carry an increased risk of male breast cancer, the identification of a BRCA2 mutation in a male without a family history would be rare. Risk factors for men include radiation exposure (e.g., Hodgkin's lymphoma), Klinefelter's syndrome, and hepatic schistosomiasis.

Because most of the breast tissue of males is within 2 cm in diameter, deep to the nipple-areolar complex, the mass generally appears here as well. Ulceration of the nipple can sometimes be seen, as can Paget's disease of the nipple. Most frequently, ductal carcinoma is identified; lobular carcinoma is rare, and lobular carcinoma in situ is generally not identified. Studies of receptor status note that males have a high frequency of ER-positive tumors.

Surgically, the standard operation is that of modified radical mastectomy, as long as the tumor is not attached to the pectoralis major muscle. For patients with more extensive involvement, the rare use of a radical mastectomy is indicated. Prospective trials of systemic therapy have not focused solely on males; therefore, the chemotherapeutic regimens offered to women have been used in men by extrapolation. Tamoxifen therapy, too, has been used successfully, although information about aromatase inhibitors and fulvestrant are lacking. Per stage, the outcomes are comparable to those of women with similar staging and prognostic factors.

Locally Advanced and Inflammatory Breast Cancer

The standard of treatment for locally advanced breast cancer was alluded to in the earlier section about systemic therapies. Certainly surgery could be performed first, but this would usually necessitate a mastectomy with axillary lymph node assessment. Adjuvant chemotherapy would follow. The choice of radiotherapy to the chest wall would depend on the size of the tumor, the number of positive lymph nodes, and other factors, as mentioned above. Neoadjuvant chemotherapy is another option, allowing for breast conservation in approximately one third of all patients who opt to undergo such therapy. Breast conservation would necessarily be linked to postoperative total breast radiation. However, in the context of neoadjuvant chemotherapy, performance of a sentinel lymph node biopsy in a patient with a previously positive lymph node can be associated with up to a 25% false-negative rate and thus is discouraged.

Inflammatory breast cancer is approached first with neoadjuvant chemotherapy, and, as long as testing to establish the extent of disease fails to reveal metastatic disease, the patient proceeds with a modified radical mastectomy followed by radiation therapy. Further chemotherapy may be considered if the patient has residual disease within the lymph nodes, but this is controversial. This sequence of therapy has been studied at length, and it has been shown to maximize both disease-free and overall survival; other sequences have not been optimal.

Key Reading

Bland KI, Copeland EM III, eds. *The breast: comprehensive management of benign and malignant diseases.* Philadelphia: WB Saunders, 2004, p. 1189.

Selected Readings

Baker R, Montague A, Childs J. A comparison of modified radical mastectomy to radical mastectomy in the treatment of operable breast cancer. *Ann Surg* 1979;189:553–559.

Clarke M, Collins R, Darby S, *et al*. Early Breast Cancer Trialists' Collaborative Group (EBCTCG). Effects of radiotherapy and of differences in the extent of surgery for early breast cancer on local recurrence and 15-year survival: an overview of the randomised trials. *Lancet* 2005;366:2087–2106.

Fentiman IS, Fourquet A, Hortobagyi GN. Male breast cancer. *Lancet* 2006;367:595–604.

Fisher B, Redmond C, Poisson R, *et al.* Eight year result of randomized clinical trial comparing total mastectomy and lumpectomy with or without radiation in the treatment of breast cancer. *N Engl J Med* 1989;320:822–828.

Fentiman IS, Fourquet A, Hortobagyi GN. Male breast cancer. *Lancet* 2006;367:595–604.Baker R, Montague A, Childs J. A comparison of modified radical mastectomy to radical mastectomy in the treatment of operable breast cancer. *Ann Surg* 1979;189:553–559.

Hanrahan EO, Valero V, Gonzalez-Angulo AM, Hortobagyi GN. Prognosis and management of patients with node-negative invasive breast carcinoma that is 1 cm or smaller in size (stage 1; T1a,bN0M0): a review of the literature. *J Clin Oncol* 2006;24:2113–2122.

Hansen NM, Grube BJ, Giuliano AE. The time has come to change the algorithm for the surgical management of early breast cancer. *Arch Surg* 2002;137:1131–1135.

Krag DN. Minimal access surgery for staging regional lymph nodes: the sentinel node concept. *Curr Probl Surg* 1998;35:951–1016.

Kuerer HM, Newman LA. Lymphatic mapping and sentinel lymph node biopsy for breast cancer: developments and resolving controversies. *J Clin Oncol* 2005;23:1698–1705.

Mamounas EP. NSABP Protocol B-27. Preoperative doxorubicin plus cyclophosphamide followed by preoperative or postoperative docetaxel. *Oncology* 1997;11: 37–40.

Newman LA. Lymphatic mapping and sentinel lymph node biopsy in breast cancer patients: a comprehensive review of variations in performance and technique. *J Am Coll Surg* 2004;199:804–816.

Newman LA, Sabel MS. Advances in breast cancer detection and management. *Med Clin North Am* 2003;87:997–1028.

Pierce LJ. The use of radiotherapy after mastectomy: a review of the literature. *J Clin Oncol* 2005;23: 1706–1717.

Singletary SE. Skin-sparing mastectomy with immediate breast reconstruction: the M.D. Anderson Cancer Center experience. *Ann Surg Oncol* 1996;3:411–416.

Turner RR, Ollila DW, Krasne DL, Giuliano AE. Histopathologic validation of the sentinel lymph node hypothesis for breast carcinoma. *Ann Surg* 1997;226:271–276.

Veronesi U, Banfi A, del Vecchio M, *et al.* Comparison of Halsted mastectomy with quadrantectomy, axillary dissection and radiotherapy in early beast cancer: long-term results. *Eur J Cancer Clin Oncol* 1986;22: 1085–1089.

Veronesi U, Paganelli G, Viale G, Luini A, *et al.* A randomized comparison of sentinel-node biopsy with routine axillary dissection in breast cancer. *N Engl J Med* 2004;349:546–553.

Veronesi U, Boyle P, Goldhirsch A, *et al.* Breast cancer. *Lancet* 2005;365:1727–1741.

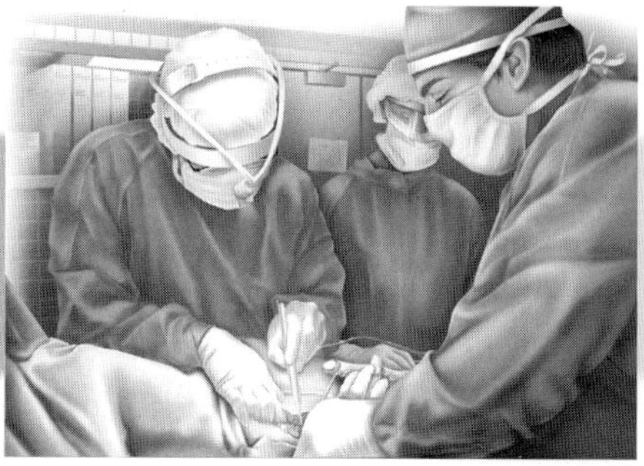

10

Melanoma and Nonmelanoma Skin Cancer

Quan P. Ly and Vernon K. Sondak

Melanoma and Nonmelanoma Skin Cancer: Key Points

- List the epidemiologic and etiologic factors pertinent to melanoma and nonmelanoma skin cancer.
- Determine the factors that contribute to the diagnosis process for melanoma and nonmelanoma skin cancer.
- Describe the pathologic processes found in melanoma and nonmelanoma skin cancer.
- Outline the most important prognostic factors in cutaneous melanoma.
- Delineate the surgical treatment options for cutaneous melanoma.
- Describe the management of regional lymph nodes.
- Outline the role of adjuvant therapy for melanoma.
- Detail the management of metastatic disease.
- List the facts about noncutaneous melanomas.

The skin is the most common site of cancer development in humans. Although melanoma accounts for only 4% of all skin cancer, it is the sixth most common malignancy in men and the seventh most common in women in the United States. Because of the relatively young age of onset, melanoma is second only to leukemia in terms of years of potential life lost.

Epidemiology and Etiology

Sites

Melanoma and nonmelanoma skin cancer can occur on any part of the skin surface as well as in the pigmented cells of the retina and on the mucous membranes of the nasopharyngeal sinuses, the vulva, and the anal canal. In general, these noncutaneous tumors present at a more advanced stage.

BOX 10–1 RISK FACTORS FOR MELANOMA

- ***Familial***
  - History of malignant melanoma
  - Skin type and color
- ***Environmental***
  - ≥3 blistering sunburns before the age of 20 years
  - Outdoor summer jobs for ≥3 years during the adolescent years
  - Use of sunlamps and tanning beds
- ***Other***
  - Actinic keratosis, elastosis
  - Marked freckling on the upper back
  - Large number of normal nevi
  - Atypical nevi, congenital giant nevi
- ***Immunosuppression***

Age

Melanoma affects all age groups, with a mean age of 55 years. More than 75% of melanomas occur in individuals younger than 70 years old. By comparison, for colon cancer, more than 40% of patients are diagnosed after they reach the age of 70 years.

Gender

Melanoma is slightly more common in men than women, with a male-to-female ratio of approximately 1.2:1.0. The most common site of melanoma development in females is the extremity, whereas the trunk is the site that is most affected in males. Most series have found that women have a slightly better prognosis, stage for stage, than men do.

Race/Skin Type

Skin type and color are more important as risk factors than race. Individuals with light-colored skin who burn easily and who do not tan are more likely to develop melanoma, regardless of ethnicity (Table 10-1). Melanoma and nonmelanoma skin cancers are much less common among dark-skinned individuals, with an annual age-adjusted incidence of only 1% of that seen among whites or those with light skin color. Asians and Hispanics are at very low risk of melanoma. Nonetheless, it is important to remember that both melanoma and nonmelanoma skin cancers do occur in all ethnic and racial groups.

The skin cancers of deeply pigmented individuals differ in their presentation. Most melanomas among these individuals occur on the relatively nonpigmented skin of the palms and soles. Interestingly, basal cells cancers, which are usually nonpigmented among whites, are almost always pigmented among dark-skinned patients. Finally, although most cases of squamous cell cancer among white patients occur on the sun-exposed skin of the head and neck or arms, the majority of the cases among black patients develop on less-exposed areas, such as the legs.

Ultraviolet Exposure

Melanoma and nonmelanoma skin cancers share a common causative factor: exposure to the ultraviolet (UV) radiation in sunlight. However, the precise mechanism of causation and the types of exposures most likely to cause each disease may vary. Most dangerous is UV-B radiation (wavelength, 290-320 nm); however, UV-A radiation (wavelength, 320-400 nm) probably also has carcinogenic potential. Overall, skin cancer incidence rates are increasing, most likely both because people spend more time in the sunlight and because the atmosphere's ability to screen out UV radiation has decreased via depletion of the ozone layer.

Different types of skin cancer are associated with different patterns of sun exposure. Almost all basal cell and squamous cell cancers of the skin occur on chronically exposed areas.

Melanoma is most common in parts of the world in which fair-skinned people live close to the equator. Australia and New Zealand have the highest incidence of invasive melanoma, reaching 50 per 100,000 individuals. South Africa has twice as many melanoma cases as Middle Africa. Asian countries such as China, Japan, and India have the lowest rates.

Genetic Predisposition

Mutations of two cyclin-dependent kinase genes, CDKN2A (also called p16) and CDK4,

TABLE 10-1 • *Skin Phototypes*

	Skin Type	Sun History	Features	Skin Reddens
I	Extremely sun sensitive	Never tans, burns easily	Redheaded, freckles	15 minutes in direct sunlight
II	Very sun sensitive	Minimal tan, burns easily	Fair skin, blonde hair, blue eyes	18–25 minutes
III	Sun sensitive	Light tan, sometimes burns	Medium skin tone	20–35 minutes
IV	Minimally sun sensitive	Minimal burns, always tans	Olive skin tone	35–40 minutes
V	Sun insensitive	Rarely burns	Light brown skin tone	40–50 minutes
VI	Insensitive	Very rarely burns	Dark brown skin	55–70 minutes

mark an individual as more susceptible to melanoma. Although these genes are linked to melanoma, there is no strong evidence to recommended genetic testing as a routine study for melanoma at this time.

The most reliable clinically identifiable risks for cutaneous melanoma are a strong family history and/or having multiple atypical moles. The genetic basis for the inheritance of atypical moles remains unclear.

Typical Moles

Typical or benign moles, which are also called *melanocytic nevi,* are small (<6 mm), round, uniformly tan or brown, and symmetrical. They are generally raised above the skin surface, as opposed to freckles. Patients with many (>25-50) melanocytic nevi are at increased risk of melanoma; most of these patients are also fair-skinned, light-haired individuals who burn easily and rarely tan.

Atypical Moles

Atypical moles, which are called clinically *atypical nevi* or *dysplastic nevi,* are larger (generally >6 mm) and irregularly shaped, and they have a pebbly surface. They are usually tan or brown, but they may have various shades of coloration within them. At least 5% of the white population of the United States has at least one clinically atypical nevus. Fair-skinned individuals with at least one clinically atypical nevus have a 6% lifetime risk of developing melanoma. This risk rises to as high as 80% among individuals who also have a family history of melanoma.

Some clinically atypical nevi eventually progress to melanoma. Even if every atypical mole is surgically removed, however, the patient remains at an increased risk of developing melanoma over the rest of the normal skin. Until such time (if ever) that genetic testing identifies those individuals with atypical moles who are at the greatest risk of melanoma development, all individuals with clinically atypical nevi should be carefully followed, especially those with a family history of melanoma.

Giant Congenital Nevi

Congenital nevi are pigmented lesions that are present at birth (as opposed to developing months or years later). Among congenital nevi, giant (>20 cm in diameter) congenital nevus, which is an extremely rare lesion, has a very high rate of malignant degeneration during childhood. Nearly all melanomas that occur in children younger than 5 years old arise within these lesions. Whenever the cosmetic result permits, giant congenital nevi should be excised during early childhood. If complete excision is impossible, even with staged procedures, close follow-up is indicated.

Xeroderma Pigmentosum

Xeroderma pigmentosum is a rare congenital disorder in which patients lack the capacity to repair UV-induced DNA damage. It is associated with the development of innumerable melanoma and nonmelanoma skin cancers at an early age.

Actinic Keratoses

Actinic keratoses are scaly, rough, erythematous patches that occur in chronically sun-exposed areas; they are both markers for and precursors to nonmelanoma skin cancer development. These lesions may progress to squamous cell cancers, or, in some cases, they may regress spontaneously in response to prolonged avoidance of sun exposure. If few in number, actinic keratoses can be removed or destroyed with liquid nitrogen. For multiple lesions, topical fluorouracil cream has been used successfully.

Burns

Squamous cell cancers occasionally arise in burns or other scars. Burn scar cancers (also called *Marjolin's ulcers*) may have a more aggressive clinical course than the usual nonmelanoma skin cancer.

Immunosuppression or Prior Hematologic Malignancy

Nonmelanoma skin cancers and, to a lesser degree, melanomas are more common among patients who are immunosuppressed or who have had previous hematologic malignancies. Furthermore, the aggressiveness of the skin tumors can be significantly greater in these patients.

Diagnosis

Although the vast majority of skin cancers are curable, a substantial number of skin-cancer–related deaths occur each year. Because these cancers are visible on the skin, early detection should be the goal in every case.

History

It is important to obtain a history with a focus on how long the lesion has been present, if and when it began changing color/texture, and whether it arose from a preexisting nevus. Also, any history of sun exposure, severe burns, previous skin cancers, hematologic malignancy, or immunosuppressive conditions should be noted.

Physical Examination

Total body skin examination is a critical step in the initial evaluation and follow-up of any patient with skin cancers or atypical nevi. Patients with one skin cancer are at significant risk for developing or harboring a second or even multiple skin cancers, often of a different histologic type. Thus, a thorough and complete skin examination in a well-lit room with the patient completely disrobed is fundamental. Some dermatologists use serial photography of individual lesions as well as whole skin areas, Wood's lamp ("black light") examination, and dermoscopy (also called *epiluminescence microscopy;* examination with a magnifying lens of an area of skin that has had oil applied to minimize reflectance).

Early melanoma can be differentiated from a benign mole using the ABCDE features. Other signs of melanoma are itching, bleeding, ulceration, or changes in a preexisting mole.

BOX 10–2 THE ABCDEs OF SKIN CANCER RECOGNITION

A Asymmetry
B Border irregularity
C Color variation
D Diameter of >6 mm
E Evolution (change in lesion)

An assessment of all regional lymph nodes is part of a complete examination at initial diagnosis and at each follow up visit, because lymphatic spread is the most common type of dissemination.

Biopsy

Most suspicious pigmented or nonpigmented skin lesions should be biopsied, because physical examination alone is often inadequate to determine the precise nature of a skin lesion. To make an accurate diagnosis, the pathologist must receive adequate tissue in good condition to assess all relevant histologic features. A properly performed biopsy should not make subsequent definitive surgical treatment more difficult. Incisions on the extremities should be oriented in the longitudinal plane so as to not alter the lymphatic drainage (for subsequent sentinel lymph node biopsy) and to allow for primary closure after reexcision should the biopsy reveal melanoma (Figure 10-1).

Cryosurgery and electrodesiccation do not allow any pathological evaluation and thus should be avoided for lesions that are suspected of being melanoma. Similarly, shallow shave biopsy is considered inadequate, because the margins and depth of invasion cannot be assessed. Whenever possible, complete excision with a 1- to 2-mm margin of normal skin down to subcutaneous fat should be performed. For large lesions or cosmetically sensitive areas such as the face, an incisional or punch biopsy would be appropriate.

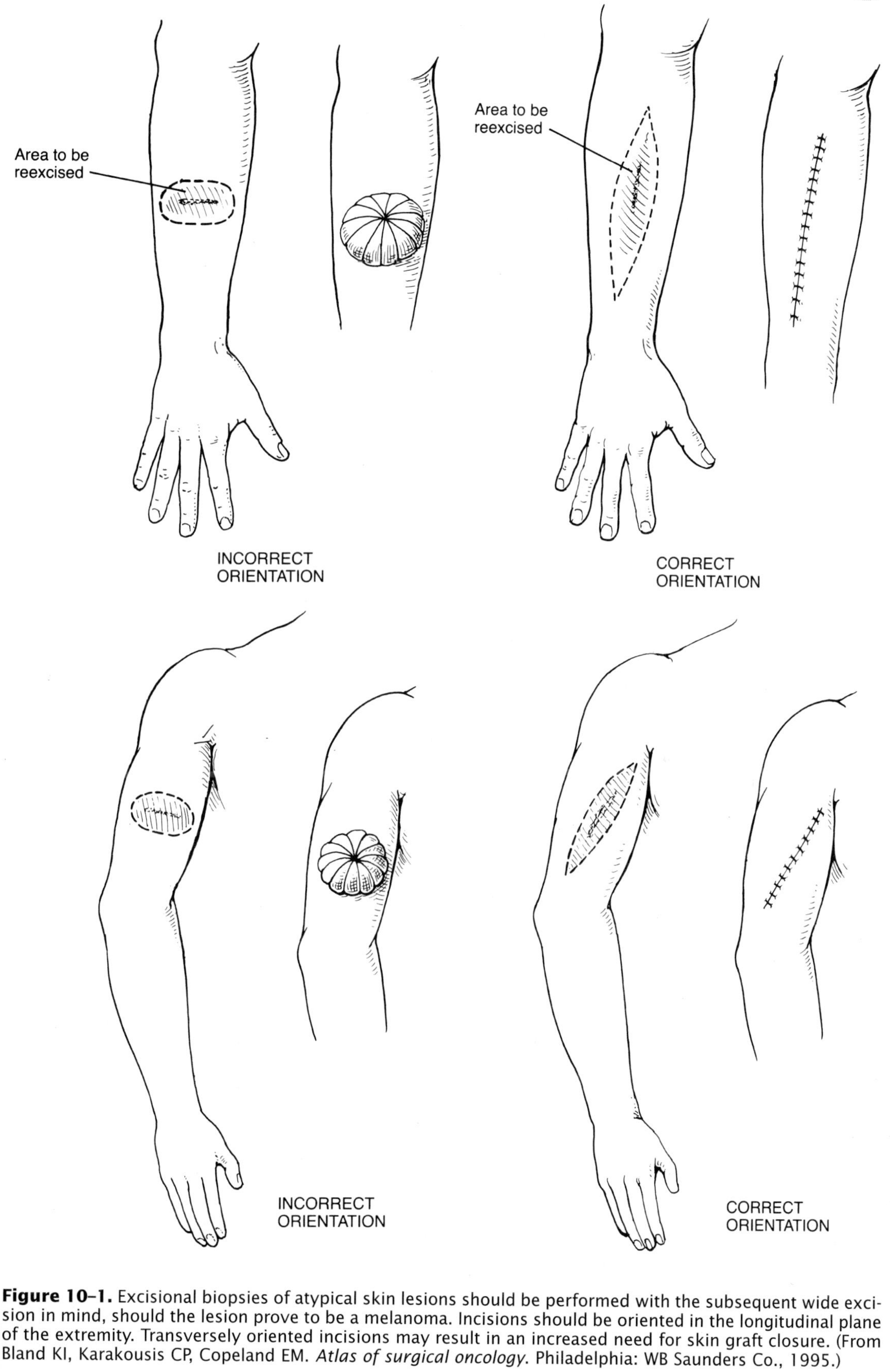

Figure 10–1. Excisional biopsies of atypical skin lesions should be performed with the subsequent wide excision in mind, should the lesion prove to be a melanoma. Incisions should be oriented in the longitudinal plane of the extremity. Transversely oriented incisions may result in an increased need for skin graft closure. (From Bland KI, Karakousis CP, Copeland EM. *Atlas of surgical oncology*. Philadelphia: WB Saunders Co., 1995.)

The area to be sampled should be the most elevated portion of the lesion. It is helpful to the pathologist if the actual size of the lesion is noted whenever a partial biopsy is performed.

When an enlarged lymph node is palpated in a patient with melanoma, the best diagnostic modality is usually a fine-needle aspiration. If the cytology is negative or nondiagnostic, an open biopsy of that enlarged node should be the next step. Frozen section during the open biopsy may allow the surgeon to proceed with definitive lymphadenectomy if the node is positive.

Pathology

Histologic Types (Figure 10-2)

Basal cell carcinoma is the most common skin tumor, and it is associated with chronic sunlight exposure. It is often an ulcerated irregular lesion with a raised pearly border. The tumor is believed to arise from the basal layer of the epidermis or hair follicle. Management of basal cell carcinoma is directed by the histologic nature of the tumor, the anatomic site, and the clinical presentation (Table 10-2).

Squamous cell carcinoma is the next most common skin cancer, and it is also associated with chronic sunlight exposure as well as chemical carcinogens (arsenic and tar) and sites of previous trauma, irradiation, or burns (Marjolin's ulcer). The lesions appear as roughened keratotic areas, ulcers, or horns.

Merkel cell carcinoma is a rare but aggressive skin cancer that is believed to arise from the neuroendocrine cells of the skin.

The most common primary sarcoma affecting the skin is *dermatofibrosarcoma protuberans* (DFSP). *Leiomyosarcoma, angiosarcoma,* and *malignant fibrous histiocytoma* can also arise entirely within the skin.

Superficial spreading melanoma is the most common type of cutaneous melanoma. It often arises within a preexisting nevus, and it is surrounded by a zone of atypical melanocytes that may extend beyond the visible borders of the lesion.

Nodular melanoma represents about 10% to 15% of cutaneous melanoma. It is generally a dark blue-black, and it is more symmetrical

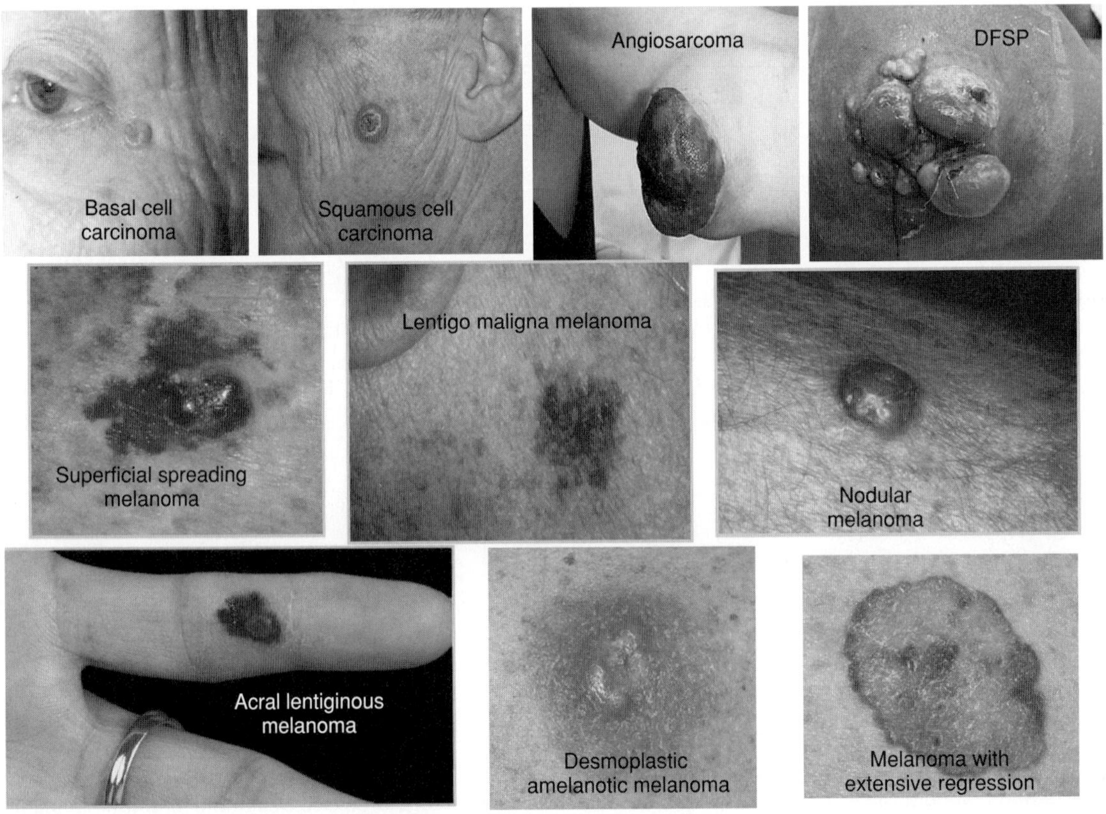

Figure 10–2. Pictures of various skin cancers.

TABLE 10-2 • *Treatment Options for Basal Cell Carcinoma*

Treatment	Description	Indications
Excision	Surgical resection with 4-mm margins where possible	BCC on trunk or extremity
Mohs micrographic surgery	Tangential excision with a minimal margin of clinically normal-appearing tissue, precisely mapped and processed immediately by frozen section for microscopic examination; reexcision as needed until negative margins are ensured	Treatment of choice for recurrent and infiltrative BCC; excellent choice for BCC on face
Curettage and electrodesiccation	Visible tumor is removed by curettage for a 2- to 4-mm margin, followed by electrodesiccation	High recurrence rates; not recommended for BCC
Cryosurgery	Liquid nitrogen is applied to the lesion	Only for very small, superficial BCC
Radiation therapy		For extensive lesions precluding surgical resection or for patients who cannot tolerate surgery

BCC, Basal cell carcinoma.

and uniform in coloration than other melanomas. Amelanotic nodular melanomas also occur and are frequently misdiagnosed.

Lentigo maligna melanoma accounts for 10% to 15% of cutaneous melanomas. It typically occurs on the sun-exposed areas of the head, neck, and hands. Clinically, it is a large (often >3 cm in diameter), flat, tan lesion with areas of dark brown or black coloration. These lesions arise from a precursor lesion known as *lentigo maligna* or *Hutchinson's freckle.*

Acral-lentiginous melanoma occurs on the palms, soles, and subungual locations. Subungual melanomas can easily be confused with subungual hematomas; the presence of pigmentation in the paronychial skin is indicative of melanoma. Acral-lentiginous melanoma occurs in equal frequency among whites and darker-pigmented races. Because of the high incidence of other types of cutaneous melanoma among light-skinned individuals, acral-lentiginous melanomas account for only 2% to 8% of melanomas among these people (as opposed to making up 40% to 60% of melanomas among darker-skinned individuals).

Growth Phases

Cutaneous melanomas are thought to begin as radial growth-phase lesions and then progress, in many cases, to vertical growth. The radial growth phase is characterized by melanoma tumor cells in the epidermis and papillary dermis, with the development of a raised irregular surface on the skin. Although pure radial growth-phase melanomas may be fully invasive lesions, they are unlikely to metastasize to the regional nodes or beyond, and have a prognosis nearly as good as that of melanoma in situ. Vertical growth phase is associated with increasing nodularity of the lesion and a much greater potential for metastasis. The depth of invasion correlates directly with prognosis.

Staging

The three most important prognostic factors in cutaneous melanoma are depth of invasion, involvement of regional lymph nodes, and presence of distant metastasis.

Tumor staging has undergone multiple revisions since 1969, when Dr. Wallace Clark and associates published a system to classify melanoma according to the level of invasion relative to histologically defined landmarks in the skin (Figure 10-3). In 1970, Dr. Alexander Breslow proposed an alternative melanoma classification based on the absolute thickness of the lesion determined by measurements obtained through a microscope from the top of the granular layer of the epidermis to the deepest contiguous tumor cell at the base of the lesion. Many studies during the past three decades demonstrated an inverse correlation between Breslow's tumor thickness and survival. In a head-to-head comparison, tumor

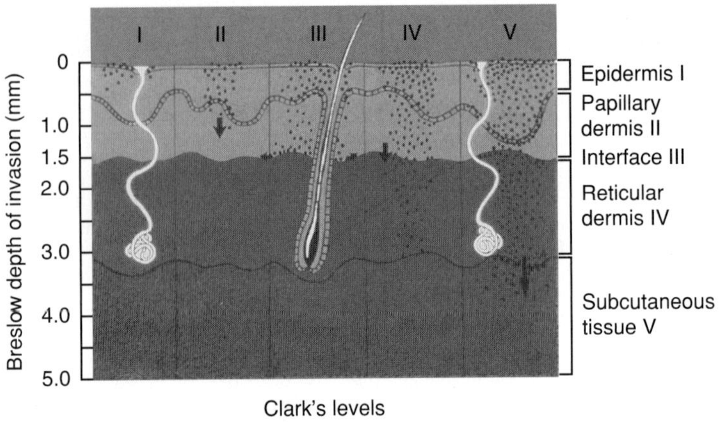

Figure 10–3. Clark's levels.

thickness proved to be a better predictor of outcome than Clark's level.

In early 2000, a new staging system was proposed based on the TNM classification. The Melanoma Staging Committee of the American Joint Committee on Cancer (AJCC), which is made up of experts in various disciplines from multiple major melanoma centers around the world, evaluated published data and gathered and analyzed 17,600 patient records. The results were published in sixth edition of the AJCC guidelines in 2002. In this newest version of melanoma staging, tumor staging is differentiated by thickness (<1 mm; 1-2 mm; 2-4 mm; and >4 mm) and by the presence of ulceration, and by Clark's level for lesions less than 1 mm (Table 10-3).

In recent years, other prognostic factors besides thickness were shown to have significant impact on recurrence rate and/or outcome. Ulceration is a highly significant predictor of outcome and has been incorporated into the AJCC staging of the primary tumor in melanoma. Mitotic rate correlates with survival as well as with the likelihood of nodal metastases. Some authors suggest that the site of the primary tumor is also an important prognostic factor; patients with melanoma on their extremities may have a better survival than those with a lesion arising on the trunk, head, or neck. The so-called BANS (*b*ack, back of upper *a*rms, *n*eck, and *s*calp) areas are believed by some to have a worse prognosis than lesions in other sites when matched for thickness.

Regional Node Involvement

Nodal involvement has always been recognized to adversely impact prognosis, regardless of the thickness of the primary lesion. However, there is a direct correlation between the primary lesion thickness and the likelihood of microscopic nodal involvement in clinically node-negative patients. As in other cancers, the number of involved lymph nodes in melanoma patients has an inverse correlation with survival. The 5-year survival rate for patients with multiple positive lymph nodes is about 20% to 25%, whereas the rate for patients with only one or two involved lymph nodes is more than 50%.

BOX 10–3 HISTOPATHOLOGIC VARIABLES OF PRIMARY MELANOMA ASSOCIATED WITH PROGNOSIS

- Tumor thickness (mm)
- Ulceration
- Phase of tumor growth (radial versus vertical)
- Mitotic rate
- Angiolymphatic invasion
- Histogenic type
- Regression
- Tumor-infiltrating lymphocytes
- Host response
- Satellitosis
- Neurotropism

BOX 10–4 LIKELIHOOD OF NODAL METASTASES BASED ON BRESLOW TUMOR THICKNESS

< 1 mm	<5%
1–4 mm	15–25%
>4 mm	35%

TABLE 10-3 • *Current Melanoma Staging*

Primary Tumor (T)	
TX	Primary tumor cannot be assessed (e.g., shave biopsy or regressed melanoma)
T0	No evidence of primary tumor
Tis	Melanoma in situ
T1	Melanoma ≤ 1.00 mm in thickness with or without ulceration
T1a	Melanoma ≤ 1.0 mm in thickness and level II or III, no ulceration
T1b	Melanoma ≤ 1.0 mm in thickness and level IV or V or with ulceration
T2	Melanoma 1.01 - 2.0 mm in thickness with or without ulceration
T2a	Melanoma 1.01-2.0 mm in thickness, no ulceration
T2b	Melanoma 1.01-2.0 mm in thickness, with ulceration
T3	Melanoma 2.01-4.0 mm in thickness with or without ulceration
T3a	Melanoma 2.01-4.0 mm in thickness, no ulceration
T3b	Melanoma 2.01-4.0 mm in thickness, with ulceration
T4	Melanoma > 4.0 mm in thickness with or without ulceration
T4a	Melanoma > 4.0 mm in thickness, no ulceration
T4b	Melanoma > 4.0 mm in thickness, with ulceration
Regional Lymph Nodes (N)	
NX	Regional lymph nodes cannot be assessed
N0	No regional lymph node metastasis
N1	Metastasis in one lymph node
N1a	Clinically occult (macroscopic) metastasis
N1b	Clinically apparent (macroscopic) metastasis
N2	Metastasis in two or three regional nodes or intralymphatic regional metastasis without nodal metastases
N2a	Clinically occult (microscopic) metastasis
N2b	Clinically apparent (microscopic) metastasis
N2c	Satellite or in transit metastasis without nodal metastasis
N3	Metastasis in four or more regional lymph nodes, or matted metastic nodes, or in-transit metastasis or satellite(s) with metastasis in regional node(s)
Distant Metastasis (M)	
MX	Distant metastasis cannot be assessed
M0	No distant metastasis
M1	Distant metastases
M1a	Metastasis to skin, subcutaneous tissue, or distant lymph nodes
M1b	Metastasis to lung
M1c	Metastasis to all other visceral sites or distant at any metastasis site associated with an elevated serum lactic dehydrogenase (LDH)

Clinical Stage Grouping

Stage	T	N	M
0	Ta	N0	M0
IA	T1a	N0	M0
IB	T1b	N0	M0
	T2a	N0	M0
IIA	T2b	N0	M0
	T3a	N0	M0
IIB	T3b	N0	M0
	T4a	N0	M0
IIC	T4b	N0	M0
III	Any T	N1	M0

(Continued)

TABLE 10-2 • *Current Melanoma Staging—Cont'd*

Stage	T	N	M
	Any T	N2	M0
	Any T	N3	M0
IV	Any T	Any N	M1
Note: Clinical staging includes microstaging of the primary melanoma and clinical/radiological evaluations for metastases. By convention it should be used after complete excision of the primary melanoma with clinical assessment for regional and distant metastases.			
Histopathologic Type			
Pathologic Stage Grouping			
Stage	T	N	M
0	Ta	N0	M0
IA	T1a	N0	M0
IB	T1b	N0	M0
	T2a	N0	M0
IIA	T2b	N0	M0
	T3a	N0	M0
IIB	T3b	N0	M0
	T4a	N0	M0
IIC	T4b	N0	M0
IIIA	T1-4a	N1a	M0
	T1-4a	N2a	M0
IIIB	T1-4b	N1a	M0
	T1-4b	N2a	M0
	T1-4a	N1a	M0
	T1-4a	N2a	M0
	T1-4a/b	N2a	M0
IIIC	T1-4b	N1a	M0
	T1-4b	N2a	M0
	Any T	N3	M0
IV	Any T	Any N	M1
Note: Pathologic staging includes microstaging of the primary melanoma and pathologic information about the regional lumph nodes after partial or complete lymphadenectomy. Pathologic Stage 0 or Stage IA patients are the excetion; they do not require pathologic evaluation of their lymph nodes			

Adapted from Greene FL *et al. AJCC cancer staging handbook,* Sixth Edition, New York: Springer-Verlag.

In general, patients with palpable nodes fare worse than those with only microscopic involvement. Furthermore, large, matted nodes or those with extracapsular extension are associated with a worse prognosis.

Distant Metastasis

Stage IV melanoma has a very poor overall prognosis. However, some patients can be long-term survivors with aggressive treatment. Melanoma can metastasize to any organ, although the most common sites are the skin, lung, and lymph nodes. The central nervous system, gastrointestinal tract, and other abdominal viscera (particularly the liver, spleen, and adrenal glands) can also be involved with melanoma metastases. Patients with metastatic disease limited to the skin and subcutaneous tissues usually fare much better than those with visceral or central nervous system involvement. A high level of lactic dehydrogenase (LDH) in the serum is also associated with a worse outcome.

Treatment

Surgical Treatment

The primary treatment of cutaneous melanoma is surgical excision. Although it was long recognized that tumor cells could extend within the skin for several centimeters beyond the visible borders of a melanoma and that the risk of local recurrence relates to the width of the normal skin excised around the primary lesion, only recently has some consensus regarding the margin of the excision based on the thickness of the lesion been reached.

Several trials have examined the surgical margins of excision (Table 10-4). In 1988 and again in 1999, Veronesi and colleagues conducted a randomized trial looking at thin primary melanoma, comparing excisional margins of 1 cm versus 3 cm. They found that patients treated with a 1-cm margin for melanomas of less than 1 mm have very low local recurrence rates (<1%), and their survival is equivalent to those treated with a 3-cm margin. For melanomas that are 1 to 2 mm in thickness, survival was the same for both margins, but the local recurrence rate was slightly higher with the 1-cm margin (about 2%).

In 1993, Balch and colleagues completed a randomized prospective trial comparing the efficacy of 2-cm versus 4-cm excision margins for intermediate thickness melanoma (1-4 mm). Both local recurrence and survival were the same regardless of whether 2-cm or 4-cm margins were taken. The differences were a lower frequency of skin grafting and a shorter hospital stay in the group with the 2-cm margin.

In 2000, Cohn-Cedermark and colleagues reported a randomized study by the Swedish Melanoma Group of 2-cm versus 5-cm resection margins for patients with cutaneous melanoma measuring 0.8 mm to 2.0 mm. They, too, found no difference in local or distant relapse rate or overall survival between a 2-cm and a wider excision margin.

For lesions more than 4-mm thick, in a retrospective review, Heaton and colleagues found no significant difference in local recurrence, disease-free survival, or overall survival

TABLE 10-4 • *Prospective Randomized Trials of Surgical Margins for Melanoma Resection*

Trial	N	Tumor Thickness	Treatment Arms (cm)	Local Recurrence	Survival
French Cooperative Trial (Khayat et al 2003)	337	<2.1 mm	2 versus 5	NSD	NSD
World Health Organization (Veronesi et al 1991)	612	<2 mm	1 versus 3	NSD for melanoma <1 mm; local recurrence slightly higher for 1- to 2-mm tumors with 1-cm margin	NSD
Swedish Melanoma Trial (Cohn-Cedermark et al 2000)	989	0.8–2.0 mm	2 versus 5	NSD	NSD
Intergroup Melanoma Surgical Trial (Balch et al 2001)	740	1.0–4.0 mm	2 versus 4	NSD	NSD
United Kingdom Study (Thomas et al 2004)	900	>2.0 mm	1 versus 3	Higher locoregional recurrence rate for 1-cm margin	NSD

NSD, No significant difference.

whether the patient received a 2-cm margin or a wider one. In 2004, Thomas and colleagues conducted a randomized clinical trial comparing 1-cm versus 3-cm margins for thick melanoma (>2 mm), and they found that a 1-cm margin conferred a greater risk of locoregional recurrence but no statistical difference in overall survival rate. The present recommendations for the margins of excision are based on the results of these trials. The excision should extend at least to the level of the fascia. Many surgeons routinely excise the fascia with the specimen.

BOX 10–5 CURRENT SURGICAL RECOMMENDATIONS BASED ON RESULTS FROM CLINICAL TRIALS

- For melanoma in situ, a margin of 0.5 cm
- For lesions <1 mm in thickness, a margin of 1 cm
- For lesions 1–4 mm in thick ness, a margin of 2 cm, when anatomically feasible
- For lesions >4 mm in thickness, a margin of at least 2 cm

BOX 10–6 IMPORTANT POINTS REGARDING THE SURGICAL EXCISION OF MELANOMA

Regardless of the recommended margin, a histologically negative margin is necessary. Thus, if a 2-cm margin is taken and the final pathology report reveals melanoma cells or atypical melanocytic hyperplasia at the margins, further excision is indicated.

When the anatomic location of the lesion precludes the excision of the desired margin (e.g., on the hands, feet, or face), at least 1 cm should be taken, as long as the margins are histologically negative.

If a minor compromise in the excision margin can allow primary closure without a skin graft, it may be worthwhile, particularly with melanomas between 1 mm and 2 mm in thickness.

Management of Regional Lymph Nodes

Melanoma patients with regional lymph node metastasis and no evidence of distant disease should undergo a complete regional lymph node dissection. Depending on the number of lymph nodes found to be involved, the prognosis for long-term survival is approximately 20% to 40% among these patients.

For decades, the management of melanoma patients with clinically normal lymph nodes has been controversial. It is clear that the likelihood of occult nodal involvement rises with increasing thickness of the primary tumor. However, the benefit of an elective node dissection—aside from more accurate staging—is debatable.

In 1977, Veronesi and colleagues evaluated the efficacy of immediate node dissection for stage I melanoma in a prospective, randomized, clinical trial and found that elective lymph node dissection (ELND) did not improve the overall survival. In 1982, the same group reexamined their database and again found no difference in survival in both treatment groups, even when the data were stratified into subsets. In a prospective, multi-institutional, randomized trial published in 1996, Balch and colleagues reported improved survival for patients younger than 60 years old with non-ulcerated melanoma of intermediate thickness (1-2 mm) treated with ELND. The survival difference was more pronounced when the data were analyzed with actual treatment received instead of intention to treat.

The controversy between ELND and observation for melanoma appeared to be resolved for some with the advent of lymphatic mapping and sentinel lymph node (SLN) biopsy. Lymphatic mapping and SLN biopsy were first described by Morton and colleagues in 1992, when it was observed that lymphatics from any given location in the skin drained to a single node (or, at most, 2 or 3 specific nodes) within the regional basin (or basins). SLN biopsy has numerous advantages over routine elective node dissection for the staging of patients with clinically negative regional nodes. One is the lower incidence of lymphedema, wound infection, seroma, and nerve injury. Furthermore, lymphatic mapping also identifies interval nodes, which are nodes that are located outside of the formal confines of the regional basins. Examples of these interval nodes are the popliteal and epitrochlear nodes, as well as those within the soft tissue of the flank, the lateral back, the upper arms, and the mid thighs. More importantly, with fewer nodes, the pathologist can carefully scrutinize the selected nodes and provide the surgeon with a more detailed and accurate staging of the pathology specimen.

Because of the low morbidity, low false-negative rate (<4%), and the above-mentioned advantages, SLN biopsy has been widely adopted as the preferred staging method for patients with clinically negative nodes. However, some controversy still exists, because there is no proof yet that SLN biopsy actually improves survival. A large multicenter trial is in progress to answer this question and to determine the rate of nodal recurrence after SLN biopsy.

Patients with regional involvement, whether detected clinically (and confirmed by fine-need aspiration biopsy) or on sentinel lymph node biopsy, should undergo a complete lymph node dissection (Figures 10-4 and 10-5).

The original lymphatic mapping technique described by Morton uses a blue lymphangiogram dye (isosulfan blue [Lymphazurin]) injected intradermally at the site of the primary lesion (or adjacent to the biopsy scar if the primary lesion has already been excised) (Figure 10-6). After waiting about 5 minutes, an incision is made over the lymph node basin to identify any blue lymphatic channel and to remove any blue-stained nodes. This technique successfully identifies the sentinel lymph node at least 80% of the time.

An alternative technique uses radiolabeled colloid solution, which is injected 2 to 4 hours before surgery. A lymphoscintigram is obtained to show all possible regional basins (Figure 10-7). For example, a lesion on the mid back could map to either or both axillae as well as to the inguinal regions. In addition, this technique also reveals the number of sentinel lymph nodes within each basin. However, the radioisotopes provide no visual clues to the nodes' locations.

The combination of dye and radiolabeled colloid allows the surgeon to identify the sentinel lymph node in more than 98% of cases; thus, it is the procedure of choice in most cancer centers around the country.

Isolated Limb Perfusion

Isolated limb perfusion or *hyperthermic isolated limb perfusion* is a surgical treatment for in-transit metastases (cutaneous or subcutaneous nodules located between an extremity's primary and the regional lymph nodes). This procedure involves the cannulation of the main artery and the vein of the affected limb, connecting these cannulas to a cardiopulmonary bypass machine, and applying a tourniquet to that extremity. Melphalan (Alkeran) is the chemotherapeutic agent that is commonly injected through this circulating system and allowed to perfuse the limb. The drug and the limb are usually heated to 41°C while being perfused for 90 minutes. The drug must be washed out of the system before reconnecting the limb with the normal circulation. Both the therapeutic effect and adverse side effects are localized to the limb of interest. Partial or complete response rates of more than 90% can be achieved with hyperthermic isolated limb perfusion. However, because of the intricacy of the approach and the complicated postoperative care, this procedure is offered only at some cancer centers. In 1994, Thompson and colleagues proposed using isolated limb infusion as an alternative approach to isolated limb perfusion. In this procedure, the vessels of interest are accessed percutaneously from the opposite limb; the limb to be treated will be isolated from circulation with a tourniquet. Some favor this approach because it has similar rates of response but is better tolerated, especially by patients more than 70 years old.

Adjuvant Therapy

The 10-year disease-free survival estimate for patients with stage I cutaneous melanoma is 85%. However, fewer than half of the patients with deep primaries or intermediate-level primaries with ulceration and/or regional lymph node involvement will experience long-term disease-free survival. At the present time, adjuvant therapy is offered to high-risk patients (i.e., those who have >4-mm thick melanomas or positive lymph nodes). For those with intermediate risk, the current recommendation is observation or enrollment in a clinical trial.

Over the past few decades, various drugs have been proposed as adjuvant therapy for melanoma. From a myriad of randomized clinical trials, interferon alfa-2b is the only treatment shown to improve both relapse-free survival (by about 20% to 30%) and overall survival (by up to 10%). In 1996, because of the positive results from the Eastern Cooperative Oncology Group trial (ECOG 1684), the US Food and Drug Administration approved the use of high-dose interferon for high-risk patients who have been rendered disease-free in the hope of reducing the risk of recurrence. Unfortunately, many patients are unable to tolerate the high-dose regimens. Over the past decade, lower-dose regimens have been investigated, but they have not been found to be effective for prolonging the disease-free interval or overall survival. In 2004, an updated analysis of the ECOG 1684 data with a longer

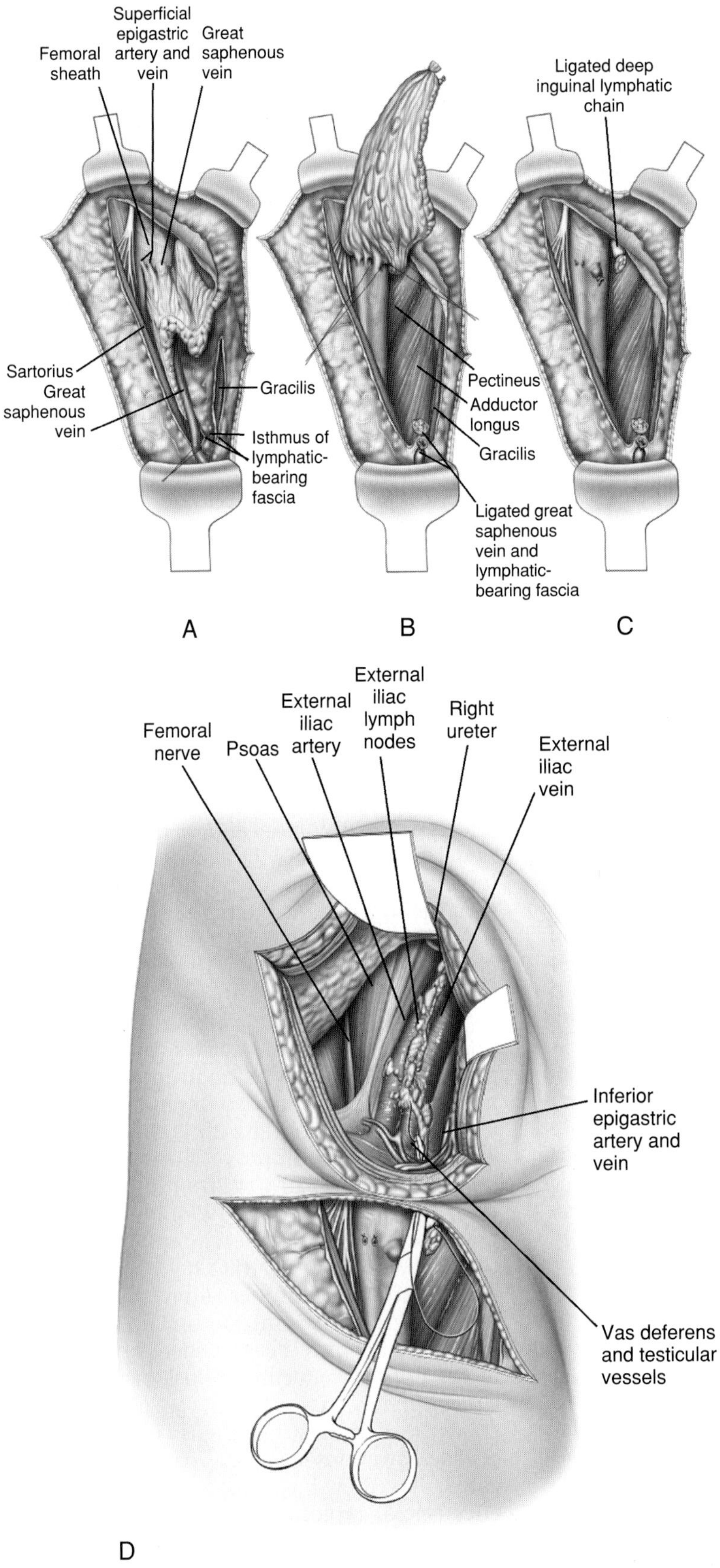

Figure 10–4. Superficial inguinal dissection. **A,** The subcutaneous tissue is dissected medially off of the gracilis and laterally off of the sartorius. **B,** The saphenous vein can be divided or preserved. All lymphatic tissue is dissected off of the femoral vessels. **C,** If a superficial node dissection only is to be performed, the operation is completed by ligating and dividing the lymphatic chain. **D,** If a deep node dissection is to be performed, this can be accomplished by dividing the inguinal ligament or through a second abdominal incision. All nodal tissue is then dissected from inferiorly to superiorly along the external iliacs. (From Bloom ND, Beattie EJ, Harvey JC. *Atlas of Cancer Surgery.* Philadelphia: WB Saunders, 2000.)

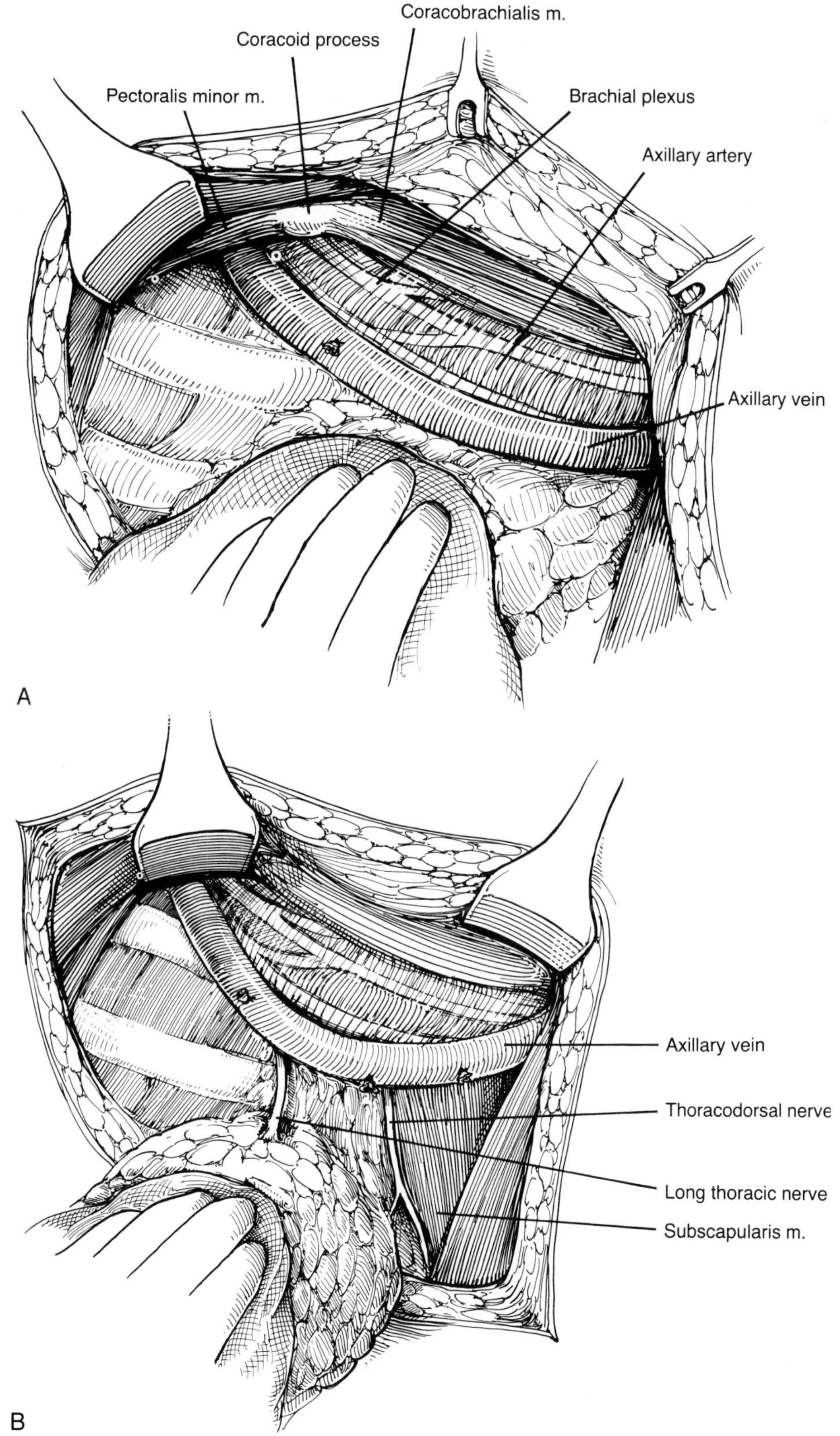

Figure 10–5. Axillary node dissection. **A,** Through a transverse incision between the pectoralis major and the latissimus dorsi muscle, both muscles and the axillary vein are identified. The fibrofatty tissue is dissected off of the axillary vein, including the tissue underneath the pectoralis minor muscle (level II lymph nodes). The pectoralis minor can be divided to gain access to the level III lymph nodes. **B,** The thoracodorsal and long thoracic nerves are preserved, and the fibrofatty tissue is dissected off of the underlying subscapularis muscle. (From Bland KI, Karakousis CP, Copeland EM. *Atlas of surgical oncology*. Philadelphia: WB Saunders Co., 1995.)

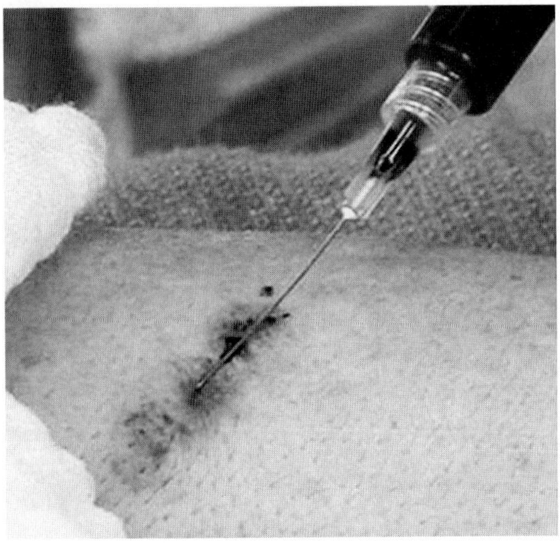

Figure 10–6. Intradermal injection with blue dye.

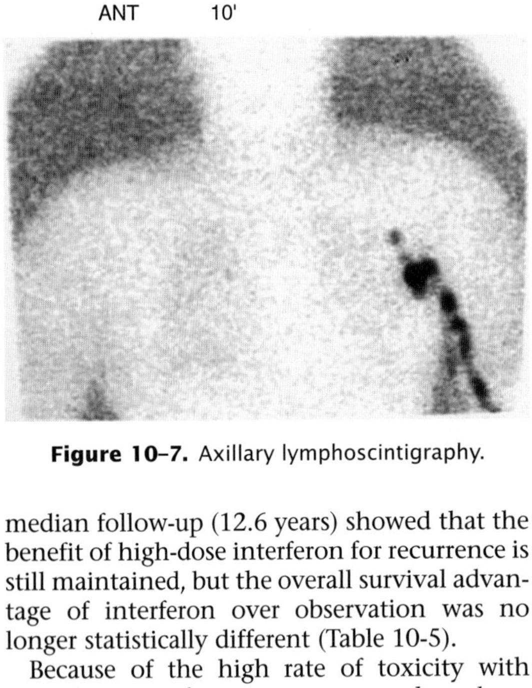

Figure 10–7. Axillary lymphoscintigraphy.

median follow-up (12.6 years) showed that the benefit of high-dose interferon for recurrence is still maintained, but the overall survival advantage of interferon over observation was no longer statistically different (Table 10-5).

Because of the high rate of toxicity with high-dose interferon, many researchers have investigated alternative treatments. Either low-dose or intermediate-dose interferon was used in combination with immunological or biochemotherapy. There are currently a number of vaccine trials available around the country. Each vaccine employs an antigen (i.e., melanoma cell lysate and polyvalent whole cell) and an immunostimulant, called an *adjuvant* (e.g., Detox, granulocyte-macrophage colony-stimulating factor, bacille Calmette-Guérin) (Table 10-6). So far, none of the vaccines has been shown to be superior to high-dose interferon in a randomized prospective trial. Nevertheless, with new vaccine regimens emerging, patients who are unable to tolerate the toxicity of interferon may benefit from enrollment in a clinical trial.

Radiation is another modality that is used as adjuvant treatment for high-risk melanoma patients. The long-standing pessimistic impression that melanoma is a "non-radioresponsive" tumor has recently been challenged by a study at MD Anderson Cancer Center using postoperative radiation therapy to the neck after radical or modified radical neck dissection. Radiation was associated with a decreased regional recurrence rate in node-positive patients, especially in those with 10 or more involved lymph nodes or gross extracapsular extension. Ongoing clinical studies will hopefully help clarify the benefit of postoperative radiation after an axillary or inguinal node dissection.

Metastatic Disease

The AJCC subdivides the metastatic classification into three groups: M1a, which includes distant skin, subcutaneous, or nodal metastasis; M1b, which involves lung metastases; and M1c, which includes all other visceral metastases or any distant metastases with an elevated serum LDH. Although there is a statistical difference in survival between the groups ($P < .0001$), the 1-year survival rate differences between the groups are quite small (59% for M1a, 57% for M1b, and 41% for M1c). Other prognostic factors—in addition to the sites of metastases and the serum LDH level—that have been found to be predictive of survival are performance status, the presence of visceral involvement, and the number of sites of involved.

The current accepted principle for metastatic melanoma is that a complete surgical resection (R0) will give the patient the best chance of survival. Unfortunately, an R0 resection is not achievable for most patients with metastatic disease due to the extent of disease. However, when the disease is limited (as in an M1a) or localized to one lobe of the lung (M1b), surgical resection, possibly followed by adjuvant therapy (as discussed earlier), may be worthwhile. Surgery is also offered as a palliative option for patients with symptomatic visceral or cerebral lesions.

When the disease is unresectable, the options are limited to systemic chemother-

TABLE 10-5 • *Summary of Interferon Trials*

ECOG 1684: High-dose interferon (HDI) versus observation; all patients in this study required to have regional lymphadenectomy. With a mean follow-up of 6.9 years, the interferon arm has a prolonged disease-free interval from 1 to 1.7 years (P = .0237) and overall survival from 2.8 to 3.8 years (P = .0023). With a mean follow-up of 12.7 years, the relapse-free survival is still significant, with a hazard ratio of 1.38 and a P value of .02 for the interferon group; however, although the overall survival hazard ratio (HR) of 1.22 favors interferon, it is no longer statistically different (P = .18). This loss of statistical difference may be the result of comorbid conditions in an aging population.
ECOG 1690: HDI versus low-dose interferon (LDI) versus observation; patients were not required to have regional lymphadenectomy. With a mean follow-up of 4.3 years, HDI conferred a better relapse-free survival ascompared with observation (HR, 1.28; P = .025), whereas LDI did not show any benefit. The overall survival was not significantly different for all three groups. Interestingly, during a retrospective analysis of the study, it was found that there were a significant number of patients who crossed over from observation to HDI when they had regional recurrence. This may explain the lack of overall survival difference between the two groups.
ECOG 1694: HDI versus ganglioside GM2 vaccine. Trial was closed early after 16 months when an interim analysis showed that HDI was significantly superior to the vaccine in terms of relapse-free survival (HR, 1.47; P = .0015) as well as overall survival (HR, 1.52; P = .009).

apy or immunotherapy. Although the US Food and Drug Administration has approved dacarbazine (DTIC) for the treatment of metastatic melanoma, overall, this regimen has a low and usually short-lived objective response rate of 10% to 15%. Trials with two-drug or three-drug combinations did not show any consistently significant advantage over DTIC alone. Biological therapy with high-dose interleukin-2 (IL-2) or interferon showed an approximate 10% to 20% response rate for each therapy. A meta-analysis of 20 randomized trials comparing DTIC alone, DTIC with chemotherapy, and DTIC and immunotherapy found that DTIC and interferon-alfa achieved 53% more responses than DTIC alone, but there was no significant overall survival difference.

IL-2 is a recombinant biological molecule that has antitumor activity against melanoma. The high-dose regimen can cause serious cardiopulmonary complications; thus, IL-2 is usually administered in a hospital setting under the care of an experienced provider. When high dose-intensity levels are achieved, up to a 20% objective response rate has been observed, and some of the responding patients enjoy a durable and complete remission that lasts for more than 5 years. This outcome may be in part the result of the selection of healthy patients who could withstand the multisystem toxicities. IL-2 modulators have been used in hope of decreasing toxicities, but they have not yet been found to be effective. Combining interferon and IL-2 has also been studied. This regimen showed increased toxicities without any increased in benefit; thus, it is not recommended.

Vaccines and other targeted immunotherapy have been proposed (Table 10-7). The idea of training a person's own immune system to combat and remember cancer cell antigen is quite attractive. To date, the effectiveness of vaccines against metastatic melanoma has been disappointing. However, recent exciting results with adoptive cell transfer therapy offer hope to patients with refractory metastatic melanoma.

TABLE 10-6 • *Summary of Vaccines and Adjuvants*

Melacine is a vaccine developed by Malcolm Mitchell using allogeneic melanoma tumor cell lysate combined with an adjuvant, Detox, which is a monophosphoryl lipid A and mycobacterial cell wall skeleton.
Canvaxin is a vaccine developed by Donald Morton at John Wayne Cancer Center using irradiated allogeneic whole melanoma cell. Bacille Calmette-Guérin (BCG) was the first adjuvant to be used with this polyvalent vaccine.
GMK is one form of gangliosides isolated from bovine brain modified with a keyhole limpet hemocyanin (a natural protein from mollusk). Both compounds are found to increase antigenic responses to haptens, and, thus, they have been used as adjuvants.
QS-21 is a natural product isolated from a soap bark tree; it has immunoadjuvant effects. When combined with a vaccine, this drug enhances the antitumoral antibody and cytotoxic T cell responses to the vaccine.
Sargramostim is a recombinant protein that is chemically identical to endogenous granulocyte-macrophage colony-stimulating factor (GM-CSF).

TABLE 10–7 • *Current Phase III Clinical Trials for Stage IV Metastatic Melanoma*

Title	Sponsor	Open
1. Extended schedule, escalated dose of temozolomide versus dacarbazine	EORTC melanoma group, Schering-Plough	August 2004
2. MDX-010 monotherapy, MDX-010 in combination with a melanoma peptide vaccine monotherapy in an HLA-A2*0201-positive patient	Medarex	September 2004
3. Sargramostim (GM CSF) and peptide	ECOG, NCI, SWOG	March 2002
4. Sorafenib in combination with paclitaxel/ carboplatin versus paclitaxel/carboplatin with a placebo	ECOG, NCI, SWOG	July 2005

(MDX-010 is an antibody to cytotoxic T cell lymphocyte antigen 4 [anti-CTLA4] designed to prevent CTLA-4 from downregulating T cell activation. Sorafenib is a small molecule inhibitor of Raf kinase, which activates the Ras oncogene pathway. Incidentally, it was found that sorafenib also inhibits vascular endothelial growth factor as well as platelet-derived growth factor.

Noncutaneous Melanoma

Ocular melanomas differ from other melanomas in that they do not have access to lymphatic channels and thus metastasize only hematogenously. Characteristically, ocular melanoma metastasizes to the liver, often many years after the initial diagnosis. Small peripheral ocular melanomas, which are defined as 1.0 to 3.0 mm in apical height and between 5.0 and 16.0 mm in diameter, can be treated with partial retinal resection. Larger lesions are treated with enucleation or implanted radiotherapy. A randomized trial conducted by the Collaborative Ocular Melanoma Study Group found no significant survival difference between these two treatments. Disease-specific 5-year survival was 72% to 74%.

Anal and vulvar melanomas often present with inguinal lymph node metastases. Radical surgical resection with abdominoperineal resection or radical vulvectomy has found to be unnecessarily deforming, because it is not associated with improved survival. Thus, the current recommendation is conservative removal of the primary and dissection of any involved regional nodal basins if there is no evidence of distant disease. Some authors suggest a role for SLN biopsy, but there currently is no clinical trial to validate or refute its use. According to the National Cancer Database melanoma study, 5-year survival was 19.8% for anal melanoma and 11.4% for vulvar melanoma.

Nasopharyngeal melanomas are difficult to excise with wide, tumor-free margins. Often, underlying bony structure must be resected to clear the surgical margins. When the margin cannot be cleared, postoperative radiation is used to improve local control. The 5-year survival for these tumors in the National Cancer Database study was 32%.

Melanoma and Pregnancy

Concerning melanoma and pregnancy, melanoma is one of few cancers that can metastasize to the placenta as well as the fetus; thus, it is best for the patient to avoid pregnancy while she has active metastatic or high-risk melanoma. Although a retrospective analysis with stage-matched controls showed that pregnancy does not appear to result in a worse outcome for a patient who was diagnosed with melanoma or developed melanoma during a pregnancy, these cases predominately had localized disease. Young female patients should be counseled regarding the risks of melanoma and pregnancy.

The primary treatment of melanoma during pregnancy remains the same as for the nonpregnant patient: wide excision of the lesion. If possible, surgery should be performed during the second or third trimester. Lymphatic mapping and sentinel node biopsy can be performed safely in the pregnant patient. In our practice, we prefer giving a low dose of radiolabeled isotope and avoiding isosulfan blue altogether to avoid the remote possibility of an anaphylactic reaction that would be harmful to the fetus.

Key Selected Reading

Blackwell PM, Balch CM, Houghton AN, eds. *Cutaneous melanoma,* 4th ed. St. Louis: Quality Medical Publishing, Inc., 2003.

Selected Readings

Balch CM, Buzaid AC, Soong SJ, *et al.* Final version of the American Joint Committee on Cancer staging system for cutaneous melanoma. *J Clin Oncol* 2001;19:3635–3648.

Balch CM, Urist MM, Karakousis CP, *et al.* Efficacy of 2-cm surgical margins for intermediate-thickness melanomas (1 to 4 mm). Results of a multi-institutional randomized surgical trial. *Ann Surg* 1993;218:262-267; discussion 267–269.

Cohn-Cedermark G, Rutqvist LE, Andersson R, *et al.* Long term results of a randomized study by the Swedish Melanoma Study Group on 2-cm versus 5-cm resection margins for patients with cutaneous melanoma with a tumor thickness of 0.8-2.0 mm. *Cancer* 2000;89:1495–1501.

Heaton KM, Sussman JJ, Gershenwald JE, *et al.* Surgical margins and prognostic factors in patients with thick (>4mm) primary melanoma. *Ann Surg Oncol* 1998;5:322–328.

Kirkwood JM, Manola J, Ibrahim J, *et al.* A pooled analysis of eastern cooperative oncology group and intergroup trials of adjuvant high-dose interferon for melanoma. *Clin Cancer Res* 2004;10:1670–1677.

Miller AJ, Mihm MC Jr. Melanoma. *N Engl J Med* 2006;355:51–65.

Rubin AI, Chen EH, Ratner D. Basal-cell carcinoma. *N Engl J Med* 2005;353:2262–2269.

Thompson JF, Scolyer RA, Kefford RF. Cutaneous melanoma. *Lancet* 2005;365: 687–701.

Thompson JF, Scolyer RA, Uren RF. Surgical management of primary cutaneous melanoma: excision margins and the role of sentinel lymph node examination. *Surg Oncol Clin N Am* 2006;15:301–318.

Tsao H, Atkins MB, Sober AJ. Management of cutaneous melanoma. *N Engl J Med* 2004;351:998–1012.

Veronesi U, Cascinelli N, Adamus J, *et al.* Thin stage I primary cutaneous malignant melanoma. Comparison of excision with margins of 1 or 3 cm. *N Engl J Med* 1988;318:1159–1162.

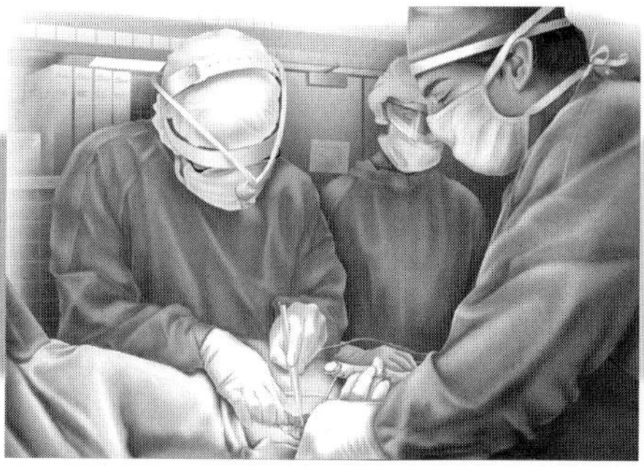

11

Sarcomas of Bone and Soft Tissues

Pamela J. Hodul and Vernon K. Sondak

SOFT-TISSUE SARCOMAS
BONE SARCOMAS
CHILDHOOD SARCOMAS
METASTATIC SARCOMA

Sarcomas of Bone and Soft Tissues: Key Points

- Describe the incidence, epidemiology, genetic connections, and diagnosis of soft-tissue sarcomas in general.
- Detail the evaluation, staging, and prognosis of soft-tissue sarcomas.
- Discuss the histologic types of soft-tissue sarcomas.
- List the therapeutic goals for the treatment of soft-tissue sarcomas.
- Review the findings and treatment for retroperitoneal sarcoma and gastrointestinal stromal tumors.
- Describe the clinical presentation, diagnosis, surgery, and staging for bone sarcomas.
- Outline the pertinent facts concerning rhabdomyosarcoma and Ewing's sarcoma in children.
- Discuss the management of metastatic sarcoma.

Sarcomas are a heterogeneous group of tumors composed of cells of mesenchymal origin. They are classified as either soft-tissue or bone sarcomas. The location in which these tumors originate contributes to their variable presentation, treatment algorithms, and outcome. Despite the fact that soft tissues and bone comprise almost two thirds of the mass of the human body, sarcomas are uncommon tumors, accounting for less than 1% of adult and about 15% of pediatric malignancies. Because of the relative rarity of sarcomas as compared with benign soft-tissue tumors, they often present as challenging cases for physicians who are less familiar with their diagnosis and management. The goal of this chapter is to familiarize the reader with the approach to and treatment of the most commonly recognized soft-tissue and bone sarcomas.

Soft-Tissue Sarcomas

Incidence and Epidemiology

The annual incidence of soft-tissue sarcomas in the United States is an estimated 9530 new cases, with 3500 deaths annually. Soft-tissue sarcomas can occur anywhere in the body, but most originate in the extremities (60%), the trunk (15%), the retroperitoneum (15%), and the head and neck region (10%). There is no obvious gender or racial predilection. In general, soft-tissue sarcomas do not result from the malignant degeneration of benign soft-tissue tumors but rather from inherited or spontaneous genetic alterations within mesenchymal cells that result in malignancy. Environmental or genetic factors may be related to the development of soft-tissue sarcomas, but the majority arise without a well-defined etiology. Risk factors associated with the development of sarcomas include exposure to ionizing radiation and occupational substances, including vinyl chloride, arsenic, and possibly herbicides (Table 11-1). Lymphedema as a result of surgery, radiation therapy, or congenital or infectious etiologies (filariasis) is associated with the development of lymphangiosarcoma. Stewart-Treves syndrome is the development of lymphangiosarcoma arising in chronic lymphedema associated with radical mastectomy. In addition, human immunodeficiency virus and human herpesvirus-8 viruses have been implicated in the pathogenesis of Kaposi's sarcoma.

The majority of sarcoma patients present with localized disease; fewer than 10% of patients demonstrate evidence of metastasis on initial evaluation. The dominant pattern of metastasis is hematogenous. Extraabdominal sarcomas most commonly metastasize to the lungs. Retroperitoneal sarcomas and gastrointestinal stromal tumors (GISTs) tend to metastasize to the liver. Lymph node metastasis is rare (<5% of cases), and it is associated with specific histologic subtypes, including epithelioid, clear cell, and embryonal sarcomas as well as rhabdomyosarcomas, synovial sarcomas, and angiosarcomas.

TABLE 11-1 • *Risk Factors for Sarcoma*

Risk Factors	Associated Sarcoma Type
Genetic	
Neurofibromatosis type I (von Recklinghausen's disease)	Malignant peripheral nerve sheath tumor
Retinoblastoma	All
Li-Fraumeni syndrome	All
Gardner's syndrome	Desmoid tumor
Werner's syndrome	Soft-tissue sarcoma
Gorlin's syndrome	Fibrosarcoma, rhabdomyosarcoma
Carney's Triad	Gastrointestinal stromal tumor
Bourneville disease (tuberous sclerosis)	Rhabdomyosarcoma
Beckwith-Wiedemann syndrome	Rhabdomyosarcoma
Cardiofaciocutaneous syndrome	Rhabdomyosarcoma
Radiation	All
Lymphedema (Stewart-Treves syndrome)	Lymphangiosarcoma
Chemical Agents	
Phenoxy herbicides (controversial)	All
Dioxin (Agent Orange) (controversial)	Soft-tissue sarcoma
Thorotrast	Hepatic angiosarcoma
Vinyl chloride	Hepatic angiosarcoma
Arsenic	Hepatic angiosarcoma
Viral	
Human immunodeficiency virus	Kaposi's sarcoma
Human herpesvirus-8	Kaposi's sarcoma

BOX 11-1 SARCOMAS ASSOCIATED WITH A HIGHER RISK OF LYMPH NODE METASTASES

- Clear cell sarcoma
- Epithelioid sarcoma
- Embryonal rhabdomyosarcoma
- Synovial sarcoma
- Lymphangiosarcoma
- Angiosarcoma

Genetics

There is a high incidence of acquired gene alterations in soft-tissue sarcomas. Sarcomas can be separated into two types, depending on the specificity of the genetic alteration. Sarcomas with specific genetic alterations are exemplified by Ewing's sarcoma and gastrointestinal stromal tumors. Ewing's sarcoma possesses a specific gene translocation (EWS-FLI-1 fusion), which is principally responsible for tumor proliferation and transformation. Gastrointestinal stromal tumors are associated with a specific point mutation in the KIT oncogene, resulting in the constitutive activation of a tyrosine kinase receptor and subsequent tumor growth. Alterations in tumor suppressor genes, such as the retinoblastoma gene (Rb) and p53, are found in multiple sarcoma types and are therefore considered nonspecific genetic alterations. Examples of sarcomas with frequent mutations in these tumor suppressor genes include osteosarcoma, malignant fibrous histiocytoma, liposarcoma, angiosarcoma, and leiomyosarcoma. Oncogenes have also been implicated in the development of soft-tissue sarcomas and include MDM2, N-myc, c-erbB2, and the ras oncogene family. For example, MDM2 amplification in tumor cells negatively regulates the function of the tumor suppressor gene, p53. Sarcomas commonly have abnormalities of either p53 or MDM2, but they almost never have abnormalities of both.

Several genetic conditions are associated with an increased risk for the development of soft-tissue sarcomas. Patients with neurofibromatosis type I (von Recklinghausen's disease) have a 2% to 10% lifetime risk of developing a neurofibrosarcoma, also called malignant peripheral nerve sheath tumor or MPNST. Familial retinoblastoma (Rb gene mutation) and Li-Fraumeni syndrome (p53 mutation) are examples of genetic susceptibility syndromes in which affected individuals are at increased risk for developing a second primary sarcoma as well as other cancers. Familial adenomatous polyposis is an autosomal dominant syndrome that results from a germline mutation in the adenomatous polyposis coli gene, and it is associated with the development of colonic polyps and colon cancer. One phenotypic variant, Gardner's syndrome, describes the additional presentation of soft-tissue tumors and bone abnormalities. Approximately 15% of individuals with familial adenomatous polyposis develop desmoid tumors, which are nonmetastatic, locally aggressive, fibroblastic tumors.

Clinical Presentation

Soft-tissue sarcomas most commonly present as an asymptomatic mass, although pain is noted in up to a third of cases. Often patients are incorrectly diagnosed as having a "pulled muscle" or "chronic hematoma," which may delay the diagnosis and treatment for several months. When a soft-tissue mass arises in a patient with no history of trauma, persists for more than 6 weeks, or changes in size or presenting symptoms, further evaluation is warranted. Tumors in the proximal extremities and the retroperitoneum can become quite large before they become symptomatic. Progressive growth of these tumors can compress surrounding normal structures, resulting in pain, swelling, and neurologic symptoms (Figure 11-1). In the case of retroperitoneal tumors, bowel obstruction and hydronephrosis may become evident (Figure 11-2).

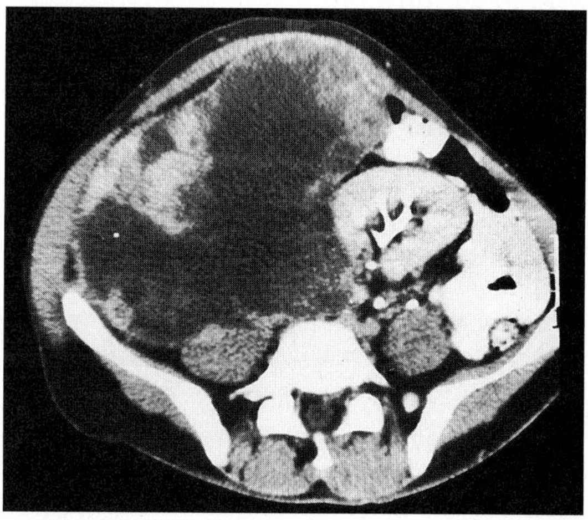

Figure 11-1. Right midabdominal sarcoma displacing the right kidney. (From Bland KI, Karakousis CP, Copeland EM III, eds. *Atlas of surgical oncology*. Philadelphia: WB Saunders, 1995.)

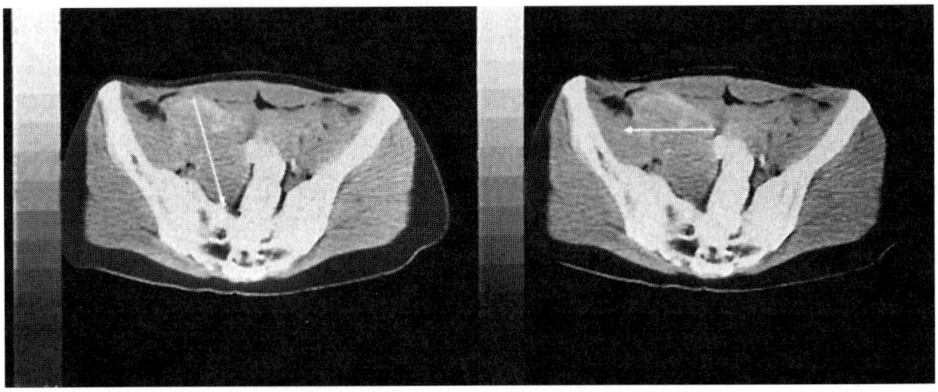

Figure 11–2. Fibrosarcoma involving the wall of the right pelvis and causing obstruction of the right ureter. (From Bland KI, Karakousis CP, Copeland EM III, eds. *Atlas of surgical oncology*. Philadelphia: WB Saunders, 1995.)

BOX 11–2 PRESENTING SYMPTOMS OF SOFT-TISSUE SARCOMAS

- Trunk/extremity
  - Mass (may be painful or asymptomatic)
  - Compressive symptoms (swelling, neurologic symptoms)
- Retroperitoneal
  - Abdominal discomfort
  - Early satiety
  - Abdominal mass
  - Bowel obstruction
  - Hydronephrosis

Biopsy Techniques

Unfortunately, physical examination is unreliable for distinguishing benign tumors from their malignant counterparts, and biopsy is often indicated. A properly performed and timely biopsy is a critical first step in ensuring early diagnosis and treatment. The choice of biopsy technique is determined by the location and size of the mass and according to the experience of the pathologist (Table 11-2).

Fine-Needle Aspiration Biopsy

Fine-needle aspiration uses a fine-gauge needle to sample tumor cells within the soft-tissue mass. Interpretation of these results requires a cytopathologist who has experience with soft-tissue sarcomas. The limited number of cells within a given sample can make a specific sarcoma diagnosis challenging. The accuracy of fine-needle aspiration ranges from 60% to 96% in the hands of an experienced cytopathologist. Fine-needle aspiration is relatively atraumatic and can be performed under ultrasound or computed tomography (CT) guidance. The fine-needle aspiration minimizes the formation of hematomas and tumor cell tracking, which are often observed with open biopsy techniques. Fine-needle aspiration is generally the preferred method for documenting a potential metastatic focus or local recurrence.

Core Needle Biopsy

Core needle biopsy yields a thin sliver of tissue that can be used for standard histopathology, electron microscopy, cytoge-

TABLE 11–2 • *Biopsy Techniques for Soft-Tissue Masses*

Biopsy Technique	Most Useful For	Comments
Fine-needle aspiration	Suspected metastasis or recurrence	Requires experienced cytopathologist; rarely enough cells to diagnose a specific subtype
Core needle biopsy	Biopsy of choice for primary soft-tissue masses	May require imaging guidance
Incisional biopsy	When core biopsy is nondiagnostic	Orient incision allowing for subsequent wide local excision; ensure hemostasis
Excisional biopsy	Small, superficial lesions	Orient incision allowing for subsequent wide local excision; ensure hemostasis

netic analysis, and flow cytometry. Histologic subtype and grade can be correctly determined in more than 90% of cases. CT-guided core needle biopsies for deep extremity or retroperitoneal sarcomas are obtained with minimal morbidity.

Incisional Biopsy

A generous sample of tissue can be acquired from an open incisional biopsy. This technique, however, should usually be reserved for cases in which fine-needle aspiration or core needle biopsy is nondiagnostic. If an incisional biopsy is indicated, several principles should be followed. The biopsy incision should be placed directly over the tumor and oriented longitudinally along the extremity to allow for subsequent wide local excision. For truncal or retroperitoneal sarcomas, incisional biopsy should be performed so that the biopsy tract can be resected along with the primary tumor after the diagnosis of sarcoma is made. Adequate hemostasis at the time of biopsy is important for preventing the spread of tumor cells along tissue planes contaminated by hematoma.

Excisional Biopsy

Removal of all gross tumor without a significant margin constitutes an excisional biopsy. This type of biopsy should generally be reserved for small or superficial lesions. Excision of larger or deeper lesions can lead to complications, including hematoma and contamination of surrounding tissue planes with microscopic tumor.

Preoperative Evaluation

Physical examination is important when planning the treatment of sarcomas. The size of the tumor, its fixation to adjacent structures, and the relationship of the tumor to the biopsy site are important to document. For extremity sarcomas in particular, a thorough functional and neurovascular examination can be crucial for determining whether limb salvage therapy or amputation is indicated (Figure 11-3). Lymph node involvement is noted in fewer than 5% of cases, but it should be assessed by physical examination.

Radiologic imaging is critical for preoperative diagnosis, for treatment planning, and for detecting recurrence after surgical resection (Figure 11-4). CT and magnetic resonance imaging (MRI) are the most important radiologic studies for assessing the extent and resectability of soft-tissue sarcomas (Figure 11-5). The choice between them is based primarily on availability, cost, and the experience of the radiologist. When considering the advantages and disadvantages of each modality, the choice of radiographic study should be tailored to each case.

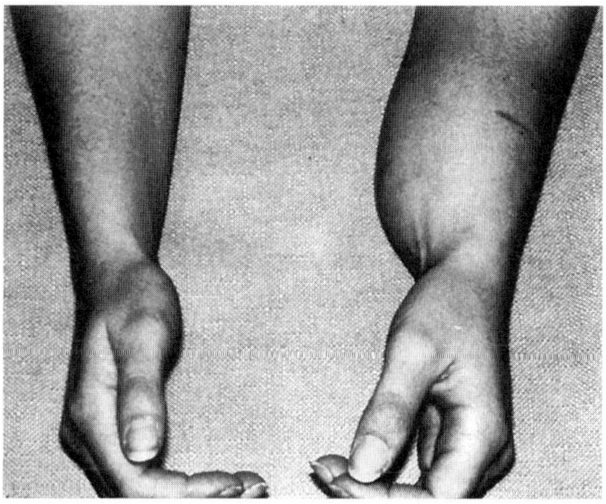

Figure 11-3. Large soft-tissue sarcoma of the volar aspect of the right forearm. (From Bland KI, Karakousis CP, Copeland EM III, eds. *Atlas of surgical oncology*. Philadelphia: WB Saunders, 1995.)

CT is the preferred imaging technique for evaluating the local extent of retroperitoneal sarcomas. Information regarding the involvement of critical vascular structures and adjacent organs aids in treatment planning before surgical intervention. Liver metastases, which are most commonly associated with retroperitoneal and intraabdominal sarcomas, are readily diagnosed using CT scanning.

MRI is the preferred imaging technique for soft-tissue sarcomas of the extremity. It accurately defines muscle compartment involvement, and it delineates tumor from bone and neurovascular structures. Furthermore, characteristics of the tumor on MRI may distinguish benign lesions such as lipoma, hemangioma, or myxoma from their malignant counterparts. MRI also has the advantage of reconstructing coronal, sagittal, and even oblique planes, which are sometimes useful when planning therapy.

The thoracic cavity is the most common location for metastases originating from primary

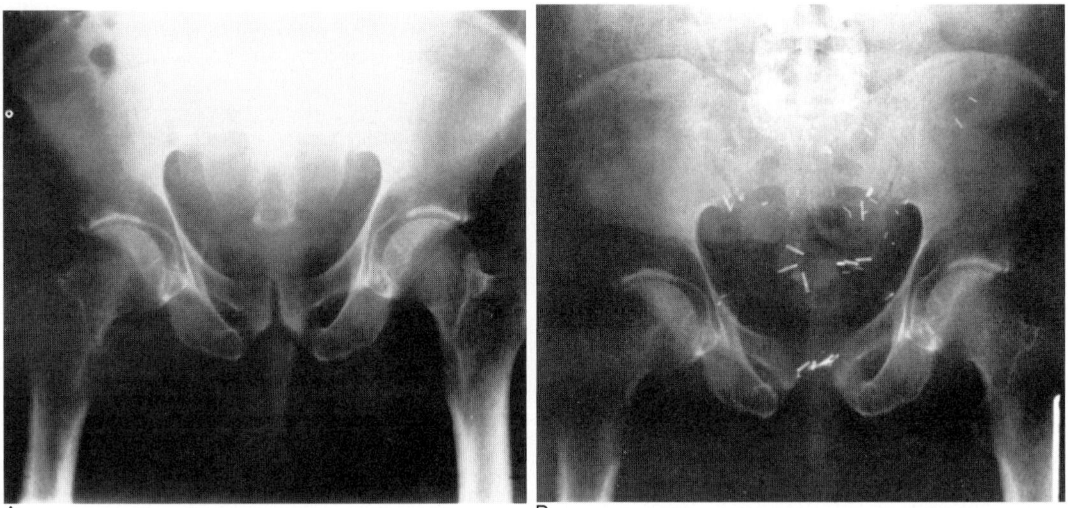
A B

Figure 11-4. A, Preoperative x-ray of the pelvis. **B,** Postoperative x-ray shows the separation of the pubic symphysis, which allows distal exposure and removal of the sarcoma. (From Bland KI, Karakousis CP, Copeland EM III, eds. *Atlas of surgical oncology*. Philadelphia: WB Saunders, 1995.)

sarcomas of the extremities. As part of the initial staging workup for distant metastases, a chest radiograph should be performed. CT of the chest should be considered for patients with high-grade lesions or tumors larger than 5 cm because these patients are at increased risk for pulmonary metastases.

Additional studies are occasionally helpful when formulating a treatment strategy. Angiography may provide useful information about the proximity of the tumor to major vessels; however, similar information can often be obtained from specially sequenced MR images. Plain radiographs or bone scans are sometimes useful for determining cortical bone destruction or bone metastasis and for differentiating a primary bone sarcoma from a soft-tissue mass.

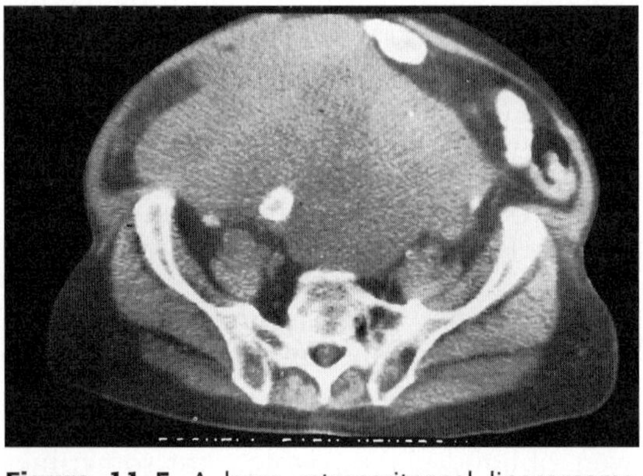

Figure 11-5. A large retroperitoneal liposarcoma. (From Bland KI, Karakousis CP, Copeland EM III, eds. *Atlas of surgical oncology*. Philadelphia: WB Saunders, 1995.)

Staging and Prognosis

The staging of soft-tissue extremity sarcomas is important for defining the extent of disease, and it helps to guide treatment and predict outcome. The current American Joint Committee on Cancer staging system for soft-tissue sarcomas is based on histologic grade, size of the primary tumor, lymph node status, and the presence or absence of metastases (Table 11-3). Of these, histologic grade is the most important prognostic factor for a clinically localized sarcoma. Grade is determined histologically on the basis of the degree of differentiation, the number of mitosis, and the extent of spontaneous tumor necrosis. Several grading systems have been developed based on a two-, three-, or four-tiered system. In the three-tier system, well-differentiated, low-grade sarcomas are designated as grade 1, moderately differentiated (intermediate-grade) sarcomas as grade 2, and poorly differentiated (high-grade) lesions as grade 3. The three-tiered system is favored by most pathologists and clinicians, because intermediate and high-grade sarcomas clearly do have different outcomes. In the four-tier system, grades 1 and 2 (well to moderately differentiated) are considered low-grade, whereas

TABLE 11-3 • American Joint Committee on Cancer Staging System for Soft-Tissue Sarcomas

Primary Tumor (T)				
T1	Tumor ≤ 5 cm			
	T1a Superficial tumor			
	T1b Deep tumor			
T2	Tumor > 5 cm			
	T2a Superficial tumor			
	T2b Deep tumor			
Regional Lymph Nodes (N)				
N0	No regional lymph node metastasis			
N1	Regional lymph node metastasis			
Distant Metastasis (M)				
M0	No distant metastasis			
M1	Distant metastasis			
Histologic Grade (G)				
G1	Well differentiated			
G2	Moderately differentiated			
G3	Poorly differentiated			
G4	Poorly differentiated or undifferentiated			
Stage Grouping				
Stage I	G1-2	T1a, 1b, 2a, 2b	N0	M0
Stage II	G3-4	G3-4T1a, 1b, 2a	N0	M0
Stage III	G3-4	T2b	N0	M0
Stage IV	Any G	Any T	N1	M0
	Any G	Any T	N0	M1

Greene FL, Page DL, Fleming FD, *et al.* eds. *American Joint Committee on Cancer: cancer staging manual,* 6th ed. New York: Springer, 2002:221–226.

grades 3 and 4 are reserved for poorly differentiated and undifferentiated lesions, respectively, and considered high-grade. The two-tiered grading system collapses the four-grade system into low-grade and high-grade tiers only. For practical purposes, most clinical decisions are made based on considering soft-tissue sarcomas to be either low- or high-grade, with intermediate-grade tumors treated in the same way as high-grade ones.

Soft-tissue sarcomas are further classified by size and relationship to the investing fascia of the extremity or trunk. A T1 lesion is a tumor that is 5 cm or smaller, whereas a T2 tumor is larger than 5 cm. Patients with larger tumors, especially those 10 cm or greater, have been found to have poorer 5-year survival rates. The "a" designation signifies a tumor superficial to muscular fascia, while the "b" designation attached to or below the fascia. Lymph node metastases are rare, occurring in less than 5% of the cases. When lymph node involvement is present, it is a poor prognostic finding, and it is classified as stage IV disease. As mentioned previously, histologic subtypes such as epithelioid sarcoma, angiosarcoma, clear cell sarcoma, rhabdomyosarcoma, and synovial cell sarcoma have a higher incidence of lymph node metastases (10% to 15%). Lung metastases are most commonly associated with sarcomas of the extremity. Other sites of metastatic disease include the bone, brain, and liver; the last is a frequent occurrence with retroperitoneal sarcomas.

Histologic Types

Malignant Fibrous Histiocytoma

Malignant fibrous histiocytoma (MFH) is the most common soft-tissue sarcoma in adults. It generally occurs later in life, and it is more frequently found in men than in women. It most commonly presents as a soft-tissue mass arising within the deep tissues. Histologically, a broad range of appearances are present, depending on the distinct subtype and degree of differentiation. The very existence of this common histologic type as a separate entity has been questioned, with some pathologists contending that tumors called MFH are really poorly differentiated examples of other sarcoma subtypes, lacking the distinctive differentiation patterns that would permit ready classification into the proper histologic type. Recent developments in genetic analysis have supported this contention, because they do not show MFH tumors to segregate as genetically distinct tumors in the way that many other types do.

Liposarcoma

Liposarcoma is the second most common soft-tissue sarcoma in adults. Liposarcomas are a heterogeneous group of tumors with several distinct subtypes, some of which may coexist in the same tumor. Well-differentiated liposarcomas are often difficult to distinguish both radiographically and histologically from benign lipomas. Findings of prominent septae formation on MRI are suggestive of malignancy in a large fatty mass. Liposarcomas are often found growing in between and through muscle compartments, and complete resection can be challenging. Dedifferentiated liposarcomas are of high grade and are frequently found in the abdominal cavity. The myxoid liposarcoma is an intermediate-grade form that is commonly associated with extrapulmonary metastases and microscopically defined by a rich, fine network of capillaries. The pleomorphic subtype of liposarcoma is a particularly aggressive sarcoma.

Leiomyosarcoma

Leiomyosarcomas commonly present as deep-seated masses or as an occasional subcutaneous nodule, most often during the fourth to sixth decade of life. The proximal extremity, the retroperitoneum, and the trunk are the most common sites of presentation. Microscopically, elongated fibroblast-like cells in a uniform growth pattern are present. These tumors may also arise in association with large blood vessels, resulting in symptoms of vascular obstruction.

Dermatofibrosarcoma Protuberans

Dermatofibrosarcoma protuberans is a nodular, subcutaneous mass that appears plaque-like, with either a bluish or violaceous hue. It infiltrates through the dermis and, if left neglected, can become fungating. Microscopically, spindle-shaped cells with low mitotic activity and storiform growth pattern are present. Malignant transformation to fibrosarcoma or MFH has been reported. Up to 50% recur after incomplete excision and may result in the extensive invasion of adjacent structures. Complete resection should be curative, however, because metastasis is an extremely rare event in nontransformed dermatofibrosarcoma protuberans.

Rhabdomyosarcoma

Rhabdomyosarcoma is the most common primary soft-tissue sarcoma in children, accounting for 20% of all solid childhood malignancies. It is most frequently found in the head and neck region, followed by the genitourinary system. Only 15% of rhabdomyosarcomas occur in the extremities. Four histologic subtypes exist, with the embryonal type being the most common. Microscopically, eosinophilic cytoplasm and cross striations are present. Cells stain positive for desmin, actin, and myogenin by immunohistochemistry. Survival data for adults are limited, but available data demonstrate a worse prognosis in adults as compared with children.

Synovial Sarcoma

Synovial sarcoma is commonly found in adolescent and younger adult patients. It can occur around joints, but it rarely originates within them. It is the most common sarcoma of the foot. Radiographically, one third of patients will have mineralization present on plain film.

Angiosarcoma

Angiosarcomas may arise in either blood or lymphatic vessels, and they have been linked to several predisposing conditions. Chronic lymphedema predisposing to lymphangiosarcoma in postmastectomy patients is known as the Stewart-Treves syndrome. Irradiation, particularly for breast cancer treatment, is also associated with the formation of angiosarcomas. Vinyl chloride and arsenic exposure have been linked to angiosarcomas in the liver. These lesions tend to be aggressive, with both lymphatic and hematogenous metastases.

Kaposi's Sarcoma

Classic Kaposi's sarcoma is an unusual vascular tumor commonly found in elderly men of Mediterranean or Jewish descent. The disease's course is usually indolent, and lesions are commonly located on the extremities; symptomatic lesions respond to palliative radiation therapy. Epidemic Kaposi's sarcoma is associated with human herpesvirus-8 infection and is a complication of human immunodeficiency virus (HIV) infection. It is a multicentric tumor that arises simultaneously in several sites. Microscopically, these tumors are characterized by a predominance of spindle-shaped cells thought to be derived from lymphatic endothelial cells. Unlike most sarcomas, surgical excision is rarely the best choice for the management of AIDS-related Kaposi's sarcoma. Local therapies such as photodynamic therapy, topical chemotherapy, and radiation therapy may be useful for localized disease; antiretrovirus therapy is considered essential for treating AIDS-related Kaposi's sarcoma.

Malignant Peripheral Nerve Sheath Tumors

Malignant peripheral nerve sheath tumors (MPNSTs), which are also known as *neurofibrosarcomas, malignant schwannomas,* or *neurogenic sarcomas,* involve nerves of the trunk and extremities, and they typically affect adults during the third to fifth decade of life. This tumor is characteristically high grade, and it likely originates from the nerve sheath rather than the nerve fiber itself. The development of neurofibromas is a characteristic of von Recklinghausen's disease neurofibromatosis type I (NF1). Up to 10% of patients with NF1 eventually develop MPNSTs.

Treatment

When considering the appropriate modality of therapy for soft-tissue sarcomas of the extremity, several therapeutic goals must be kept in mind: optimal functional outcome, limited morbidity, improved survival, and avoidance of local recurrence. A multimodality approach is often required to maximize the benefit as compared with surgical resection alone (Figure 11-6).

Surgery

Surgery is the primary treatment modality for nearly all patients with localized sarcomas of the extremity or elsewhere. Their risk of local recurrence increases nearly threefold with inadequate margins. Thus, complete en bloc resection of the primary tumor with adjacent normal tissue is the goal whenever possible.

Limb-sparing surgery consisting of wide local excision with or without radiation therapy is the standard treatment for patients with extremity soft-tissue sarcoma. Local control rates with limb-sparing surgery are comparable with amputation, and survival is equivalent. Wide excision requires en bloc resection through normal tissue beyond the reactive zone but within the muscular compartment of origin. A margin of 3 to 5 cm of normal tissue is obtained both proximally and distally. This resection involves the removal of some overlying skin so as to include all previous biopsy sites or incisional scars. To achieve adequate lateral and deep margins, at least one grossly uninvolved fascial plane is resected with the tumor. If necessary, major neurovascular structures may be resected and appropriately reconstructed to preserve limb function. Titanium clips are strategically placed to outline the limits of excision to assist the radiation oncologist with adjuvant treatment.

Compartmental excisions are reserved for those tumors occupying an anatomically defined muscular compartment or for some cases in which radiation therapy is contraindicated. Resection comprises an en bloc removal of the tumor with excision of the compartmental muscles from origin to insertion. The resection of major neurovascular structures may be required, and a functional deficit can be expected depending on the compartment sacrificed.

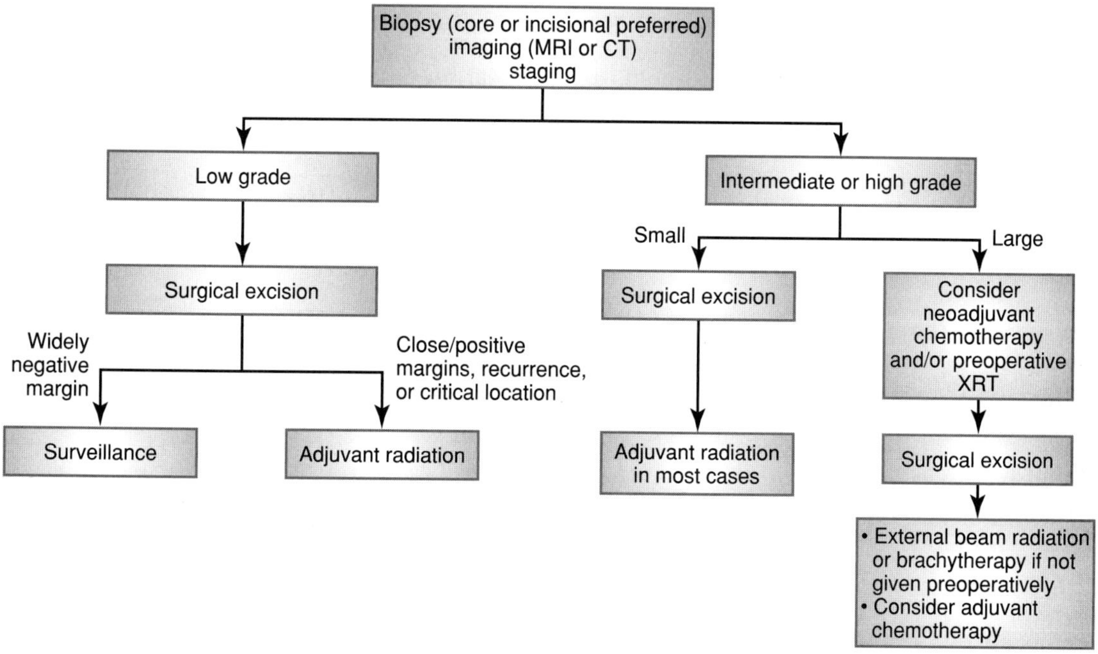

Figure 11-6. Management of soft-tissue sarcomas.

Amputation for the treatment of extremity sarcomas is indicated for less than 5% of cases. Resection usually requires the disarticulation of the joint proximal to the involved compartment with removal of the entire compartment at risk. Radical amputation is currently reserved for patients who are not suitable candidates for limb-sparing surgery. General indications for amputation include anticipated inadequate limb function after wide local excision or compartmental resection, large size or multicompartmental involvement of the tumor, and encasement of bone or major neurovascular structures without potential for reconstruction. In general, patients requiring amputation for adequate resection and local control tend to have sarcomas with poor prognostic features and tumors that are not amenable to alternative surgical options.

Fundamental surgical principles apply to the resection of extremity soft-tissue sarcomas. Tumors are resected en bloc with an adjacent margin of normal tissue, with special attention given to not disrupting the tumor pseudocapsule. Disruption of the pseudocapsule increases the risk of local recurrence. Rarely does nerve or bone involvement require the removal of these vital structures. Incisions are made along the length of the extremity and localized over the soft-tissue mass. Patients who have been resected but have known positive margins should undergo re-resection if at all possible. Re-resection should include excision of the existing scar with en bloc resection of the underlying soft-tissue cavity. Local recurrences should be treated with surgical resection when possible.

Radiation Therapy

Radiation in combination with surgical resection achieves better outcomes than either modality alone. Similar rates of disease-free and overall survival have been reported for patients treated with amputation or the combination of limb-sparing surgery and radiation therapy for extremity soft-tissue sarcomas.

External beam radiation therapy can be administered in either the neoadjuvant (preoperative) or adjuvant (postoperative) setting (Table 11-4). Retrospective series report similar rates of local control and disease-specific survival. Preoperative radiation therapy is often favored for large (>5 cm), high-grade, or deep extremity sarcomas. Complications related to radiation therapy can occur both early and late in relation to treatment. Acute wound healing complications and late toxicity and fibrosis are commonly encountered and can adversely affect long-term functional outcome and quality of life.

Brachytherapy involves the placement of afterloading catheters at 1-cm intervals within the operative tumor bed. Maximal radiation can be directed within a particular region with minimal effects on surrounding tissues. This approach is technically complex and requires that an experienced radiation specialist be present in the operating room. No randomized trials comparing the efficacy of brachytherapy and external beam radiation therapy have been reported, but the addition of either brachytherapy or external beam radiation to surgery appears to improve local control rates in high-grade sarcomas to a similar degree. Brachytherapy, with its short overall exposure time of the tumor to the radiation, may be less efficacious for low-grade sarcomas.

Chemotherapy

Controversy surrounds the use of systemic chemotherapy for the treatment of extremity

TABLE 11-4 • *Preoperative Versus Postoperative Radiation Therapy*

Advantages	Disadvantages
Preoperative	
• Facilitates planning and tissue sparing • May minimize visceral injury for retroperitoneal sarcomas • May increase chance of limb sparing	• Requires careful coordination • More wound complications • May require flap closure
Postoperative	
• Better wound healing • X-ray therapy dose can be based on margin status	• Larger volumes need to be treated • Possible increased late tissue morbidity

soft-tissue sarcomas. Several reports suggest that doxorubicin-based therapies such as MAID (mesna, doxorubicin, ifosfamide, and dacarbazine) may improve local control and distant recurrence-free and overall survival. Some other studies, however, report no significant differences between patients treated with adjuvant doxorubicin-based chemotherapy and those treated with local therapy alone. Patients with large, high-grade, soft-tissue sarcomas or those facing amputation should be considered for aggressive neoadjuvant chemotherapy. Significant responses may occur, with the potential for limb-sparing surgery. Additionally, patients with locally aggressive tumors and increased risk for recurrence and metastases should be considered for clinical trials.

Special Situations

Retroperitoneal Sarcoma Retroperitoneal sarcomas account for about 15% of all sarcomas. The most common histologic types include liposarcoma and leiomyosarcoma. Abdominal fullness and vague gastrointestinal complaints typically prompt workup by CT scanning, and findings of a large soft-tissue extravisceral mass are generally evident. Differential diagnosis of retroperitoneal sarcoma includes lymphoma or a primary or metastatic germ cell tumor. Laboratory tests including a β-hCG and an α-fetoprotein level may be indicated to exclude germ-cell tumors, particularly in young males.

Complete resection is the first-line treatment for retroperitoneal sarcomas, either primary or recurrent. Complete resection entails the removal of all gross tumor, including an intact pseudocapsule, and en bloc resection of adherent organs. The most frequently removed organs include the kidney, the colon, and the pancreas. Partial resection or debulking procedures do not lead to a survival benefit for the patient and should generally be avoided. Primary lesions are more likely to be completely resectable than recurrent disease. Up to 80% of primary lesions can be completely resected, as compared with around 50% of first recurrences and 30% of second recurrences. Limiting factors of surgical resection include the involvement of major vascular structures, peritoneal seeding, and distant metastases.

The use of chemotherapy and radiation for retroperitoneal sarcomas is even more controversial than in extremity primaries. In circumstances in which large primary sarcomas are being considered for surgical resection, neoadjuvant chemoradiation has been used in an attempt to improve chances for complete resection. Several chemotherapy agents, including doxorubicin, ifosfamide, and cisplatin, have been used in this setting. Chemoradiation in the adjuvant setting is advocated for patients with a high likelihood for local recurrence. Overall prognosis for patients with nonmetastatic disease is strongly influenced by the completeness of the surgical resection and the histologic grade of the tumor. Some investigators have also found that large tumors (>10 cm) and fixation to adjacent organs adversely affect survival. Five-year actuarial survival rates for patients with completely resected retroperitoneal sarcomas are 54% to 64%. Patients with locally recurrent and metastatic disease have median disease-specific survivals of 28 months and 10 months, respectively.

Gastrointestinal Stromal Tumor GIST is the most common mesenchymal tumor of the gastrointestinal tract. Traditionally, spindle-cell tumors of the gastrointestinal tract were referred to as *leiomyomas, leiomyosarcomas,* or *autonomic nerve tumors*. More recently, the discovery of a shared cellular antigen (KIT protein) has refined the classification of these tumors. GISTs express KIT protein and CD34, both of which are also associated with the interstitial cells of Cajal in the gastrointestinal tract. Mutations in the KIT oncogene result in constitutive activation of the KIT receptor tyrosine kinase and uncontrolled cellular growth. KIT positivity as detected by immunohistochemical staining is a defining characteristic establishing diagnosis, although KIT-negative GISTs do exist.

GISTs account for less than 3% of all gastrointestinal tract neoplasms and 5% of all sarcomas. Because most GISTs develop submucosally, diagnosis can be difficult before surgery.

GISTs exhibit highly variable behavior, and their characteristics at diagnosis are important with regard to prognosis. Aggressive tumors with an increased risk for recurrence and metastases include those that are symptomatic, those that are larger than 5 cm, and those that demonstrate a high mitotic rate (>1-5 per 10 high-power fields). Although they are often called "benign," small GISTs tumors with low mitotic rates have been found to recur or to metastasize after resection. Metastases develop most frequently in the liver, the peritoneum, or the omentum, and local recurrences are common. Therefore, long-term follow-up is warranted for all patients, and it is not clear whether any GISTs are truly "benign" as opposed to being low-grade malignancies.

Surgical resection is the first-line treatment for GISTs. Complete resection with negative margins is the most significant factor for determining outcome and overall prognosis. En bloc resection of the tumor and its pseudocapsule should be performed when feasible; wide margins are not necessary. Surgical resection may vary from a simple wedge resection for a gastric GIST to radical resection of a GIST with the removal of contiguous organs. Because GISTs metastasize either hematogenously or by tumor seeding and not through the lymphatic system, extensive lymphadenectomy is not indicated. Avoidance of tumor rupture is crucial for the performance of curative resection. Five-year survival rates of 42% and 9% have been reported for patients who had complete resections as compared with those who had incomplete resections, respectively.

Establishing the molecular pathogenesis of GISTs has paved the way for the development of new chemotherapeutic agents with specific cellular targets. Imatinib is an orally bioavailable compound that effectively and selectively inhibits the KIT receptor, thereby inhibiting proliferation and provoking apoptosis. Imatinib is currently available for use in the treatment of KIT-positive malignant metastatic or unresectable GISTs. Trials are presently underway to evaluate the usefulness of imatinib in the neoadjuvant and adjuvant settings.

Bone Sarcomas

Clinical Presentation and Diagnosis

Primary bone sarcomas are uncommon, and they present unique challenges in terms of diagnosis and treatment. Osteosarcomas and chondrosarcomas are the most frequently occurring bone sarcomas and will be the focus of further discussion.

Pain is the usual presenting symptom among patients with large aggressive and destructive bone tumors. Pain at night or at rest is particularly concerning and mandates further investigation. Deformity or limited range of motion may be present with lesions near or involving a joint. Pathologic fractures occur in up to 10% of patients with osteosarcoma during the course of their disease.

BOX 11–3 CLINICAL SYMPTOMS ASSOCIATED WITH BONE TUMORS

- Pain and swelling
- Deformity
- Limited range of motion
- Pathologic fracture

Preoperative evaluation is important for establishing a tissue diagnosis and assessing the extent of disease. Although plain radiographs often confirm the findings diagnosed on physical examination, such as soft-tissue swelling and mass, MRI is superior for determining the size of the tumor and the extent of intraosseous or extraosseous involvement; it is particularly helpful for planning surgical treatment. Radionuclide bone scanning is an important adjunct for determining distant metastases to other bones and for defining skip lesions within the bone of origin; bone scans, however, are limited by a lack of specificity and sensitivity. CT scans of the thorax are important for determining the presence or absence of metastatic lung disease, because 80% of metastatic lesions in osteosarcoma occur in the lungs.

Biopsy of a bone tumor is required in cases in which histologic distinction may alter the planned course of treatment or when radiographic diagnosis cannot determine the benign or malignant nature of the lesion. If a biopsy is to be undertaken, similar principles to those used for soft-tissue sarcomas are followed. Open biopsies should be performed with an incision oriented longitudinally and in a manner such that the entire biopsy tract

BOX 11–4 FEATURES USED TO EVALUATE BONE TUMORS ON IMAGING

- Anatomic site (e.g., metaphyseal vs. diaphyseal)
- Borders (well-defined vs. poorly delineated)
- Soft-tissue extension
- Bone destruction (geographic vs. moth-eaten vs. permeative)
- Matrix formation (calcification, ossification)
- Periosteal reaction

can be excised during later definitive surgery. The importance of obtaining adequate hemostasis must be stressed, because hematoma can permit the spread of tumor cells into adjacent compartments. Core biopsies are preferable to open biopsies and can be performed at the bedside or with the aid of ultrasonic or CT guidance. Biopsy tracks should traverse only one compartment, they should avoid neurovascular structures and joints, and they should be placed along the planned course of resection. Biopsies require interpretation by an experienced pathologist for accurate diagnosis, and they should ideally be performed at the institution at which definitive treatment will be performed.

Staging

The preferred staging system for primary bone sarcomas is the Enneking staging system, which is based on surgical principles (Table 11-5). Patients with malignant bone tumors are stratified into three groups based on tumor grade, location within or outside of a compartment, and the presence or absence of metastatic disease, including lymph node involvement. The American Joint Committee on Cancer staging system used for the staging of soft-tissue sarcomas is less commonly referred to for the staging of primary bone sarcomas.

Surgery

The surgical management of bone sarcomas emphasizes local control with compete excision of the tumor. To achieve this goal, wide local resection of the primary tumor with an adjacent cuff of normal tissue outside the pseudocapsule is required. Occasionally, radical resection with joint disarticulation is mandated to obtain negative margins.

Limb-salvage surgery has gained popularity with the advent of chemotherapy, particularly for the treatment of osteosarcoma. Tumor location and extent of disease are important determinants when considering limb salvage. Although there are no absolute contraindications to limb-salvage surgery, there are situations in which amputation may be preferred. Pathologic fractures occur in a small subset of patients during the course of their disease and are associated with the microscopic spread of tumor as a result of hematoma formation. Recent studies have demonstrated a significant difference in survival between patients who present with a pathological fracture and those without. Neurovascular involvement and significant limb length discrepancies frequently signal the need for amputation. Reconstruction after tumor resection depends on the type and extent of the defect, the anticipated function, and the experience of the surgeon. Allografts are frequently used to reconstruct large bone defects and joints after tumor resection. Ligamentous attachments allow joint function and stability, and they can be incorporated into the patient's own tissues over time. As an alternative to allograft reconstruction, metal prostheses can be implanted. Prosthetic breakage and infection are less frequent with newer metal components, but soft-tissue attachment remains problematic. New designs are undergoing clinical trials to improve the functional outcomes for reconstructive surgery.

Osteosarcoma

Osteosarcomas are the most common primary bone sarcoma. Although a number of variants have been determined, all osteosarcomas are malignant spindle-cell tumors that form osteoid. Most commonly, osteosarcoma originates from the medullary region of bone and is of a high histologic grade. A bimodal age frequency is found, with the majority of cases occurring in adolescent males and a smaller number of cases occurring in older patients with a history of radiation therapy, chronic osteomyelitis, or Paget's disease. Bones of the proximal humerus and knee joint are the most common sites of osteosarcoma.

TABLE 11-5 • *Enneking Staging System for Bone Sarcomas*

Stage	Grade	Site
IA	Low (G1)	Intracompartmental (T1)
IB	Low (G1)	Extracompartmental (T2)
IIA	High (G2)	Intracompartmental (T1)
IIB	High (G2)	Extracompartmental (T2)
III	Any G	Any T
	Regional or distant metastasis (M1)	

G, Grade; *G1*, any low-grade tumor; *G2*, any high-grade tumor; *M*, regional or distal metastases; *M0*, no metastases; *M1*, any metastases; *T*, site; *T1*, intracompartmental location of tumor; *T2*, extracompartmental location of tumor.

From Enneking WF, Spanier SS, Goodman MA. A system for the surgical staging of musculoskeletal sarcoma. *Clin Orthop* 1980;153:106.

Generally, 80% to 90% of osteosarcomas occur in the long bones, with the axial skeleton rarely being affected.

Principal treatment involves multiagent chemotherapy in conjunction with surgical resection. Typically, patients receive preoperative chemotherapy (doxorubicin, cisplatin, ifosfamide, and sometimes high-dose methotrexate); they are then are restaged, and they undergo surgery for local disease control. Metallic prostheses can be custom-built during the time that preoperative chemotherapy is being administered. This treatment plan has made limb salvage possible in up to 90% of patients.

Tumor size, location, and extent of tumor necrosis in response to chemotherapy are important factors for determining prognosis; patients with tumors of the pelvis and spine and those with less than 90% necrosis after induction chemotherapy have a worse prognosis. Osteosarcomas commonly metastasize to the lung. Patients with synchronous pulmonary metastases have a 17% 5-year survival as compared with 79% for patients with localized disease. Pulmonary metastasectomy with chemotherapy can improve survival for patients with limited lung disease and a controlled primary tumor.

Chondrosarcoma

Chondrosarcomas are the second most common primary malignant spindle-cell tumor of bone. They are a heterogenous group of tumors sharing the commonality of cartilaginous tissue without direct evidence of osteoid formation. Overall, 60% of chondrosarcomas are located in the axial skeleton (chest wall, sternum, pelvic/shoulder girdle), and 40% arise in the extremities; the most common sites are the pelvis and femur. They can occur de novo or arise in a benign tumor, such as an osteochondroma or enchondroma. Chondrosarcomas are most common after the fourth decade of life, and they affect males more than females.

In contrast with osteosarcomas, chondrosarcomas are relatively resistant to chemotherapy and radiation, and surgical resection remains the best and often only chance for cure. For low-grade lesions confirmed by radiographic assessment and histologic diagnosis, intralesional curettage and cryosurgery is an acceptable treatment. Internal fixation with plates and screws may be necessary to prevent pathologic fracture after surgery. By contrast, patients with evidence of cortical penetration as determined by the degree of scalloping of the endosteum and/or histologic grade II or III on biopsy require aggressive surgical management with wide excision and appropriate reconstruction.

Childhood Sarcomas

Soft-tissue sarcomas are the sixth most common cancer in children and account for 15% of all cancer cases in patients under the age of 20 years. Pediatric soft-tissue sarcomas are thought of as belonging to one of two groups: rhabdomyosarcomas, which are the most common soft-tissue sarcoma of childhood, and non-rhabdomyosarcoma soft-tissue tumors. The most common non-rhabdomyosarcoma tumors include synovial sarcoma, malignant peripheral nerve sheath tumor, and fibrosarcoma. In general, the most commonly occurring soft-tissue sarcomas in adults are exceedingly rare in children. Ewing's sarcoma is the second most common primary bone tumor in pediatric patients, with osteosarcoma being the most common. These tumors can occur as either osseous or soft-tissue tumors. Both rhabdomyosarcoma and Ewing's sarcoma will be the focus of further discussion.

Rhabdomyosarcoma

Rhabdomyosarcoma is the most common primary soft-tissue tumor in childhood, and it accounts for 4% to 8% of all pediatric malignancies. Among the extracranial solid tumors of childhood, rhabdomyosarcoma is the third most common neoplasm after neuroblastoma and Wilms' tumor. Nearly 50% of cases are diagnosed in children 5 years old and younger, and there is a slight male predominance (1.3 to 1.4 times more common).

These tumors are most commonly found in the head and neck region (37%), followed by the genitourinary system (25%); less than 20% of rhabdomyosarcomas occur in the extremities. This anatomic distribution is in contrast with the occurrence of soft-tissue sarcomas in adults, among whom almost two thirds arise in the extremities, followed by the trunk and the retroperitoneum. Lymph-node metastases are also more commonly found in childhood rhabdomyosarcoma than in adults, occurring in 20% to 40% of cases.

Although the majority of these tumors arise sporadically, associations with several familial cancer syndromes have been made. Rhabdomyosarcomas have been reported in association with neurofibromatosis type 1, Beckwith-Wiedemann syndrome, cardiofaciocutaneous syndrome, and particularly Li-Fraumeni syndrome (involving a germline mutation in the p53 tumor-suppressor gene).

Histologic diagnosis of rhabdomyosarcoma is made on the findings of a small, round, blue-cell neoplasm and malignant skeletal muscle differentiation. Four basic histologic subtypes are identified. The embryonal subtype is the most common form of rhabdomyosarcoma, and it is frequently diagnosed within the first decade of life. The botryoid type is typically seen in the genitourinary tract. The alveolar subtype is the second most common form of rhabdomyosarcoma, and it has a high incidence among adolescents. The fourth subtype is pleomorphic.

Treatment generally consists of surgical resection and multiagent chemotherapy. However, fewer than 20% of patients have tumors that are completely excised with negative margins as a result of tumor location, particularly in the head and neck region. Patients who have undergone complete surgical resection, with tumors arising in favorable sites, and who are without regional lymph node involvement will have the most favorable outcome, with an expected 5-year survival of 95%. Those with alveolar histology and metastatic disease have significantly poorer outcomes, with 5-year survival rates of less than 30%. For patients with microscopic or gross residual disease after surgery and for those with embryonal or alveolar histology, radiation therapy plays an important role in successful local tumor control.

Ewing's Sarcoma

This is a high-grade malignant bone tumor that most commonly occurs within the first two decades of life. It is commonly described as a small, round, blue-cell tumor. Ewing's sarcoma is more commonly found in boys than girls, and it is rare among children of African-American descent. Cytogenetic studies have consistently found a translocation of chromosomes 11 and 22, t(11:22).

Patients typically present with pain at the affected site that progresses from intermittent to constant, often awakening them from sleep. Local swelling is a common finding, and fever can also occur. The femur is the most frequent primary site, accounting for 20% to 25% of all cases. The pelvis is the second most common primary site, accounting for an additional 20% of new cases. Metastases are present in approximately 25% of patients at initial diagnosis. The most frequent sites include the lungs and other bones, including the bone marrow. On plain films, the primary tumor is often diagnosed as a large circumferential soft-tissue mass accompanied by bone destruction having a characteristic onion-skinning periosteal reaction.

Treatment consists of multiagent chemotherapy both before and after surgical resection. Radiation therapy after surgery is effective for providing local control for large tumors and in cases in which tumor margins are close or positive. Current survival rates are good for patients with nonmetastatic locally resectable disease, and approximately 50% of patients with metastatic disease may have long-term survival. Patients with genetic aberrations consisting of the type 2 fusion transcript for the FLI-1 oncogene (exon 7 EWS joins exon 5 of FLI-1) or the p53 mutation appear to define a small group of patients with markedly poor prognosis.

Metastatic Sarcoma

For soft-tissue sarcomas of the extremity and primary bone sarcomas, hematogenous metastasis to the lung parenchyma is the primary form of distant spread. Patients with pulmonary nodules are considered candidates for metastasectomy if the lungs are the only site of disease. In retrospective series, 20% to 40% of patients who undergo metastasectomy are alive at 5 years. Patients most likely to achieve long-term survival after metastasectomy include those with complete resection of all metastases (especially in cases in which the number of metastases is limited to 4 or less), a disease-free interval of more than 12 months from primary treatment to the development of pulmonary metastases, and those with low-grade primary tumors. Combination chemotherapy may add additional survival benefit as compared with resection alone. The resection of liver metastases for sarcoma has been far less successful, with recurrent disease developing in nearly all patients.

Conclusions

Sarcomas are a rare, heterogeneous group of tumors that exhibit variable behavior based on histologic subtype, grade, size, location, and propensity for metastatic disease; therein lies the challenge in diagnosing and treating these tumors. The patient's best chance for survival and functional outcome often depends on a thorough preoperative evaluation, a carefully planned surgical resection, and consideration for all reconstructive options. Whenever possible, patients with suspected malignant soft-tissue or bone tumors should be referred to highly experienced centers for complete evaluation and treatment.

Key Selected Readings

Clark MA, Fisher C, Judson I, *et al.* Soft-tissue sarcomas in adults. *N Engl J Med* 2005;353:701–711.

Karakousis CP. Surgery for soft-tissue sarcomas. In: Bland KI, Karakousis CP, Copeland EM III, eds. *Atlas of surgical oncology*. Philadelphia: WB Saunders, 1995:283–400.

Selected Readings

Blay JY, Bonvalot S, Casali P, *et al.* Consensus meeting for the management of gastrointestinal stromal tumors: report of the GIST Consensus Conference of 20-21 March 2004, under the auspices of ESMO. *Ann Oncol* 2005;16:566–578.

Borden EC, Baker LH, Bell RS, *et al.* Soft-tissue sarcomas of adults: state of the translational science. *Clin Cancer Res* 2003;9:1941–1956.

Clark MA, Fisher C, Judson I, Thomas JM. Soft-tissue sarcomas in adults. *N Engl J Med* 2005;353:701–711.

Corless CL, Fletcher JA, Heinrich MC. Biology of gastrointestinal stromal tumors. *J Clin Oncol* 2004; 22:3813–3825.

Feig BW. Retroperitoneal sarcomas. *Surg Oncol Clin N Am* 2003;12:369–378.

Helman LJ, Meltzer P. Mechanisms of sarcoma development. *Nature Rev* 2003;3:685–694.

Herzog CE, Stewart JM, Blakely ML. Pediatric soft-tissue sarcomas. *Surg Oncol Clin N Am* 2003;12:369–378.

Nielsen TO, West RB, Linn SC, *et al.* Molecular characterization of soft-tissue tumours: a gene expression study. *Lancet* 2002;359:1301–1307.

O'Sullivan B, Davis AM, Turcotte R, *et al.* Preoperative versus postoperative radiotherapy in soft-tissue sarcoma of the limbs: a randomized trial. *Lancet* 2002;359:2235–2241.

Raut CP, Pisters PW. Retroperitoneal sarcomas: combined-modality treatment approaches. *J Surg Oncol* 2006;94:81–87.

Scoggins CR, Pollock RE. Extremity soft tissue sarcoma: evidence-based multidisciplinary managment. *J Surg Oncol* 2005;90:10–13.

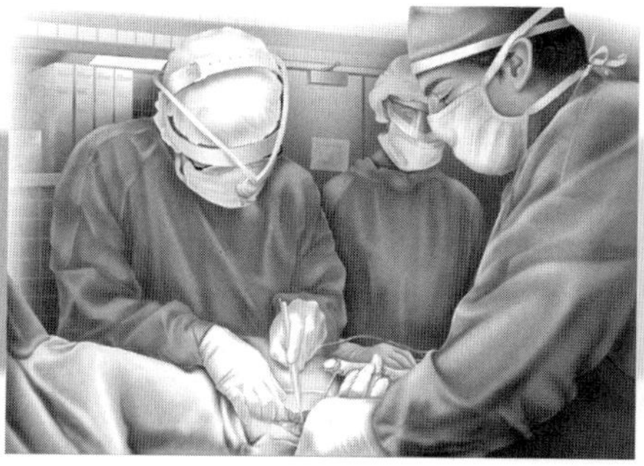

12

Surgical Thyroid and Parathyroid Disease

Sonia L. Sugg

Surgical Thyroid and Parathyroid Disease: Key Points

- Detail the role of the surgeon in managing thyroid disease.
- List the types of benign thyroid conditions and their management options.
- Outline the pros and cons of the medical and surgical approaches to managing hyperthyroidism.
- Describe the anatomic considerations and techniques for performing thyroid surgery.
- Compare the types of thyroid cancers.
- Compare the effectiveness of the various adjuvant treatments for thyroid cancer.
- Describe how to monitor for recurrence after treatment for thyroid cancer.
- Differentiate the types of hyperparathyroidism.
- Outline the process of diagnosing primary hyperparathyroidism.
- List the treatment options for hyperparathyroidism.
- Describe the surgical approaches to parathyroid disease.
- Describe the treatment for parathyroid carcinoma.

The treatment of thyroid and parathyroid disease requires a multidisciplinary approach with the knowledge of both the surgical and medical management of these diseases. The surgical anatomy and technical aspects are challenging, requiring meticulous technique to avoid complications.

The Solitary Thyroid Nodule

The majority of thyroid cancers will present as a solitary thyroid nodule; however, thyroid nodules are very common, occurring in up to 50% of individuals examined, depending on their age and the method of ascertainment. When examined by ultrasound, 30% of healthy volunteers had thyroid nodules detected. Overall, only 10% of thyroid nodules are malignant.

The role of the surgeon in the management of thyroid disease is to do the following: (1) to obtain a definitive diagnosis of a thyroid nodule; (2) to relieve symptoms from a mass effect, hyperthyroidism, or cosmetic deformity for benign disease; and (3) to provide definitive management of a thyroid malignancy. Workup should begin with a detailed history, including any neck-related symptoms, any history of prior neck surgery or head and neck irradiation, and family history. Symptoms concerning for thyroid carcinoma include hoarseness or rapid mass growth. Other symptoms may include a change in cosmetic appearance, dyspnea, dysphagia, and systemic signs or symptoms of hypothyroidism or hyperthyroidism. A history of prior neck surgery, especially if the recurrent laryngeal nerve has been placed at risk, mandates a vocal cord examination to rule out previous nerve injury, even if the voice sounds normal.

BOX 12–1 SYMPTOMS OF HYPERTHYROIDISM

- Tachycardia
- Restlessness
- Delirium
- Hyperreflexia
- Diarrhea
- Heat intolerance
- Insomnia
- Weight loss
- Warm, moist skin
- Tremors

BOX 12–2 SYMPTOMS OF HYPOTHYROIDISM

- Fatigue/weakness
- Bradycardia
- Constipation/ileus
- Dementia
- Cold intolerance
- Dry skin/hair loss
- Edema/effusions
- Menstrual irregularities
- Hoarseness

A history of head and neck irradiation is a significant risk factor for thyroid carcinoma. A detailed family history may reveal an inherited syndrome. Familial forms of medullary thyroid carcinoma are associated with the multiple endocrine neoplasia syndromes, and familial papillary thyroid carcinoma is being increasingly recognized. Goiters often occur in families, and patients with Graves' disease have a higher family incidence of autoimmune diseases.

A detailed physical examination should include evaluating the submandibular, jugular, central, and supraclavicular lymphatic basins (Figure 12-1). The thyroid is thoroughly palpated, with assessment of its texture, overall size, location and size of nodules, and mobility. The oropharynx, the ability to extend the neck, voice assessment with consideration of flexible laryngoscopy, and systemic signs of hypothyroidism and hyperthyroidism should also be evaluated.

A thyroid stimulating hormone (TSH) level is the best single test to determine the functional status of the thyroid (low = hyperthy-

BOX 12–3 THE THYROID EXAMINATION

- Palpate thyroid thoroughly.
- Assess texture, overall size, location and size of nodules, and mobility.
- Assess voice quality; consider preoperative laryngoscopy.
- Palpate submandibular, central, and lateral neck nodal basins.
- Assess oropharynx and neck extension; look for systemic signs of hypothyroidism and hyperthyroidism.

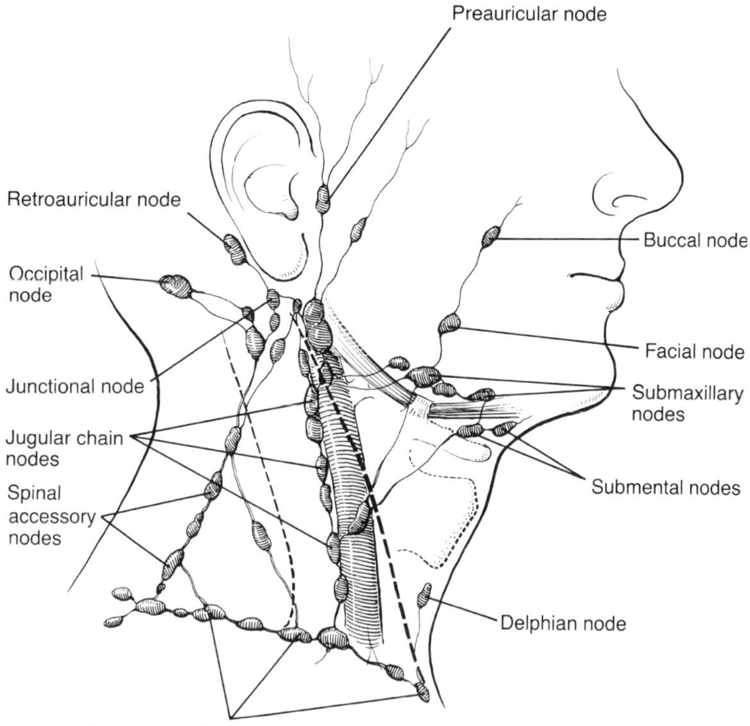

Figure 12-1. Anatomy of the cervical lymph nodes for physical examination. (From Bland KI, Karakousis CP, Copeland EM. *Atlas of surgical oncology*. Philadelphia: 1995, WB Saunders.)

roidism, high = hypothyroidism). There is no role for I^{131} or I^{123} scanning. A thyroid scan is valuable for identifying hyperfunctioning nodules, but it is not helpful for distinguishing benign from malignant disease. Ultrasound is often used for detection, biopsy, and follow-up of thyroid nodules. (Figure 12-2). Imaging features that may be associated with malignancy include hypoechogenicity, internal microcalcification, poorly defined or irregular borders, and hypervascularity. Fine-needle aspiration (FNA) has changed the management of thyroid nodules, decreasing the number of thyroid surgeries performed for diagnosis and increasing the surgical yield of carcinoma (Figure 12-3). The specificity for

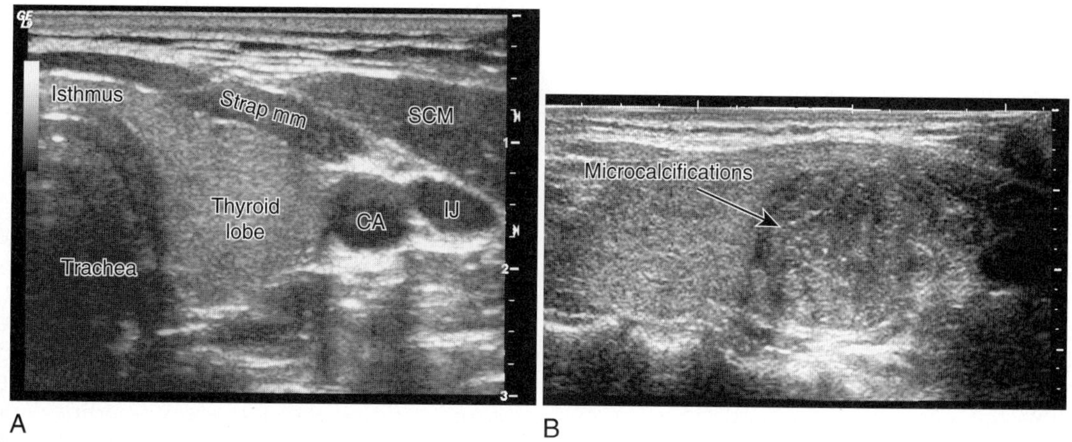

Figure 12-2. A, Ultrasound image of normal thyroid anatomy. Note the homogeneous echotexture of a normal thyroid lobe. **B,** Longitudinal ultrasound image of papillary thyroid cancer. Note the fine microcalcifications and the irregular, ill-defined borders of this malignant thyroid nodule. *CA*, Carotid artery; *IJ*, internal jugular vein; *SCM*, sternocleidomastoid muscle. (Courtesy of Dr. Francisco Quiroz.)

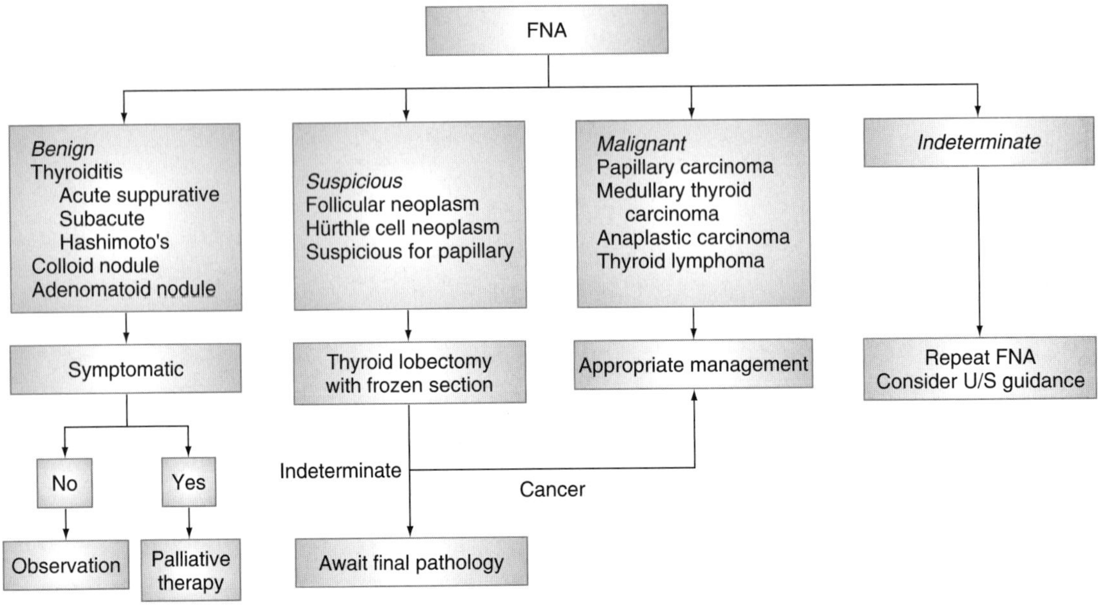

Figure 12-3. Management of the thyroid nodule based on fine-needle aspiration biopsy. (From Weigel R. Thyroid. In: Norton JA, Barie PS, Bollinger RR, *et al.*, eds. *Surgery: basic science and clinical evidence.* New York: Springer, 2001:833.)

the detection of malignancy ranges from 72% to 100%, and the sensitivity ranges from 65% to 98%. It requires an expert cytopathologist for interpretation. FNA may be repeated if insufficient diagnostic material is obtained. On the basis of diagnoses made by FNA, a definitely benign condition such as a colloid nodule may be diagnosed. A malignancy may also be diagnosed, allowing for definitive treatment to be arranged. In some cases, an indeterminate FNA may be obtained that will require either repeat biopsy or additional tissue. For example, follicular neoplasms cannot be determined to be benign or malignant based on FNA cytology, because formal pathology of the whole specimen is required to detect the capsular and vascular invasion that is characteristic of malignancy. All dominant nodules (the largest nodule within a lobe) greater than 1 cm should undergo FNA. Ultrasound guidance may be required if the nodule is difficult to palpate. An *incidentaloma* is an otherwise asymptomatic thyroid nodule discovered on imaging studies, such as carotid ultrasounds, nuclear medicine, or CT scanning. The risk for cancer in an incidentaloma is low, but current recommendations are to investigate those larger than 1 cm or with imaging characteristics that are suspicious for malignancy with FNA.

Management of Benign Thyroid Disease

Colloid nodules are very common and are usually asymptomatic, unless they are large. On FNA, uniform-appearing thyroid epithelial cells are seen in a background of colloid (Figure 12-4), the proteinaceous material that contains stores of thyroglobulin. Asymptomatic, FNA proven benign nodules that are stable in size may be safely observed. Long-term follow-up demonstrates a less than 1% incidence of cancer in such nodules. The natural history of thyroid nodules observed over a 10-year period is that 40% will decrease in size or disappear and that 20% will enlarge. Size alone is occasionally an indication for surgery, although it is usually in the context of symptoms, cosmesis, or concern regarding potential sampling error by FNA. Thyroxine suppression therapy to curb the TSH stimulation of thyroid nodules remains controversial, despite widespread use. Clinical trials have not demonstrated a clear benefit for thyroid suppressive therapy for solitary or multiple thyroid nodules, except in areas of iodine deficiency. There is a subgroup (about 20%) of patients who do respond, but this must be weighed against the possible adverse side

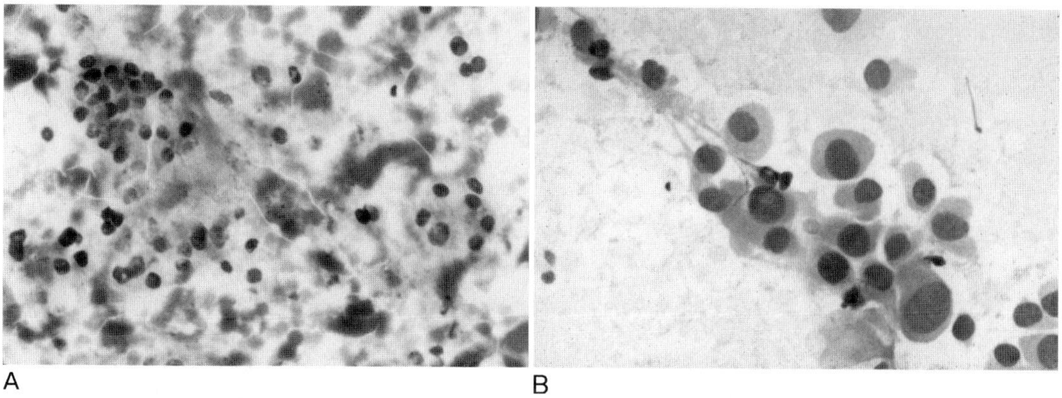

Figure 12–4. A, Fine-needle aspirate of a colloid nodule showing abundant colloid in the background, with cohesive thyroid epithelial cells of similar size and shape. **B,** Fine-needle aspirate of a papillary thyroid cancer showing intranuclear cytoplasmic inclusion bodies, nuclear grooving, and cells and nuclei of differing sizes. (Courtesy of Dr. Edwin L. Kaplan.)

effects of suppression, including osteoporosis and cardiac arrhythmias.

Nodules may also be present in *lymphocytic thyroiditis* (Hashimoto's disease). These patients may present with or develop hypothyroidism over time, but they usually do not require surgical therapy. Other inflammatory thyroid disorders include *acute thyroiditis,* which may present as a thyroid abscess in children, *subacute thyroiditis* or *de Quervain's disease,* which often presents with self-limited hyperthyroidism and is usually treated medically with nonsteroidal antiinflammatory drugs or steroids in severe cases, and *Reidel's thyroiditis,* which is a rare disorder that is similar to retroperitoneal fibrosis. In Reidel's thyroiditis, an isthmusectomy is often performed to provide airway control and confirm the diagnosis.

Multinodular goiter is benign enlargement of the thyroid containing multiple nodules, and it is especially common in iodine-deficient areas. Symptoms include those related to compression of the trachea or esophagus and to cosmesis. Dominant nodules should undergo FNA, and unless they are symptomatic, they can be followed if stable. *Toxic multinodular goiter (Plummer's disease)* is characterized by the autonomous function of at least some of the nodules within a goiter causing clinical hyperthyroidism. It is best managed surgically after medical control of the hyperthyroidism is achieved.

Graves' disease is an autoimmune disorder caused by antibodies against the TSH receptor, manifesting with hyperthyroidism and a diffuse goiter. It is often associated with eye disease (exophthalmos) and, less commonly, with pretibial edema and acropachy. Thyroid acropachy is an extreme manifestation of autoimmune thyroid disease. It presents with digital clubbing, swelling of digits and toes, and periosteal reaction of extremity bones. In the United States, it is usually managed with radioactive iodine (RAI). Graves' disease is initially controlled by antithyroid medications, but long-term remission after the discontinuation of medical therapy occurs in only 25% of cases. A second RAI treatment is required in at least 25% of patients, and hypothyroidism occurs in 50% to 70%. Indications for surgery include a contraindication to RAI (e.g., pregnancy), persistent disease after RAI, patient preference, a cold and suspicious nodule, a large goiter, and aggressive hyperthyroidism that is unresponsive to medical therapy.

Follicular adenomas are cellular on FNA, and they cannot be distinguished from follicular carcinomas by cytologic examination; therefore, they require lobectomy for diagnosis. A *toxic adenoma* or hot nodule is an autonomously functional variant of follicular adenoma that may lead to a diagnosis without an operation (Figure 12-5). These nodules are rarely (<5%) malignant, but they may cause subclinical hyperthyroidism with the suppression of TSH levels. Clinical hyperthyroidism develops at a rate of 4% per year, and iodine exposure may provoke the development of toxicity. Treatment options are surgical removal, RAI ablation, or medical management.

Treatment of Hyperthyroidism

Radioactive Iodine

RAI is delivered by Iodine-131, which emits mostly beta particles and some gamma radiation (10% of total). The depth penetration of

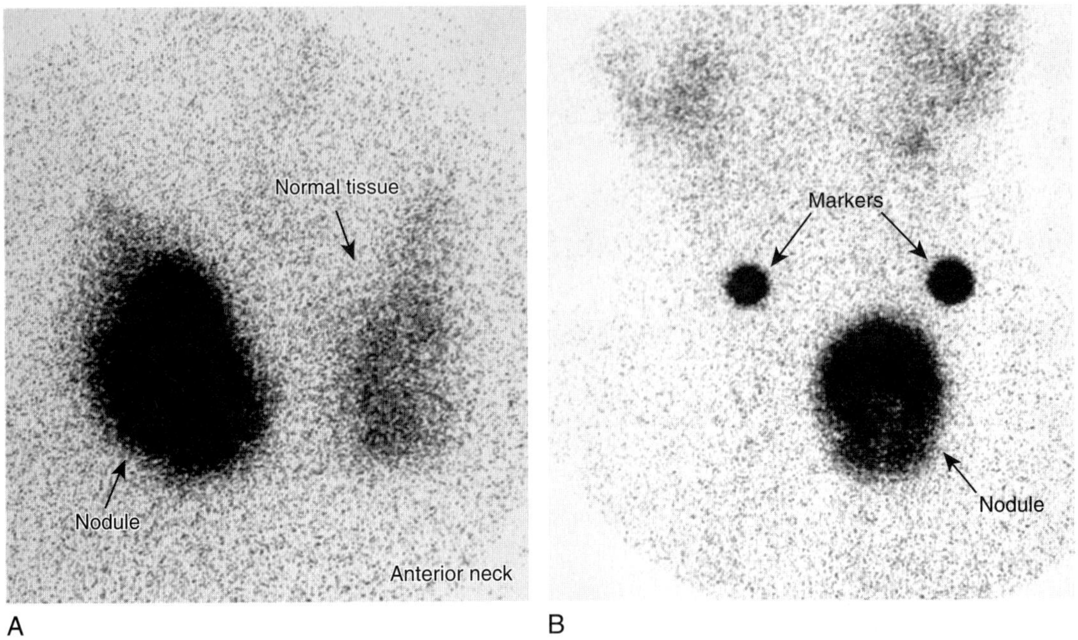

Figure 12–5. A, B, Radioactive iodine scan of a toxic adenoma. The toxic adenoma has taken up most of the radioactive iodine. The remaining thyroid is suppressed and has very little uptake. (Courtesy of Dr. Robert Hellman.)

beta particles in tissue is 2 mm. RAI is preferentially taken up by thyrocytes, and it destroys thyroid cells and their function. Other sites that take up RAI are the salivary glands and bone marrow. RAI is used to treat hyperfunctioning thyroid diseases such as toxic adenomas, toxic multinodular goiter, and Graves' disease. The doses used to treat benign, hyperfunctioning thyroid glands range from 15 mCi for patients with Graves' disease to larger doses for patients with toxic adenomas (20 mCi or higher) and toxic multinodular goiters (>50 mCi). RAI causes complete regression of toxic thyroid nodules in up to half of cases, and it is associated with a 5% to 10% incidence of hypothyroidism. Repeated doses are required in 10% to 20% of patients. Administration of RAI is easy, avoids the complications of surgery, and has a good success rate. Many clinicians are reluctant to treat young (up to teenage years) patients with RAI, because of a concern for the development of future malignancy, but studies to date have not demonstrated a clinically significant increased risk.

Medical Management

Antithyroid medications are the thionamide drugs methimazole and propylthiouracil. Biochemical euthyroidism is usually established within 6 to 8 weeks after initiating therapy. Side effects include pruritus and rash in up to 25% of patients, nausea, jaundice, and, rarely, agranulocytosis and liver failure. These drugs may lose effectiveness over time, and they usually will not shrink an enlarged gland. Propranolol or beta-blockers are used to control tachycardia and other hyperthyroid-induced arrhythmias. Dexamethasone has been used to rapidly correct hyperthyroidism preoperatively. Lugol's iodine solution will help reduce the vascularity of the thyroid when it is given for 5 to 6 days preoperatively, but it can lead to worsening hyperthyroidism if it is given for longer periods.

Surgical Management

The advantages of the surgical management of hyperthyroidism include a rapid resolution of symptoms, no recurrence, and complete removal of the nodule for pathologic evaluation. Disadvantages include increased cost and risks associated with surgery. The extent of surgery depends on the extent of disease and on the surgeon's expertise with performing a total/near-total operation. Unilateral disease, such as single or even multiple thyroid nodules, may be treated with a lobectomy and isthmusectomy. Bilateral disease, such as a multinodular goiter or Graves' disease, is treated with near-total/total thyroidectomy or bilateral subtotal thyroidectomy. In bilateral disease, a larger thyroid remnant increases the rate of recurrence and lowers the rate of hypothyroidism. Most experienced thyroid surgeons advocate a total or near-total operation, because hypothyroidism is easier to treat than recurrence. Reoperative thyroid surgery is associated with at least a doubling of complications.

Thyroid Anatomy and Surgery

Surgical treatment of the thyroid is technically demanding and requires a thorough understanding of the relevant anatomy (Figures 12-6 and 12-7). The thyroid gland is enveloped by the deep cervical fascia of the neck under the sternohyoid and sternothyroid strap muscles. It is composed of the right and left lobes joined by the isthmus. There is often (30–40% of cases) a pyramidal lobe extending up toward the hyoid bone. The ligament of Berry, which is also known as the posterior suspensory ligament of the thyroid, is a condensation of the thyroid capsule that attaches to the larynx at the level of the cricoid, first and second tracheal rings. The tubercle of Zuckerkandl is a lobule of thyroid tissue that can extend posteriorly just below the ligament of Berry. The vascular supply of the thyroid gland is from the superior thyroid artery, which branches from the external carotid artery, and the inferior thyroid artery, which is a branch of the thyrocervical trunk of the subclavian artery. The inferior thyroid artery is often the sole arterial supply to the parathyroid glands, and, therefore, it requires preservation when the thyroid is removed if these glands are to remain viable. The venous drainage is through the superior, middle, and inferior thyroid veins. The thyroid's innervation is from the autonomic nervous system. Two pairs of laryngeal motor nerves lie in close proximity to the thyroid gland. The recurrent laryngeal nerve is the motor nerve to the intrinsic muscles of the larynx, and it travels in the tracheoesophageal groove and enters the larynx posterior to the lower margin of the cricothyroid muscle at the cricoid cartilage (Figure 12-7). The right recurrent nerve has a more oblique course than the left as a result of its looping around the subclavian artery instead of the ligamentum arteriosum on the left. The nerve anatomy is variable, and it branches before entering the larynx in 30% to 76% of cases. It usually travels posterior to the inferior thyroid artery, but occasionally it is anterior to the artery. Its relationship to the ligament of Berry and the tubercle of Zuckerkandl is variable. The nerve may be lateral to, beneath, or lying across the ligament of Berry. The relationship of the nerve to the tubercle is variable, and, if the tubercle is enlarged, it can obscure the course of the nerve. The external branch of the superior laryngeal nerve enervates the cricothyroid muscle. The nerve runs within the pharyngeal constrictor muscle 20% of the time, and it is not visible to the surgeon. However, it can be found running in the cricothyroid space, and, in 20% of cases, it is intertwined among branches of the superior thyroid artery, where it is most vulnerable to injury.

The extent of surgery is discussed with the patient preoperatively. The possibility of requiring long-term thyroxine replacement is mentioned, even if only a lobectomy is planned. In general, a total or near-total lobectomy removes all or most of the thyroid lobe, leaving behind less than 1 gram of thyroid tissue. A subtotal lobectomy removes more than 50% of the thyroid lobe, leaving behind a variable extent of thyroid tissue at the tubercle of Zuckerkandl and the ligament of Berry. The isthmus is generally removed with a lobectomy to facilitate potential reoperation. A bilateral operation can consist of bilateral total/near-total thyroidectomy, a combination of total/near-total on one side and subtotal on the other, or bilateral subtotal thyroidectomy.

Technical Aspects

The neck incision is usually placed 2 to 3 cm above the sternal notch or in a suitable skin crease. A higher incision facilitates exposure of the superior lobe. The length of the incision is variable, from 4 to 12 cm, depending on the patient's body habitus, the size of the gland to be removed, and the surgeon's fondness for small incisions. The platysma muscle is divided, and subplatysmal flaps are raised to the thyroid and sternal notches. The superficial layer of deep cervical fascia is divided in the midline to separate the strap muscles, and the overlying strap muscles are dissected away from the thyroid gland. The middle thyroid vein is ligated and divided. The pyramidal lobe, if present, is

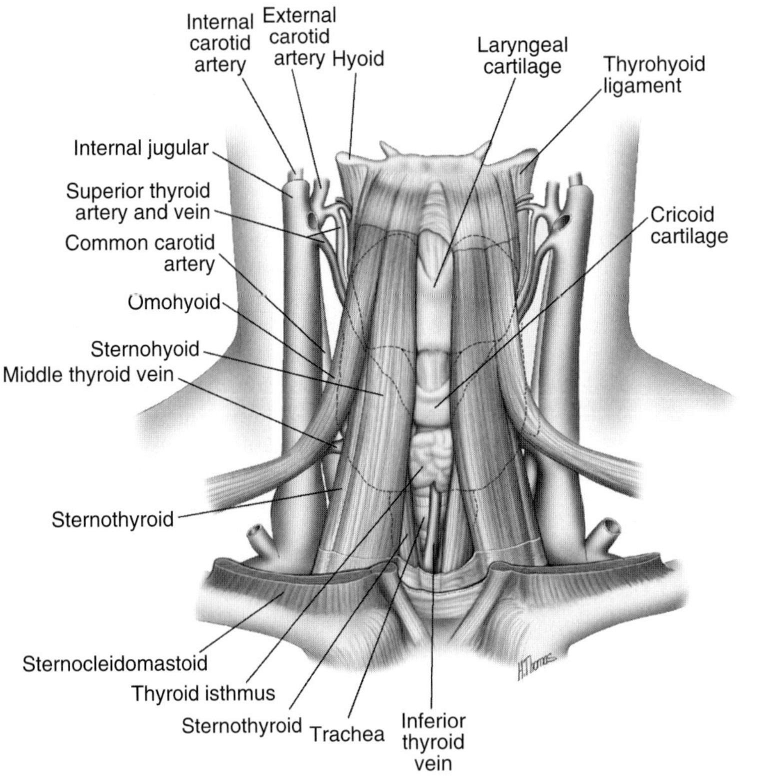

Figure 12–6. Surgical anatomy of the thyroid gland. (From Bloom ND, Beattie EJ, Harvey JC: *Atlas of cancer surgery*. Philadelphia: WB Saunders, 2000.)

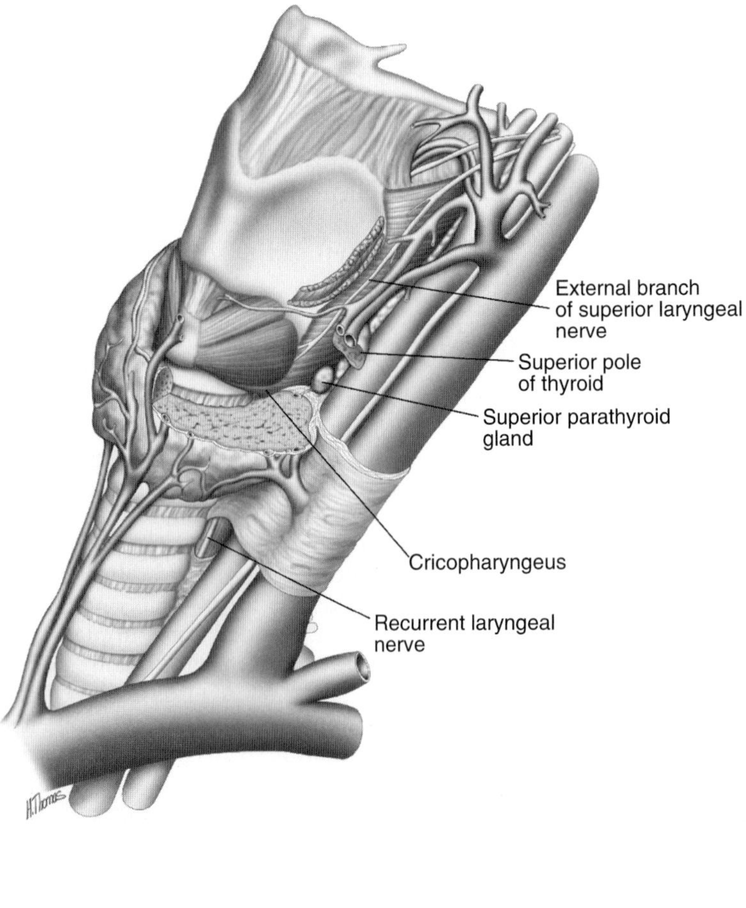

Figure 12–7. Anatomy of nerves showing the left recurrent laryngeal nerve. (From Bloom ND, Beattie EJ, Harvey JC: *Atlas of cancer surgery*. Philadelphia: WB Saunders, 2000.)

mobilized and divided at its highest extent, sometimes up to the hyoid bone. The cricothyroid space (between the cricoid cartilage and the superior lobe) is opened, and the external branch of the superior laryngeal nerve may be identified. Branches of the superior thyroid artery and vein are individually ligated on the thyroid capsule to avoid injury to the superior laryngeal nerve. Placing the index finger into the cricothyroid space helps pull down the superior thyroid lobe for better exposure. At the posterior aspect of the superior lobe, the superior parathyroid may be identified. If so, it should be mobilized off of the thyroid gland, starting medially to preserve its blood supply, which comes from a lateral direction. In this area, the recurrent laryngeal nerve may also be close by, where it is about to enter into the larynx. The inferior parathyroid gland is identified, usually lying on the capsule of the inferior thyroid lobe or along the thyrothymic tract, and it is dissected off of the thyroid gland and preserved. The recurrent laryngeal nerve may be identified low in the neck and traced toward its entry into the larynx or at the level of the cricoid cartilage. Although there is some debate about whether or not the nerve needs to be identified, most studies indicate a lower complication rate—especially among less-experienced surgeons—when the nerve is searched for and identified. Branches of the inferior thyroid artery are ligated and divided on the thyroid capsule, preserving the blood supply to the parathyroid glands. The tubercle of Zuckerkandl, if present, is mobilized. The ligament of Berry, which contains small blood vessels and sometimes thyroid tissue, is divided between snaps and ligated. The recurrent laryngeal nerve needs to be visualized and protected during this dissection. The lobe is then removed off of the anterior surface of the trachea. For a unilateral operation, the thyroid is divided above a clamp placed between the isthmus and the opposite lobe, and a hemostatic stitch is placed into the cut surface of the remaining thyroid lobe. For a bilateral operation, the procedure is repeated on the opposite side. Meticulous hemostasis allows for visual identification of the parathyroid glands and nerves. At the conclusion of the case, the operative field should be dry. The strap muscles are reapproximated in the midline, and the platysma or subcutaneous layer closed; this is followed by skin closure. The routine use of drains after thyroid surgery is unnecessary, and it may lead to an increased rate of infection. However, drains may be useful after the removal of large goiters, when seromas tend to accumulate in the dead space.

Nerve monitoring has been proposed as a method to reduce superior and recurrent laryngeal nerve injury, especially in cases with a higher risk to the recurrent laryngeal nerve, such as reoperative surgery, and surgery performed on the side of the only functioning recurrent laryngeal nerve. Conclusive evidence that nerve monitoring results in a reduction in nerve injury rates is still pending due to the low rate of recurrent laryngeal nerve injury in general.

Postoperative Complications

After thyroid surgery, the patient can develop seromas, hematomas, transient or permanent recurrent or superior laryngeal nerve injury, and transient or permanent hypoparathyroidism.

Seromas occur in up to 6% of cases, especially after a subtotal bilateral thyroid operation or the removal of a substernal goiter. They may be safely observed in most cases, and they will spontaneously resolve in several weeks; percutaneous aspiration is performed if the seroma is tense or symptomatic.

Hematomas requiring surgical drainage are rare (1%), but they can cause mortality from airway compromise. Most occur during the first 4 to 6 hours after surgery, but they can occur up to 5 days postoperatively.

Superior laryngeal nerve injury results in the inability to tense the vocal cord, and it is often unnoticed by the physician or patient. However, among patients who are singers or public speakers, superior laryngeal nerve injury may result in permanent disability. The incidence ranges from 9% to 14%. This injury may be detected by electromyogram testing of the cricothyroid muscle or by changes in vocal cord morphology and function on laryngoscopy. Superior laryngeal nerve injuries are not repaired, and they are treated with voice rehabilitation.

Recurrent laryngeal nerve injury results in vocal cord paralysis in up to 6% of patients. The vocal cord on the injured side is usually fixed in the median position, and the voice is usually—but not always—hoarse. Bilateral nerve injury results in both cords being fixed in the median position and a compromised airway, usually requiring a tracheostomy. The nerve injury may be transient or permanent. Controversy exists with regard to repair of a transected recurrent laryngeal nerve. Regrowth of the nerve fibers in the repaired nerve may be disorderly and may result in vocal cord malfunction.

Hypoparathyroidism may result from inadvertent removal of parathyroid glands located on the thyroid capsule or even of intrathyroidal glands, especially during goiter surgery. The removed thyroid gland should always be inspected for parathyroid glands before being sent for pathology, especially if the parathyroids were not identified during the thyroidectomy. Hypoparathyroidism may also result from devascularization of the parathyroid glands. It is difficult to identify devascularized glands, which may have a normal color but not bleed when incised. Compromised glands should be reimplanted to prevent permanent hypoparathyroidism. The reported incidence of permanent hypoparathyroidism ranges from 0% to 13% after a bilateral operation. The reported incidence of transient hypoparathyroidism is 0.3% to 49%, which reflects the technique and the extent of surgery. After a unilateral operation, there will not be any hypoparathyroidism unless there was prior surgery on the opposite side, with unknown and possibly compromised function of the glands. Hypoparathyroidism is manifested by low calcium and parathyroid hormone (PTH) levels. Hypoparathyroidism is treated by calcium and, if required, vitamin D. Calcitriol (1,25-dihydroxy vitamin D) has a shorter half-life than other forms of vitamin D. It is useful for the treatment of refractory hypocalcemia, but it must be used judiciously because of the narrow therapeutic window to toxicity.

Thyroid storm is an unusual intraoperative or early postoperative complication that can occur in hyperthyroid patients undergoing surgery. It represents a massive release of thyroid hormones that results in tachycardia, fever, and hemodynamic instability. It is unusual, because most hyperthyroid patients are medically controlled before surgery. Occasionally, patients with unsuspected hyperthyroidism will manifest thyroid storm while undergoing procedures or being treated for other illnesses or trauma. Thyroid storm is treated by beta blockade, measures to decrease body temperature, and hemodynamic support. The mortality rate is 28% to 100%.

Technique of Parathyroid Reimplantation

The excised gland requires confirmation by a frozen section to be a parathyroid, because it is possible to misidentify a metastatic lymph node for a parathyroid gland. It is kept in iced saline until reimplantation. A pocket is developed within the sternocleidomastoid muscle after incising its fascia. It is important to have good hemostasis, because a hematoma will compromise parathyroid engraftment. The parathyroid gland is minced into 1-mm^3 pieces and placed into the pocket. An alternate technique is to reimplant the pieces in multiple small pockets. We prefer to mince the gland using scissors in a medicine cup containing a small amount of saline and to then dispense the parathyroid saline mixture into the muscle pocket using a glass medicine dropper. The pocket is closed with a permanent suture to mark its position. Immediate reimplantation has a success rate of around 80%, and the graft should start functioning in 2 weeks.

Thyroid Cancer

Thyroid cancer is the most common endocrine cancer; it is diagnosed in approximately 25,000 new patients annually. It is three times more common in women, making it the eighth most common cancer among women. In the United States, its incidence is 10 per 100,000, and mortality is 5 to 6 per million. Worldwide, the incidence of thyroid cancer is rising. Genetic predisposition is important in the etiology of medullary thyroid carcinomas and in a small proportion of papillary thyroid cancer. However, environmental exposures, such as radiation and diet, are all factors in the development of thyroid cancer. Exposure to radiation is a well-known risk factor for thyroid cancer. Exposure, especially in childhood, is associated with the development of thyroid cancer 5 to 35 years later. Examples include children who were radiated for benign conditions such as "enlarged thymus" and acne in the 1930s and 1940s and those who were exposed to the fallout from the atomic bombs

BOX 12-4 RISK FACTORS FOR THYROID CANCER

- Radiation exposure to the thyroid gland, particularly at a young age
  - Medically administered external-beam irradiation
  - Environmental exposure (nuclear fallout)
  - Ingestion of radioisotopes of iodine (medical treatment or contamination)
- Iodine-deficient diet
  - Low intake of iodine
  - High intake of cruciferous vegetables (which block iodine uptake)
- Family history: multiple endocrine neoplasia type II, familial medullary thyroid cancer, familial adenomatous polyposis, Cowden's disease, familial papillary thyroid cancer
- Female gender

in Japan during World War II or the Chernobyl nuclear disaster.

Thyroid Cancers of Follicular Origin

Thyroid cancers of follicular origin are carcinomas that originate from the follicular cell type; this includes both papillary and follicular thyroid cancers (Table 12-2). *Papillary thyroid carcinoma* is the most common type (80% in iodine-rich environments), and it is characterized by nuclear features such as nuclear clearing and grooves. *Psammoma bodies,* which are laminated calcific spherules found in the stroma or lymphatics, are also a feature of papillary thyroid cancer. Cytology obtained by FNA is often diagnostic. Clinically, papillary thyroid cancers present in younger patients, and they metastasize more frequently to lymph nodes than follicular cancers.

Variants of papillary cancer include the follicular subtype, which grows in a follicular pattern but has the nuclear features and clinical behavior of papillary thyroid cancer. The unusual histologic subtypes of thyroid cancer have a worse prognosis. The *tall cell variant* of papillary thyroid cancer is defined as having a greater than 2-to-1 height-to-width ratio. *Insular carcinomas* are often large, with areas of necrosis, and many cases include areas of differentiated papillary thyroid cancer. Clinically, patients with these two variants have higher local and distant recurrence rates.

Follicular thyroid cancer cannot be diagnosed via FNA. Histologically, these cancers resemble follicular adenomas, but they are characterized by vascular or capsular invasion. They usually spread hematogenously rather than to lymph nodes, and, in general, they have a worse survival rate than papillary thyroid cancers. *Hürthle cell adenomas* are considered a variant of follicular adenomas, and they are composed of cells with abundant eosinophilic cytoplasm. Although most Hürthle cell adenomas behave in a benign fashion, there are some that present later with metastases or recurrence, pointing to the difficulty of differentiating benign from malignant tumors. Therefore, some pathologists prefer to use the term *Hürthle cell tumor* to designate their uncertain biologic behavior. *Hürthle cell carcinomas,* unlike well-differentiated papillary and follicular neoplasms, generally do not take up RAI, making this form of treatment for advanced disease largely ineffective.

TABLE 12-2 • *Clinical Features of Papillary and Follicular Thyroid Cancer*

	Papillary	Follicular
Environment	Iodine sufficient	Iodine deficient
Peak age	Third and fourth decades	Fourth and fifth decades
Nodal metastases	30–40%	5–10%
Distant metastases	2–14%	10–20%
Multicentric	30–80%	Rare
Extrathyroidal extension	10%	25%
Cytology	Diagnostic	Not helpful

Staging and Classification of Differentiated Thyroid Cancer

The prognosis for differentiated thyroid cancer of follicular origin is generally good, with 10-year survival rates of 96% for papillary and 80% for follicular thyroid cancer. Clinical characteristics associated with worse survival are age of more than 45 years, male gender, larger tumor size, extrathyroidal extension, and presence of distant metastases. Lymph node metastases and multifocal disease are associated with an increased local recurrence rate. Various groups have created risk-group classifications based on review of these characteristics in a retrospective manner. These include the European Organisation for Research and Treatment of Cancer (EORTC), AMES, AGES, MACIS, and the University of Chicago (Table 12-3). Studies comparing the classification systems demonstrate the ability to separate patients into high- and low-risk groups with accurate prediction of prognosis. Most centers are now using the newly revised TNM system (Table 12-4), which seems to have fairly good correlation with clinical outcomes.

Extent of Surgery for Differentiated Thyroid Cancer

There is little debate among experts regarding the appropriateness of total or near-total thyroidectomy for high-risk thyroid carcinoma. In these cases, a bilateral resection is associated with significantly lower local recurrence rate (20–26% versus 40–59%) and lower cause-specific mortality in most studies. There is also general agreement about minimal thyroid cancer: it is defined as an incidentally found papillary thyroid cancer of 1 cm or less or a follicular thyroid cancer with minimal capsular or vascular invasion; these tumors are adequately treated with lobectomy alone. The controversy lies with low-risk but clinically significant cancers, for which the retrospective data are less clear (Table 12-5). In most studies, there does appear to be a lower recurrence rate with bilateral as compared with unilateral thyroidectomy (4–6% versus 14–20%), but cause-specific mortality is not altered. Follow-up with thyroglobulin and radioiodine scans is simplified with total or near-total thyroidectomy. The ability to optimally ablate residual normal thyroid tissue and treat with RAI is improved with a more complete resection. After ablation of any normal thyroid remnant, thyroglobulin levels are easier to interpret. A total thyroidectomy has higher complication rates, especially when it is performed by less-experienced surgeons. Therefore, the extent of surgery must be tailored to the patient's disease as well as to the surgeon's expertise and complication rate.

Lymph Node Dissection

Thyroid cancer metastasizes most commonly to the level VI or central nodes, followed by

TABLE 12-3 • *Components of Prognostic Schemes Used for Defining Risk-Group Categories in Patients with Follicular and Papillary Thyroid Cancer*

	Staging or Scoring System						
Prognostic Variable	**EORTC (1979)**	**AGES (1987)**	**AMES (1988)**	**U of C (1990)**	**MACIS (1993)**	**OSU (1994)**	**MSKCC (1995)**
Patient Factors							
Age	X	X	X	...	X	...	X
Sex	X	...	X	...	...	...	...
Tumor Factors							
Size	...	X	X	X	X	X	X
Multicentricity	...	...	...	...	...	X	...
Histologic grade	...	...	...	...	...	...	X
Histologic type	X	(P)*	...	...	(P)*	...	X
Extrathyroid invasion	X	X	X	X	X	X	X
Nodal metastatic lesion	...	...	...	X	...	X	X
Distant metastatic lesion	X	X	X	X	X	X	X
Operative Factors							
Incomplete resection	...	...	...	...	X	...	...

AGES, Patient age and tumor grade-extent, and size; *AMES,* patient age, presence of distant metastatic lesions, and extent and size of primary cancer; *EORTC*, European Organisation for Research and Treatment of Cancer; *FCDC*, follicular cell-derived cancer; *MACIS,* metastatic lesions, patient age, completeness of resection, invasion, and size of tumor; *MSKCC,* Memorial Sloan-Kettering Cancer Center; *OSU,* Ohio State University; *U of C,* University of Chicago; *X,* variable used in defining risk group; ..., variable not used.

*Schemes devised only for papillary thyroid carcinoma.

Reproduced from Thyroid Carcinoma Guidelines, *Endocr Pract.* 2001;7(No.3) 208.

TABLE 12-4 • *TNM Staging for Thyroid Carcinoma*

Stage	Papillary or Follicular Age <45 Years	Papillary or Follicular Age ≥45 Years	Medullary, Any Age	Anaplastic, Any Age
I	M0	T1	T1	...
II	M1	T2	T2	...
III	...	T3 or N1a	T3 or N1a	...
IVA	...	T4a or N1b	T4a or N1b	T4a
IVB		T4b	T4b	T4b
IVC		M1	M1	M1
Primary Tumor (T)				
TX	Primary tumor cannot be assessed			
T0	No evidence of primary tumor			
T1	Tumor 2 cm or less in greatest dimension limited to the thyroid			
T2	Tumor >2 cm but ≤4 cm in greatest dimension limited to the thyroid			
T3	Tumor >4 cm in greatest dimension limited to the thyroid or any tumor with minimal extrathyroid extension (e.g., extension to sternothyroid muscle or perithyroid soft tissue)			
T4a	Tumor of any size extending beyond the thyroid capsule to invade subcutaneous soft tissues, larynx, trachea, esophagus, or recurrent laryngeal nerve			
T4b	Tumor invades prevertebral fascia or encases carotid artery or mediastinal vessels			
Note: All anaplastic carcinomas are considered T4 tumors.				
T4a	Intrathyroidal anaplastic carcinoma, surgically resectable			
T4b	Extrathyroidal anaplastic carcinoma, surgically resectable			
Regional Lymph Nodes (N)				
Note: Regional lymph nodes are the central compartment and lateral, cervical, and upper mediastinal lymph nodes.				
NX	Regional lymph nodes cannot be assessed			
N0	No regional lymph node metastasis			
N1	Regional lymph node metastasis			
N1a	Metastasis to level VI (pretracheal, paratracheal, and prelaryngeal/Delphian lymph nodes)			
N1b	Metastasis to unilateral, bilateral, or contralateral cervical lymph nodes			
Distant Metastasis (M)				
MX	Distant metastasis cannot be assessed			
M0	No distant metastasis			
M1	Distant metastasis			

Adapted from Greene FL, Page DL, Fleming ID, *et al.*, eds. *AJCC cancer staging handbook,* 6th ed. New York: Springer-Verlag, 2002.

TABLE 12-5 • *Controversies Regarding Extent of Surgery in Patients with Moderate to Low Risk Thyroid Cancer:*

Listed Below Are Reasons Cited for Each Position: Total Thyroidectomy (TT)	Less Than TT
Bilateral disease occurs in 30–85% of patients	Multicentricity not clinically significant
Recurrent disease occurs in 5–24% of <TT patients	<5% recurrences in thyroid bed
50% of patients die from recurrence	50% local recurrences surgically curable
Survival is improved for tumors >1.5 cm	Data are retrospective and controversial
Improved efficacy for Iodine-131	Low risk patients may not benefit from I_{131}
Improved efficacy of thyroglobulin levels as marker	Thyroglobulin may still be used as a marker with native thyroid in place
Avoid reoperative thyroid surgery and its complications	TT has higher complication rate

Adapted from Udelsman R, Lakatos E, Ladenson P. Optimal surgery for papillary thyroid carcinoma. *World J Surg* 1996;20:88–93.

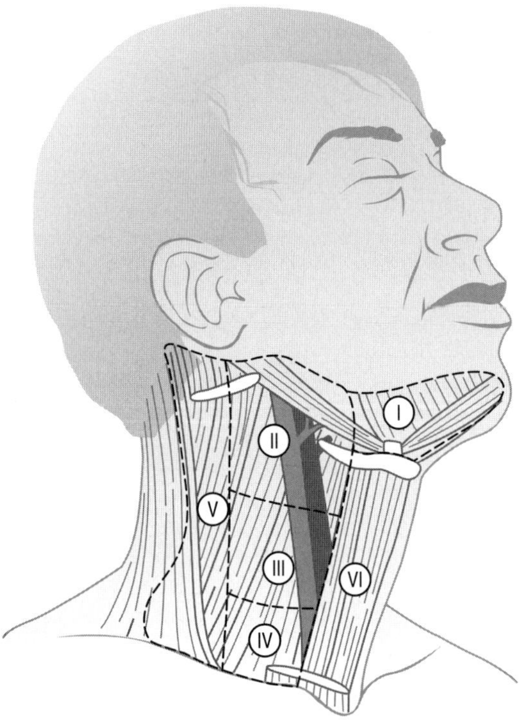

Figure 12–8. Lymph node compartments of the neck. (From Greenfield LJ, Mulholland MW, Oldham KT, *et al.*, eds. *Surgery: scientific principles and practice*, 3rd ed. Philadelphia: Lippincott Williams & Wilkins, 2001:1265.)

the internal jugular nodes at levels II, III, and IV (Figure 12-8). A preoperative ultrasound for patients with known thyroid cancer is useful for evaluating the lateral neck for lymphadenopathy. It is less sensitive for the detection of central nodal metastases. Routine lymph node dissection reveals metastases in up to 80% of cases, and it has not been demonstrated to decrease recurrence or improve survival. The current practice of most endocrine surgeons with regard to well-differentiated thyroid cancer is to only perform a neck dissection in the setting of clinically evident nodal disease. However, because reoperative surgery to remove metastatic central nodes puts the recurrent laryngeal nerves and parathyroid glands at increased risk, some surgeons have recommended a prophylactic central neck dissection at the time of thyroidectomy for known thyroid cancer. The lateral neck nodes are not removed unless they are clinically involved, in which cases a compartment-oriented node dissection had lower recurrence rates as compared with selective node picking (10% versus 25%). The preferred approach is a modified neck dissection that preserves the internal jugular vein, the sternocleidomastoid muscle, and the spinal accessory nerve.

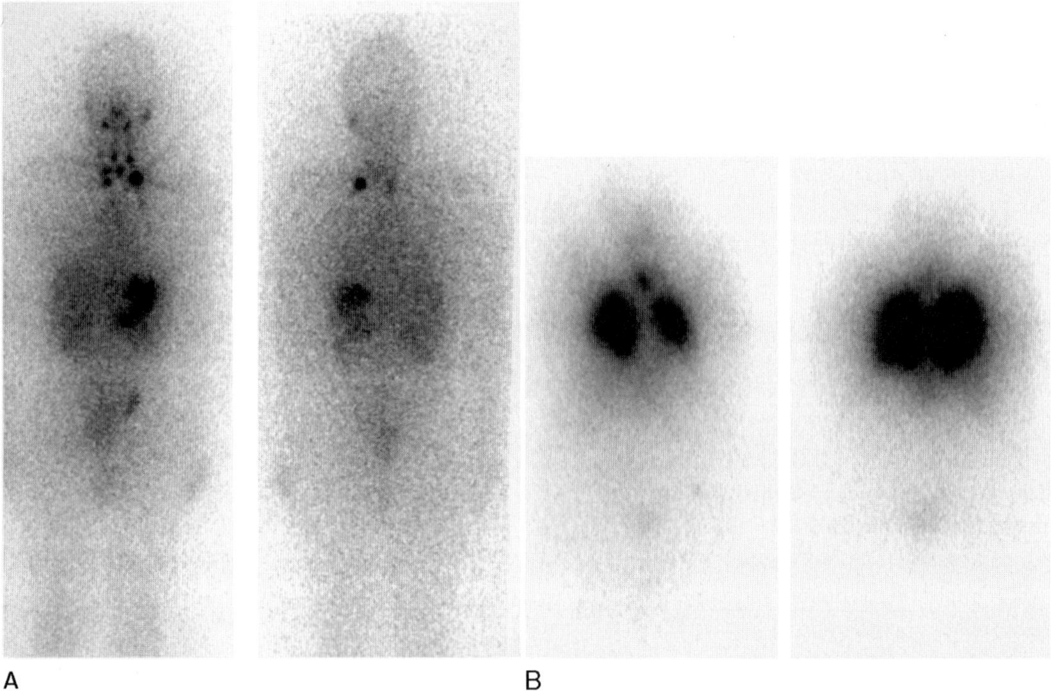

Figure 12–9. A, Whole-body scan showing multiple cervical metastases from papillary thyroid cancer. **B,** Whole-body scan showing diffuse pulmonary metastases from thyroid cancer. (Courtesy of Dr. Robert Hellman.)

Adjuvant Treatment

RAI is the mainstay of adjuvant treatment for differentiated thyroid cancer. It is used to ablate residual thyroid tissue after surgery and to treat metastatic differentiated thyroid carcinoma. A post-therapy scan may reveal unsuspected metastatic disease (Figure 12-9). The dose used for postsurgical ablation depends on the residual thyroid tissue present and on the risk of recurrence. It ranges from 30 to 50 mCi for ablation of a small amount of residual thyroid to 100 to 200 mCi to treat patients with high-risk disease or known metastases. It is not recommended to ablate an entire lobe because of a higher incidence of side effects, such as thyroiditis. In most centers, a standard dose is given, but some centers perform dosimetry to calculate the optimal dose. The use of RAI for remnant ablation for low-risk patients is controversial. Remnant ablation has been shown in several retrospective analyses to decrease recurrence rates and death, but other studies have not confirmed this, especially in low-risk patients. For high-risk patients, remnant ablation is recommended. Patients with metastatic carcinoma may be treated with repeated doses of RAI. Toxicity at high cumulative doses includes pulmonary fibrosis (from treatment of lung metastases), bone marrow suppression, and dry mouth. Above 500 mCi, there is an increased risk of leukemia. TSH is a growth factor for differentiated thyroid cancer. TSH suppression by supraphysiologic dosing of thyroxine decreases the risk of recurrence and death in retrospective analyses. The detrimental side effects of high doses of thyroid hormone include cardiac arrhythmias and osteoporosis, which must be weighed against the risk of recurrence and the patient's comorbid conditions. For patients with a high risk of recurrence, serum TSH should be maintained below 0.1 mIU/L; in for low-risk patients, the serum TSH can be maintained in the 0.1 to 0.4 mIU/L range.

External beam radiation may be useful for cases with minimal iodine uptake, with aggressive local invasion, or with gross or microscopic residual disease. *Chemotherapy* is not effective, and it is not usually used as adjuvant therapy.

Follow-Up

After initial treatment with surgery and RAI, TSH should be monitored to ensure that suppression is adequate. Thyroglobulin (Tg) monitoring can be used to detect recurrence. Tg is a highly specific tumor marker in patients with differentiated thyroid cancer. After bilateral thyroidectomy and ablation, serum Tg should be undetectable. Tg is usually less than 10 ng/mL after a unilateral lobectomy on suppression. On TSH suppression, a serum Tg lower than 2 ng/mL failed to identify 23% of patients with metastatic disease. A stimulated (TSH >30) Tg is a more sensitive test, and it may be used alone to monitor patients at low risk for recurrence. The stimulated TSH level may be obtained by either thyroxine withdrawal for 3 to 6 weeks or with the administration of recombinant human TSH (Thyrogen). If the stimulated TSH is greater than 2 ng/mL, further workup is recommended, with evaluation of the neck with ultrasound and a chest radiograph. Stimulated whole body Iodine-123 or Iodine-131 scanning detects thyroid cancer recurrence in up to 75% of cases, whether locoregional or distant, and it is useful for planning additional doses of RAI treatment. Ultrasound is useful for the determination of recurrent disease in the thyroid bed or cervical lymph nodes. An FNA may be obtained for tissue confirmation. Computed tomography scanning is very useful for anatomical details; however, use of the iodinated intravenous contrast will prevent RAI uptake for a period of up to 4 to 6 weeks. Positron emission tomography scanning has recently been approved for the detection of Tg-positive but scan negative patients.

Treatment of Recurrent Disease

Recurrent disease may present as an elevated Tg, a positive whole body scan, a palpable mass (e.g., in the neck), bony pain indicating metastases, or, less commonly, respiratory symptoms or symptoms of brain metastases. Local disease is best treated with surgical excision, if it can be identified. Isolated or symptomatic distant metastases may also be treated surgically. Otherwise, RAI is the treatment of choice. Unfortunately, some differentiated thyroid cancers are unresponsive to RAI, including Hürthle cell cancers, and some fail to take up RAI after repeated courses of treatment. Radiation therapy may also be used for palliative treatment, particularly with unresectable bony metastases.

Medullary Thyroid Cancer

Medullary thyroid cancer (MTC) represents 6% to 12% of thyroid cancers. It originates from the C cells, which are neuroendocrine cells derived from ectodermal neural crest precursors. Embryologically, the C cells derive from the ultimobranchial body, which incorporates into the lateral thyroid and is usually concentrated between the first and second third of the posterolateral thyroid lobe. These cells produce calcitonin, which is a calcium-regulating hormone of uncertain importance in humans. On FNA, MTC demonstrates plasmacytoid cells with stroma consisting of collagen and amyloid. MTC can be easily distinguished from differentiated thyroid cancer by immunohistochemical staining for calcitonin. Serum calcitonin and carcinoembrygonic antigen (CEA) levels will be elevated in most patients. Medullary thyroid cancer is the predominant phenotype of multiple endocrine neoplasia (MEN) types IIA and IIB and familial medullary thyroid cancer (FMTC). Approximately 25% to 30% of patients presenting with sporadic medullary thyroid cancer have a genetic syndrome; therefore, genetic counseling and testing is recommended for all patients with MTC, especially those with multifocal tumors. If positive, family members should also undergo genetic counseling.

MEN IIA, MEN IIB, and FMTC all harbor activating mutations in the *ret* gene, which is located on chromosome 10 and which encodes a membrane-bound tyrosine kinase receptor. The majority of patients with MEN IIA and FMTC have point mutations in the 634 codon in exon 11; fewer have mutations in the 609, 611, 618, and 620 codons in exon 10. MEN IIB is characterized by a single mutation at the 918 codon in exon 16. The syndromes are inherited in an autosomal-dominant fashion, and MTC is common to all of them. MEN IIA has the additional phenotype of pheochromocytoma, hyperparathyroidism, and cutaneous lichen amyloidosis; MEN IIB also is characterized by pheochromocytomas, but, in addition, it has a distinct clinical phenotype. These patients have a marfanoid habitus, mucosal neuromas of the tongue and lips (Figure 12-10), optic nerve hypertrophy, and gut ganglioneuromatosis. The penetrance of the various components are variable (Table 12-6), and there are no genotype/phenotype correlations identified so far. With genetic testing, it is now possible to identify mutation carriers at an early age and to offer thyroidectomy before the development of MTC, which is the usual cause of mortality in these patients. Recommendation for prophylactic surgery in children with the MEN IIA mutation is before the age of 5 years; for those with MEN IIB, it is during the first year of life.

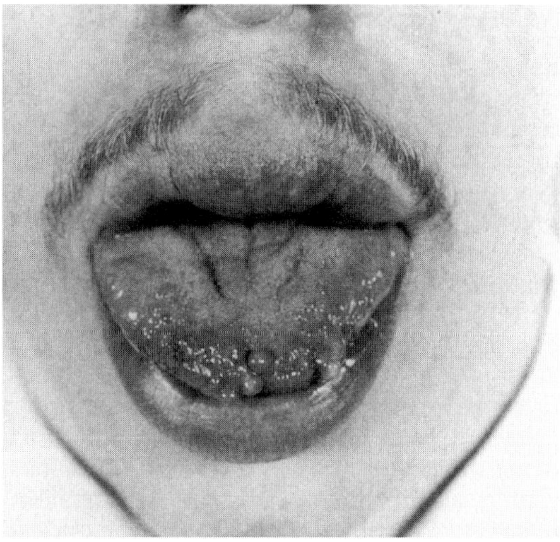

Figure 12–10. Multiple endocrine neoplasia IIB patient with mucosal neuromas of the tongue and lips.

Surgical Treatment

If a patient is known to have a MEN II mutation or has a family history that is suspicious for MEN II, pheochromocytoma must be ruled out before any surgery by 24-hour urinary catecholamines and metanephrines or plasma metanephrines. Baseline calcitonin and CEA levels are valuable for follow-up. A total thyroidectomy with central node dissection is recommended for both sporadic and familial MTC. In sporadic, palpable MTC, functional neck dissection (levels II to V) should be considered, because there is a high rate of lymph node metastases in ipsilateral (around 80%) and contralateral (40–50%) lymph nodes. Prophylactic surgery for MEN/FMTC patients need not include a functional neck dissection.

Follow-Up

The prognosis for MTC is age and stage dependent. Calcitonin and CEA are tumor markers for MTC recurrence. A biochemical cure portends an excellent survival (97.7% at 10 years), whereas survival is still good at 10 years (70–86%) for those with elevated calcitonin levels. The identification of recurrent or residual disease may be difficult. Imaging with somatostatin-receptor scintigraphy is sensitive, but it will miss lesions that are less than 1 cm and hepatic metastases. Laparoscopy may identify occult intraperitoneal disease. Regional venous sampling with pentagastrin stimulation is very sensitive. If recurrence is identified and resectable, surgery is the preferred treatment, because MTC is not very responsive to radiation or chemotherapy. Anti-CEA antibod-

TABLE 12–6 • *Clinical and Genetic Features of Multiple Endocrine Neoplasia Syndromes*

Multiple Endocrine Neoplasia Type	Syndrome	Penetrance	Genetic Mutation
I	Parathyroid hyperplasia Pancreatic islet cell tumors Pituitary	95% 40% 30%	Menin gene • Chromosome 11 • Distributed throughout gene
IIA	Medullary thyroid cancer Pheochromocytoma Parathyroid hyperplasia	95% 50% 15%	RET gene • Chromosome 10 • Codons 609, 611, 618, 620, and 634
IIB	Medullary thyroid cancer Pheochromocytoma Phenotype: • Mucosal neuromas • Marfanoid habitus • Myelinated corneal nerves • Gut ganglioneuromatosis	95% 50% 90%	RET gene • Chromosome 10 • Codon 918

ies and a combination of interferon-α and octreotide have shown some responses as evaluated by tumor markers in clinical trials involving patients with advanced MTC.

Anaplastic Thyroid Cancer

Anaplastic thyroid cancer is characterized by poorly differentiated, bizarre, and pleomorphic cell morphology that is sometimes seen arising in an area of well-differentiated follicular thyroid cancer. Clinically, it usually occurs in the elderly. A typical case history is an elderly individual with a longstanding thyroid nodule or goiter that rapidly increases in size. A tissue diagnosis by FNA, core needle, or incisional biopsy is required to rule out thyroid lymphoma, which has a better prognosis. At diagnosis, anaplastic thyroid cancer is frequently unresectable, having invaded into vital structures of the neck. An isthmusectomy may be required to relieve airway compression or for placement of a tracheostomy. If still localized within the thyroid, complete resection with adjuvant therapy may provide long-term survival. Combination chemotherapy and hyperfractionated radiotherapy followed by surgical debulking can lead to successful local control in a minority of selected patients.

Thyroid Lymphoma

Thyroid lymphoma, which now accounts for around 5% of all thyroid malignancies, usually presents in older patients. There is often a history of rapid growth, and it is usually associated with Hashimoto's thyroiditis. The diagnosis can be made with FNA with staining of lymphoid markers. Disease confined to the thyroid responds well to local treatments, such as surgical resection with or without radiation. Lymphomas are very radiosensitive and therefore the current role of surgery is limited to obtaining tissue diagnosis, if required, and establishing airway control, if necessary. Patients with extrathyroidal extension or residual disease have a high relapse rate. In a review from Yale in 1994, overall and distant relapse rates are significantly decreased with combined chemotherapy and radiotherapy for both stage I or II thyroid lymphoma. Chemotherapy is done with anthracycline-based regimens, such as CHOP (cyclophosphamide, doxorubicin, vincristine, and prednisone). Therefore, the current recommendation is multimodality treatment for patients with no contraindications for systemic chemotherapy.

The thyroid may be a site of distant metastases from adenocarcinomas, but these are rarely clinically significant. Other rare tumors that occur in the thyroid gland are paragangliomas, sarcomas, tumors related to thymic or branchial pouch differentiation, and mucoepidermoid carcinoma.

Parathyroid Disease

The parathyroid glands produce parathyroid hormone, which regulates calcium and phosphate metabolism. Parathyroid hormone causes an increase in serum calcium by activating osteoclasts to release calcium from bone stores, thereby reducing the renal clearance of calcium and increasing the intestinal absorption of calcium via the renal production of vitamin D. Hypoparathyroidism is usually iatrogenic, occurring as a result of thyroid or parathyroid surgery; however, rare cases of congenital hypoparathyroidism have occurred.

Primary hyperparathyroidism is caused by increased secretion of PTH by the parathyroid gland(s), which leads to an elevated serum calcium level. Single gland disease, caused by an adenoma, is found in 85% to 90% of cases. Multiple gland disease occurs in 10% to 15% of cases and may result from double (and rarely triple) adenomas but more commonly from four-gland hyperplasia. It may be difficult to distinguish between hyperplasia and multiple adenomas, because asymmetric hyperplasia is common.

Secondary hyperparathyroidism is the overproduction of PTH as the result of a non-parathyroid cause, usually renal failure. Renal failure decreases the production of $1,25(OH)_2D_3$, thereby impairing intestinal absorption of calcium and leading to hypocalcemia, which increases PTH secretion by the parathyroid glands. Hyperphosphatemia from decreased renal excretion also contributes to PTH secretion. The calcium level is low or normal.

Tertiary hyperparathyroidism occurs when the hyperplastic glands of secondary hyperparathyroidism become autonomous, and it is characterized by hypercalcemia.

Parathyroid carcinoma is rare, accounting for less than 1% of all cases of hyperparathyroidism. It usually presents with very high calcium and PTH levels, and it is recognized intraoperatively by local invasion, usually into the thyroid. En bloc resection of the ipsilateral thyroid lobe is recommended. Multiple reoperations and metastasectomies may lead to prolonged survival.

Hypercalcemic crisis occurs when the serum calcium level is markedly elevated, often presenting with symptoms of mental status changes. Treatment starts with intravenous hydration with or without forced diuresis, and this is followed by bisphosphonates. Some patients may require calcitonin, glucocorticoids, or dialysis.

Diagnosis of Primary Hyperparathyroidism

Primary hyperparathyroidism in the United States usually presents incidentally when hypercalcemia is noted during routine laboratory testing. Symptoms may include nephrolithiasis, decreased bone density, and other, less specific symptoms, such as fatigue, constipation, nocturia, and pruritus. Although many patients may be asymptomatic, a detailed history will often uncover unrecognized symptoms. A family history of endocrine disorders should be sought, because hyperparathyroidism is a component of MEN I and MEN IIA (see Table 12-6).

BOX 12–5 SYMPTOMS OF HYPERCALCEMIA

- Fatigue/weakness
- Polydipsia/polyuria
- Bone pain
- Constipation
- Depression
- Abdominal pain/nausea
- Pancreatitis
- Pruritus
- Nephrolithiasis
- Osteopenia
- Gout
- Ulcer disease
- Hypertension
- Nocturia

During the laboratory examination, an inappropriately elevated PTH level is the hallmark. Calcium and PTH levels are tightly regulated, and they are evaluated concurrently when considering hyperparathyroidism. For example, in a patient with hypercalcemia, a PTH level at the upper normal range is inappropriately elevated; this is indicative of primary hyperparathyroidism. A 24-hour urine is obtained to rule out familial hypocalciuric hypercalcemia, which is a benign condition that can mimic the diagnosis of primary hyperparathyroidism. A bone density study may be useful for determining the need for surgery.

Indications for Surgery

Currently there is no effective medical treatment for primary hyperparathyroidism. Bisphosphonates and estrogen therapy may be effective for preventing bone loss. Calcimimetics (compounds that mimic the effect of extracellular calcium on the calcium-sensing receptor) are currently under investigation. Thus, the treatment options are observation or surgery. Because many patients are diagnosed during the early stages and may exhibit few obvious symptoms, there continues to be debate about when to refer patients for surgery. Approximately 25% of patients followed without surgery will develop complications. Major concerns for untreated primary hyperparathyroidism are the long-term effects on decreased bone density and cardiovascular mortality. The advent of minimally invasive parathyroidectomy has encouraged earlier referrals; this is reflected in the recent changes in the National Institutes of Health consensus guidelines for asymptomatic hyperparathyroidism (Table 12-7). If observation is chosen, the recommended follow-up regimen is the semiannual monitoring of calcium and annual bone density studies. The primary treatment for secondary hyperparathyroidism is medical, using calcium supplementation, phosphate binders, vitamin D, calcitriol, and calcimimetics. When medical treatment fails to control secondary hyperparathyroidism, which is demonstrated by the development of tertiary hyperparathyroidism with persistent hypercalcemia, intractable pruritus, skeletal pain or fractures, or progressive extraskeletal calcifications or calciphylaxis (a potentially fatal disease due to calcification of cutaneous blood vessels), then surgery is indicated.

Anatomy of the Parathyroid Glands

The challenge of parathyroid surgery lies in their anatomic variation (Figure 12-11). The inferior parathyroid gland, which originates together with the thymus from the third branchial pouch, descends toward the mediastinum. The most common location is at the lower pole of the thyroid and along the thyrothymic tract, although ectopic glands can be found anywhere along the embryologic path, from the angle of the mandible to the anterior mediastinum. The superior glands originate from the fourth branchial pouch, and most can be found within 2 cm of the intersection of the recurrent laryngeal nerve and the inferior thyroid artery. Enlarged superior glands preferentially descend posteriorly along the tracheoesophageal groove. Ectopic glands may also be found within the thyroid gland (Table 12-8). The recurrent laryngeal nerve serves as a landmark, with the superior gland found within the posterior or dorsal triangle and the inferior gland within the anterior or ventral triangle (Figure 12-12). The vascular supply of the parathyroid glands is from the inferior and superior thyroid arteries.

Surgery for Primary Hyperparathyroidism

The standard operation for primary hyperparathyroidism is a four-gland exploration with cure rates of up to 98%. However, with the increasing use of preoperative imaging and intraoperative PTH monitoring, minimally invasive parathyroidectomy is increasingly performed.

Preoperative imaging should only be performed if a minimally invasive approach is offered, because it is unnecessary if both sides of the neck are to be explored. The most widely used imaging study is the sestamibi scan (Figure 12-13), which identifies an abnormal parathyroid gland in 60% to 90% of cases. The radioisotope is taken up by both the thyroid and the parathyroid glands, but it washes out of the thyroid gland at a more rapid rate, leaving activity visible in the enlarged parathyroid gland(s). Variations of the technique include single photon emission computed tomography and subtraction scanning. The study is also useful for detecting ectopic mediastinal adenomas, and it can obviate a neck exploration in the small number of patients with mediastinal adenomas. Limitations of sestamibi include low sensitivity for small adenomas and multiple gland disease. Neck ultrasound is a complementary

TABLE 12-7 • *2002 National Institute of Diabetes and Digestive and Kidney Diseases Workshop Criteria for Surgery in "Asymptomatic" Primary Hyperparathyroidism*

• Serum calcium 1 mg/dL above upper limit of normal
• 30% reduction of creatinine clearance
• Urinary calcium >400 mg in 24 hours
• Bone density T score >–2.5 at any site
• Less than 50 years old
• Other symptoms: neuropsychiatric, gastrointestinal, increased bone turnover

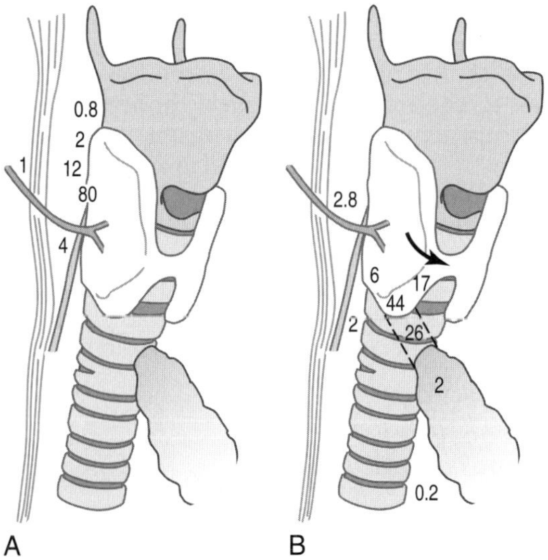

Figure 12-11. **A,** Potential superior and **B,** inferior parathyroid gland locations. Numbers refer to the percentage of glands found at each location. (From DeGroot LJ, Jameson JL, eds. *Endocrinology,* fourth edition. Philadelphia: WB Saunders, 2001.)

imaging study that requires an experienced operator. The sensitivity ranges from 60% to 80%, and it provides more detailed anatomic information for operative planning. If both sestamibi and ultrasound localizes a single abnormally enlarged gland at the same location, there is a very high probability that the patient has a single adenoma that will be identified at that site during the operation.

TABLE 12-8 • *Location of Ectopic Parathyroid Glands*

Missing superior parathyroid gland	Above superior pole
	Retrolaryngeal/esophageal areas
	Tracheoesophageal groove
	On prevertebral fascia
	Intrathyroidal
	Carotid sheath
	Lateral scalene fat pad
Missing inferior parathyroid gland	Thymus or superior mediastinum
	Undescended: carotid sheath from hyoid to thoracic inlet
	Intrathyroidal
	Medial, by trachea

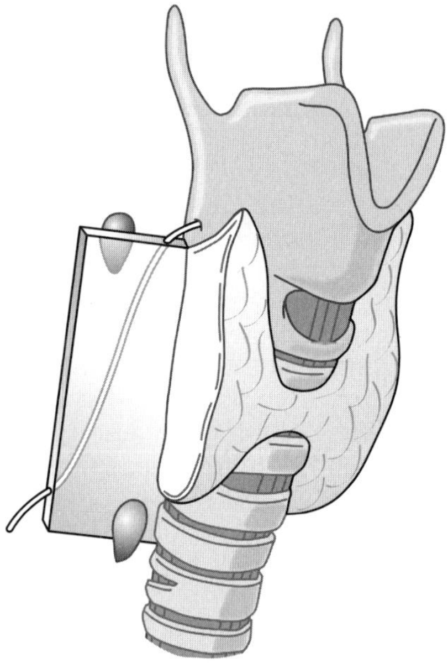

Figure 12-12. The recurrent laryngeal nerve and its relationship to the superior and inferior parathyroid gland. The superior gland is dorsal and the inferior gland is ventral to the plane of the recurrent laryngeal nerve. (From Randolph GW. *Surgery of the thyroid and parathyroid glands.* Philadelphia: WB Saunders, 2003.)

Technical Aspects of Parathyroid Surgery

The standard four-gland exploration is performed through a 4 to 6 cm incision. The thyroid gland is exposed, the middle thyroid vein is divided and ligated, and the thyroid gland rotated medially. The space between the carotid artery and the thyroid gland is exposed, the intervening loose areolar tissue is divided into layers, and the recurrent laryngeal nerve is identified. An effort is made to identify all four glands. Normal appearing glands are left undisturbed. Normal parathyroid glands are between 40 and 60 mg in weight; they are 3 to 8 mm in one dimension, and they are usually ellipsoid. They are golden brown in color, they are often associated with a tiny fat pad, and they may lie just beneath the thyroid capsule, where they are often ballotable. Care must be taken during dissection to not devascularize the tiny glands. Small biopsies may be performed if the identification is in question, although the routine biopsy of normal parathyroid glands will lead to an increased incidence of transient hypocalcemia. If multiple-gland disease is suspected, then the excision of any glands should be delayed until all four glands are evaluated.

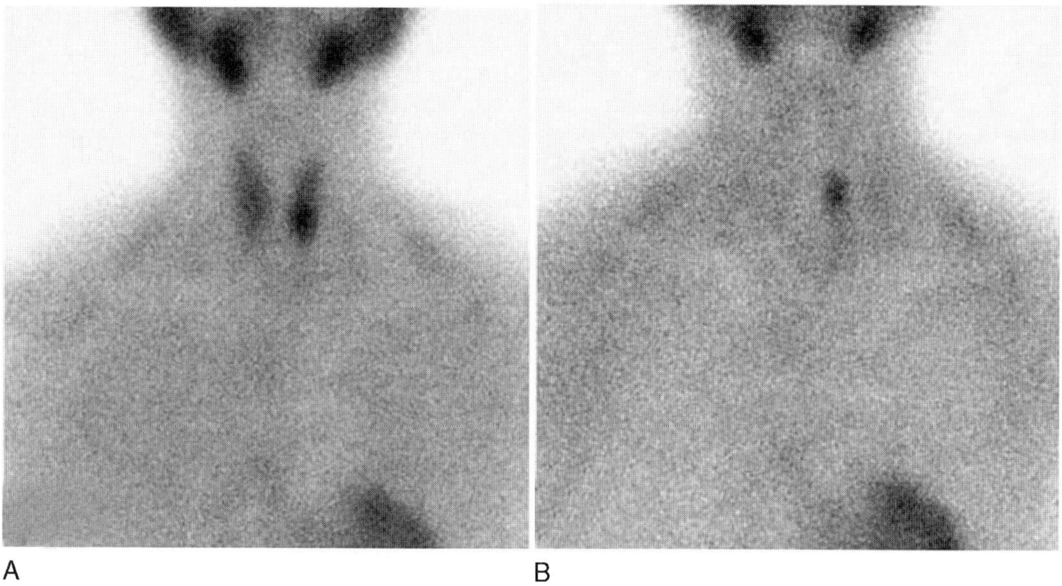

Figure 12-13. Sestamibi scan. **A,** Immediate scan showing uptake in both the thyroid and parathyroid glands. **B,** Delayed scan (1.5 hours) showing uptake only in the parathyroid adenoma.

All abnormally enlarged gland(s) are carefully dissected and excised after the vascular pedicle is ligated. In the case of four gland hyperplasia, a 40 to 60 mg remnant is fashioned from the gland with the best vascular supply before the removal of the three other enlarged glands. The recurrent laryngeal nerve is often adjacent to—or, in some cases, draped over—the parathyroid glands and must be protected.

A *minimally invasive parathyroidectomy* can be performed if a single gland is localized preoperatively, and intraoperative PTH monitoring is available to rule out multiple-gland disease (Table 12-9). The abnormal gland is excised through a small (1.5-4 cm) incision, with minimal dissection. The recurrent laryngeal nerve is often not identified. The surgeon must be prepared to perform a four gland exploration if the localization studies were inaccurate or if the intraoperative PTH levels fail to drop appropriately.

Intraoperative PTH monitoring is possible as a result of the short half-life (<5 minutes) of PTH. After excision of all hyperfunctioning parathyroid tissue, the PTH level should drop rapidly, and no further exploration is needed. A number of different criteria have been proposed to define a sufficient drop in

TABLE 12-9 • *Adjuncts Used with Minimally Invasive Parathyroidectomy*

	Advantages	Disadvantages	Role in Minimally Invasive Parathyroidectomy
Sestamibi	Excellent specificity Evaluate mediastinum Easily obtained	Not sensitive for multiple gland disease and small adenomas	Required
Ultrasound	Detects thyroid pathology Good specificity	Operator dependent Less specific than sestamibi	Increases number of patients eligible for minimally invasive parathyroidectomy
Intraoperative parathyroid hormone	Detects multiple gland disease (50–90%)	Requires special equipment	Required
Gamma probe	Facilitates use of smaller incision May be useful in reoperations	Requires special equipment	Not widely used

intraoperative PTH level to ensure that this drop is sufficient to terminate the operation. The most commonly used criterion is a 50% drop below baseline at 10 minutes after excision of the last abnormal gland (Figure 12-14). The ability of this test to detect multiple-gland disease ranges from 50% to 90%. Another adjunct in minimally invasive parathyroidectomy is the use of a *gamma probe*. Technetium-labeled sestamibi is given before surgery, and the probe is used intraoperatively to help locate the parathyroid adenoma. About 75% to 90% of patients will localize preoperatively and will be eligible for a minimally invasive approach. Advantages include a smaller incision, a shorter operative time, and possible avoidance of general anesthesia. The ability to detect multiple-gland disease is lower using this approach, and the long-term success rate remains to be determined.

Surgery in Patients with Multiple Endocrine Neoplasia Syndromes

Primary hyperparathyroidism is a feature of the MEN I and MEN IIA syndromes. In MEN I, the hyperparathyroidism is often quite aggressive, with high rates of recurrence. A 3.5-gland parathyroidectomy is the recommended surgical treatment, although some experts recommend a total parathyroidectomy with reimplantation of one gland equivalent (40-60 mg) of tissue, generally into the forearm. This allows monitoring of parathyroid function through antecubital venous blood sampling as well as easy access to remove excess parathyroid tissue if persistent disease is identified. The risk of injury to the recurrent laryngeal nerves is avoided as compared with cases in which neck re-exploration is required. In MEN IIA, the hyperparathyroidism is less aggressive and may be treated with resection of only the enlarged glands after a four-gland exploration.

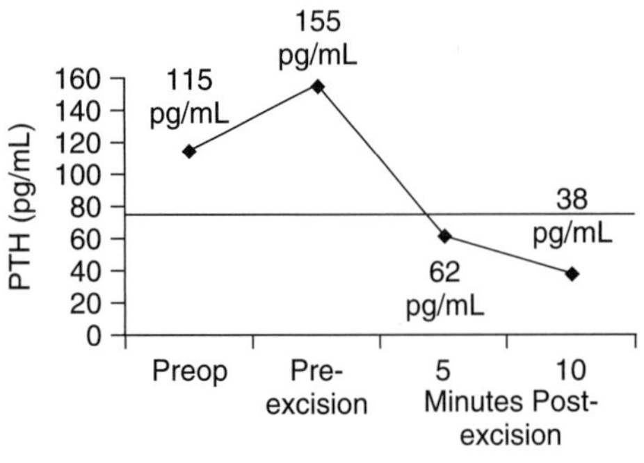

Figure 12-14. Intraoperative parathyroid hormone monitoring. The parathyroid hormone level rises from baseline just before excision of the adenoma as a result of gland manipulation. It then falls rapidly after adenoma removal to less than 50% of baseline or time zero, indicating removal of all hyperfunctioning parathyroid tissue.

Surgery for Secondary and Tertiary Hyperparathyroidism

In secondary hyperparathyroidism, all of the parathyroid glands are hyperplastic as a result of external stimuli, and they are often quite large. Parathyroid rests may manifest as supernumerary glands, which occur more frequently in patients with secondary hyperparathyroidism. They are frequently found in the thymic tongues; therefore, the thymic tongues are routinely removed in these cases. Surgical strategy is a 3.5-gland parathyroidectomy or complete parathyroidectomy with reimplantation of a small remnant, usually in the forearm.

Postoperative Complications

Recurrent laryngeal nerve injury after parathyroid surgery is reported to occur at the rate of 1% to 2%, and permanent hypoparathyroidism occurs at the rate of 2%. The incidence of these complications is at least doubled in the setting of reoperation, emphasizing the importance of a successful initial operation. Persistent hyperparathyroidism occurs in 2% to 4% of cases in experienced hands, and it is likely to be higher for surgeons who do not perform parathyroidectomy routinely. Recurrent hyperparathyroidism (occurring 6 months after surgery) is unusual. Transient hypoparathyroidism with hypocalcemia occurs more frequently among patients undergoing more extensive exploration and resection and among those patients with extensive bone disease or those with an elevated alkaline phosphatase. This can be treated with careful use of calcium and vitamin D supplementation until residual parathyroid function normalizes.

Selected Readings

Bilezikian JP, Brandi ML, Rubin M, Silverberg SJ. Primary hyperparathyroidism: new concepts in clinical, densitometric and biochemical features. *J Intern Med* 2005;257:6–17.

Bilezikian JP, Potts JT Jr, Fuleihan Gel-H, *et al*. Summary statement from a workshop on asymptomatic primary hyperparathyroidism: a perspective for the 21st century. *J Clin Endocrinol Metab* 2002;87:5353–5361.

Brandi ML, Gagel RF, Angeli A, *et al.* Guidelines for diagnosis and therapy of MEN type 1 and type 2. *J Clin Endocrinol Metab* 2001;86:5658–5671.

Castro MR, Gharib H. Continuing controversies in the management of thyroid nodules. *Ann Intern Med* 2005;142:926–931.

Doherty GM. Multiple endocrine neoplasia type 1. *J Surg Oncol* 2005;89:143–150.

Hegedus L. The thyroid nodule. *N Engl J Med* 2004;351:1764–1771.

Mazzaferri EL, Kloos RT. Current approaches to primary therapy for papillary and follicular thyroid cancer. *J Clin Endocrinol Metab* 2001;86:1447–1463.

Mazzaferri EL, Robbins RJ, Spencer CA, *et al.* A consensus report of the role of serum thyroglobulin as a monitoring method for low-risk patients with papillary thyroid carcinoma. *J Clin Endocrinol Metab* 2003;88:1433–1441.

Mittendorf E, McHenry C. Parathyroid carcinoma. *J Surg Oncol* 2005;89:136–142.

Quayle FJ, Moley JF. Medullary thyroid carcinoma: including MEN 2A and MEN 2B syndromes. *J Surg Oncol* 2005;89:122–129.

Rawat N, Khetan N, Williams DW, Baxter JN. Parathyroid carcinoma. *Br J Surg* 2005;92:1345–1353.

Robbins RJ, Robbins AK. Recombinant human thyrotropin and thyroid cancer management. *J Clin Endocrinol Metab* 2003;88:1933–1938.

Sawka AM, Thephamongkhol K, Brouwers M, *et al.* Clinical review 170: A systematic review and meta-analysis of the effectiveness of radioactive iodine remnant ablation for well-differentiated thyroid cancer. *J Clin Endocrinol Metab* 2004;89:3668–3676.

Schlumberger MJ. Papillary and follicular thyroid carcinoma. *N Engl J Med* 1998;338:297–306.

Udelsman R, Lakatos E, Ladenson P. Optimal surgery for papillary thyroid carcinoma. *World J Surg* 1996;20:88–93.

Woodrum DT, Gauger PG. Role of ^{131}I in the treatment of well differentiated thyroid cancer. *J Surg Oncol* 2005;89:114–121.

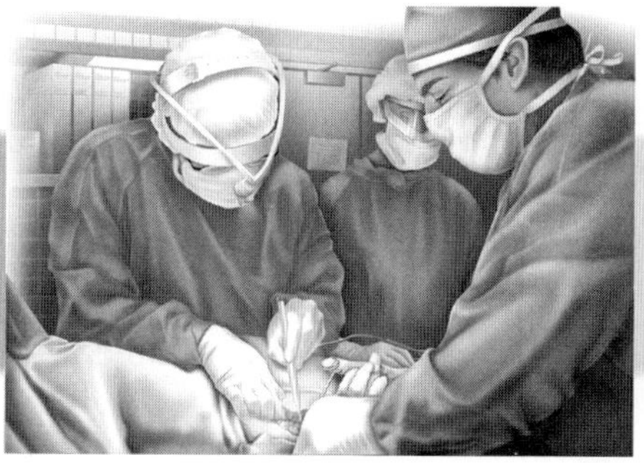

13

Benign and Malignant Tumors of the Adrenal Gland

Derek T. Woodrum and Paul G. Gauger

Benign and Malignant Tumors of the Adrenal Gland: Key Points

- Describe the anatomy of the adrenal glands.
- Outline the diagnostic process for benign conditions related to a functioning adrenocortical adenoma.
- Detail the clinical features, diagnostic procedures, and treatment of benign pheochromocytoma.
- Outline the workup of an incidentaloma.
- Describe the workup and staging of adrenocortical cancers.
- Compare the treatments for adrenocortical cancers.
- List the indications for and advantages of laparoscopic adrenalectomy.
- Describe the postoperative care of patients who have malignant adrenal tumors.

Tumors of the adrenal gland are common. Their true incidence is unknown, but autopsy surveys have found small (approximately 2 mm or greater) adrenal tumors in as many as 10% of patients, and abdominal computed tomography (CT) scans may reveal larger tumors approximately 2% to 3% of the time. Adrenal tumors are found in several different ways. They may be encountered during the workup for essential hypertension or when attempting to diagnose a patient with a history and symptoms referable to a syndrome of adrenal hormone hypersecretion (e.g., pheochromocytoma). Additionally, as a result of the increasing number of abdominal CT and magnetic resonance imaging (MRI) scans being performed in all areas of medicine, more clinically inapparent tumors of the adrenal glands are being discovered. These tumors are referred to as *incidentalomas,* which are defined as otherwise unsuspected adrenal tumors of more than 1 cm in the greatest diameter. Patients may have symptoms or signs attributable to the adrenal lesion on subsequent history and workup, but most lesions are clinically silent before incidental discovery.

The goal of the workup for an incidentaloma is to place it into one of three categories: (1) clearly benign; (2) clearly cancer; or (3) clearly a pheochromocytoma (Table 13-1). A small percentage of tumors will remain unspecified after workup, but most lesions can be placed into one of these three groups by using a combination of biochemical testing, modern imaging, and, very rarely, percutaneous biopsy of selected lesions. Benign lesions include adrenocortical adenomas (regardless of functional status or hormone produced) and most pheochromocytomas. Malignant lesions include primary adrenocortical carcinomas, a small percentage of pheochromocytomas, and metastatic lesions from a different primary cancer. Because pheochromocytomas may behave in a malignant fashion, they conceptually bridge both the benign and malignant diagnostic categories.

During the process of evaluating an adrenal tumor, it is critical to determine whether or not the tumor is hyperfunctioning. By definition, aldosteronomas and pheochromocytomas are hyperfunctioning, whereas cancers and the remaining benign lesions may either be hyperfunctioning or nonfunctioning. This chapter will review Cushing's syndrome, Conn's syndrome, pheochromocytoma, and adrenal cancers. Additionally, attention will be given to the evaluation of the increasingly common incidentaloma. The consulting surgeon is commonly faced with an adrenal tumor of unknown etiology and an inconclusive history; therefore, a standardized approach to the biochemical and radiologic workup of incidentalomas is described in detail.

Anatomy

The adrenal glands are crescent- or triangular-shaped glands that sit atop each kidney. They have a rich blood supply befitting their central role in the endocrine system (Figure 13-1). The adrenal gland can be thought of as being made up of two separate units: the cortex and the medulla (Table 13-2). The cortex is involved with steroid (e.g., aldosterone, cortisol, and androgen) synthesis, whereas the medulla synthesizes catecholamines (e.g., epinephrine and norepinephrine). The cortex comprises three zones from superficial to deep: the zona glomerulosa, the zona fasciculata, and the zona reticularis. The zona glomerulosa produces aldosterone but no cortisol, whereas the inner two zones contain the enzyme 17-alpha-hydroxylase, which enables cortisol production. The inner two zones are also involved in adrenal androgen (i.e., sex steroid) production.

Benign Lesions

The goal when imaging adrenal tumors is to recognize characteristics of likely benign or likely malignant lesions. On cross-sectional imaging, benign lesions have smooth round or oval edges, homogeneous texture, and well-defined margins. On noncontrast CT, a cutoff of less than 10 Hounsfield units (HU) carries a

TABLE 13–1 • *Benign and Malignant Tumors of the Adrenal Gland*

Benign	Malignant	May Be Either
Nonfunctioning cortical adenoma	Primary adrenocortical carcinoma	Pheochromocytoma
Cortisol-producing cortical adenoma	Metastatic lesion	
Aldosteronoma		
Myelolipoma and hematoma		

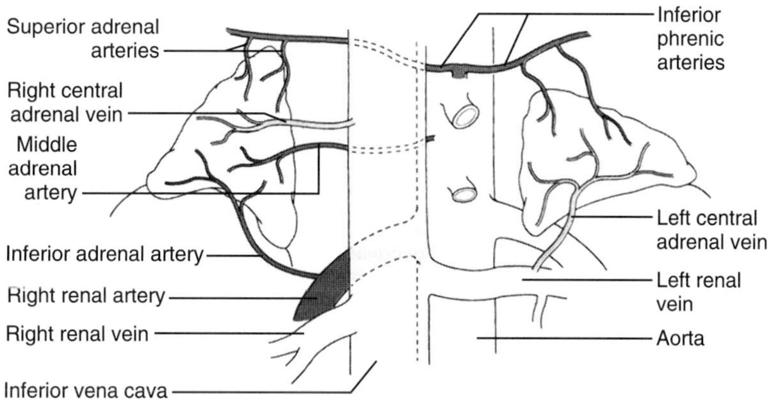

Figure 13–1. Vascular anatomy of the adrenal glands.

TABLE 13–2 • *Adrenal Gland Anatomy and Hormones Produced*

Anatomic Unit	Zones	Hormone Produced
Cortex	Zona glomerulosa	Aldosterone
	Zona fasciculata and reticularis	Cortisol and sex steroids
Medulla		Catecholamines

sensitivity of 74% and a specificity of 96% for benign adenoma. Lipid-rich benign tumors have a low HU value and are easily recognized in this manner, but lipid-poor benign tumors are not easily separated from non-benign tumors with noncontrast CT alone. To address this problem, a contrast-enhanced CT is obtained, and a simple *enhancement washout percentage* (EW%) is determined: contrast-enhanced adrenal images are obtained immediately after an intravenous contrast bolus and again 15 minutes later for delayed contrast-enhanced images. Enhancement measurements (in HU) are obtained in the enhanced and delayed-enhanced images. An EW% is calculated using the following equation:

$$EW\% = [(\text{Enhanced HU} - \text{Delayed enhanced HU})/(\text{Enhanced HU} - \text{Unenhanced HU})] \times 100$$

An EW% of 60% or greater carries a sensitivity of 98% and a specificity of 92% for benign adrenal tumor. MRI is also used to evaluate adrenal lesions by calculating an adrenal-to-spleen signal ratio. The ratios are less sensitive and specific than the HU criteria above, and CT remains the standard for tumor evaluation. Finally, NP-59 scintigraphy can be used to image the adrenal glands. The scan shows functioning adrenal tissue, so it has somewhat limited utility for classifying an adrenal lesion as benign or malignant, because both may either be functional or nonfunctional. Most adrenal cancers do not concentrate NP-59, thereby giving a discordant image as compared with CT, which suggests malignancy.

Cushing's Syndrome

About 5% of incidentalomas will be functioning adenomas of the zona fasciculata or reticularis causing subclinical hypercortisolism. *Cushing's syndrome* is a general term that refers to a state of excess blood cortisol levels, regardless of etiology (endogenous production or exogenous corticosteroid intake). This section will address Cushing's syndrome caused by a benign, hyperfunctioning adrenocortical adenoma. Adrenocortical carcinoma can also cause Cushing's syndrome, as will is discussed later, and Cushing's syndrome can also be

BOX 13–1 CAUSES OF CUSHING'S SYNDROME

- Benign hyperfunctioning adrenocortical adenoma
- Adrenocortical carcinoma
- Adrenocorticotrophic-hormone–producing pituitary adenomas (Cushing's disease)
- Other adrenocorticotrophic-hormone producing tumors

seen with conditions such as adrenocorticotrophic-hormone (ACTH)–producing pituitary adenomas (Cushing's disease) and other ACTH-producing tumors. Patients with Cushing's syndrome often have multiple nonspecific symptoms and signs, including obesity, abdominal striae, hypertension, glucose intolerance, and weakness. Although none of these are specific to Cushing's syndrome, the new onset or the progressive worsening of the symptom complex should alert the physician to the possibility of glucocorticoid excess.

The diagnosis of Cushing's syndrome is made with an elevated 24-hour urine cortisol level. Although ACTH is typically suppressed by the excess cortisol made by a hypersecreting adrenal tumor, ACTH is sporadically secreted, and a non-suppressed level does not rule out the disease. Therefore, an overnight dexamethasone suppression test (DMST) is performed to confirm the diagnosis. The patient is given 1 mg of dexamethasone orally at 11 pm, and an 8 am serum cortisol level is measured the next morning. In patients with Cushing's syndrome—including that caused by a functioning adrenal adenoma—the cortisol level will be non-suppressed (>5 ug/dL). There has been recent consideration of lowering that limit even further (approximately 2 μg/dL) in an effort to increase sensitivity and diagnose more patients with subclinical Cushing's syndrome.

Conn's Syndrome

Only 1% of incidentalomas will be functioning adenomas causing Conn's syndrome. Nevertheless, they are important, because they are a surgically correctable cause of hypertension. Primary hyperaldosteronism classically manifests as clinical triad of hypertension, hypokalemia, and sodium/ water retention leading to fluid overload. However, the absence of hypokalemia is relatively common and does not exclude the diagnosis. In approximately 60% of cases, the hyperaldosteronism is caused by a so-called aldosteronoma located in the zona glomerulosa that inappropriately overproduces aldosterone (Conn's syndrome). The remaining 40% of primary hyperaldosteronism is caused by bilateral adrenal hyperplasia (also known as *idiopathic hyperaldosteronism*).

Any patient with an adrenal tumor and hypertension should undergo screening for an aldosteronoma. Plasma aldosterone and renin levels are obtained, and serum is sent for potassium and creatinine levels. An aldosterone level:renin activity ratio is elevated in patients with Conn's syndrome (normal is less than 20:1). If necessary, confirmation of the diagnosis may be aided by a 24-hour urine collection for aldosterone and by the documentation of nonsuppressible aldosterone levels after salt loading.

As stated above, as many as 40% of cases of primary hyperaldosteronism may be the result of bilateral adrenal hyperplasia rather than a unilateral functioning adenoma. This distinction becomes very important when determining if the patient is an operative candidate: a single-gland resection is not curative and is generally not appropriate in the setting of bilateral hyperplasia, where the contribution of hypersecretion is essentially equal between the adrenal glands. CT images in hyperplasia reveal bilaterally enlarged glands that maintain an adreniform shape and a smooth surface without focal enlargement. If both adrenals are diffusely nodular, there is a 25% incidence of underlying adenoma. Traditionally, the NP-59 scan has been used in some centers to determine if a patient has evidence of bilateral hyperplasia. However, with improvements in CT quality, it is generally possible to determine if both glands are diffusely enlarged or if the hyperaldosteronism is the result of a unilateral adenoma. If diagnostic uncertainty remains after CT imaging, selective venous blood sampling may be performed to directly sample aldosterone levels from the veins draining both glands, thereby providing an alternative to NP-59 scintigraphy. In fact, this test is becoming a more common feature of the preoperative workup of these patients to better select those patients with unilateral disease that will respond best to adrenalectomy. Selective adrenal vein sampling may demonstrate hyperfunction that consistent with bilateral—but asymmetrical—hyperplasia, in which case unilateral adrenalectomy may have an impact.

Nonfunctioning Adrenocortical Adenoma

More than 80% of incidentalomas will ultimately prove to be nonfunctioning adenomas. They cause no problems by themselves, and their presence alone is not an indication for resection. Although these tumors are nonfunctioning and appear to be benign, a small percentage (especially in larger tumors) may harbor occult cancer or a subclinical functional benign tumor. Therefore, resection is considered based on size criteria and imaging characteristics, as discussed later. The remainder may be observed with serial imaging and clinical reassessment.

Other Benign Lesions

A very small number of benign adrenal lesions will be myelolipomas or organized adrenal hematomas (pseudocysts). CT and MRI are both very good for showing gross fat or blood, respectively. These lesions are generally not of clinical significance, and they are not removed. However, if they are exceptionally large and not distinguishable from a simple adrenal cyst or myelolipoma (usually the result of heterogenous density in the more solid portions of the mass), resection may be indicated.

Pheochromocytoma

Pheochromocytoma is a rare tumor of the adrenal medulla that can have malignant potential. The incidence is approximately 2 new cases per 1 million people, and less than 0.1% of all hypertensive patients have a pheochromocytoma. The tumors produce excess catecholamines (e.g., epinephrine, norepinephrine, and, rarely, dopamine). Most—but not all—patients with pheochromocytoma have hypertension, and 50% of patients will have additional paroxysms of severe hypertension. The classic symptoms of pheochromocytoma include headache, palpitations, and perspiration that correspond with spikes of catecholamine hypersecretion. Other common symptoms can also be present, such as tremor, anxiety, or vague abdominal or chest pain. Of course, none of the symptoms are specific, and unfortunately up to one third of pheochromocytomas cause death before the tumor is found.

Despite uncertain origins, the "rule of tens" is often quoted when describing the epidemiology of pheochromocytoma: 10% are bilateral, 10% occur in children, 10% are familial (either isolated or as part of a multiple endocrine neoplasia syndrome), 10% are ectopic, and 10% are malignant. Recent reports have shown, however, that the incidence of bilateral tumors may be as high as 20%, particularly among children, and the incidence of malignant behavior may be higher than previously appreciated as well.

The diagnosis of pheochromocytoma is largely biochemical. Traditionally, a 24-hour urine sample was collected for vanillylmandelic acid (VMA) and metanephrines (catecholamine breakdown products). This is time consuming, costly, and subject to inaccuracies resulting from incomplete collection. As an alternative to 24-hour urine collection, plasma free metanephrine levels may be measured; they are sensitive and specific when elevated at least 100% above normal.

BOX 13–2 THE "RULE OF TENS" OF PHEOCHROMOCYTOMA

- 10% bilateral (up to 20% in children)
- 10% in children
- 10% familial (isolated or part of multiple endocrine neoplasia syndrome)
- 10% extra-adrenal
- 10% malignant (although it may be higher)

On noncontrast CT imaging, most pheochromocytomas have density measurements of more than 10 HU. They can be quite large, with areas of central necrosis. MRI will show a characteristic bright enhancement in T2 sequences. Although this finding can be very characteristic of a pheochromocytoma in the proper clinical setting, T2 enhancement alone is not specific for pheochromocytoma. In general, MRI is equivalent to CT for the imaging of a primary adrenal tumor, but it is better than CT for extra-adrenal tumors.

Meta-iodobenzylguanidine nuclear medicine scanning has traditionally been performed as a confirmatory test when the diagnosis is supported by anatomic imaging and biochemical testing. However, recent studies have shown that MIBG imaging may not be necessary during the evaluation of patients with a biochemical diagnosis and a unilateral lesion on CT. It should be used if the patient is at high risk for bilateral or extra-adrenal lesions (i.e., familial pheochromocytoma, multiple endocrine neoplasia type 2, Von Hippel–Lindau syndrome, neurofibromatosis) or in cases of suspected recurrent or metastatic disease.

Recent research has revealed additional genes (including those associated with multiple endocrine neoplasia type 2 or Von Hippel–Lindau syndrome) that may predispose a patient to the development of a pheochromocytoma. As many as 25% of apparently spontaneous, nonsyndromic pheochromocytomas may show mutations in these genes. Because of this finding, most patients that appear to have an isolated, nonfamilial case of pheochromocytoma should still be offered genetic testing. If the patient has a predisposing mutation, consideration should be given to testing all first-degree relatives.

To help prevent wide and dangerous swings in blood pressure during operative resection, preoperative α-receptor blockade should be used for at least 10 days preoperatively. Phenoxybenzamine, prazosin, or doxazosin are the most frequently used α-blockers (Table 13-3). The initial dose should be moderate (phenoxybenzamine 10 mg by mouth 1 or 2 times daily) and increased every 2 or 3 days (as guided by frequent blood pressure and pulse measurements as an outpatient) until the effect is therapeutic. Typically, this is when the patient has normal blood pressure and occasionally some mild symptoms of orthostasis upon standing. If tachycardia accompanies the therapeutic α-blockade, a β-blocker (generally propranolol) should be added. Other regimens have been described, including single-drug therapy with a calcium-channel blocker (nicardipine), which may be used for both preoperative preparation and intraoperative blood pressure management.

Traditionally, pheochromocytomas were removed in an open fashion. Over the past decade, however, laparoscopic adrenalectomy for pheochromocytoma has become common. A multi-institution, decade-long retrospective case series with mean 41-month follow up has shown the laparoscopic approach to be safe and effective while at the same time decreasing morbidity and shortening hospital stays. It is generally agreed that the laparoscopic approach is preferred for most pheochromocytomas, provided that they are small enough to allow for adequate visualization and that there is no suggestion of a malignant tumor, such as local invasion into surrounding tissues or organs.

The prognosis is excellent for patients with a benign pheochromocytoma, with 5-year survival rates of approximately 95%. However, the survival is approximately 45% for patients with malignant pheochromocytoma. Because patients may benefit from the resection of metastases, close evaluation with blood pressure monitoring and secondary biochemical screening is recommended at 6-month intervals. For malignant pheochromocytoma, anatomic imaging is also obtained at the same intervals.

Incidentaloma: The Standard Approach

Surgical consultation is becoming more frequent with the increased discovery of adrenal incidentalomas. Although the clinical syndromes above (Cushing's, Conn's, pheochromocytoma) should be understood, the consulting resident and attending surgeon most frequently will be referred patients with an undiagnosed adrenal tumor found on other imaging studies (e.g., during abdominal CT for trauma). Rather than routinely ordering the specific studies for aldosteronoma or pheochromocytoma, it is useful to have a standard initial approach to all patients referred for evaluation of an adrenal tumor. The thought process is generally a logical sequence of investigations intended to determine whether the incidental mass is (1) a cancer; (2) a pheochromocytoma; or (3) a benign cortical adenoma (and, if so, whether it is related to a hormonally mediated syndrome) (Table 13-4). A thorough history and physical examination are performed, with particular attention paid to blood pressure, symptoms of hormonal excess, and any signs of hypercortisolism or virilization (in females). Minimal biochemical testing for all patients

TABLE 13-3 • *Preoperative Pharmacologic Preparation for Pheochromocytoma*

Medication Class	Drug	Starting Dose	Frequency of Dosage Increase
α-blockade, initial treatment	Phenoxybenzamine	5–10 mg/day	Every 48–72 hours
	Prazosin	1–2 mg/day	Every 48–72 hours
	Doxazosin	1–2 mg/day	Every 48–72 hours
β-blockade, if needed	Propranolol	5 mg/day	Every day
Calcium-channel blocker, alternative treatment	Nicardipine	60–120 mg/day	Not required

TABLE 13-4 • *Pathology of Incidentalomas After Workup and Resection*

Tumor Pathology	Approximate Percentage of Total
Nonfunctioning adenoma	80%
Cortisol hypersecreting adenoma (subclinical Cushing's syndrome)	5%
Pheochromocytoma	5%
Primary malignancy (adrenocortical cancer)	4%
Secondary malignancy (metastasis)	2.5%
Aldosteronoma	1.0%

includes a serum potassium level, a 1-mg overnight dexamethasone suppression test (or 24-hour urinary free cortisol), and a 24-hour urine sample for metanephrines and VMA. As an alternative to this 24-hour urine test, it has become increasingly common to measure free plasma metanephrines if a reference laboratory is available. Finally, in the hypertensive patient, a plasma aldosterone level and a plasma renin activity level should be measured to determine the ratio of these numbers.

BOX 13-3 THE INITIAL WORKUP OF AN INCIDENTALOMA

- 1-mg overnight dexamethasone suppression test
- 24-hour urinary metanephrines and vanillylmandelic acid (or random plasma metanephrines)
- If hypertensive, a plasma aldos terone:renin activity ratio
- Adrenal protocol computed tomography scan with unenhanced, contrast-enhanced, and delayed contrast-enhanced images

Anatomic Imaging: Overview

If this information is not available from the original study that incidentally discovered the adrenal tumor, a dedicated CT scan with and without timed-intravenous contrast may be performed to provide additional information. Cuts between 2 mm and 5 mm in size through the adrenal glands are performed both immediately after the contrast bolus and after a short elapsed time to obtain delayed contrast-enhanced images. CT will accurately determine the tumor's size, and it will provide phenotypic information to help predict the nature of the tumor. Although MRI scans may provide similar diagnostic information, CT is probably the imaging modality of choice for the workup of adrenal tumors. The imaging characteristics of each tumor are discussed elsewhere in this chapter, but generalizations can be made about tumor size. In retrospective studies, 90% of adrenocortical carcinomas will be greater than 4 cm in size at the time of diagnosis, and 75% will be greater than 6 cm. These isolated facts are not particularly helpful in clinical decision making, however, because the physician will be faced with a size measurement and an unknown tumor pathology. A 4-cm cutoff is highly sensitive for adrenal cancers, but it carries a poor specificity as a result of many false positives. When analyzing the number needed to treat, the removal of eight benign tumors at this size would have to be performed to resect a single adrenal cancer. For this reason, size is a factor that is central to decision making, but it is not used as the sole factor when deciding whether or not to resect an incidentaloma.

Scintigraphic Imaging: Overview

In addition to cross-sectional anatomic imaging, scintigraphic functional imaging of adrenal tumors is often employed. Scintigraphy should not be used as part of the primary screening or diagnosis of an adrenal tumor. Rather, its utility lies in additional confirmation of the diagnosis and as an aid in staging and preoperative planning. Nuclear medicine scanning has the advantage of whole-body imaging after a single tracer injection, and it is often used to determine if a patient has unilateral or bilateral disease and if there is evidence of metastatic disease (in the case of pheochromocytoma). There are two main nuclear medicine scans used when imaging the adrenal gland: cortical scintigraphy is accomplished using Iodine-131 odomethylnorcholesterol (NP-59), whereas adrenomedullary tumors are imaged with Iodine-131 MIBG or Iodine-123 MIBG.

For scintigraphy of the functioning adrenal cortex, intravenously administered NP-59 is taken up by the adrenal glands and stored in intracellular lipid droplets. Imaging takes place beginning the third day after NP-59 administration, and imaging on subsequent days is common. Thyroid uptake of any free Iodine-131 is blocked by giving oral potassium iodide before the procedure. When scanning for aldosteronoma, preprocedural dexamethasone may be given to block baseline cortisol secretion, thereby increasing the ability to image bilateral disease. After the images are obtained, it is generally possible to appreciate differences between unilateral adenoma and bilateral cortical hyperplasia.

I-131 and MIBG-123 is used for the scintigraphic imaging of tumors with extensive sympathetic innervation: pheochromocytoma and paraganglionoma (extra-adrenal pheochromocytoma). MIBG is an analog of norepinephrine, and it is taken up as an amine precursor and stored in cytoplasmic vesicles. In addition to the illumination of medullary tumors and paraganglionoma, MIBG also distributes to the heart, spleen, and salivary glands. Images are obtained 24 hours after the injection of MIBG. As with NP-59 scanning, radioactive iodine uptake by the thyroid should be blocked with oral potassium iodide.

The Role of Biopsy in the Workup of Incidentaloma

CT-guided percutaneous biopsy has very little utility in the workup of an incidentaloma. As discussed previously, most incidentalomas can be classified as benign cortical lesions, malignant cortical lesions, or pheochromocytoma with biochemical testing and radiographic imaging alone. Additionally, it is exceedingly rare (approximately 0.2% of the time) for an incidentaloma to represent the solitary metastasis from a cancer of an unknown primary site; this should not be used as a reason to routinely biopsy adrenal lesions. Percutaneous biopsy can be dangerous in the case of pheochromocytoma as a result of hypertensive crisis or in a primary cancer by spilling tumor cells and spreading cancer to the biopsy tract. Finally, percutaneous biopsy results are confounded by frequent false negatives, thereby giving a low sensitivity to the test, with limited ability to discriminate benign from malignant cortical lesions. Therefore, biopsy is only useful when the patient is suspected of having recurrent disease or metastasis to the adrenal gland from a separate cancer of a known primary site. Percutaneous biopsy is safe and warranted in these settings alone, in which the nature of the lesion can have therapeutic implications.

BOX 13–4 INDICATIONS FOR PERCUTANEOUS BIOPSY OF INCIDENTALOMA

Indications

- Suspected recurrent disease
- Metastases to adrenal gland from known primary cancer if results would alter therapeutic plan

Limitations

- Difficulty differentiating between benign and malignant lesions
- Danger in precipitating hypertensive crisis in pheochromoctyoma
- Risk of tumor seeding from primary adrenal cancers

Selection of Surgical Candidates

The judicious selection of surgical candidates is critical when dealing with adrenal tumors (Table 13-5). Resection is warranted for nearly all tumors when the biochemical evaluation and imaging studies suggest either a functioning benign tumor (aldosteronoma or benign cortical adenoma causing Cushing's syndrome), a malignant lesion (adrenocortical carcinoma; see below), or a pheochromocytoma. When the tumor is nonfunctioning and has benign imaging characteristics, its size is used to guide the decision for resection. If greater than 6 cm, all tumors should be removed, regardless of the results of further workup; a significant percentage of these lesions are adrenocortical cancers. As discussed below, a 4-cm cutoff for resection carries a high sensitivity but a relatively low specificity, which will lead to the removal of several benign, nonfunctioning adenomas for each cancer removed. Nevertheless, this is felt to be an acceptable risk given the morbidity and mortality (mean survival, 3 months) of an untreated adrenal cancer. Therefore, the removal of all tumors measuring between 4 cm and 6 cm should be considered.

Observation and Follow-Up of Benign Adrenal Tumors

Observation is preferred over resection when the adrenal tumor appears benign, is nonfunctioning, and measures 4 cm or less in size. The patient may be reassured that 75% to 95% of tumors less than 4 cm in size will not enlarge, and a few may even decrease in size. Nevertheless, some tumors do enlarge; there-

TABLE 13-5 • *Surgery Versus Observation*

Surgery	Observation
All functioning tumors	Nonfunctioning, benign-appearing tumors <4 cm
Tumors >4 cm, regardless of functional status	Any tumor in a patient with medical contraindications to surgery
Any tumor with imaging characteristics of cancer	
Any tumor that enlarges or develops hormone hypersecretion during observation	
Solitary metastases to the adrenal gland	
Surgically resectable local recurrences of adrenal cancer	

fore, a CT scan should be performed between 6 and 12 months after the initial diagnosis. If the lesion enlarges during follow up, it should be removed, regardless of functional status. Many clinicians will continue to monitor patients on a yearly basis, but few data suggest that an adrenal tumor will grow if it has not done so during the initial 12-month follow-up period. A hypersecretory state (usually overproduction of cortisol) will develop in approximately 20% of patients during observation, but this rarely happens when the tumor is less than 3 cm in size. Secondary screening with an overnight DMST and the measurement of urinary VMA and metanephrines (or serum metanephrines) should be performed yearly for 3 to 4 years.

Malignant Lesions

Adrenocortical Carcinoma

Adrenocortical carcinomas are rare, with an annual incidence of 2 to 3 per 1 million people. Nevertheless, approximately 4% of all incidentalomas represent cancer; however, the number can be considerably higher for incidentalomas greater than 4 cm in diameter. The prognosis is poor for patients with adrenocortical cancer, with 5-year actuarial survival rates between 32% and 48% following a potentially curative resection (total removal of all grossly visible tumor). The TNM staging system for adrenocortical carcinoma is in Table 13-6.

As with all adrenal tumors, there has been an increase in the number of adrenocortical cancers found incidentally during other studies. Although most incidentalomas are relatively small at discovery, more than 75% of cancers are larger than 6 cm at presentation (90% are larger than 4 cm), and the mean diameter is more than 12 cm. In contrast with pheochromocytomas, only approximately 2% are bilateral. The incidence by age shows a bimodal distribution, with a pediatric peak at the age of 5 years and an adult peak during the fourth and fifth decades of life.

The workup for a suspected adrenocortical cancer bears some similarity to that for an incidentaloma; the goals of accurate imaging and the determination of secretory status remain the same. In cases in which virilization is present, adrenal androgens may be measured in the serum. In addition, it is very important to evaluate any involvement of surrounding structures (e.g., the vena cava) to determine the feasibility and extent of the

TABLE 13-6 • *TNM Classification and Staging System for Adrenocortical Cancer*

Tumor (T)			
T1	≤5 cm, no invasion		
T2	>5 cm, no invasion		
T3	Any size tumor with local invasion into fat		
T4	Any size tumor with invasion into adjacent organs		
Regional Nodal Metastases (N)			
N0	No positive lymph nodes		
N1	Positive lymph nodes		
Distant Metastases (M)			
M0	No (known) distant metastases		
M1	Distant metastases present		
Stage Grouping			
Stage	T	N	M
I	T1	N0	M0
II	T2	N0	M0
III	T1 or T2 T3	N1 N0	M0 M0
IV	T3 or T4 Any T	N1 Any N	M0 M1

planned resection. Cushing's syndrome will be present in 50% of cancers, and virilization (in females) is evident in a third of adult cancers. Only rarely will a cancer present with mineralocorticoid excess. Tumors that oversecrete multiple hormones (e.g., aldosterone, cortisol) and estrogen-secreting tumors in males are likely to be cancers. In children less than 5 years old, most (95%) cancers will present with rapid virilization or precocious puberty.

The imaging characteristics of an adrenocortical carcinoma are often (but not always) striking, because most are 12 cm or larger at the time of diagnosis. CT will reveal irregular margins, areas of patchy central necrosis, and frequent (20%) evidence of local invasion into the kidney or the inferior vena cava. As already noted, cancers are typically lipid-poor as compared with their adenoma counterparts, giving HU measurements of more than 10 on noncontrast CT and less than 60% enhancement washout percent at 15 minutes. More than 50% of patients will have radiographically demonstrable metastases at the time of diagnosis; the most common sites are the liver (approximately 50%), the lungs (approximately 40%), and the bone (approximately 15%). Imaging by noncontrast MR may be nonspecific on T1 and T2 sequences if hemorrhage is present. With the addition of contrast, the most commonly seen characteristics are peripheral enhancement and central hypoperfusion. The greatest utility of MR is to determine local invasion or tumor thrombus, particularly when evaluating for inferior vena cava invasion by a right-sided tumor, and especially when images are reconstructed in the sagittal and coronal planes.

The primary treatment for adrenocortical cancers is surgical resection by an open transabdominal or thoracoabdominal approach. Patients have the best chance of survival when a gross total resection is accomplished with negative margins. Involved organs (kidney, spleen, or parts of liver, pancreas, colon) are removed if necessary to facilitate an en bloc removal of the cancer. Laparoscopic approaches are not currently recognized as appropriate management of adrenal tumors that are preoperatively known (or suspected) to be cancer, and neoadjuvant therapies are not routinely used. Although there is disagreement about whether a debulking operation should be performed for patients with unresectable disease, it is known that patients have improved outcomes if all

BOX 13–5 TREATMENT OF ADRENOCORTICAL CANCERS

- Surgery
  - Thoracoabdominal approach
  - Cortex-sparing adrenalectomy
- Medical therapy
  - Mitotane or chemotherapy on a research protocol
- Combined mitotane and re-resection for recurrences
- Mitotane adjuvant therapy after complete initial resection
- Palliative external beam radiotherapy

gross tumor is removed at the initial operation as compared with those with incomplete resections. Tumor thrombus in the renal vein or inferior vena cava is not a contraindication to surgery, and cardiac bypass can be employed to facilitate the removal of tumor from the inferior vena cava or the right atrium. Unfortunately, most tumors will ultimately recur, regardless of the completeness of resection at the initial operation. Although it has been reported that re-resection may prolong survival, all treatment for recurrent or metastatic disease is palliative. Isolated hepatic or pulmonary metastases, as well as local recurrences, are re-resected when surgically feasible.

In terms of medical therapy, the only chemotherapeutic agent commonly used is the adrenocorticolytic drug mitotane (a compound closely related to the insecticide DDT). Generally, mitotane is used to treat tumor recurrences, metastatic disease, and incomplete initial resections. In rare cases in which the primary tumor is inoperable or the patient's medical condition mitigates against surgery, mitotane may be used as a palliative primary therapy. Usually, mitotane for recurrences is combined with re-resection, but it is not definitively known that this approach improves survival. Although only approximately 50% of patients will have tumor response to mitotane, rare complete remissions have been reported.

The use of mitotane as adjuvant therapy after a complete initial resection is controversial. Some small, nonrandomized case series have suggested that, when it is given immediately and indefinitely after a primary operation that removes all gross disease, mitotane may improve survival for some patients. Side effects of mitotane are common and dose-related, and they can be severe (diarrhea, nausea/vomiting, adrenal insufficiency, hepatotoxicity, dizziness, confusion). In summary, studies that report on the adjuvant use of mitotane are far from conclusive, and strong consideration should be given to enrollment of these patients in clinical trials.

After resection of an adrenocortical cancer, patients are seen every 3 months for a complete physical examination and to obtain an interval history regarding recurrent symptoms. Biochemical screening is carried out if the original tumor produced hormones. Cross-sectional imaging is performed at 3-month intervals and to look for local or distant (e.g., hepatic) recurrences. Positron emission tomography scanning is also useful for the follow-up of these patients, who are prone to recurrent disease.

Secondary Adrenal Malignancy

Metastases to the adrenal gland from other primary tumors are common, occurring in up to 27% of cases of patients with other primary malignant epithelial tumors (particularly lung, breast, melanoma). If a patient with another primary cancer is found to have an adrenal lesion, it will be a metastasis approximately 50% of the time. The imaging characteristics are similar to other malignancies: on noncontrast CT, the lesions are larger and more heterogeneous, they have less distinct margins, and the HU level is generally greater than 10. Nuclear medicine studies (e.g., NP-59) will show a photopenic area (imaging that is discordant with cross-sectional imaging), whereas positron emission tomography scanning with fluorine-18 fluorodeoxyglucose will often show activity that is concordant with anatomic images. Fluorine-18 fluorodeoxyglucose is a glucose analog that indicates tissues (e.g., metastases) that take up glucose more avidly than surrounding structures. As mentioned previously, it is reasonable to biopsy these tumors if there is no suspicion of a primary adrenal cancer or pheochromocytoma, but only if the biopsy results will have an impact on the therapeutic algorithm.

Surgical Approaches

In general, any patient with a benign-appearing, functional adrenal tumor should be offered a laparoscopic adrenalectomy unless it is larger than 6 cm or otherwise specifically contraindicated (Table 13-7). The advantages of the laparoscopic approach include less postoperative pain, shorter hospitalization, and decreased incidence of late complications (e.g., hernia). In situations of extensive previous abdominal surgery or exceptional obesity, in which the laparoscopic approach is not possible, a posterior approach may be useful. If there is any significant suspicion that a tumor may be an adrenocortical carcinoma, all patients should undergo an open anterior adrenalectomy. There is no role for the laparoscopic resection of known adrenal cancers. In very large tumors for which vascular control may be more difficult, a thoracoabdominal approach can be used for increased exposure.

Some tumors will not fall into the "clearly benign" or "clearly cancer" categories. Resection of tumors between 4 cm and 6 cm should be considered, but the approach to use is not always clear. Tumors larger than 4 cm are removed because they "might be" cancer, but this uncovers a therapeutic dilemma: do all of these patients need to undergo an open adrenalectomy? Certainly this should not be the case, because most benign-appearing tumors larger than 4 cm are not cancer. In addition, the benefits of laparoscopy are clear and will be realized by most patients. Conversely, the negative influence of the inadvertent laparoscopic removal of a very small adrenocortical cancer is not yet known, and it will probably affect only a very few

TABLE 13-7 • *Comparison of Surgical Approaches*

Laparoscopic	Open Anterior	Open Posterior	Thoracoabdominal
Benign, functioning tumors	Tumors suspicious for cancer of any size	If laparoscopic approach is contraindicated, such as by extensive prior upper abdominal sugery	For additional vascular control
Benign, nonfunctioning tumors, 4-6 cm	Benign, nonfunctioning tumors, >6 cm	Extreme obesity	Large cancers to be resected with surrounding organs

patients. In summary, if the benign-appearing, nonfunctional lesion is 4 cm to 6 cm in size, a laparoscopic approach is suggested, if there are no imaging or clinical characteristics that suggest that primary adrenal malignancy is likely. For larger tumors, consideration should be given to an open anterior resection.

Laparoscopic Approach

The most common laparoscopic approach is transabdominal, with the patient in an 80-degree lateral decubitus position with the table flexed (Figure 13-2, *A*). Three or four 10-mm trocars are placed between the midclavicular line medially and the midaxillary line laterally. The medial port is for retraction, the next port is for the camera, and the two lateral ports are for dissection. For a right adrenalectomy, the right triangular ligament is taken down to mobilize the liver (Figure 13-2, *B*). The adrenal gland is dissected in a superior to inferior manner, and the central adrenal vein is identified and ligated with clips or a stapler. For a left adrenalectomy, exposure is obtained by mobilizing the splenic flexure of the colon and dividing the lateral attachments of the spleen and pancreas, which allows these organs to fall medially, thereby exposing the kidney and the adrenal gland (Figure 13-2, *C*). The left adrenal vein is longer than the right adrenal vein and can be more easily secured. The periadrenal tissue should be resected with the adrenal gland.

Open Anterior Approach

This is generally accomplished via a bilateral subcostal incision, which affords excellent exposure to the adrenals (particularly laterally and superiorly), the inferior vena cava, the aorta, and the renal vessels while minimizing the risk for tumor spillage from direct manipulation (Figure 13-3, *A*). A midline incision may be used if there is concern for extra-adrenal disease, particularly lower in the abdomen. The right adrenal gland is approached by mobilizing the hepatic flexure of the colon and then performing a Kocher maneuver. The right lobe of the liver is retracted medially after division of the right triangular ligament (Figure 13-4). The adrenal gland and the inferior vena cava are then separated to visualize and ligate the central adrenal vein. For a left adrenalectomy, it is important to consider the location of the gland with relation to the pancreas. If it is inferior to the pancreas, the gland is approached through the lesser sac, where the pancreas is retracted superiorly after division of its inferior peritoneal attachments (Figure 13-5, *A*). If the adrenal is superior to the pancreas, a visceral rotation is performed to mobilize the spleen and the pancreas toward the midline (Figure 13-5, *B*).

Open Posterior Approach

This approach has many of the same benefits of laparoscopy, with the main drawbacks being those of limited exposure and inability to explore the contralateral adrenal gland under the same incision. Fewer surgeons are familiar with this approach, and its use is generally limited. The patient is prone, and the table is flexed at the twelfth rib (Figure 13-3, *B*). Under a hockey-stick–shaped incision, the latissimus is divided, and the twelfth rib is excised. The pleura and the diaphragm are retracted superiorly, and the adrenal gland is mobilized in a superior to inferior manner.

Thoracoabdominal Approach

A thoracoabdominal approach may be used if the tumor is very large and additional vascular control is needed or if a cancer must be resected en bloc with several surrounding organs or a portion of the diaphragm (Figure 13-3, *C*). The patient is positioned in the near-lateral position with flexion of the table at the eleventh rib, and a thoracic incision is made from the end of the eleventh (left) or the tenth (right) rib and carried down onto the abdominal wall to as far as the midline, if needed. The incision is deepened through the ribs and the abdominal musculature. The lung is then retracted superiorly and the liver anteriorly (on the right side), which provides a wide exposure for the adrenalectomy.

Cortex-Sparing Adrenalectomy

As an alternative to the complete removal of one or both adrenal glands, some surgeons employ a so-called "cortex-sparing" adrenalectomy. This operation is simply a subtotal adrenalectomy and not an extirpation of a medullary tumor, as the name might imply. Historically, subtotal adrenalectomy has been used for Cushing's disease, but more recently the strategy has been extended to the treatment of adrenal neoplasms, either by an open or a laparoscopic approach. For bilateral tumors, a subtotal resection may avoid the

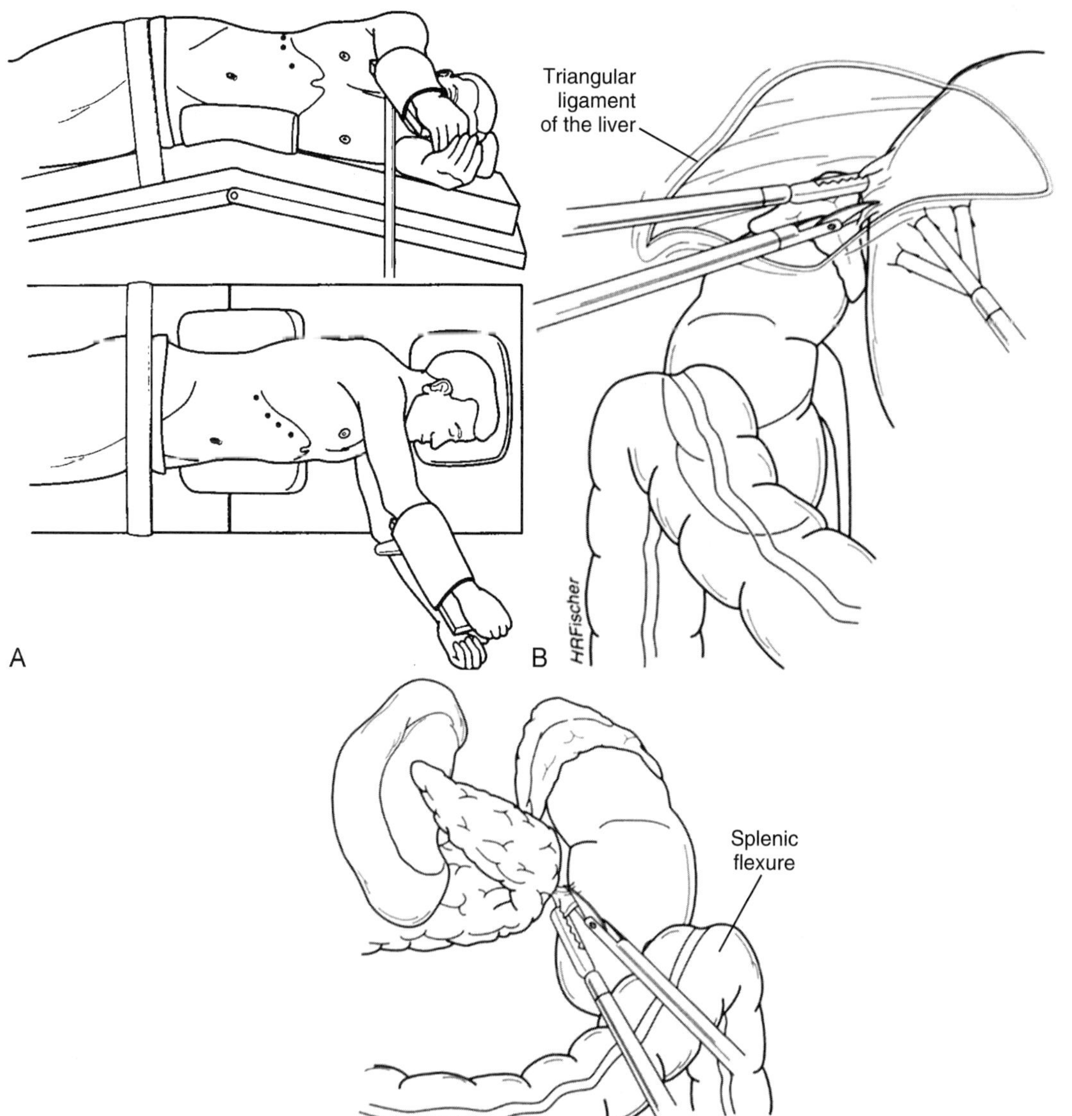

Figure 13–2. A, Patient position and port site placement for a right-sided laparoscopic adrenalectomy. **B,** Laparoscopic dissection of the right adrenal gland. Note that the liver has been rotated medially after division of the right triangular ligament. **C,** Laparoscopic dissection of the lateral and inferior pancreatic attachments for exposure of the left adrenal gland.

need for lifelong corticosteroid replacement. For unilateral tumors, a subtotal resection preserves adrenal tissue to allow for future events that may further reduce the volume of adrenal tissue (e.g., trauma necessitating removal, subsequent surgery for recurrent tumor). In all cases, intraoperative ultrasound should be employed to ensure that residual tumor is not left behind at the initial operation. A recent review of this topic by Walz found that, although complete adrenalectomy remains the standard of care for patients with bilateral inherited pheochromocytomas, a clinical and biochemical cure can be achieved by subtotal adrenalectomy. For this condition, a cortex-sparing approach is acceptable, provided that the tumor is not invasive and that at least one third of one gland can be preserved. Short-term follow up in small studies has shown that results for the subtotal resection of unilateral benign tumors (e.g., Conn's or Cushing's adenomas) have been

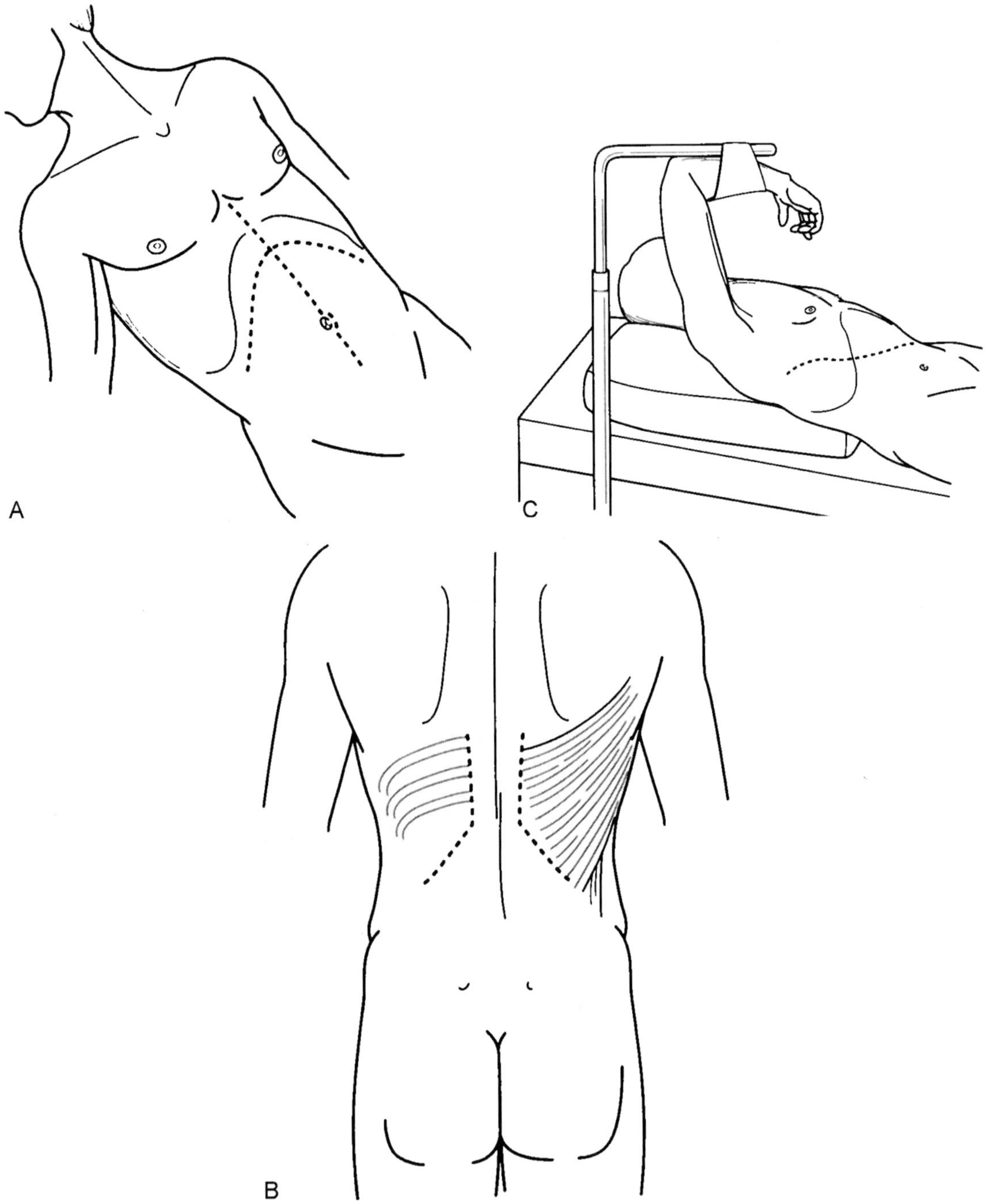

Figure 13–3. Incisions for open adrenalectomy. **A,** Bilateral subcostal and midline incisions. **B,** Open posterior approach. **C,** Right-sided thoracoabdominal approach.

comparable to those of total adrenalectomy. However, until long-term results are available, it is not definitively known if cortex-sparing/subtotal resections are as safe and effective as complete, unilateral adrenalectomy.

Postoperative Care

Steroid Replacement

The daily secretion of cortisol ranges between 15 mg and 30 mg per day, but it may rise to

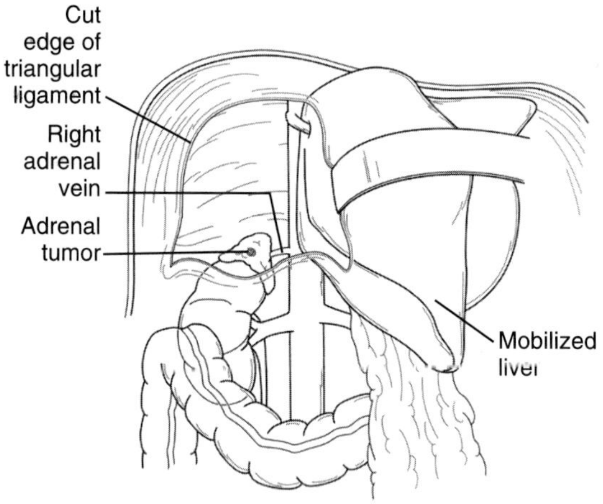

Figure 13-4. Exposure of the right adrenal gland during open anterior adrenalectomy.

200 mg to 300 mg per day under stress. Patients who have undergone a unilateral adrenalectomy for Conn's syndrome or pheochromocytoma do not need hormone supplementation, because the remaining (contralateral) adrenal gland will provide sufficient hormone production in nearly all patients if the contralateral gland is largely normal. However, patients with bilateral adrenalectomy for any reason or with a unilateral adrenalectomy for Cushing's syndrome (even if subclinical) need hormone replacement (Table 13-8). A standard practice is to give "stress-dose" steroids at the time of operation, followed by a rapid taper to general physiologic requirements in 5 days (see Table 13-8). If an adrenal gland remains, the baseline dose is continued for approximately 6 to 8 weeks, at which time the pituitary-adrenal axis is stimulated to test for the return of hormone production by the remaining adrenal gland: 25 units of corticotrophin is administered intramuscularly, and plasma cortisol (hydrocortisone) levels are determined both before and 45 minutes after the injection. An increase by 7 μg/dL or any increase to 20 μg/dL is considered sufficient, and exogenous hydrocortisone treatment is weaned and discontinued.

Summary

Adrenal tumors are being discovered with increasing frequency, which often leads to consultation with a surgeon. A consistent approach using a standard biochemical workup and directed imaging will generally allow the adrenal tumors to be classified as benign, cancer, or pheochromocytoma. Many tumors will warrant excision, and the laparoscopic approach will be beneficial for many patients who are appropriately selected.

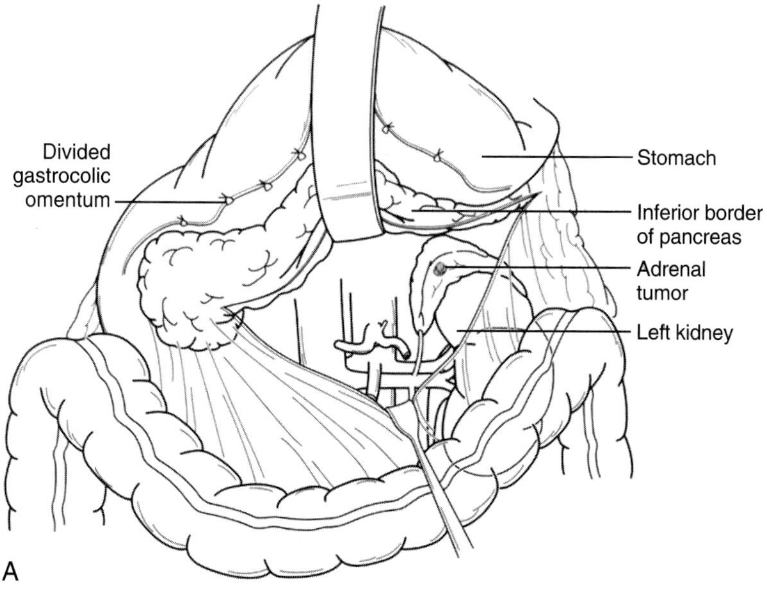

Figure 13-5. Exposure of the left adrenal gland during open anterior adrenalectomy. **A,** Approach to the superiorly positioned adrenal gland, where the pancreas is retracted superiorly.

(Continued)

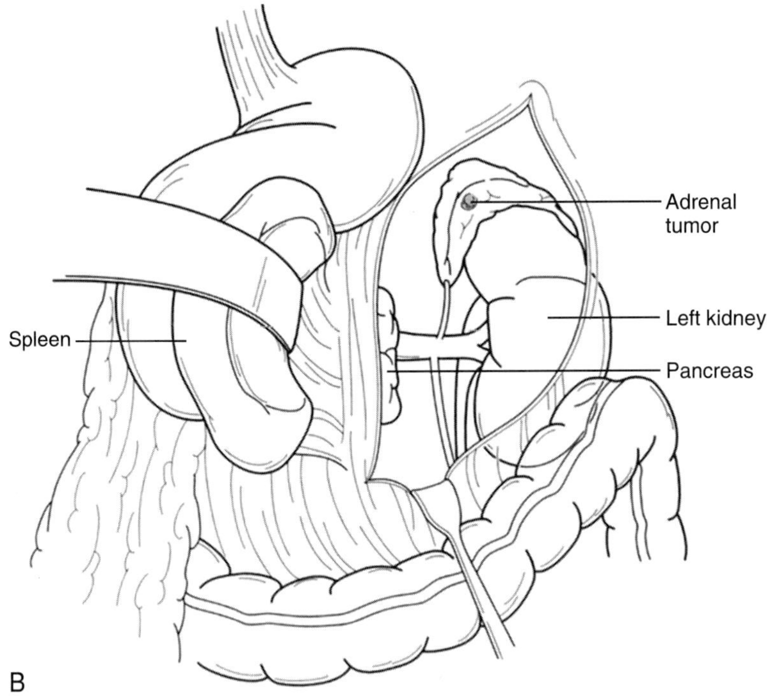

Figure 13–5. Cont'd. **B,** The spleen and the pancreas are retracted medially for a more inferiorly positioned adrenal gland.

TABLE 13–8 • *Postoperative Steroid Dosing Regimen*

Day	Hydrocortisone (Solu-Cortef) Given Intravenously	Hydrocortisone (Cortef) Given by Mouth*			Fludrocortisone (Florinef) Given by Mouth
		7 am	12 noon	8 pm	
On call to operating room	100 mg				
Day of operation	50 mg twice postoperative, divided doses				
Day 1	50 mg every 8 hours × 3				
Day 2	25 mg every 8 hours × 3				0.1 mg
Day 3		20 mg	20 mg	10 mg	0.1 mg
Day 4		20 mg	10 mg	5 mg	0.1 mg
Day 5 and after		15 mg	10 mg	5 mg	0.1 mg

*For patients who have undergone bilateral adrenalectomy, mineralocorticoid replacement (fludrocortisone, given daily at 7 am) is required unless the hydrocortisone dose is greater than 100 mg/day. At doses of more than 100 mg/day, hydrocortisone exerts an adequate mineralocorticoid effect.

Key Selected Reading

NIH State-of-the-Science Statement on management of the clinically inapparent adrenal mass ("incidentaloma"). *NIH Consens State Sci Statements* 2002;19:1–25.

Selected Readings

Barry MK, van Heerden JA, Farley DR, *et al.* Can adrenal incidentalomas be safely observed? *World J Surg* 1998;22:599–604.

Kebebew E, Siperstein AE, Clark OH, Duh Q-Y. Results of laparoscopic adrenalectomy for suspected and unsuspected malignant neoplasms. *Arch Surg* 2002;137:948–953.

Kirschner LS. Review: emerging treatment strategies for adrenocortical carcinoma: a new hope. *J clin Endocrinol Metab* 2006;91:41–21.

Kurtaran A, Traub T, Shapiro B. Scintigraphic imaging of the adrenal glands. *Eur J Radiol* 2002;41:123–130.

Lee JE, Evans DB, Hickey RC, *et al.* Unknown primary cancer presenting as an adrenal mass: Frequency and implications for diagnostic evaluation of adrenal incidentalomas. *Surgery* 1998;124:1115–1122.

Lenders JW, Eisenhofer G, Mannelli M, Pacak K. Phaeochromocytoma. *Lancet* 2005;366:665–675.

Lin DD, Loughlin KR. Diagnosis and management of surgical adrenal diseases. *Urology* 2005;66:476–483.

Liu H, Crapo L. Update on the diagnosis of cushing syndrome. *Endocrinologist* 2005;15:165–179.

Lochart ME, Smith JK, Kenney PJ. Imaging of adrenal masses. *Eur J Radiol* 2002;41:95–112.

Miskulin J, Shulkin BL, Doherty GM, *et al.* Is preoperative iodine 123 metaiodobenzylguanidine scintigraphy routinely necessary before initial adrenalectomy for pheochromocytoma? *Surgery* 2003;134:918–922.

Neumann HPH, Bausch B, McWhinney SR, *et al.* Germline mutations in nonsyndromic pheochromocytoma. *N Engl J Med* 2002;346:1459–1466.

Shen WT, Sturgeon C, Duh QY. From incidentaloma to adrenocortical carcinoma: the surgical management of adrenal tumors. *J Surg Oncol* 2005;89:186–192.

Thompson GB, Young WF Jr. Adrenal incidentaloma. *Curr Opin Oncol* 2003;15:84–90.

14

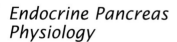

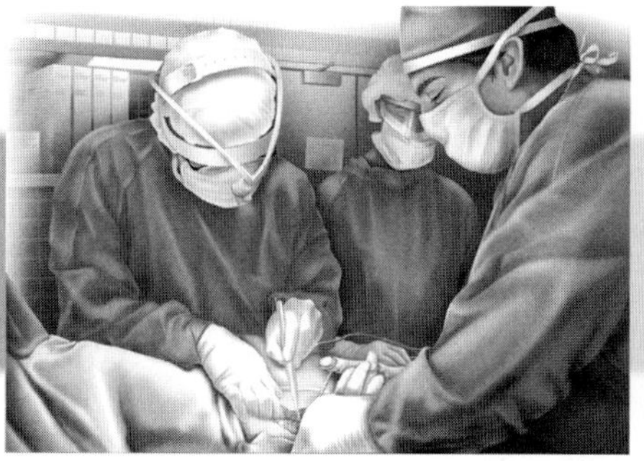

Tumors of the Endocrine Pancreas

Candace Y. Williams-Covington and Gerard M. Doherty

Tumors of the Endocrine Pancreas: Key Points

- Outline the principles of the management of endocrine tumors.
- Describe the symptoms, the diagnostic considerations, and the management of insulinomas.
- Describe the symptoms, the diagnostic considerations, and the management of gastrinomas.
- Describe the symptoms, the diagnostic considerations, and the management of glucagonomas.
- Recognize the characteristics of somatostatinoma, VIPoma, and multiple endocrine neoplasia I syndromes.

Endocrine Pancreas Physiology

The endocrine pancreas consists of a variety of neuroendocrine cell types that are interspersed in small clusters (islets) within the structure of the exocrine pancreas. The cells make a variety of hormone products (Table 14-1) that have important roles in the control of normal physiology. The tumors that form from these cell types frequently produce the hormone made by the cell of origin (Table 14-2), often with defects in the normal feedback control of the hormone

TABLE 14–1 • *Pancreatic Islet Cells and Function*

Cell	Hormone Secreted	Hormone Function	Stimulation	Suppression
A cells	Glucagon	Gluconeogenesis; glycogenolysis; increase serum glucose	Sympathetic nervous system; low blood glucose	Insulin; somatostatin; elevated blood glucose
Beta cells	Insulin	Glyconeogenesis; protein and fatty acid synthesis; decrease serum glucose	Parasympathetic nervous system; gastrin; cholecystokinin; gastric inhibitory peptide; vasoactive intestinal polypeptide; enkephalin; gastrin-releasing peptide; elevated blood glucose	Sympathetic nervous system; somatostatin; neurotensin; substance P; pancreastatin; amylin; leptin; decreased blood glucose
D cells	Somatostatin	Inhibits islet cell secretion, amino acid absorption, and pancreatic enzyme secretion; decreases gut motility	Food and acid in stomach	Unknown
PP cells	Pancreatic polypeptide	Unknown; role for correction of hepatic resistance to insulin	Unknown	Unknown

release. For example, insulinomas are functional tumors that produce insulin without the normal feedback control of hypoglycemia; despite life-threatening hypoglycemia, the tumor continues to release hormone into the circulation, thus producing the associated syndrome. The functional tumors described below can be characterized by certain important features:

- the hormone produced and the endocrine syndrome that accompanies the hormone overproduction;
- the location of the tumor occurrence, which can be outside of the pancreatic parenchyma; and
- the frequency of the tumor subtype occurring as a malignancy.

The medical measures that can be used to control the endocrinopathy and the relative effectiveness of this management vary for the different tumor types.

Tumor Types

The most common types of these rare tumors are insulinoma and gastrinoma. Tumors of the endocrine pancreas can also be nonfunctional. Nonfunctional tumors are frequently larger, and they have malignant features at the time of presentation. This may be the result of the fact that these tumors present because of local mass effects (e.g., pain, compression of adjacent organs or bile ducts, splenic vein thrombosis). The nonfunctional tumors are managed in similar ways as low-grade pancreatic exocrine malignancies, because they do not have the added issue of a hormonal syndrome requiring control.

General Management Principles

The first general principle is to assess the biochemistry unequivocally before embarking on localization studies. This applies particularly to the situation in which the patient is thought to present with functional syndrome (e.g., patients who present with hypoglycemia and who may be thought to have an insulinoma). Failure to adhere to this can lead to some very distressing consequences. For example, many patients with ulcer disease have an elevated gastrin level while receiving acid-suppression therapy. Careful documentation of their hypergastrinemia in the presence of simultaneous

BOX 14–1 MANAGEMENT PRINCIPLES OF ENDOCRINE TUMORS

- Assess the biochemistry before localization studies are performed.
- Separate control of the hormonal syndrome from control of the malignancy.
- Tailor the risk of surgery to the severity of the disease.

TABLE 14-2 • Overview of Endocrine Pancreas Tumors

Type	Typical Age of Onset	Gender Predominance	Hormone Secreted
Insulinoma	Fourth decade	Female	Insulin
Glucagonoma	Fifth decade	Equal male-to-female ratio	Glucagon
Gastrinoma	20–50 years	Male	Gastrin
Somatostatinoma	Fifth decade	Equal male-to-female ratio	Somatostatin
VIPoma	30–50 years	Equal male-to-female ratio	Vasoactive intestinal polypeptide

VIP, Vasoactive intestinal polypeptide.

elevated gastric acid output is critical if subtle localizing findings are to be correctly interpreted. After the diagnosis is established, it is then important, early in the management, to deliberately assess the possibility that the patient has a familial cause for the tumor (usually multiple endocrine neoplasia type 1). The presence of an endocrine neoplasia syndrome will affect the overall treatment planning.

The second general principle is to separate, as much as possible, the control of the hormonal syndrome from the control of the potential malignancy. For patients with functional hormonal syndromes, the syndrome itself is frequently more life threatening than the tumor. Current medical management of the hormonal syndromes can often be used to great effect to palliate the syndrome and to allow deliberate treatment planning for the management of the potential malignancy. Gastrinoma is an example of a functional tumor syndrome that can always be controlled with nonsurgical management. All patients with gastrinoma can have complete control of their hormonal syndrome with current medical management. All patients with gastrinomas should have nonoperative control of the syndrome, which will allow for preoperative investigation, including imaging and medical optimization, before exploration. Insulinoma is a syndrome that is not easily treated medically. Unfortunately, there is not good suppression therapy for the insulin release or effective end-organ blockade of the hormone effects; thus, nonoperative management of the syndrome is generally poor.

The third general principle is to tailor the risk of the operative approach to the severity of the disease. Although this may seem obvious during all operative planning, the relative risks of various pancreatic endocrine tumors are often overlooked. For example, most insulinomas are small benign tumors, and the risk to the patient comes from the hormonal syndrome. For this reason, all patients will require exploration and complete resection of the tumor. However, they do not require a radical resection of the pancreas or peripancreatic lymph node dissection. By contrast, gastrinoma is more frequently malignant than not, and it often spreads to the locoregional lymph nodes. Attempts to cure this disease operatively require a very thorough exploration and regional lymph node dissection. However, even for gastrinoma, the natural history for patients who are not cured is quite long. Thus, the level of aggressiveness of the patient and the surgeon must be tempered by a thorough knowledge of the natural history of both the syndrome and the disease.

Insulinoma

Insulinoma is the most common of the functional pancreatic endocrine tumors and is usually benign (Table 14-3). The treatment planning for this tumor is affected by the lack of effective management for insulinoma syndrome other than tumor resection. The tumor itself is usually small, noninvasive, and benign.

Symptoms

Patients who have insulinoma suffer from recurrent episodes of hypoglycemia brought on by periods of fasting. They have relatively constant secretion of insulin into their system

TABLE 14-3 • Insulinoma

Location	Pancreas
Percentage of malignancy	5–10%
Endocrinopathy	Hypoglycemia
Medical control of endocrinopathy	Diazoxide; verapamil; phenytoin; octreotide
Quality of medical control	Poor

and circulation. It is possible for them to maintain normal blood glucose levels by eating in response to their hypoglycemic symptoms; however, when intervals of fasting occur, the patients develop acute and life-threatening symptoms. The most prominent symptom is central nervous system glucose deficit, which is called *neuroglycopenia*. Symptoms of this condition include diplopia and blurred vision, confusion, inability to rouse from sleep, seizure, and coma. Prolonged hypoglycemia can lead to permanent central nervous system injury. Patients may also have catecholamine-release–associated symptoms. These may include tremor, nausea, anxiety, palpitations, sweating, or weakness. Frequently, symptoms occur early in the morning, after the patient has been fasting during sleep.

Many patients are symptomatic for long periods of time before their diagnosis is considered or confirmed. Patients are often misdiagnosed and treated for anxiety disorder, seizure disorder, or drug abuse.

Diagnosis

Fasting hypoglycemia is the hallmark of insulinoma. To definitively demonstrate this, however, it is necessary to fulfill Whipple's Triad.

BOX 14–2 INSULINOMA CLINICAL FEATURES

Whipple's Triad:

1. Hypoglycemia (glucose <50 mg/dL)
2. Central nervous system effects and other symptoms present at time of hypoglycemia
3. Glucose relieves symptoms

The biochemical diagnosis of insulinoma requires the demonstration of hyperinsulinism associated with the hypoglycemia as well as a lack of evidence of exogenous factors that could cause the hyperinsulinism (Table 14-4).

The clinical setting that best demonstrates insulinoma is the 48-hour fast. During this supervised fast, patients are allowed to have clear liquids that do not contain glucose by mouth; they otherwise take nothing by mouth. An intravenous line or a heparin-flushed catheter is placed to allow for the rapid administration of glucose (should that be necessary) and also to allow for the drawing of blood to document the serum glucose level. The patient fasts for as long as 48 hours, although symptoms typically develop in a much shorter period of time. After the patient develops symptoms of hypoglycemia, the serum glucose level is documented. The fast is concluded when the plasma glucose level drops to less than 45 mg/dL and is associated with symptoms. At that time, blood samples are also obtained for insulin levels, C-peptide levels, and proinsulin levels. A urine specimen is obtained for sulfonylurea products.

The proper interpretation of the results of the 48-hour fast is important but not always straightforward. Patients with glucose levels below 45 mg/dL should not have any measurable insulin. Thus, patients who have insulin levels greater than 6 mU/mL are abnormal. The insulin-to-glucose ratio of greater than 0.3 can be used as a guideline to separate the obviously positive fasts from those that should be accessed more carefully. However, it is clear that a substantial minority population of patients with insulinoma will have an insulin-to-glucose ratio of less than 0.3.

TABLE 14–4 • *Diagnostic and Localization Tests for Insulinoma*

Test	Findings	Accuracy
Hypoglycemic serum insulin	>6 microU/mL	Nearly 100%
48-hour fast	Hypoglycemic symptoms prompting biochemical assessment	Nearly 100%
Computed tomographic scanning with contrast or magnetic resonance imaging	Pancreatic mass	50–60%
Selective arteriography	Pancreatic mass	50–90%
Octreotide scintigraphy	Octreotide uptake in area of tumor	60%
Endoscopic ultrasonography	Pancreatic mass	82%
HVS or PVS after arterial stimulation	Elevated HV or PV insulin after injection of calcium gluconate to specific regional arteries	75%

HV, Hepatic vein; *HVS,* hepatic vein sampling; *PV,* portal vein; *PVS,* portal vein sampling.

The C-peptide and proinsulin levels are measured to show that levels of insulin in the blood are from an endogenous source. Exogenously administered insulin will not contain C-peptide or proinsulin in the mix. However, the administration of oral hyperglycemic agents that cause the release of insulin could cause hypoglycemia, and they could have measurable levels of C-peptide and proinsulin. It is important to rule out the possibility of exogenously administered sulfonylureas with urine testing.

Localization

After the biochemical diagnosis of insulinoma is secured, the surgeon can be 100% certain that the tumor is located in the pancreas. There are two critical questions that the surgeon should address in treating the patient. The first is whether this patient is among the minority (5%-10%) of patients who have large tumors with metastases in the liver. The second issue is where in the pancreas the tumor is located. The first question is critical, because the management of patients with malignant insulinoma and metastatic disease is different from that of the majority of patients who have benign localized disease. These patients may require pancreatic and/or liver resections or other types of hepatic tumor ablation. Occasionally, there is no surgical option for palliating these patients, who must rely on the suboptimal nonsurgical management that is available. After it is established for the majority of patients, however, that there is no metastatic disease, the only remaining issue is to identify and remove the tumor.

Many different localization techniques can be used to seek pancreatic insulinomas before operation. These studies include ultrasound, computed tomographic (CT) scan, magnetic resonance imaging (MRI), angiography, portal or hepatic venous sampling, and nuclear medicine scanning. In selected centers, the best preoperative imaging study appears to be endoscopic ultrasonography. This requires an experienced practitioner who can perform and interpret this technically demanding study. However, it is extremely sensitive and specific for these often-small hypoechoic lesions in the pancreas.

The choice of preoperative imaging studies must be tempered by the surgeon's knowledge that the tumor is within the pancreatic parenchyma somewhere and that he or she can use intraoperative ultrasonography to gain significant information. Overall, the single most sensitive test for insulinoma is intraoperative ultrasound performed by the surgeon at the time of exploration. In our practice, the best localizing scheme for these patients is a CT scan of the abdomen to look for lesions in the pancreas as well as to rule out malignant insulinoma with metastases. The patient then has an endoscopic ultrasound, which can nearly always identify or confirm the lesion within the pancreas. Regardless of the endoscopic ultrasound results, however, the patient should be explored with intraoperative ultrasound to both positively identify the tumor and to guide enucleation, as will be noted below. We do not feel that it is justified to proceed with multiple preoperative imaging tests to demonstrate a tumor before operation after the biochemical diagnosis is clear.

Surgical Management

The operative management of insulinoma depends on the location of the lesion within the pancreas. For lesions that have been identified preoperatively by CT scan, endoscopic ultrasound, or some other modality, a minimally invasive surgical resection may be an excellent option. Either enucleation of the tumor or resection of the distal pancreas can be performed. Laparoscopic ultrasound can be used to help guide that resection. In all but the simplest cases, the exploration involves mobilization of the head of the pancreas by Kocher maneuver or the tail of the pancreas by incising the retroperitoneum inferior to the pancreas and dissecting the avascular plane posterior to the pancreatic body and tail (Figure 14-1). This allows for bimanual palpation of the gland and intraoperative ultrasound of the organ. After the lesion is identified, it is resected with the safest low-morbidity resection that is practical. Enucleation is usually best for tumors in the pancreatic head. Unless the main pancreatic duct appears to be directly involved, a formal resection is generally unnecessary in this location. The enucleation of tumors in the pancreatic head involves incision on the anterior or posterior surface of the pancreas, whichever is closest to the surface of the tumor and that will keep the operation furthest from the main pancreatic duct. Ultrasound is used to help guide the surgeon directly to the tumor capsule. The tumor is then enucleated from the surrounding pancreatic parenchyma (Figure 14-2). Small bleeding vessels are controlled with clips or bipolar electrocautery. Any small ducts that are encountered can be oversewn

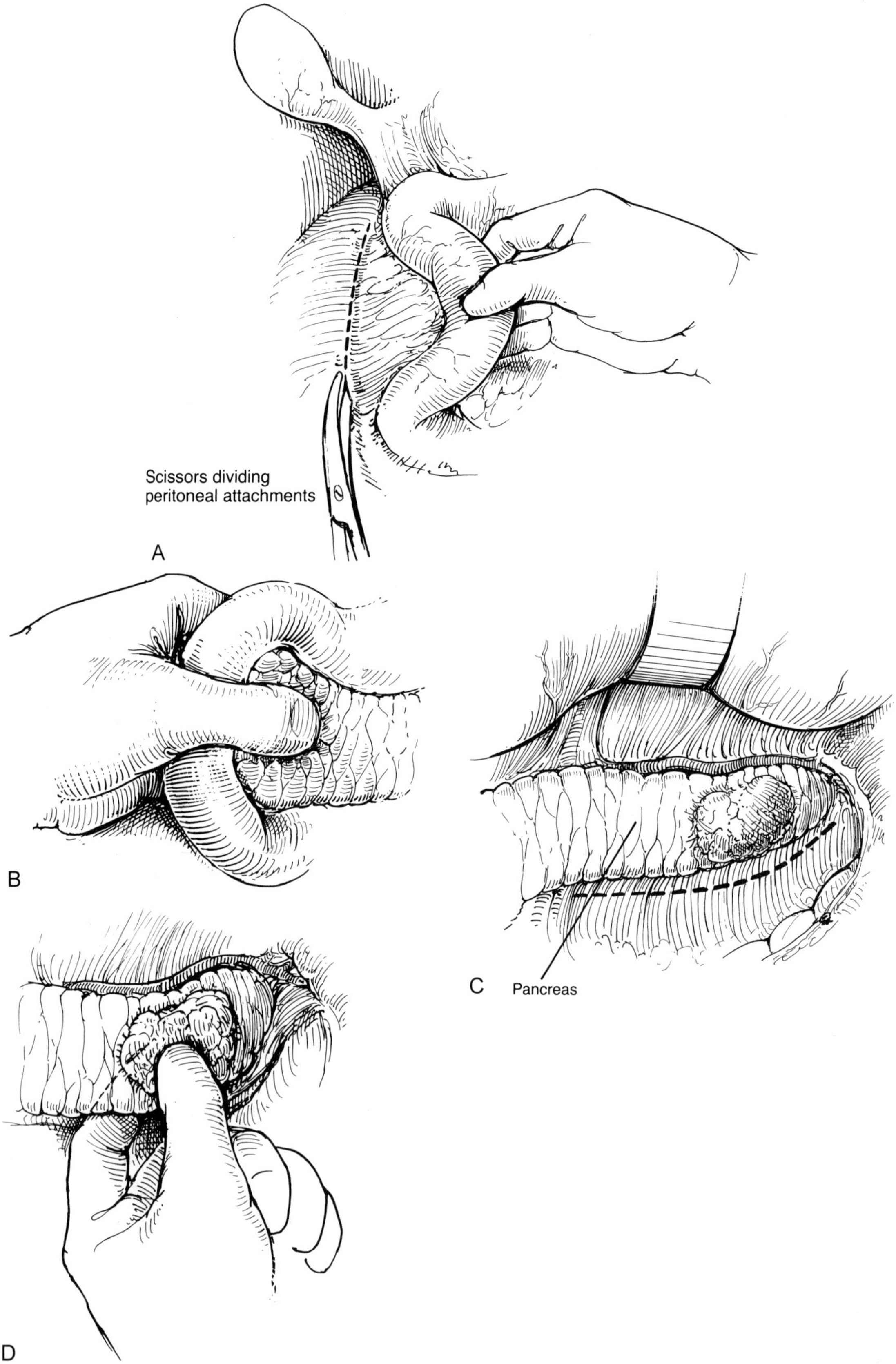

Figure 14–1. Exploration of pancreas. **A,** Mobilization of the head of the pancreas. **B,** Palpation of the head of the pancreas. **C,** Mobilization of the tail of the pancreas. **D,** Palpation of the tail of the pancreas. (From Bland KI, Karakousis CP, Copeland EM III. *Atlas of surgical oncology*. Philadelphia: WB Saunders, 1995.)

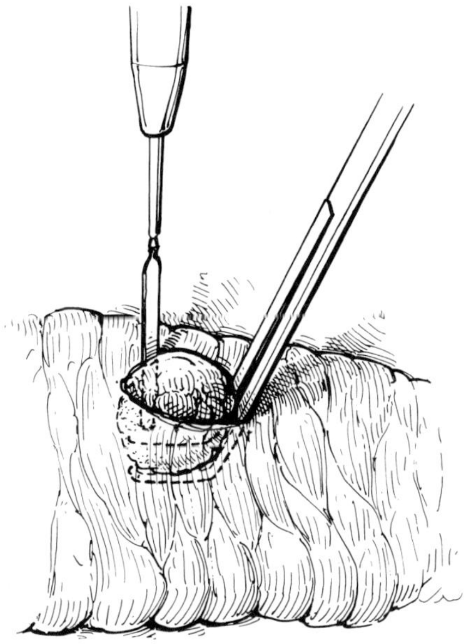

Figure 14–2. Shelling out lesion. (From Bland KI, Karakousis CP, Copeland EM III. *Atlas of surgical oncology*. Philadelphia: WB Saunders, 1995.)

with a 6-0 monofilament absorbable suture. After the lesion has been enucleated, a portion of the omentum can be placed within the defect if possible. Some surgeons place a drainage catheter nearby.

Lesions in the very distal pancreas are often better treated by a spleen-sparing distal pancreatectomy (Figure 14-3). The lesion is again identified by intraoperative ultrasound, and the pancreatic tail is mobilized, beginning in the splenic hilum and working proximally. Small vessels are divided between clips or fine ligatures. After the pancreatic tail has been mobilized to a point right of the tumor, the parenchyma can be divided. The remaining portion of the pancreas and the pancreatic duct are controlled with direct ligature either with or without staple control of the cut end of the pancreas.

The resected tumor should always be confirmed by intraoperative pathology assessment to be certain that the surgeon is not being misled by some other benign hypoechoic lesion within the pancreas. Lymph-node dissection is not necessary for insulinoma patients.

For patients with malignant insulinoma, the procedure should be planned to attempt to encompass all of the disease. This may require major pancreatic resection by itself or in combination with liver resection. Radiofrequency ablation can also be used to address unresectable lesions in the liver. If 90% of the insulin-producing tumor can be addressed by a single procedure, then this may benefit the patient in terms of long-term symptomatic control of the functional tumor.

Postoperative Management

After tumor resection, the blood glucose level typically rebounds into the 160 to 200 mg/DL range for the initial 48 hours. It is somewhat unusual for the patient to require insulin supplementation to control blood glucose after resection of the insulinoma, although this may occur, especially if a major pancreatic resection has been performed. The glucose level should be monitored for the first several days after operation to ensure that it returns to the normal range. The remainder of the recovery is the same as that for any other pancreatic procedure.

Gastrinoma

Epidemiology

Gastrinomas are neuroendocrine tumors that secrete gastrin and that produce the Zollinger–Ellison syndrome (Table 14-5). Gastrinomas were previously considered to be less frequent than insulinomas; however, more recent reports indicate that the frequency appears to be nearly equivalent, at about 1 patient per year per 1 million population. The management for gastrinoma differs significantly from insulinoma because of three facts: (1) there is nonoperative therapy that can completely control the syndrome associated with the gastrinoma; (2) gastrinoma tumors can occur outside of the pancreas in the duodenum or, more rarely, in other sites, such as the ovary or the hepatic ducts, and (3) gastrinomas are frequently malignant, and patients often harbor lymph node or liver metastases at the time of the diagnosis. These facts dictate the management of these patients and the utility of imaging studies for planning an operation.

TABLE 14–5 • *Gastrinoma*

Location	Pancreas, duodenum
Percentage of malignancy	70%
Endocrinopathy	Hypergastrinemia
Medical control of endocrinopathy	Proton-pump inhibitor
Quality of medical control	Virtually 100% effective

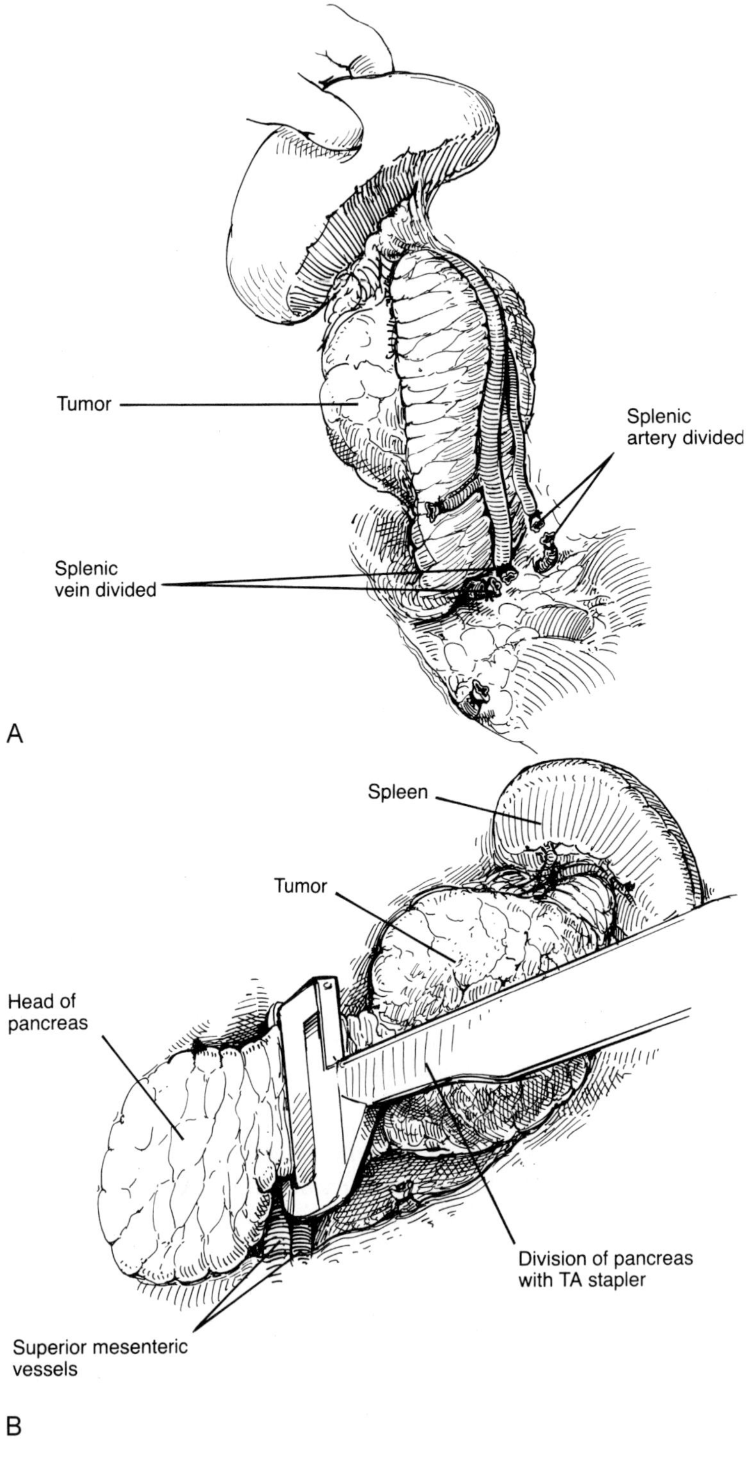

Figure 14–3. Distal pancreatectomy. **A,** Mobilization of the distal pancreas and spleen. **B,** Division of the pancreas to the anatomic right of the tumor. (From Bland KI, Karakousis CP, Copeland EM III. *Atlas of surgical oncology*. Philadelphia: WB Saunders, 1995.)

Clinical Presentation

Patients with Zollinger–Ellison syndrome suffer from the effects of their elevated gastrin levels. Abdominal pain caused either by peptic ulcer disease or gastroesophageal reflux disease is the most common presentation. These symptoms may prove refractory to routine doses of acid-suppression agents. Diarrhea is also a very frequent symptom, and it occurs

BOX 14–3 GASTRINOMA MNEMONIC

Gastrinoma = Peptic Ulcer Disease

Plentiful: multiple ulcers
Unusual sites: distal duodenum or jejunum
Difficult: resistant to therapy, recurrent, complicated by perforation or bleeding

because of the excess acid presented to the small bowel, which cannot absorb it. Proper treatment with high doses of acid-suppression agents resolves both the peptic ulcer disease and the diarrhea. In some patients, severe gastroesophageal reflux disease can be the dominant symptom at presentation.

Diagnosis

The situations in which Zollinger–Ellison syndrome should be considered are those of unusual ulcer disease. There are many more patients with peptic ulcer disease than there are patients with gastrinoma. Among patients with a duodenal ulcer, the presence of diarrhea, the presence of a pancreatic tumor, and the failure of standard medical therapy to control the disease are indications for further investigation. Patients who have particularly severe peptic ulcer disease that leads to complications such as perforation or bleeding should be investigated, as should patients who have multiple duodenal ulcers or ulcers in unusual locations, such as the proximal jejunum. Finally, patients who have evidence of other components of multiple endocrine neoplasia type 1, such as hyperparathyroidism or pituitary disease, should be investigated for gastrinoma. The diagnosis of Zollinger–Ellison syndrome requires the demonstration of an elevated fasting serum gastrin level and the simultaneous presence of acid in the stomach (Table 14-6). The presence merely of hypergastrinemia is most frequently a physiologic response to hypochlorhydria. The most common reason for this is pernicious anemia with atrophic gastritis, although patients taking acid-suppressant medications can also develop an elevated gastrin level. These situations can be excluded by measuring the gastric pH. If the gastric pH is above 2.5, then Zollinger–Ellison syndrome is unlikely to be the cause of the hypergastrinemia. For patients who are being treated with acid-suppressant agents, the diagnosis of gastrinoma can be somewhat difficult. The most straightforward way to make the diagnosis is to discontinue the agents for 1 week before the study and then to evaluate the patient with a serum gastrin and gastric fluid pH level. If the patient has a history of severe symptoms when not taking the proton-pump inhibitors, it may be necessary to switch the patient to histamine H2-receptor antagonists for 1 week, which can be discontinued for just 30 hours before measuring gastric acid output and serum gastrin levels.

If the gastric pH is less than 2.5 and the serum gastrin level is above 1,000 pg/mL, then the only diagnosis remaining to be differentiated from gastrinoma is retained antrum syndrome. This can generally be distinguished on the basis of history. If the pH is less than

TABLE 14–6 • *Diagnostic and Localization Tests for Gastrinomas*

Test	Findings	Accuracy
Fasting serum gastrin level	>1,000 pg/mL	Nearly 100%
Secretin stimulation test	Serum gastrin rise of 200 pg/mL	90% sensitive and specific
Serum chromogranin A	Elevation is correlated with tumor volume	Nonspecific neuroendocrine tumor marker
Calcium infusion study	50% increase in serum gastrin	74% sensitive
Octreotide scintigraphy	Octreotide uptake in area of tumor	For tumors >1.1 cm, 90% sensitive; for tumors <1.1 cm, 70% sensitive
Computed tomographic scanning	Pancreatic mass, duodenal mass, or metastases	Octreotide scintigraphy better for primary tumor localization
Endoscopic ultrasonography	Pancreatic mass, duodenal mass, regional adenopathy	Localization in 90–98%
HVS after arterial stimulation	Elevated HV gastrin after injection of secretin to specific regional arteries	Not as effective for gastrinoma as for insulinoma

HV, Hepatic vein; *HVS*, hepatic vein sampling.

2.5 and the gastrin level is elevated but less than 1,000 pg/mL, then the patient should have more thorough studies performed, including a secretin stimulation test to evaluate the response of gastrin and a formal gastric acid output test to determine whether the basal acid output is above 15 mEq/hr. These patients with borderline levels can be very difficult to diagnosis accurately, and they will require careful study by a group that is familiar with the potential results.

Medical Treatment

The first step in the treatment of Zollinger–Ellison syndrome is the complete control of the end-organ effect of hypergastrinemia. This can always be accomplished with adequate medical therapy. The availability of proton-pump inhibitors has made this achievable with a minimum number of daily doses for all patients. The initial dose of omeprazole for a patient with uncomplicated gastrinoma should be 60 mg daily. The efficacy of this dose can be documented by acid-secretion studies. If the basal acid output remains above 10 mEq/hr, the dose should be changed to 40 mg twice daily. The dose can be increased further, if necessary. The median dose of omeprazole required for control of acid output is 100 mg per day.

It is critical to control the patient's acid output and diarrhea before surgical intervention. Because of the complete efficacy of the medical management, the localization of the tumor and operative intervention can thus be elective.

Localization

The localization of gastrinomas is performed to determine whether resection for cure is possible, whether incomplete resection for present or impending complications is indicated, and whether medical therapy should be attempted to control the malignancy. Localization studies are also then used to evaluate the results of these interventions.

There are a large variety of localization studies that are available for patients with Zollinger–Ellison syndrome. These include anatomic studies such as ultrasound, CT scanning, and MRI of the abdomen. Functional studies include octreotide scintigraphy. Angiography has also been used as an invasive imaging test, and it can be combined with intra-arterial secretin injection and the measurement of hepatic vein gastrin levels to regionalize the site of the tumor.

Of all of the available studies, we have found it most useful to proceed with a cross-sectional imaging test such as CT scan or MRI to gain anatomic information. In addition, octreotide scintigraphy adds functional imaging to correlate with the CT. The other imaging tests can be used to try to settle questions or to search for occult tumors in unusual situations.

Intraoperatively, in addition to careful exploration, ultrasound of the regions of interest is extremely helpful. This is always used in our experience. In addition, the handheld gamma probe assessment of gastrinoma sites can be performed using a preoperative octreotide scintigraphy study and then operating within 72 hours. The handheld gamma probe can then be used to identify sites of occult disease in the abdomen.

Because of the facts that gastrinomas can occur outside of the pancreas and that they can be malignant, it is important to try to localize all of the disease before exploration; this is in contrast with insulinoma. This is particularly important with gastrinoma because of the extrapancreatic sites of disease. The most important extrapancreatic site at which gastrinomas can occur is in the wall of the duodenum. This was not recognized widely until the last 15 years, when it became clear that at least 40% of gastrinomas begin in the wall of the duodenum. For this reason, special measures must be taken to localize tumors in that area. Preoperative measures have not been particularly successful. The best localization is intraoperative duodenotomy and palpation of the wall of the duodenum (Figure 14-4). Other potential sites of disease include primary liver tumors and ovarian tumors.

Surgical Approach

The goal of the surgical management of gastrinoma is cure of the malignancy. At least 70% of gastrinomas are malignant in their behavior. Because the syndrome is completely controllable with medications, the critical goal of operations is to remove all of the disease to cure the patient.

Operation for cure involves resection of the primary disease and the regional metastases as well as any distant metastases. Preoperative localization studies will help the surgeon to determine what sites need to be addressed. Most gastrinomas occur in the gastrinoma triangle, which is located in and around the head of the pancreas and the duodenum. Intraoperative ultrasound and duodenotomy with palpation of the duodenal wall are mandatory for patients with gastrinoma. This can help with the identification of the primary disease in the head of the pancreas or the wall of the duodenum and also the recognition of deep-seated lymph nodes in or around the head or the pancreas and the duodenal sweep. In addition to removing the primary disease, the regional lymph nodes extending from the hilum of the liver to the celiac axis should all be excised. There are frequently also metastatic lymph nodes within the base of the small bowel mesentery, which require excision as well. Metastatic deposits, including liver metastases, should be resected if this is possible.

The outcome of surgical resection is that approximately two thirds of patients are initially biochemically cured; however, over time, this number drops to about one third of patients enjoying long-term disease control after resection.

For patients who cannot be resected for cure, there are occasionally those who can have long-term disease control by other means of disease destruction. This includes a combination of resection and radiofrequency ablation for liver metastases. Again, this is not necessary for control of the hormonal syndrome, but it may slow the progression of tumor and allow for longer survival. This is very difficult to demonstrate because of the small number of these patients and the indolent nature of the disease.

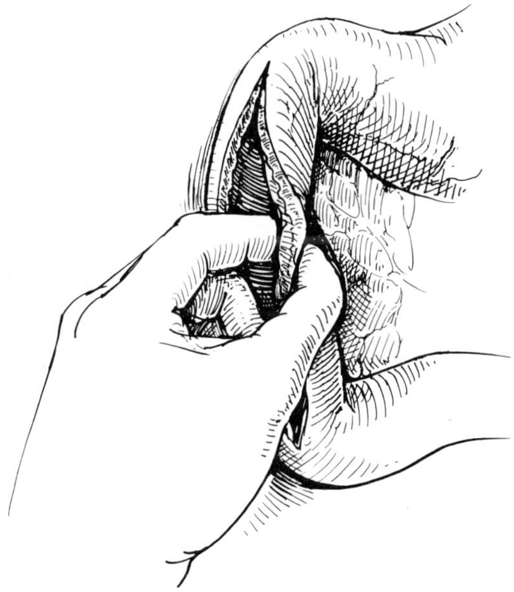

Figure 14-4. Longitudinal duodenotomy with palpation of the wall. (From Bland KI, Karakousis CP, Copeland EM III. *Atlas of surgical oncology.* Philadelphia: WB Saunders, 1995.)

Metastatic Treatment Options

Systemic therapy for metastatic islet cell tumor is of somewhat marginal benefit. Patients who have clear progression or symptoms of mass effect may benefit from cytotoxic chemotherapy; however, only the minority of patients respond.

Glucagonoma

Glucagon is a peptide that is produced by alpha cells of the pancreatic islets. Tumors that produce excessive glucagon cause a syndrome of diabetes, necrolytic migratory erythema (a skin rash), and a tendency toward deep venous thrombosis (Table 14-7). These patients may also have stomatitis, glossitis, cheilosis, and hypoaminoacidemia. All of the skin manifestations appear to be a consequence of malnutrition. These resolve with treatment using total parenteral nutrition.

This syndrome is diagnosed by an elevated plasma level of glucagon (Table 14-8). Levels above 1,000 pg/mL are diagnostic of the syndrome, whereas levels between 150 and 1,000 pg/mL are suggestive of the syndrome. The biochemical management of the hormonal syndrome with somatostatin analog is excellent. These patients also require nutritional supplementation.

TABLE 14-7 • *Glucagonoma*

Location	Tail of pancreas more frequent than head of pancreas
Percentage of malignancy	50–100%
Endocrinopathy	Hyperglycemia, necrolytic migratory erythema
Medical control of endocrinopathy	Octreotide, total parenteral nutrition
Quality of medical control	Excellent

These tumors are always located in the pancreas, and they are typically large at presentation, so localization is not a difficult issue. Imaging with a CT scan and octreotide scintigraphy are effective for identifying the disease in the abdomen and also for identifying potential metastatic sites. Intraoperatively, ultrasound can be useful for defining disease around the pancreas. Glucagonomas are usually malignant, and they may have lymph node and liver metastases.

The operative management of glucagonoma consists of attempts at complete resection. This includes resection of the primary disease, regional lymph nodes, and metastatic sites. These tumors are typically malignant; however, even with unresectable metastatic disease, the progression of the tumor is slow and may allow the patient to live for years.

BOX 14–4 GLUCAGONOMA CLINICAL FEATURES

- Necrolytic migratory erythema
- Weight loss
- Diabetes mellitus
- Associated symptoms: venous thrombosis, diarrhea, cheilitis, weakness, mental status changes

Somatostatinoma

Somatostatinoma is a rare neuroendocrine tumor that can occur in the pancreas or, occasionally, in the duodenum. The duodenal tumors are typically near the ampulla, and they are often quite small (Table 14-9). The duodenal tumors are rarely life threatening.

The endocrine syndrome produced by somatostatin release is subtle. The issue in the control of somatostatinoma is usually control of the potential or actual malignancy. The diagnosis is based on the demonstration of elevated somatostatin levels and the presence of a tumor (Table 14-10). Resection planning is dictated by the extent of tumor.

VIPoma

Tumors producing vasoactive intestinal polypeptide (VIP) almost always occur in the pancreas, although a few may arise in the duo-

BOX 14–5 SOMATOSTATINOMA CLINICAL FEATURES

- Diabetes mellitus
- Cholelithiasis
- Diarrhea with steatorrhea

TABLE 14–8 • *Diagnostic and Localization Tests for Glucagonoma*

Test	Findings	Accuracy
Serum glucagon level	>500 pg/mL; multiple molecular weight forms of glucagon	Nearly 100% sensitive and specific
Computed tomographic scanning	Pancreatic mass	86% sensitive
Endoscopic ultrasound	Pancreatic mass	82% sensitive, 95% specific
Angiography	Hypervascular pancreatic mass	Highly sensitive; rarely needed
Octreotide scintigraphy	Octreotide uptake in area of tumor	Highly sensitive and specific; useful for delineation of metastases
Biopsy	Tissue showing islet cell tumor with positive stain for glucagon	Highly specific

TABLE 14–9 • *Somatostatinoma*

Location	Pancreas, 70%; duodenum, small bowel, ampulla, 30%
Percentage of malignancy	75%
Endocrinopathy	Hyperglycemia, hypochlorhydria, hyposecretion of pancreatic enzymes and cholecystokinin
Medical control of endocrinopathy	Octreotide ± interferon alpha
Quality of medical control	Fair

denum. With the production of excess VIP, a syndrome characterized by watery diarrhea, hypokalemia, and achlorhydria can develop. These patients have a severe, watery secretory diarrhea that persists even during fasting (Table 14-11). VIP also directly inhibits gastric acid secretion, thereby causing hypochlorhydria or even achlorhydria.

BOX 14–6 VIPOMA CLINICAL FEATURES

"Pancreatic cholera syndrome"

- Watery secretory diarrhea (>700 mL per day)
- Hypokalemia
- Hypochlorhydria

Associated symptoms

- Flushing
- Lethargy
- Nausea
- Vomiting
- Muscle cramps
- Weakness

The diagnosis of VIPoma is made by documenting an elevated plasma VIP level in the presence of a secretory diarrhea (Table 14-12). The volume of the diarrhea is typically more than 3 liters a day, and it should not resolve when a patient is fasting. The VIPoma syndrome can be completely treated with somatostatin analog therapy; by this means, the patient's dehydration and hypokalemia can be completely corrected before operation.

The localization of these tumors is typically not difficult. They are generally large, and they can be easily imaged by CT scanning or ultrasound. Somatostatin-receptor scintigraphy is useful to confirm the nature of the CT abnormality and to evaluate for metastatic disease.

The only potential curative option for the treatment of these patients is complete resection. All patients who are fit for operation and

TABLE 14–10 • *Diagnostic and Localization Tests for Somatostatinoma*

Test	Findings	Accuracy
Fasting plasma; somatostatin level	>160 pg/mL	Suggestive
Computed tomographic scanning	Pancreatic mass	Highly sensitive
Magnetic resonance imaging	Pancreatic mass	Sensitive
Endoscopic ultrasound	Pancreatic mass	Sensitive
Angiography	Hypervascular pancreatic mass	Sensitive
Octreotide scintigraphy	Octreotide uptake in area of tumor	Highly sensitive, functional somatostatin receptors present

TABLE 14–11 • *VIPoma*

Location	Pancreas, bronchi, colon, adrenal, liver, sympathetic ganglia
Percentage of malignancy	60–80%
Endocrinopathy	Hypokalemia, hypochlorhydria
Medical control of endocrinopathy	Octreotide ± glucocorticoid
Quality of medical control	Highly effective

TABLE 14–12 • *Diagnostic and Localization Tests for VIPoma*

Test	Findings	Accuracy
Serum vasoactive intestinal polypeptide level	>75 pg/mL	Sensitive and specific
Stool osmolal gap	Low stool osmolal gap	Sensitive for secretory diarrhea
Abdominal computed tomographic scanning	Pancreatic mass	Highly sensitive
Octreotide scintigraphy	Octreotide uptake in area of tumor	Sensitive

whose imaged disease appears to be resectable should have abdominal exploration with resection of the appropriate portion of the pancreas, regional lymph node dissection, and resection of any metastatic disease. In addition, each patient should have a cholecystectomy, regardless of the disease stage, to facilitate later treatment with somatostatin analog. Somatostatin analog can cause patients to develop gallstones as one of the side effects.

Multiple Endocrine Neoplasia Type 1 Syndrome

Multiple endocrine neoplasia type 1 (MEN-1) is an autosomal dominant genetic syndrome that predisposes a person to multiple tumors in the endocrine glands and also to nonendocrine tumors. Pancreatic islet tumors arise in 30% to 80% of patients with MEN-1, and most patients will have multiple tumors. The majority of patients will have nonfunctional tumors (>80%). The most common functional tumor is gastrinoma, which occurs in 50% of patients; this is followed by insulinoma, which occurs in 10% of patients (Table 14-13). Up to 50% of patients with pancreatic neuroendocrine tumors have submucosal neuroendocrine tumors throughout the duodenum that secrete gastrin. These neuroendocrine tumors may manifest as Zollinger–Ellison syndrome, and they are potentially malignant.

BOX 14–7 MULTIPLE ENDOCRINE NEOPLASIA I CLINICAL FEATURES

Classic three "P" components:
1. Pituitary tumors
2. Parathyroid tumors
3. Pancreatic tumors

TABLE 14–13 • *Incidence of Pancreatic Endocrine Tumors in Multiple Endocrine Neoplasia Type 1 Patients*

Tumor	Incidence
Nonfunctional	>80%
Gastrinoma	50%
Insulinoma	10%
Glucagonoma	<2%
VIPoma	<2%

The diagnosis of pancreatic endocrine tumors in patients who are known to be members of families with MEN-1 is possible before the development of the clinical syndrome. Plasma markers, such as insulin, proinsulin, gastrin, pancreatic polypeptide, glucagon, and chromogranin A, are the most consistent markers of pancreatic endocrine lesions, and they have sensitivities ranging from 37% to 60%. A 48-hour fast may be useful to diagnose insulinoma. Radiologic screening of suspected MEN-1 carriers should be performed every 3 to 5 years. Somatostatin-receptor scintigraphy, spiral CT scanning, MRI, and positron emission tomographic scanning can be used to identify tumor.

There is general agreement that patients with MEN-1 presenting with hypoglycemia as a result of insulinoma should have resection rather than enucleation. Hypoglycemia is typically resolved, and diabetes rarely develops with this extent of resection. The presence of a VIPoma or glucagonoma is managed similarly to insulinoma. The treatment of other functional pancreatic endocrine tumors (mainly Zollinger–Ellison syndrome) for patients with MEN-1 is also resection. Surgical resection must consider the high frequency of duodenal tumors that can underlie Zollinger–Ellison syndrome. Thus, duodenotomy with the resection of identified duodenal tumors, resection of the involved areas of the pancreas, and regional lymph node resection are appropriate. The extensive resection of the pancreas is based on the frequency of multicentric tumors and the risk of postoperative recurrence. We recommend the operative management of all functional tumors that can be imaged on preoperative studies.

The management of nonfunctional pancreatic tumors among patients with MEN-1 is similar to that for patients without MEN-1. Operation is considered when the tumor is radiologically demonstrated. Surgical methods are similar to those used for patients with nonfunctional tumors without MEN-1, but they should include the resection of all affected pancreas, with the preservation of normal pancreatic parenchyma to limit glucose intolerance.

Conclusion

Tumors arising from the endocrine pancreas present unique and interesting problems. A thorough understanding of their pathophysiology, anatomy, and prognosis is necessary so that proper medical care may be provided.

Key Selected Reading

Howard J, Idezuki Y, Ihse I, Prinz R. Section XIV: the endocrine pancreas. In: *Surgical diseases of the pancreas,* 3rd ed. Baltimore: Williams & Wilkins, 1998.

Selected Readings

Ardengh JC, Rosenbaum P, Ganc AJ, *et al.* Role of EUS in the preoperative localization of insulinomas compared with spiral CT. *Gastrointest Endosc* 2000;51: 552–555.

Boden G, Ryan IG, Eisenschmid BL, *et al.* Treatment of inoperable glucagonoma with the long-acting somatostatin analog SMS-201-995. *N Engl J Med* 1986;314:1686–1689.

Boden G. Glucagonomas and insulinomas. *Gastroenterol Clin North Am* 1989;18:831–845.

Boden G, Shimoyama R. Somatostatinoma. In: Cohen S, Soloway RD, eds. *Hormone-producing tumors of the gastrointestinal tract.* New York: Churchill Livingstone, 1985:85.

Cohen MS, Picus D, Lairmore TC, *et al.* Prospective study of provocative angiograms to localize functional islet cell tumors of the pancreas. *Surgery* 1997;122:1091–1100.

Doherty GM. Multiple endocrine neoplasia type 1. *J Surg Oncol* 2005;89:143–150.

Doherty GM, Olson JA, Frisella MM, *et al.* Lethality of multiple endocrine neoplasia type I. *World J Surg* 1998;22:581–586; discussion 586–587.

Doherty GM, Doppman JL, Shawker TH, *et al.* Results of a prospective strategy to diagnose, localize, and resect insulinomas. *Surgery* 1991;110:989–996; discussion 996–997.

Fernandez-Cruz L, Saenz A, Astudillo E, *et al.* Outcome of laparoscopic pancreatic surgery: endocrine and nonendocrine tumors. *World J Surg* 2002;26: 1057–1065.

Gramatica L Jr, Herrera MF, Mercado-Luna A, *et al.* Videolaparoscopic resection of insulinomas: experience in two institutions. *World J Surg* 2002;26: 1297–1300.

Grant CS, van Heerden J, Charboneau JW, *et al.* Insulinoma. The value of intraoperative ultrasonography. *Arch Surg* 1988;123:843–848.

Hashimoto L, Walsh R. Preoperative localization of insulinomas is not necessary. *J Am Coll Surg* 1999; 189:368–373.

Hiramoto JS, Feldstein VA, LaBerge JM, Norton JA. Intraoperative ultrasound and preoperative localization detects all occult insulinomas. *Arch Surg* 2001;136:1020–1025; discussion 1025–1026.

Hirshberg B, Livi A, Bartlett DL, *et al.* Forty-eight-hour fast: the diagnostic test for insulinoma. *J Clin Endocrinol Metab* 2000;85:3222–3226.

Kouvaraki MA, Solorzano CC, Shapiro SE, *et al.* Surgical treatment of non-functioning pancreatic islet cell tumors. *J Surg Oncol* 2005;89:170–185.

Lairmore TC, Chen VY, DeBenedetti MK, *et al.* Duodenopancreatic resections in patients with multiple endocrine neoplasia type 1. *Ann Surg* 2000; 231:909–918.

Mekhjian HS, O'Dorisio TM. VIPoma syndrome. *Semin Oncol* 1987;14:282–291.

Meko JB, Doherty GM, Siegel BA, Norton JA. Evaluation of somatostatin-receptor scintigraphy for detecting neuroendocrine tumors. *Surgery* 1996;120:975–983; discussion 983–984.

Norton JA, Jensen RT. Resolved and unresloved controversies in the surgical management of patients with Zollinger-Ellison syndrome. *Ann Surg* 2004;240: 757–773.

Norton JA, Fraker DL, Alexander HR, *et al.* Surgery to cure the Zollinger-Ellison syndrome. *N Engl J Med* 1999;341:635–644.

Norton JA, Alexander HR, Fraker DL, *et al.* Comparison of surgical results in patients with advanced and limited disease with multiple endocrine neoplasia type 1 and Zollinger-Ellison syndrome. *Ann Surg* 2001;234:495–505; discussion 505–506.

Norton JA, Doppman JL, Jensen RT. Curative resection in Zollinger-Ellison syndrome: results of a 10 year prospective study. *Ann Surg* 1992;215:8–18.

O'Dorisio TM, Mekhjian HS. VIPoma syndrome. In: Cohen S, Soloway RD, eds. *Hormone producing tumors of the pancreas.* New York: Churchill Livingstone, 1985:101–110.

O'Dorisio TM, Mehkjian HS, Gaginella TS. Medical therapy of VIPomas. *Endocrinol Metab Clin North Am* 1989;18:545–556.

Roy PK, Venzon DJ, Feigenbaum KM, *et al.* Gastric secretion in Zollinger-Ellison syndrome. Correlation with clinical expression, tumor extent and role in diagnosis—a prospective NIH study of 235 patients and a review of 984 cases in the literature. *Medicine (Baltimore)* 2001;80:189–222.

Roy PK, Venzon DJ, Shojamanesh H, *et al.* Zollinger-Ellison syndrome. Clinical presentation in 261 patients. *Medicine (Baltimore)* 2000;79:379–411.

Service FJ. Hypoglycemic disorders. *N Engl J Med* 1995;332:1144–1152.

Skogseid B, Doherty GM. Multiple endocrine neoplasia type 1: clinical and genetic features. *Dig Liver Dis* 1999;31(Suppl 2):S131–S134.

Stabile BE, Morrow DJ, Passaro E. The gastrinoma triangle: operative implications. *Am J Surg* 1984;147:25–31.

Sugg SL, Norton JA, Fraker DL, *et al.* A prospective study of intraoperative methods to diagnose and resect duodenal gastrinomas. *Ann Surg* 1993;218:138–144.

Takamatsu S, Teramoto K, Inoue H, *et al.* Laparoscopic enucleation of an insulinoma of the pancreas tail. *Surg Endosc* 2002;16:217.

Tucker ON, Crotty PL, Conlon KC. The management of insulinoma. *Br J Surg* 2006;93:264–275.

van Heerden JA, Grant CS, Czako PF, *et al.* Occult functioning insulinomas: which localizing studies are indicated? *Surgery* 1992;112:1010–1014; discussion 1014–1015.

Vinik AI, Strodel WE, Eckhauser FE, *et al.* Somatostatinomas, PPomas, neurotensinomas. *Semin Oncol* 1987;14:263–281.

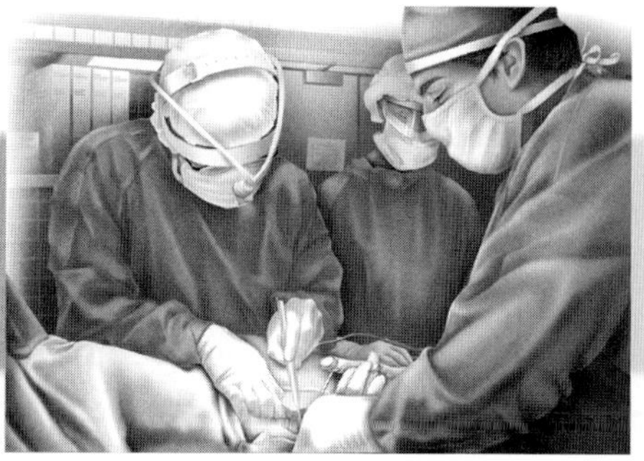

15

Esophageal Cancer

Jules Lin and Mark D. Iannettoni

Esophageal Cancer: Key Points

- List the factors that increase the risk for esophageal squamous cell carcinoma and those that help to determine patient prognosis.
- Identify predisposing conditions and risk factors for esophageal adenocarcinoma.
- Outline the signs and symptoms of esophageal adenocarcinoma and the diagnostic steps required.
- List the radiographic studies needed to diagnose and stage esophageal cancer.
- Compare the surgical treatment options for esophageal cancer.
- Describe the management of high-grade dysplasia.
- List the major prognostic factors for esophageal adenocarcinoma.

The estimated incidence of esophageal cancer in the United States for 2006 was 14,550, with approximately 13,770 cancer-related deaths. Adenocarcinoma of the esophagus is now more frequent in the United States than esophageal squamous cell carcinoma (ESCC), and the incidence continues to rise. Although resection offers the best chance for cure, most patients who present with symptoms already have systemic disease and are incurable. The most important prognostic factor for esophageal cancer remains the stage of disease at the time of diagnosis. Currently, the best strategy for improving survival is early diagnosis with resection, although various multimodality therapies are being investigated for the treatment of advanced disease.

Esophageal Squamous Cell Carcinoma

Epidemiology

In the United States, the annual incidence of ESCC is 2.6 per 100,000. The incidence is four to five times higher among blacks than whites, and men are affected three to four times as often as women. Regions with a high incidence are generally located in poorer areas of the world, including parts of China, Central Asia, and Latin America. The overall 5-year survival rate is approximately 5%, but it may be improving slightly.

BOX 15-1 EPIDEMIOLOGY OF ESOPHAGEAL CANCER

Esophageal cancer was diagnosed in 14,550 patients in 2006.

Esophageal Squamous Cell Cancer

- The incidence of ESCC in the United States is 2.6 per 100,000.
- Men are affected three to four times as often as women.
- The incidence is four to five times higher among blacks than whites.
- There is a higher incidence in poorer parts of the world.

Esophageal Adenocarcinoma

- It is the seventh leading cause of cancer-related deaths.
- Men are affected six to eight times as often as women.
- The incidence is three to four times higher among whites than blacks.
- There is a higher incidence in developed countries.

Etiology

Nutritional deficiencies, including low levels of vitamins A, C, and riboflavin, as well as of mineral elements such as selenium, zinc, and molybdenum, have been found to contribute to the pathogenesis of ESCC. High levels of nitrates and nitrites, which are converted to N-nitrosamines, have also been associated with ESCC. Numerous studies have linked alcohol and tobacco use to the development of esophageal cancer, with the risk increasing with the amount of alcohol and tobacco consumed. One study found ethanol to be associated with nearly 80% of esophageal cancers, and another found a synergistic effect between alcohol and tobacco use. Predisposing conditions include achalasia, caustic injury, tylosis (a genetic disorder characterized by hyperkeratosis of the palms and soles, oral leukoplakia, and a very high risk of esophageal cancer), and Plummer–Vinson syndrome (postcricoid dysphagia, upper esophageal webs, and iron-deficiency anemia).

BOX 15-2 RICK FACTORS FOR ESOPHAGEAL SQUAMOUS CELL CARCINOMA

- Nutritional deficiencies
- Vitamins A and C and riboflavin
- Zinc, selenium, molybdenum, trace elements
- Injury
- Thermal or caustic injury
- Carcinogens
- Alcohol
- Tobacco
- Nitrosamines
- Fungal toxins
- Predisposing conditions
- Achalasia
- Celiac sprue
- Tylosis
- Plummer–Vinson syndrome

Pathology

ESCC is most commonly located (50% of lesions) in the middle third of the thoracic esophagus. Early cancers appear as plaque-like, erosive, or papillary lesions, and they are more frequently seen in endemic areas, where routine screening is performed. More advanced cancers are described as scirrhous, medullary, or fungating (Figure 15-1), and a desmoplastic response can result in a tight esophageal stricture. Microscopically, early squamous cell tumors are classified as intraepithelial, intramucosal, or submucosal tumors (Figure 15-2). Unfortunately, most tumors have spread more extensively than their gross appearance would indicate, with invasion through the muscular layers of the esophagus and the adventitia. Lymphatic metastases are found in 30% to 70% of surgical specimens, and they are related to the depth of invasion. Tumors may also invade adjacent structures, and visceral metastases may

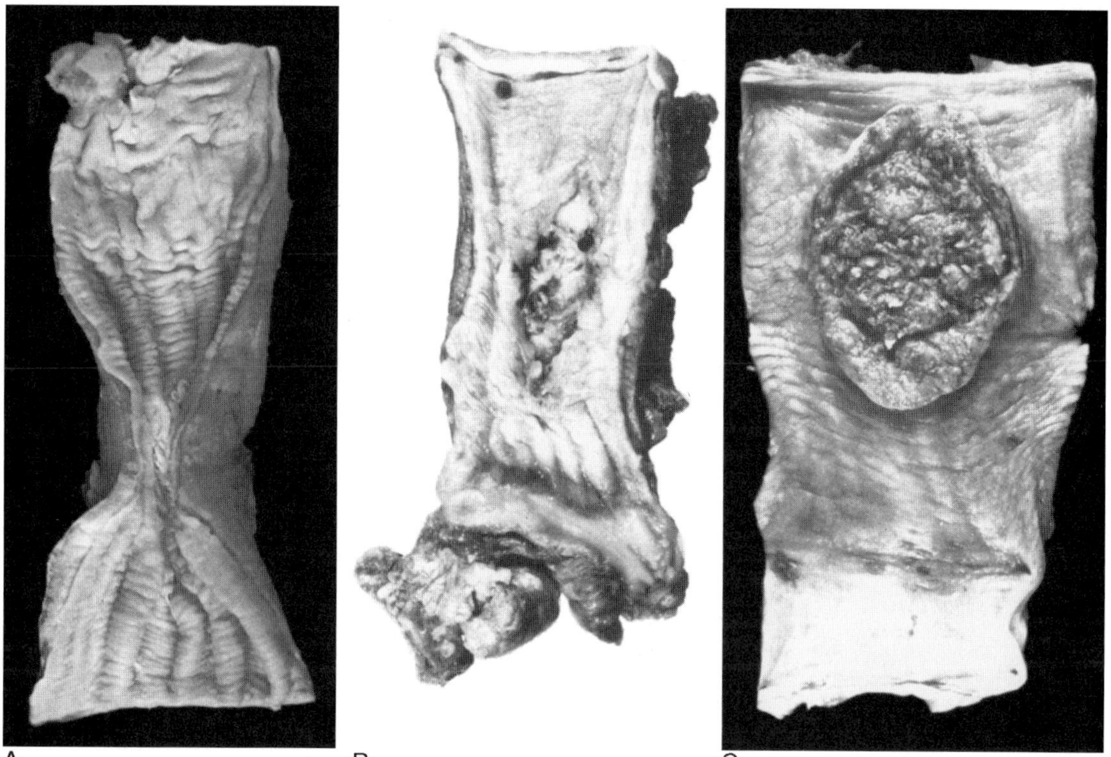

A B C

Figure 15-1. Advanced esophageal squamous cell carcinoma. **A,** Scirrhous type. **B,** Medullary type. **C,** Fungating type. (From Liu FS, *et al.* Pathology of carcinoma of the esophagus. In Huang GJ, Wu YK, eds. *Carcinoma of the esophagus and gastric cardia.* Berlin: Springer, 1994:83–85.)

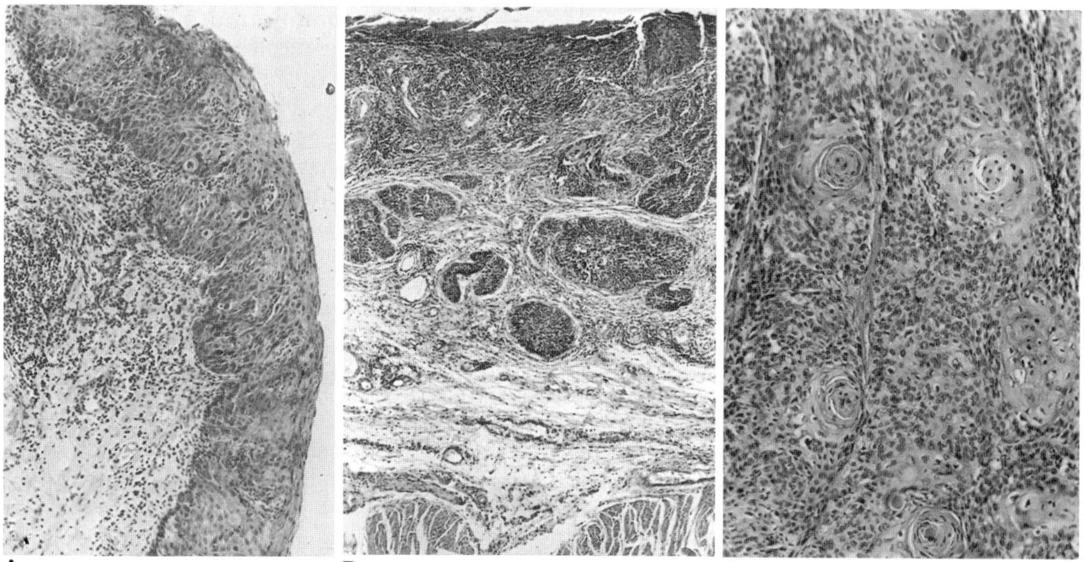

A B C

Figure 15-2. Esophageal squamous cell carcinoma. **A,** In situ, with an intact basement membrane. **B,** Submucosal carcinoma. **C,** Well-differentiated carcinoma with pearl formations. (From Liu FS, *et al.* Pathology of carcinoma of the esophagus. In Huang GJ, Wu YK, eds. *Carcinoma of the esophagus and gastric cardia.* Berlin: Springer, 1994:88, 90, 91.)

be present in up to 30% of patients at the time of diagnosis. The extent of invasion and the presence or absence of lymph-node metastases are critical for determining patient prognosis.

BOX 15-3 ADJACENT STRUCTURES THAT MAY BE INVADED BY ESOPHAGEAL CANCER

- Trachea
- Left mainstem bronchus
- Pleura
- Great vessels, pericardium
- Thoracic duct
- Anterior ligaments of the vertebral column

Upper Esophagus

- Recurrent laryngeal nerves

Lower Esophagus

- Stomach
- Diaphragm
- Liver

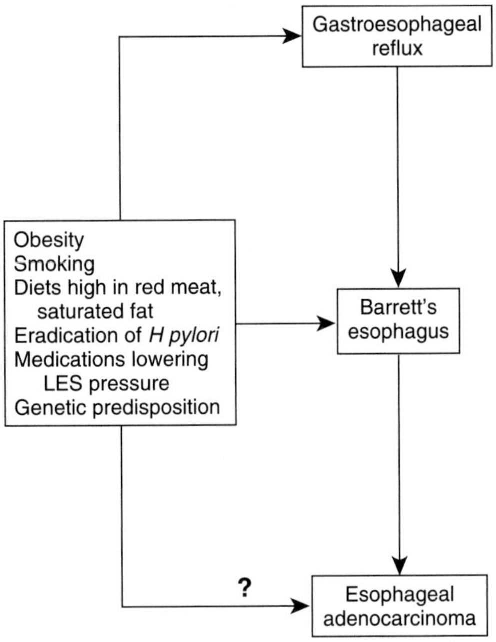

Figure 15-3. Risk factors leading to esophageal adenocarcinoma. *LES*, Lower esophageal sphincter.

Esophageal Adenocarcinoma

Epidemiology

The incidence of esophageal adenocarcinoma (EAC) has increased progressively since the 1970s. It overtook squamous cell carcinoma as the most common cancer of the esophagus in America in the mid-1990s, and it is the seventh leading cause of cancer-related deaths. The median age of diagnosis is 68 years. Men are affected six to eight times more frequently than women, and whites are affected three to four times as often as blacks. The incidence rate is also higher in developed countries.

Etiology

Barrett's Metaplasia

Barrett's metaplasia—and, specifically, intestinal-type columnar mucosa—is the precursor lesion to EAC (Figure 15-3). Among patients with Barrett's metaplasia, the risk of adenocarcinoma is increased by 30 to 125 times as compared with that of the age-matched population, and adenocarcinoma develops in 7% to 20% of patients. Barrett's esophagus appears to be an acquired condition that results from chronic inflammation caused by gastroesophageal reflux. At endoscopy, Barrett's mucosa is found in 12% to 18% of patents with reflux. Although the esophageal mucosa is relatively resistant to acid, mixed reflux with bile acids, pepsin, trypsin, lysolecithin, and gastric acid appears to be more harmful (Figure 15-4), and up to 67% of patients with Barrett's metaplasia have bile-stained duodenogastric reflux.

On endoscopy, Barrett's mucosa appears as red, velvety areas between smooth, pale esophageal squamous mucosa (Figure 15-5, *A* and *B*). Microscopically, columnar epithelium is seen, with mucosal glands that often contain intestinal goblet cells (Figure 15-6, *A*). Barrett's mucosa has been described in the past as intestinal-type columnar epithelium extending more than 3 cm above the gastroesophageal junction. However, it is being increasingly recognized that patients with short-segment Barrett's esophagus of less than 3 cm in length are also at risk of developing dysplasia and adenocarcinoma.

Surveillance During Preclinical Phase

EAC is believed to have a 4- to 5-year preclinical phase, which suggests that surveillance may be effective. Cancers detected during surveillance tend to be less advanced, and the American College of Gastroenterology has suggested that patients with chronic reflux undergo upper endoscopy. Abnormal mucosa is biopsied to diagnose Barrett's metaplasia and to detect the presence of dysplasia. Continued endoscopic surveillance of patients with Barrett's mucosa is determined by the grade of

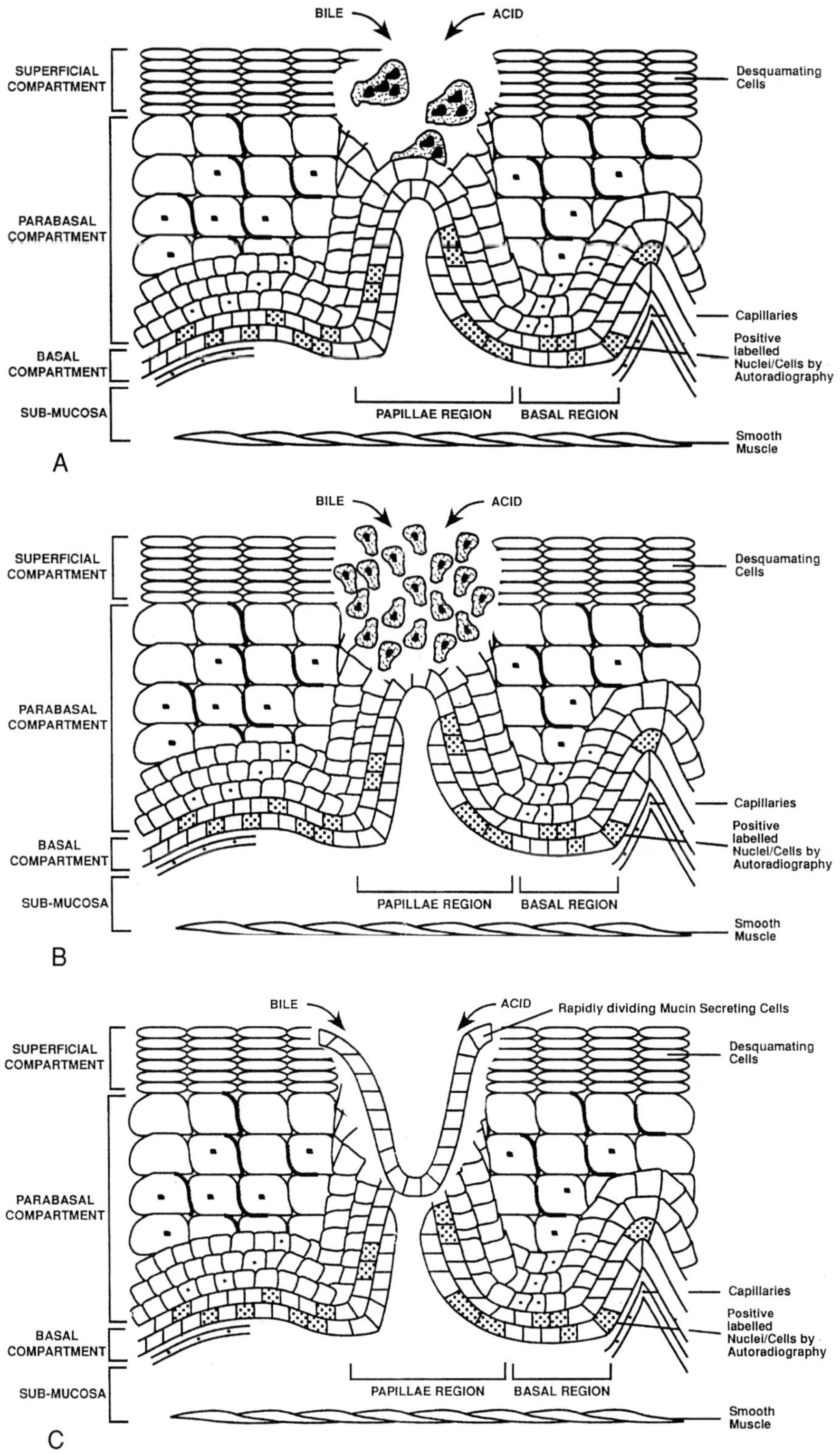

Figure 15-4. Illustration of the development of Barrett's mucosa. **A,** Damage to esophageal cells in the superficial and parabasal compartments. **B,** Damage to the epithelial stem cells (speckled nuclei) in the basal compartment. **C,** Generation of mucin-secreting acid/bile-resistant clones. (From Jankowski JA, Wright NA, Meltzer SJ, *et al.* Molecular evolution of the metaplasia-dysplasia-adenocarcinoma sequence in the esophagus. *Am J Pathol* 1999;154:968.)

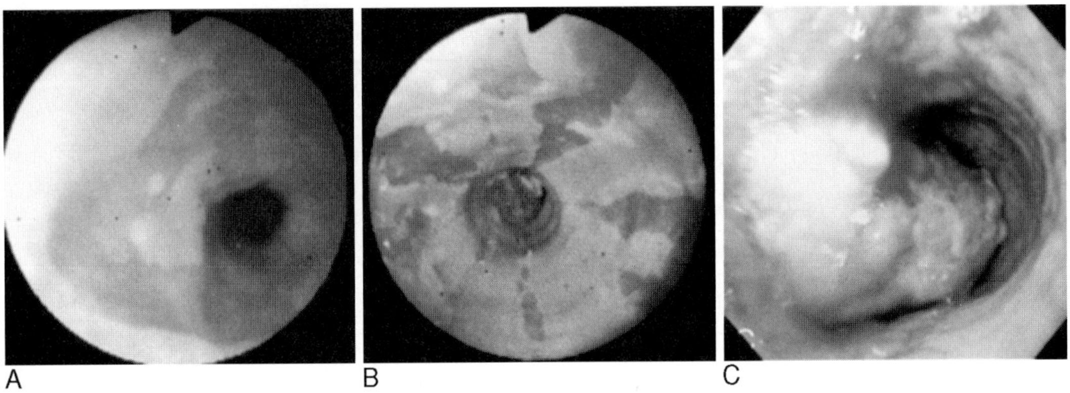

Figure 15-5. **A** and **B,** Endoscopic view of Barrett's metaplasia. **C,** Endoscopic view of esophageal adenocarcinoma. (From Lin J, Iannettoni MD: Carcinoma of the esophagus. In Shields TW, Locicero J III, Ponn RB, eds. *General thoracic surgery*, 6th ed, vol 2. Philadelphia: Lippincott Williams and Wilkins, 2005.)

dysplastic mucosa, as outlined in Figure 15-7. Four-quadrant biopsies are taken every 2 cm, along with biopsies of any visible lesions. After two consecutive biopsies are negative for dysplasia, surveillance intervals can be increased in length to every 3 years. The management of high-grade dysplasia remains controversial (see below), with some advocating for continued surveillance for focal lesions and others recommending esophagectomy as a result of the elevated risk of adenocarcinoma.

Other Risk Factors

Other risk factors for adenocarcinoma include ectopic gastric mucosa and esophageal diverticula. There may also be an association with obesity, smoking, diets high in saturated fat and red meat, and medications that reduce lower esophageal sphincter pressure (see Figure 15-3). In addition, concerns have been raised that the eradication of *Helicobacter pylori*—particularly the acid-suppressing effects of the Cag A+ strain—may actually increase the incidence of EAC.

Pathogenesis

After the squamous epithelium is injured by reflux, there is an inflammation-stimulated hyperplasia and a metaplastic change to the columnar epithelium. One hypothesis suggests that pluripotent stem cells in the basal layers undergo metaplasia after repeated stimulation from reflux. Other possible origins of columnar cells are the gastric cardia and the propagation

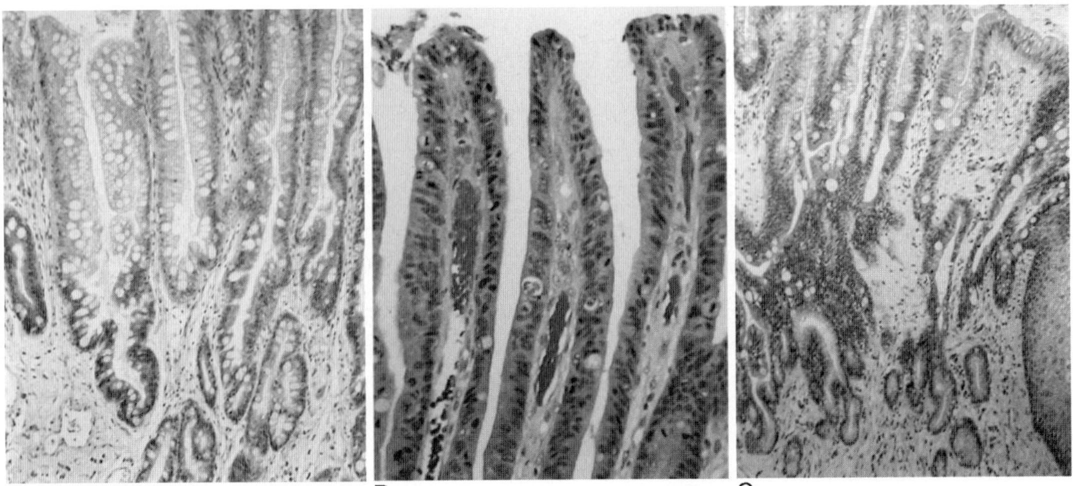

Figure 15-6. Microscopic views of **A,** Barrett's metaplasia, **B,** high-grade dysplasia, and **C,** invasive adenocarcinoma. (From Lin J, Iannettoni MD: Carcinoma of the esophagus. In Shields TW, Locicero J III, Ponn RB, eds. *General thoracic surgery*, 6th ed, vol 2. Philadelphia: Lippincott Williams and Wilkins, 2005.)

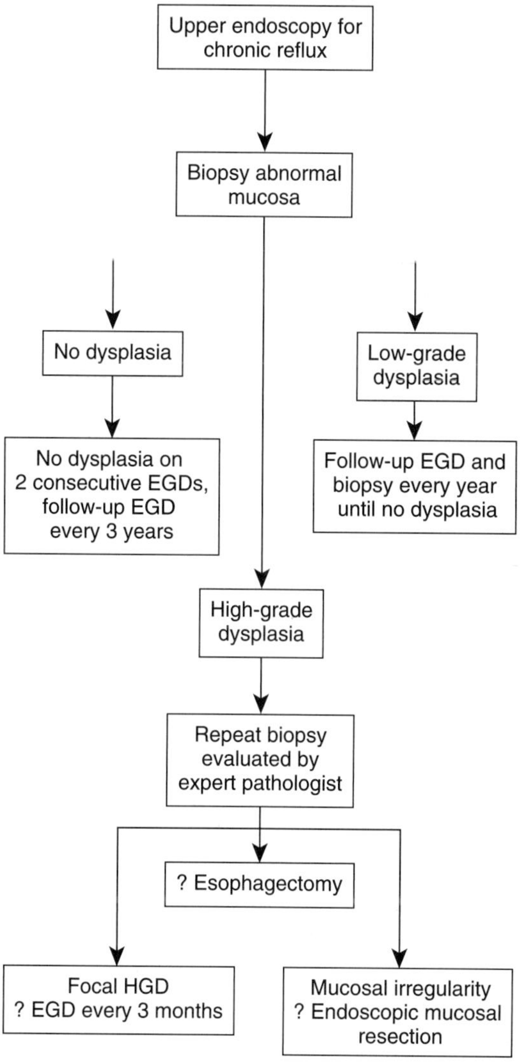

Figure 15-7. Surveillance for Barrett's mucosa in patients with chronic gastroesophageal reflux. *EGD,* Esophagogastroduodenoscopy; *HGD,* high-grade dysplasia.

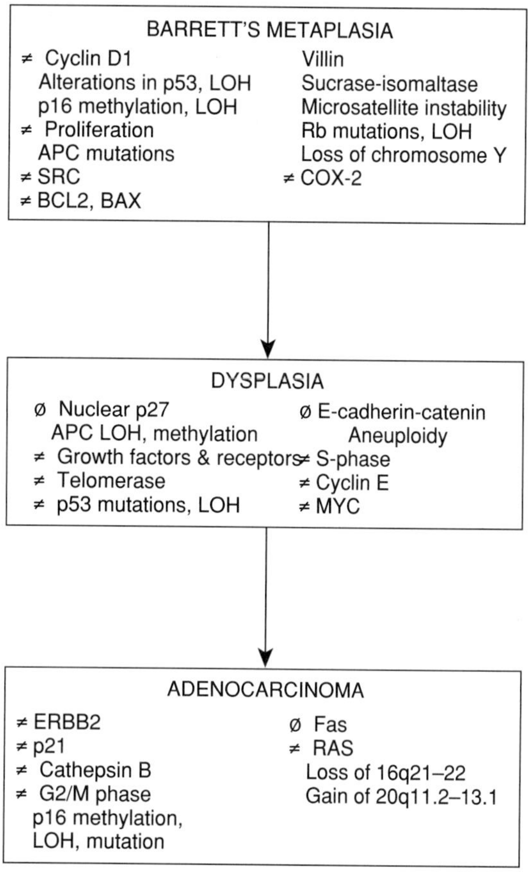

Figure 15-8. Genetic changes involved in the progression from Barrett's metaplasia to esophageal adenocarcinoma. Many of the early changes persist as the lesions progress to dysplasia and adenocarcinoma. *APC,* Adenomatous polyposis coli; *LOH,* loss of heterozygosity. (From Lin J, Beerm DG. Molecular biology of upper gastrointestinal malignancies. *Semin Oncol* 2004;31:476–486.)

of columnar cells from the esophageal gland ducts. With further injury and multiple genetic changes (Figure 15-8), progression occurs in a stepwise fashion in a metaplasia-dysplasia-adenocarcinoma sequence. Studies of the genetic changes involved in the pathogenesis of adenocarcinoma will not only improve understanding of this cancer, but they may also provide novel methods of diagnosis, staging, and treatment.

Pathology

EAC usually arises in the distal esophagus (approximately 80%). Lesions are initially flat or raised patches of mucosa that may become infiltrative or deeply ulcerated lesions. High-grade dysplasia on histopathology remains the best predictor of progression to adenocarcinoma (see Figure 15-6, *B*). Lesions are classified as low- or high-grade dysplasia, and they are distinguished by the nuclear orientation along the base of the epithelium, as well as by other characteristics (Table 15-1). Microscopically, most tumors are composed of mucin-producing intestinal-type glands (see Figure 15-6, *C*). The esophagus has an extensive submucosal lymphatic network. Even when tumors are confined by the muscularis mucosa, 8% to 30% of patients have nodal disease. This number increases to 30% to 58% when the submucosa is involved. Sites of lymph-node metastases in transmural EAC are shown in Figure 15-9. The most common sites of distant metastases include the liver, lungs, bone, brain, and adrenal glands (Table 15-2).

TABLE 15–1 • *Grading Barrett's Dysplasia*

Dysplasia	Cytology	Architecture	Surface Maturation
None	Normal or reactive	Normal	Present
Indeterminate	Mild changes; focal atypia with inflammation	Normal or mild changes	Present
Low grade	Mild changes; cellular polarity maintained: diffuse or focal marked atypia	Mild changes	Absent
High grade	Severe changes; loss of cellular polarity	Severe changes	Absent

Diagnostic Evaluation

Presentation

Dysphagia is the most common initial symptom. Typically, difficulty swallowing is noted with solid foods, which may progress eventually to include semisolids and liquids over a period of weeks to months. Odynophagia (pain with swallowing) is the next most common symptom, which may be caused by an ulcerated lesion or invasion of surrounding mediastinal structures. Constant pain in the mid back or mid chest also suggests mediastinal invasion. Hoarseness may occur with proximal tumors, and it indicates the involvement of the recurrent laryngeal nerves. The regurgitation of food immediately after swallowing may occur as the growing neoplasm narrows the esophageal lumen, and anorexia and weight loss are often present by the time the patient seeks medical attention. Although patients often have a history of reflux symptoms, clinical features do not distinguish patients with or without Barrett's mucosa, which is frequently asymptomatic.

BOX 15–4 SIGNS AND SYMPTOMS OF ADVANCED ESOPHAGEAL CARCINOMA

- Dysphagia, odynophagia
- Weight loss
- Supraclavicular lymphadenopathy
- Dyspnea due to phrenic nerve involvement
- Cough from tracheoesophageal fistula
- Hoarseness from recurrent laryngeal nerve invasion
- Upper body edema from superior vena cava syndrome
- Malignant pleural effusion
- Bone pain

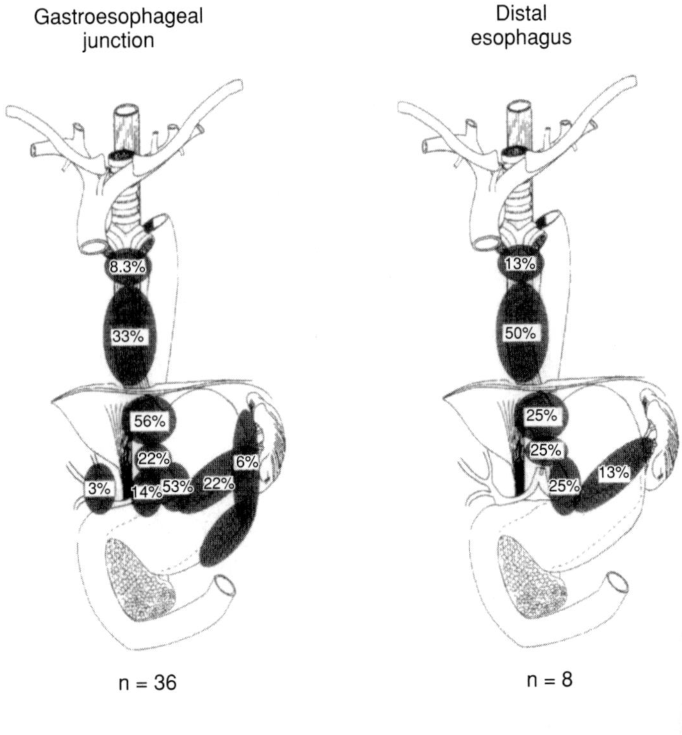

Figure 15–9. Sites of lymph-node metastases in patients with transmural esophageal adenocarcinoma. (From Nigro JJ, DeMeester SR, Hagen JA, *et al.* Node status in transmural esophageal adenocarcinoma and outcome after en bloc esophagectomy. *J Thorac Cardiovasc Surg* 1999;117:962.)

TABLE 15-2 • *Distribution of Metastases in Patients with Esophageal Cancer*

Sites	Frequency (%)
Liver	35%
Lung	20%
Bone	9%
Adrenal glands	2%
Brain	2%
Pericardium	1%
Pleura	1%
Stomach	1%
Pancreas	1%
Spleen	1%

From Quint LE, Hepburn LM, Francis IR, *et al.* Incidence and distribution of distant metastases in newly diagnosed esophageal carcinoma. *Cancer* 1995;76:1120–1125.

Dysphagia should be evaluated systematically (Figure 15-10). Although the physical examination is generally normal, it is important to look for physical findings that may alter the therapeutic approach, including supraclavicular or cervical lymphadenopathy and a discrete abdominal mass or fullness suggesting involvement of the celiac nodes or metastatic disease to the liver. Temporal wasting, weight loss, and dehydration are commonly seen. Laboratory examination may reveal anemia from chronic blood loss, hypoproteinemia from malnutrition, and hypercalcemia or abnormal liver function tests as a result of distant metastases.

Endoscopy

Endoscopic evaluation is essential for all patients who are suspected of having esophageal cancer. The location of the lesion, the degree of obstruction, and the extent of the lesion should be determined for all patients. Biopsy and cytologic smears should be performed routinely for all visible lesions. The endoscopic features of advanced carcinoma are generally easily recognized. However, during surveillance endoscopy, the mucosal changes of early cancer may be subtle and difficult to distinguish. Changes include mucosal erosion, focal congestion, and roughness of the mucosa.

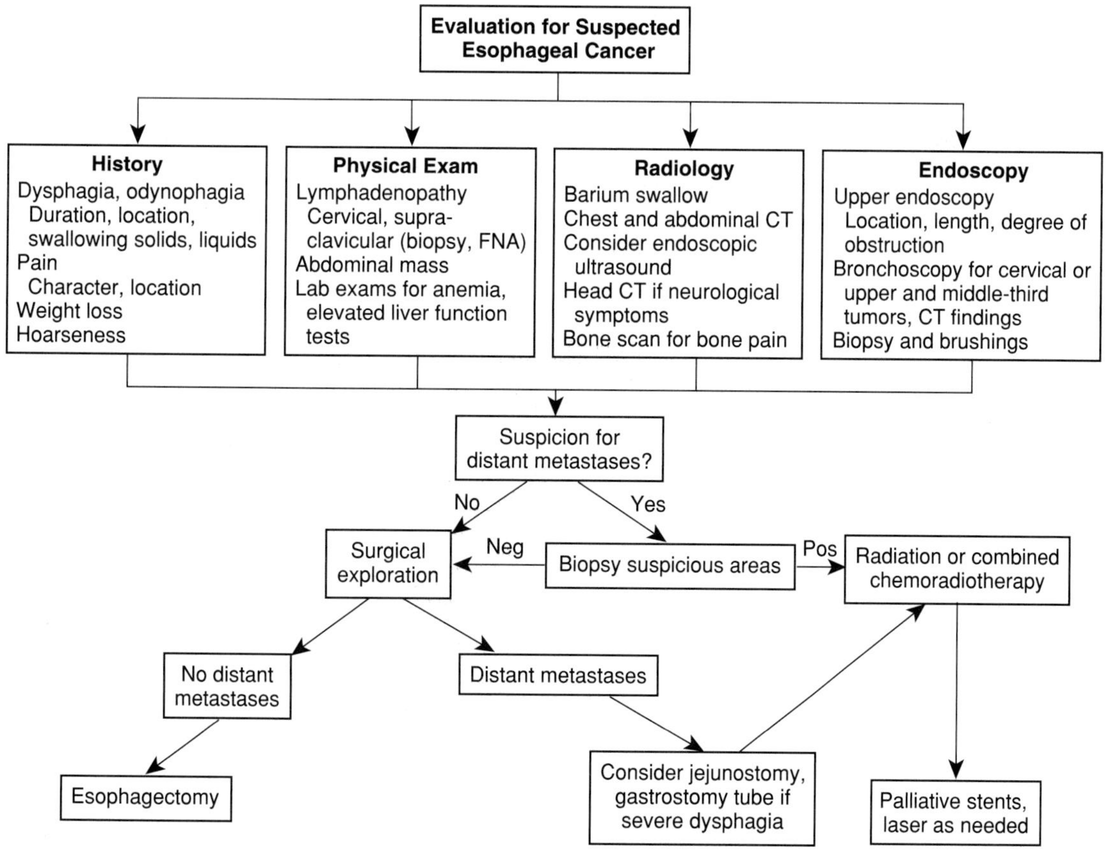

Figure 15-10. Diagnostic evaluation of a patient with suspected esophageal carcinoma. *FNA*, Fine-needle aspiration.

A nodule, an ulcer, or a small tumor mass may also be seen (see Figure 15-5, *C*).

Bronchoscopy is important to evaluate possible tracheal or bronchial invasion by esophageal carcinomas in the cervical and the upper or middle thirds of the thoracic esophagus. Patients with infracarinal bulky tumors or subcarinal lymphadenopathy on computed tomography (CT) scanning should also undergo bronchoscopy. Findings may range from simple bulging to loss of striations, fixation of the posterior wall of the trachea or the left main bronchus, frank tumor invasion, or the presence of a fistula. The carina may also appear widened as a result of subcarinal lymphadenopathy. Bronchial brushings or biopsies are obtained to confirm the diagnosis.

Radiographic Studies

Contrast Studies Barium swallow is a crucial diagnostic study in the evaluation of dysphagia to visualize the esophageal mucosa, luminal distensibility, motility, and any anatomic abnormalities (Figure 15-11). Early cancers appear as small intraluminal plaques, polypoid lesions, or areas of discrete ulceration, and they are best seen on double-contrast esophagram.

Computed Tomography Staging CT scans of the chest and upper abdomen are important studies during the initial evaluation of esophageal carcinoma and when assessing the response to neoadjuvant therapy. CT scanning is used to determine the local extent of the tumor, the relationship to adjacent structures, and distant metastases (Figure 15-12). Sensitivity for detecting abnormal lymph nodes (>1 cm) is approximately 30% to 60% in the mediastinum and 50% to 75% in the abdomen. CT scans cannot distinguish the layers of the esophageal wall, and they are not useful for determining the T stage (Table 15-3). Indentation of the trachea or a bronchus and thickening of the wall of the tracheobronchial tree adjacent to the tumor are suspicious for airway involvement (Figure 15-13).

Endoscopic Ultrasound Endoscopic ultrasound (EUS) provides more accurate T staging (see Table 15-3), and it is able to identify five distinct layers in the esophageal wall, thus providing an assessment of the depth of tumor invasion (Figure 15-14). EUS can also detect local, perigastric, and celiac lymph nodes, and it has resulted in improved staging. It is most useful during the staging of early carcinoma and in the evaluation of the extent of periesophageal invasion. Curvilinear arrays also assist in the

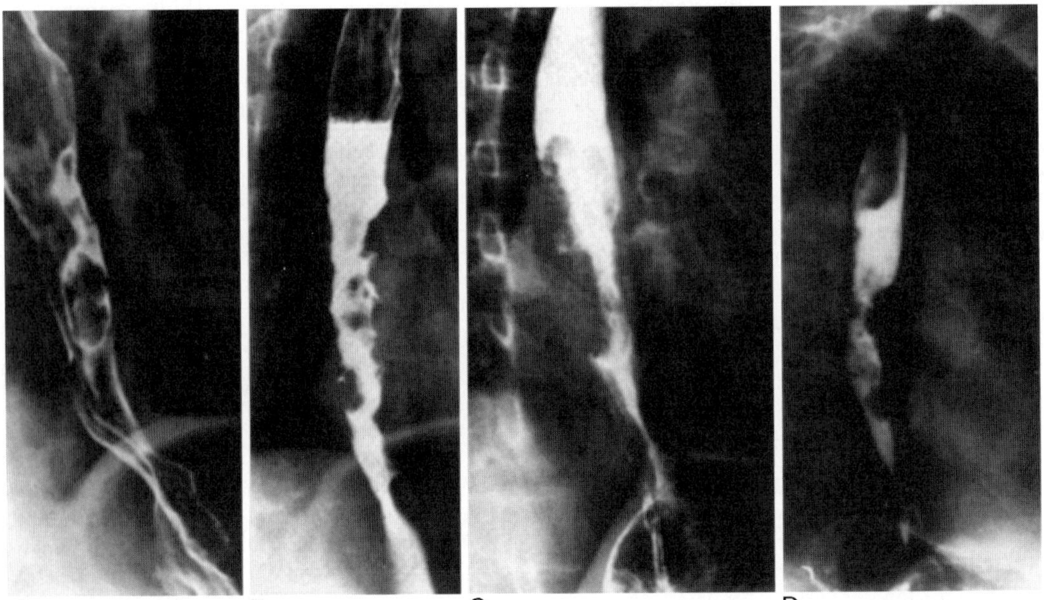

A B C D

Figure 15-11. Barium esophagram demonstrating an advanced esophageal carcinoma. **A,** Polypoid lesion. **B,** Multiple polypoid tumors. **C,** Long, ulcerative tumor. **D,** Stenotic, infiltrative tumor. (From Lin J, Iannettoni MD: Carcinoma of the esophagus. In Shields TW, Locicero J III, Ponn RB, eds. *General thoracic surgery*, 6th ed, vol 2. Philadelphia: Lippincott Williams and Wilkins, 2005.)

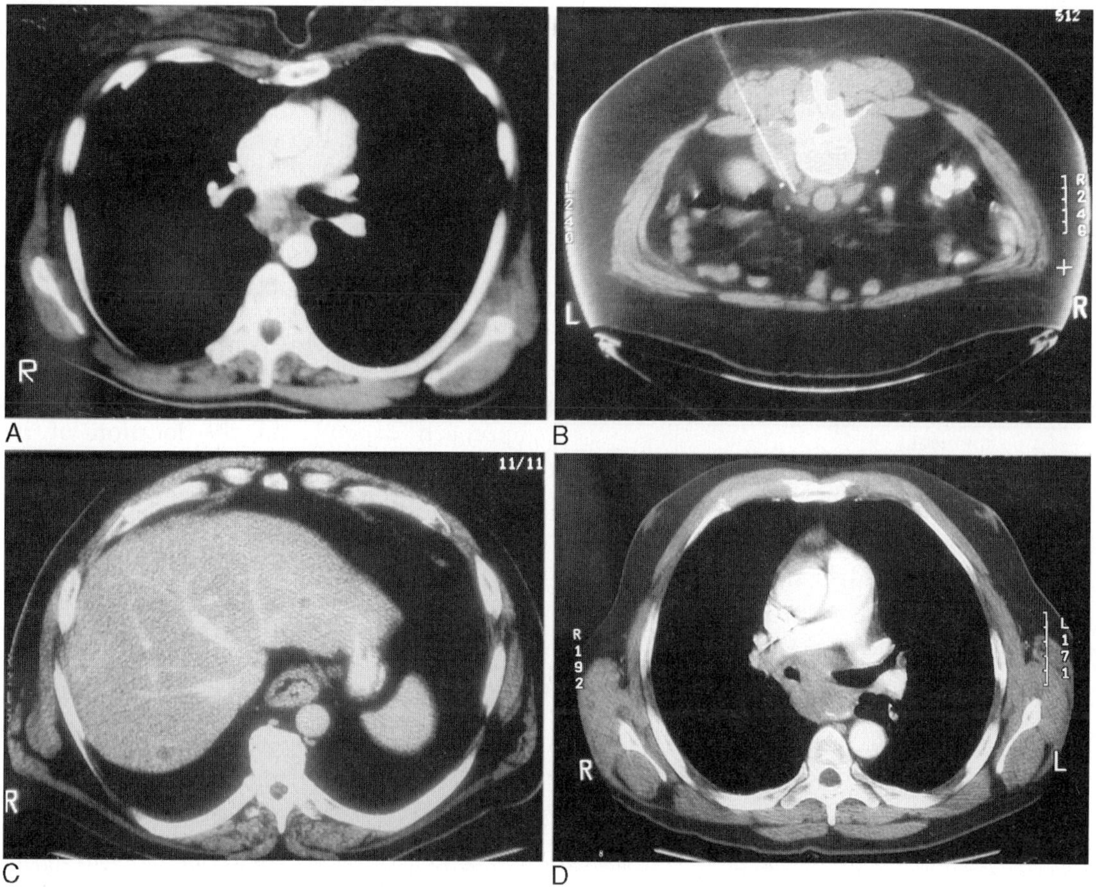

Figure 15-12. CT scans of patients with esophageal carcinoma. **A,** Tumor in contact with the thoracic aorta. **B,** CT-guided biopsy of nodal disease. **C,** Metastatic hepatic nodules. **D,** Local invasion of the right mainstem bronchus. (From Lin J, Iannettoni MD: Carcinoma of the esophagus. In Shields TW, Locicero J III, Ponn RB, eds. *General thoracic surgery*, 6th ed, vol 2. Philadelphia: Lippincott Williams and Wilkins, 2005.)

performance of fine-needle aspiration, which is up to 98% sensitive and 100% specific. EUS may also be useful for assessing the response to neoadjuvant therapy.

Thoracoscopy and Laparoscopy

Thoracoscopic and laparoscopic staging offers direct visualization and the ability to provide tissue for a pathologic diagnosis for determining the nodal status as well as for evaluating the extent of local invasion and metastatic disease. Laparoscopy should be considered for patients with locally advanced esophageal cancers or suspected intraperitoneal metastases to assess the celiac and left gastric lymph nodes, the liver, and the peritoneum for tumor implants. Laparoscopic ultrasound is also being investigated as a staging modality, and it may improve the accuracy of T and N staging. Laparoscopic ultrasound may be more accurate for staging celiac nodes than EUS, providing closer access for the ultrasound probe as well as direct inspection. For the average patient with carcinoma of the esophagus, it remains unclear whether this strategy is cost effective.

Staging

Accurate staging is important for selecting treatment and determining prognosis. The evaluation of patients with suspected esophageal cancer should include appropriate diagnostic studies as well as biopsies of any suspected metastatic lesions. Patients with biopsy-proven distant metastatic disease have a mean survival of only 6 months, and they are considered poor candidates for resection, because the risk of esophagectomy generally outweighs the short-term benefits. Both ESCC and EAC are staged according to the American Joint Committee for Cancer TNM system (see Table 15-3).

TABLE 15-3 • *Staging of Esophageal Cancer*

Primary Tumor (T)			
T_x	Primary tumor cannot be assessed		
T_0	No evidence of primary tumor		
T_{is}	Carcinoma in situ		
T_1	Tumor invades lamina propria or submucosa		
T_2	Tumor invades muscularis propria		
T_3	Tumor invades adventitia		
T_4	Tumor invades adjacent structures		
Regional Lymph Nodes (N)			
N_x	Regional lymph nodes cannot be assessed		
N_0	No regional lymph node metastasis		
N_1	Regional lymph node metastasis		
Distant Metastasis (M)			
M_x	Distant metastasis cannot be assessed		
M_0	No distant metastasis		
M_1	Distant metastasis		
Tumors of the Lower Thoracic Esophagus			
M_{1a}	Metastasis to celiac lymph nodes		
M_{1b}	Other distant metastasis		
Tumors of the Midthoracic Esophagus			
M_{1a}	Not applicable		
M_{1b}	Nonregional lymph nodes and/or other distant metastasis		
Tumors of the Upper Thoracic Esophagus			
M_{1a}	Metastasis in cervical nodes		
M_{1b}	Other distant metastasis		
Staging			
Stage 0	T_{is}	N_0	M_0
Stage I	$\mathbf{T_1}$	N_0	M_0
Stage IIA	T_2	N_0	M_0
	T_3	N_0	M_0
Stage IIB	T_1	N_1	M_0
	T_2	N_1	M_0
Stage III	T_3	N_1	M_0
	T_4	Any N	M_0
Stage IV	Any T	Any N	M_1
Stage IVA	Any T	Any N	M_{1a}
Stage IVB	Any T	Any N	M_{1b}

From Greene FL, Page DL, Fleming ID, *et al,* eds. *AJCC Cancer Staging Manual,* 6th ed. New York: Springer-Verlag, 2002:93–94.

Therapy

Surgical Treatment

Surgical therapy currently offers the best chance for cure and provides effective palliation with relief of dysphagia. Although mortality rates have decreased significantly over the past few decades, relatively high postoperative morbidity remains. Controversy continues to surround the optimal surgical approach to esophagectomy as well as the extent and necessity of regional lymph-node dissection. Currently no data exist to prove one approach clearly superior to the other. The choice of approach depends on the location of the tumor, the planned extent of lymphadenectomy, and the preference of the surgeon.

Transthoracic Esophagectomy

Some surgeons have had excellent results with the transthoracic approach to esophagectomy. The combined thoracotomy and laparotomy approach described by Ivor Lewis is safe, and proponents emphasize the direct visualization during mediastinal dissection, an en bloc resection, and a wider lymphadenectomy, thereby resulting in improved staging. A recent randomized trial suggested a trend toward improved 5-year survival when comparing transthoracic with transhiatal esophagectomy (THE), although the difference was not statistically significant. However, THE was associated with a lower postoperative morbidity.

Transhiatal Esophagectomy

The transhiatal approach may avoid the morbidity of a thoracotomy in debilitated patients as well as the potential of a disastrous intrathoracic anastomotic disruption. Although accessible subcarinal, periesophageal, and celiac lymph nodes are sampled, no attempt is made to perform an en bloc resection. Although critics have questioned the oncologic principles arguing for the need to perform an aggressive mediastinal lymph-node resection, survival has been reported in several series to be equivalent to that seen after a transthoracic resection (Figure 15-15). THE is technically possible in the majority of patients, even those with a history of prior operations, esophageal perforation, or radiation treatment, and it provides maximal vertical resection margins. In addition, the stapled side-to-side cervical anastomosis (Figure 15-16) has decreased the anastomotic leak rate to less than 3% at the University of

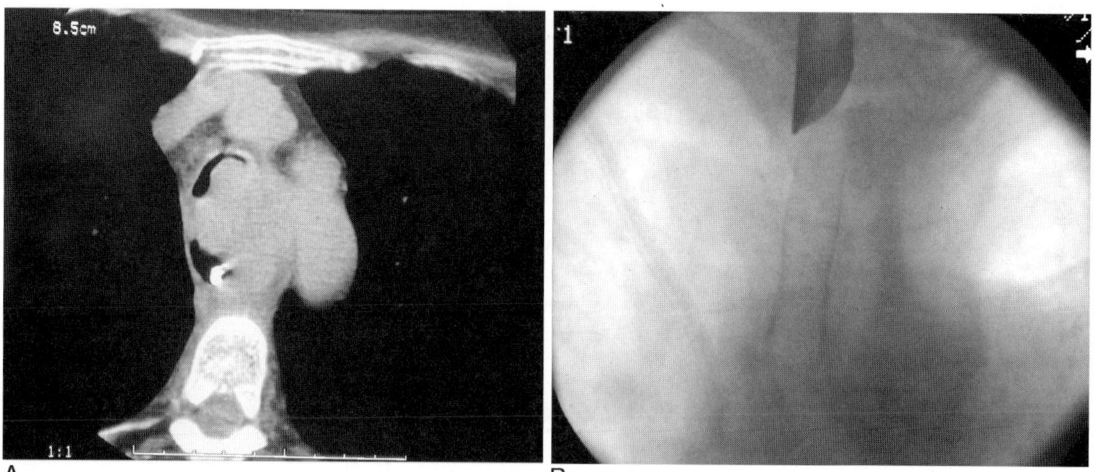

A B

Figure 15-13. **A,** CT scan of a patient with esophageal adenocarcinoma invading the trachea. **B,** Palliative placement of a tracheal stent. (From Lin J, Iannettoni MD: Carcinoma of the esophagus. In Shields TW, Locicero J III, Ponn RB, eds. *General thoracic surgery*, 6th ed, vol 2. Philadelphia: Lippincott Williams and Wilkins, 2005.)

Michigan, and most cervical leaks are treated conservatively by opening the wound at the bedside and providing saline dressing changes. Less-frequent complications include intrathoracic hemorrhage, recurrent nerve paralysis, and tracheal laceration.

High-Grade Dys plasia

The management of high-grade dysplasia is controversial. Although there is an increased risk of adenocarcinoma, with approximately 20% to 60% of patients with high-grade dysplasia developing cancer on surveillance, the natural history is unknown. Many surgeons advocate an esophagectomy because of the elevated risk of cancer. Recently, others have suggested continued surveillance, and they believe that aggressive biopsies can detect adenocarcinoma. However, there are inherent false negatives, because biopsies may miss dysplasia and carcinomas separated by large areas of Barrett's epithelium. Several retrospective studies have shown difficulty when it comes to differentiating high-grade dysplasia from adenocarcinoma using endoscopic surveillance. Currently, histopathology is the most reliable way to identify patients with adenocarcinoma. Although surveillance may be a reasonable approach in selected patients and certain centers, it carries the risk of missing an early adenocarcinoma. Until more accurate surveillance methods, molecular markers, and effective ablative techniques are available, esophagectomy remains the gold standard for the treatment of high-grade dysplasia.

Chemoradiation Therapy

Combined chemoradiotherapy is now the standard for the nonsurgical management of locally advanced disease. The combination of chemoradiation with surgery has resulted in significant down-staging of disease, but a consistent survival advantage has not yet been demonstrated. Most regimens are cisplatin-based, and they are frequently combined with 5-fluorouracil. Newer agents, including taxanes and irinotecan, are being evaluated in chemoradiotherapy trials, and they may have promising antitumor activity as well as improved tolerance. At this time, surgery remains the standard treatment for resectable esophageal cancer. For patients with locally advanced disease or for those unfit for surgery, chemoradiation therapy appears to be a reasonable alternative. For patients with advanced resectable disease, neooadjuvant chemoradiation is an increasingly popular approach. Patients who have had a complete pathologic response have an excellent prospect for long-term survival.

Prognostic Factors

Five-year survival for patients with esophageal carcinoma remains poor, at 5% to 12%. Tumor stage is the strongest predictor of survival (Figure 15-17), and number of lymph nodes

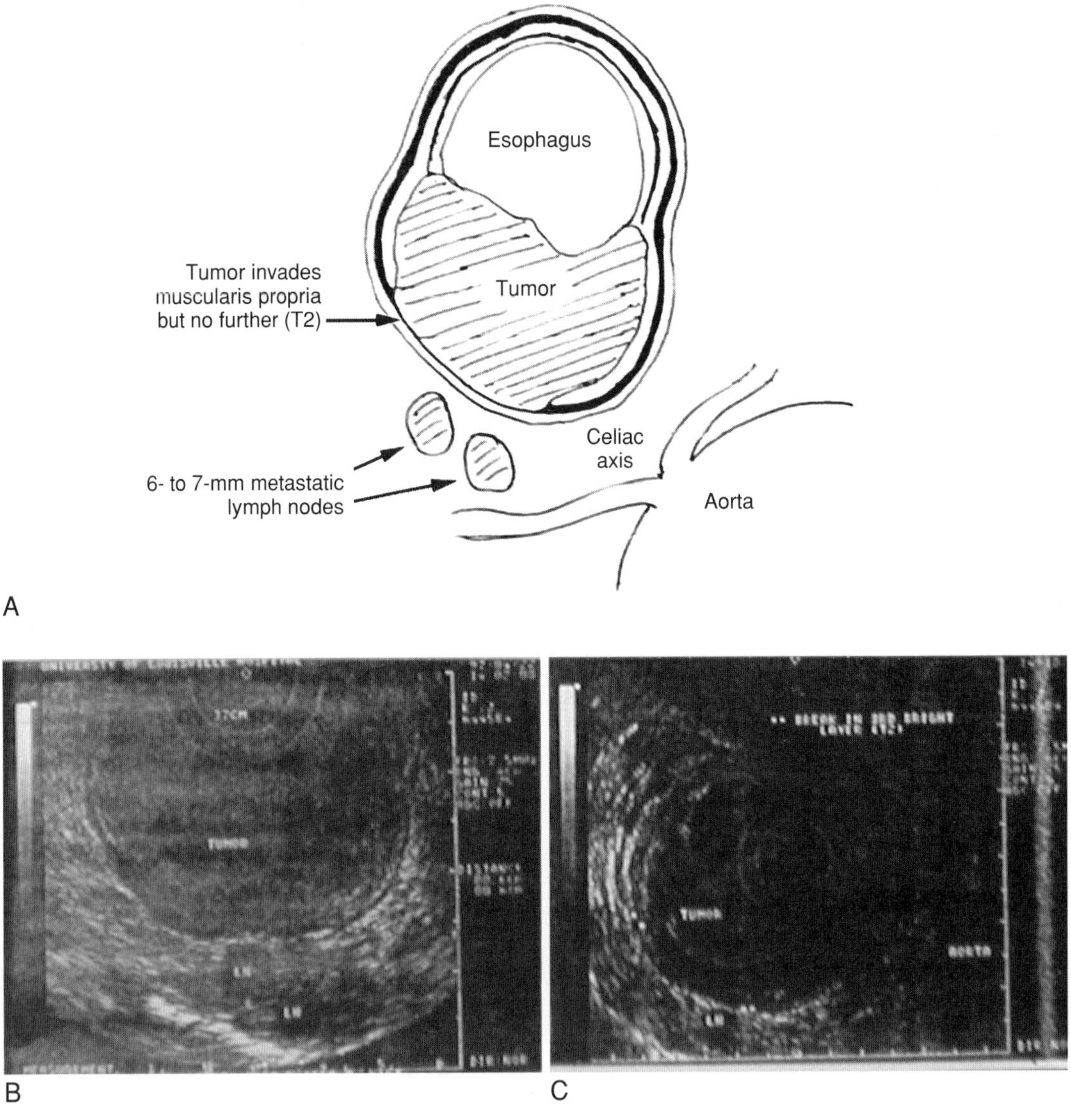

Figure 15–14. A, Illustration of the endoscopic sonographic views shown in **B** and **C** of a T2 esophageal adenocarcinoma with metastatic celiac nodes. (From Lin J, Iannettoni MD: Carcinoma of the esophagus. In Shields TW, Locicero J III, Ponn RB, eds. *General thoracic surgery*, 6th ed, vol 2. Philadelphia: Lippincott Williams and Wilkins, 2005.)

involved is also a major prognostic factor (Figure 15-18). Other factors associated with a poor prognosis include increased age, African-American race, lower esophageal tumors, and increasing length and depth of the lesion. Esophagectomy is a technically demanding procedure, and outcomes have also been correlated with hospital volume and the experience of the individual surgeon. Five-year survival greater than 80% can be seen after surgical resection among patients with early lesions limited to the mucosa. Early diagnosis continues to be the best strategy for improving survival.

Conclusions

The evaluation and management of esophageal cancer continues to present significant challenges to the thoracic surgeon. The incidence of EAC has increased rapidly over the past three decades, and it represents the fastest-growing solid malignancy in the United States. Advances have been made in surgical techniques and patient care that have resulted in significantly improved perioperative mortality rates, although morbidity remains relatively high. Despite these advances, the prognosis for both ESCC and EAC remains poor. Improved

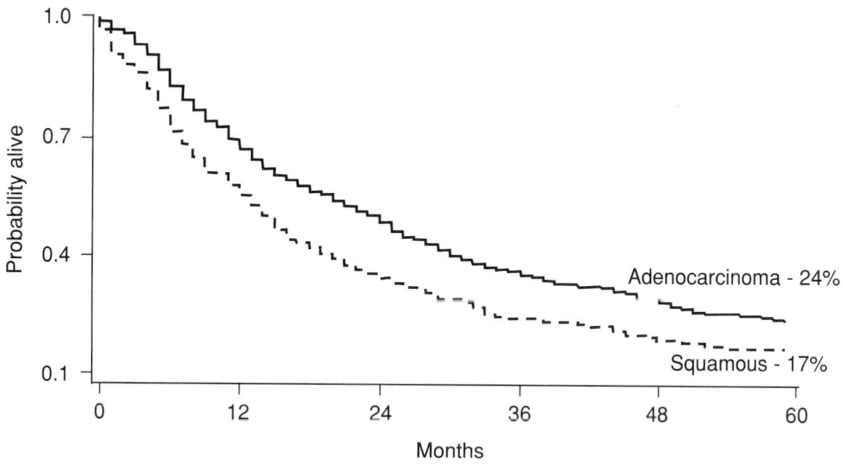

Type		Number of patients followed through interval				
Adenocarcinoma	545	338	210	135	92	67
Squamous	218	115	64	39	28	21

Figure 15-15. Survival after transhiatal esophagectomy without thoracotomy, stratified by histologic diagnosis. (From Orringer MB, Marshall B, Iannettoni MD. Transhiatal esophagectomy: clinical experience and refinements. *Ann Surg* 1999;230:398.)

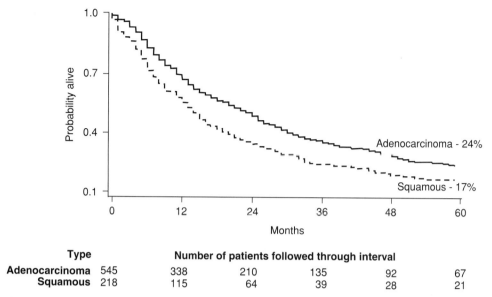

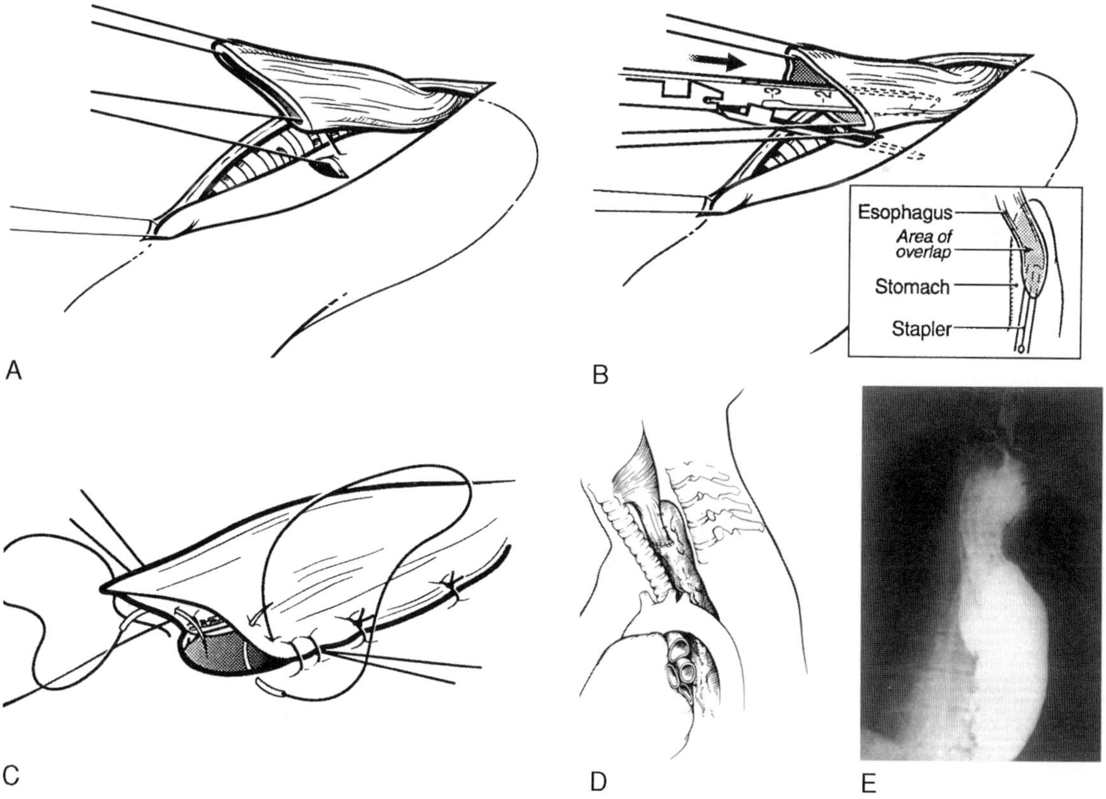

Figure 15-16. Cervical stapled side-to-side anastomosis after transhiatal esophagectomy. **A,** The esophagogastrostomy is aligned using stay sutures. **B,** An Endo-GIA is inserted. **C,** The semi-mechanical anastomosis is completed. **D,** The completed cervical side-to-side anastomosis. **E,** Postoperative barium swallow. (From Orringer MB, Marshall B, Iannettoni MD. Eliminating the cervical esophagogastric anastomotic leak with a side-to-side stapled anastomosis. *J Thorac Cardiovasc Surg* 2000;119:277.)

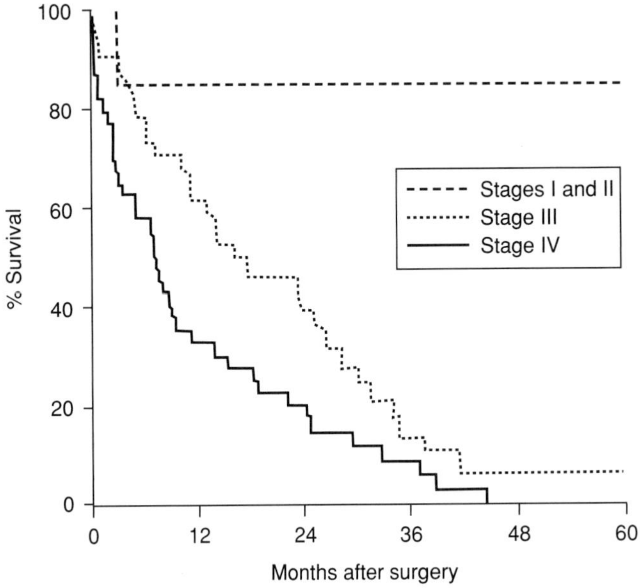

Figure 15-17. Survival stratified by stage after esophagectomy for esophageal adenocarcinoma in 88 patients. (From Moon MR, Schulte WJ, Haasler GB, Condon RE. Transhiatal and transthoracic esophagectomy for esophageal adenocarcinoma. *Arch Surg* 1992;127:953.)

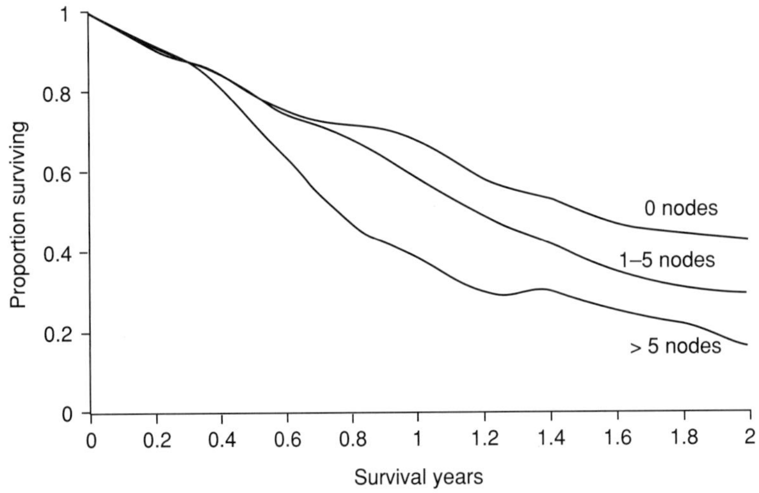

Figure 15-18. Kaplan-Meier survival plots for 1,340 patients stratified by the number of positive lymph nodes. (From Eloubeidi MA, Desmond R, Arguedas MR, *et al.* Prognostic factors for the survival of patients with esophageal carcinoma in the U.S.: the importance of tumor length and lymph node status. *Cancer* 2002;95:1440.)

understanding of the molecular changes involved will improve understanding of the pathogenesis of esophageal cancer, and it will provide novel methods of diagnosis, staging, and treatment that will allow surgeons to identify patients who may benefit from early surgical resection or neoadjuvant therapy.

Key Selected Reading

Lin J, Iannettoni MD: Carcinoma of the esophagus. In Shields TW, Locicero J III, Ponn RB, eds. *General thoracic surgery*, 6th ed, vol 2. Philadelphia: Lippincott Williams and Wilkins, 2005.

Selected Readings

Blot WJ, McLaughlin JK. The changing epidemiology of esophageal cancer. *Semin Oncol* 1999;26:2–8.

Cooper JS, Guo MD, Herskovic A, *et al.* Chemoradiotherapy of locally advanced esophageal cancer: long-term follow-up of a prospective randomized trial (RTOG 85-01). Radiation Therapy Oncology Group. *JAMA* 1999;281:1623–1627.

Dellon ES, Shaheen NJ. Does screening for Barrett's esophagus and adenocarcinoma of the esophagus prolong survival? *J Clin Oncol* 2005;23:4478–4482.

DeMeester SR. Adenocarcinoma of the esophagus and cardia: a review of the disease and its tretment. *Ann Surg Oncol* 2006;13:12–30.

Enzinger PC, Mayer RJ. Esophageal cancer. *N Engl J Med* 2003;349:2241–2252.

Hulscher JB, van Sandick JW, de Boer AG, *et al.* Extended transthoracic resection compared with limited transhiatal resection for adenocarcinoma of the esophagus. *N Engl J Med* 2002;347:1662–1669.

Kent MS, Schuchert M, Fernando H, Luketich JD. Minimally invasive esophagectomy: state of the art. *Dis Esophagus* 2006;19:137–145.

Lin J, Iannettoni MD. Transhiatal esophagectomy. *Surg Clin North Am* 2005;85:593–610.

Nichols FC 3rd, Allen MS, Deschamps C, *et al.* Ivor Lewis esophagogastrectomy. *Surg Clin North Am* 2005;85:583–592.

Orringer MB, Marshall B, Iannettoni MD. Eliminating the cervical esophagogastric anastomotic leak with a side-to-side stapled anastomosis. *J Thorac Cardiovasc Surg* 2000;119:277–288.

Orringer MB, Marshall B, Iannettoni MD. Transhiatal esophagectomy: clinical experience and refinements. *Ann Surg* 1999;230:392–400.

Sampliner RE. Long-term endoscopic surveillance of Barrett's esophagus. *Am J Gastroenterol* 2003;98: 1912–1913.

Thomas CR Jr. Current and ongoing progress in the therapy for resectable esophageal cancer. *Dis Esophagus* 2005;18:211–214.

16

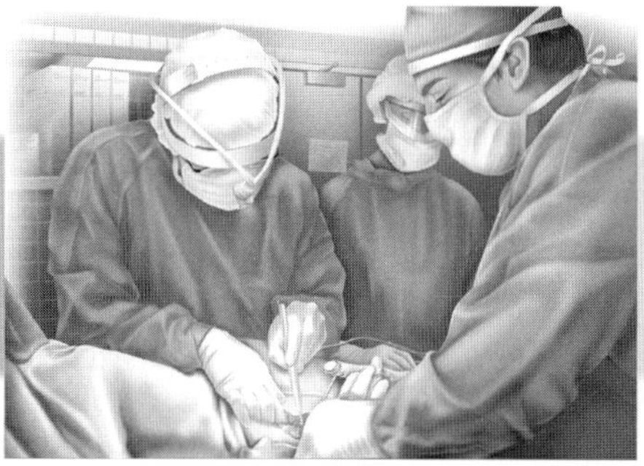

Neoplasms of the Stomach and Small Intestine

Vincent M. Cimmino and Michael S. Sabel

Neoplasms of the Stomach and the Small Intestine: Key Points

- List the risk factors and epidemiologic specifics related to gastric cancer.
- Outline the diagnostic steps taken, the staging workup, and the treatment options for gastric cancer.
- Discuss the evidence concerning extent of resection, lymph-node dissection, and adjuvant therapy for the curative resection of gastric cancer.
- List the types of benign and malignant small-bowel tumors and the risk factors for developing these lesions.
- Outline the diagnostic steps taken and the treatment options for small-bowel tumors specific to the type of lesion.
- Outline the diagnostic steps taken, the staging workup, and the treatment options for gastric lymphoma.

Gastric Cancer

The incidence of gastric carcinoma is on the decline. This is primarily the result of a decrease in lesions of the fundus and the antrum; there has actually been a slight increase in the incidence of cancers of the cardia. Despite the decreased incidence, gastric cancer remains a significant health problem because of the extremely poor prognosis associated with it. In the United States, the 5-year survival rate for stomach cancer ranges from 5% to 15%. This is primarily related to the fact that most patients present with advanced disease. In some countries with a high incidence of gastric cancer, screening programs have been used to identify early lesions; however, this strategy is not cost-efficient in the United States. Although surgical resection remains the mainstay of therapy for gastric cancer, both locoregional and distant recurrence after gastrectomy occurs in at least 80% of patients. This has prompted significant interest in multimodality therapy.

Epidemiology

Although stomach cancer is relatively rare in the United States, it is the second most frequent cancer in the world, after lung cancer. Data from selected population-based cancer registries indicate that the highest rates (>40 per 100,000 males) are reported in Japan, China, the former Union of Soviet Socialist Republics, and certain countries in South and Central America. The lowest rates (<15 per 100,000) are seen in North America (specifically among the white population), India, the Philippines, most African countries, some countries in Western Europe, and Australia.

This represents a dramatic change. In 1930, gastric cancer was the leading cause of deaths in the United States; however, over the last six decades, the incidence rates for gastric cancer have dropped dramatically. At present, there are approximately 22,500 new cases of gastric cancer per year in the United States. The exact causes of the decline are not well understood, but they likely include improvements in diet, better food storage, and possibly the decline of *Helicobacter pylori* infection.

Gastric cancer rarely occurs before the fourth decade, but its incidence rises thereafter, peaking in those between the ages of 60 and 70 years. Gastric cancer is twice as common among men as women. In the United States, African Americans, Hispanics, and Native Americans are 1.5 to 2.5 times more likely to have gastric cancer than whites. Gastric cancer tends to be more prominent among populations of lower socioeconomic status, most likely reflecting dietary habits and environmental exposures.

Pathology

More than 90% of all tumors of the stomach are adenocarcinomas. The remaining 10% comprise mostly non-Hodgkin's lymphoma, sarcomas, or gastrointestinal stromal tumors. Gastric adenocarcinomas can be divided into two histological subtypes: intestinal type and diffuse type. The intestinal type has a glandular structure that is well delineated, whereas the diffuse type is composed of small cells that grow diffusely into the surrounding gastric wall.

BOX 16–1 FACTORS ASSOCIATED WITH AN INCREASED RISK OF STOMACH CANCER

- Diet high in nitrates (e.g., preserved, smoked, and cured foods)
- Diet low in vitamins A and C
- Diet high in salt
- Lack of refrigeration
- Poor drinking water
- *Helicobacter pylori* infection
- Previous gastric surgery
- Atrophic gastritis
- Cigarette smoking
- Adenomatous gastric polyps
- Ménétrièr's disease
- Pernicious anemia
- Type A blood

BOX 16–2 INTESTINAL-TYPE VERSUS DIFFUSE-TYPE GASTRIC CANCER

Intestinal Type

- More common in less-developed nations
- Predominant subtype in high-risk populations
- Located in distal stomach and often ulcerative
- Preceded by a prolonged precancerous phase

Diffuse Type

- Presents at a younger age
- Less associated with environment; more associated with genetics
- Located in cardia
- Associated with worse prognosis

The intestinal subtype is more commonly seen in less-developed nations, and it is the predominant histological subtype among high-risk populations. These typically occur in the distal stomach; they are often ulcerative, and they are typically preceded by a prolonged precancerous phase. They have a better prognosis than the diffuse type, which tends to present at a younger age and which appears to be more associated with genetics than environmental factors. Diffuse lesions occur throughout the stomach, but they are more common in the cardia, and they are associated with a worse prognosis. *Linitis plastica* is an entity that is characterized by extensive infiltration of the entire stomach with cancer of the diffuse type. The decline in the incidence of gastric cancer is largely attributable to a decrease in the intestinal-type tumors.

Carcinoma arising in the gastric cardia appears to have different etiologic factors and a different biologic behavior from distal non-cardia carcinoma. Whereas the incidence of non-cardia gastric carcinoma is decreasing, the incidence of cardia carcinoma has been increasing in many countries. Carcinoma arising in the gastric cardia behaves similarly to esophageal cancer, including a strong association with reflux esophagitis (see Chapter 15: Esophageal Cancer).

Risk Factors

Several gastric conditions are associated with an increased risk for the development of gastric cancer. When gastric atrophy is present, intestinal metaplasia can develop, which can ultimately progress to dysplasia and then to carcinoma. Risk factors for both atrophic gastritis and gastric cancer are similar, and areas of the world in which atrophic gastritis is common also have a high incidence of gastric cancer. *Ménétrièr's disease* is a disease of the stomach that is characterized by giant hypertrophy of the mucosa of the gastric fundus, with cystic changes in the crypts. It is associated with protein loss, sometimes to the point of peripheral edema. Although rare, approximately 10% of patients with Ménétrièr's disease will ultimately develop carcinoma. Pernicious anemia increases the risk of gastric cancer, but recent studies have shown that the proportion of gastric cancer associated with pernicious anemia has remained very low in recent years.

Multiple studies have demonstrated a link between the incidence of stomach cancer and *H pylori*. Although suggestive, this is not straightforward, and most patients with *H pylori* will not develop gastric carcinoma. *H pylori* is most likely a cofactor in gastric carcinogenesis, increasing the risk by less than twofold. The precise role of *H pylori* in the genesis of gastric cancer is unclear, and whether *H pylori* eradication will affect the incidence of gastric cancer remains to be seen.

Numerous dietary factors have been implicated as having the potential to increase the risk of the development of gastric adenocarcinoma. High salt intake is associated with an increased risk, probably via the induction of chronic gastritis. It is also possible that a high intake of smoked, grilled, or barbecued meats (high in nitrites) may be associated with an increased risk. Several epidemiologic studies have suggested a protective effect for diets high in fruits and vegetables and that involve a higher intake of vitamins A, C, and E, possibly because of their antioxidant properties. There is also evidence that the long-term use of refrigeration to preserve food is associated with a reduced risk and that this may be associated with the decreased incidence of gastric cancer in Western countries.

Multiple cohort and case-control studies have demonstrated a relationship between cigarette smoking and gastric carcinoma. Several of these also show a positive dose-response relationship. An inverse socioeconomic gradient has been observed in most populations: the rate among lower socioeconomic groups is two to three times higher than that seen among the more affluent classes. An excess risk has also been linked to certain industries, such as coal mining, fishing, and agriculture. Because occupations are related to socioeconomic background, some of the excess risk observed might be attributed to patterns of lifestyle, such as dietary habits.

A role for genetic factors is suggested by the study of blood groups as determinants of chronic gastritis. It has been known for some time that individuals with type A blood have an approximately 20% excess incidence of gastric cancer as compared with those with types O, B, or AB blood. Carriers of mismatch repair gene mutations like hMSH2, which is associated with hereditary non-polyposis colorectal carcinoma syndrome, have an increased risk of stomach cancer. Germ-line mutations in a gene encoding the cell adhesion protein E-cadherin may lead to an autosomal-dominated predisposition to diffuse gastric cancer.

Patients who have previously undergone partial gastrectomy for benign peptic ulcer disease have a small but statistically significant increased risk for gastric remnant carcinoma. These typically occur more than 25 years after the original gastric resection.

Presentation and Diagnostic Evaluation

Abdominal pain, weight loss, and upper gastrointestinal (GI) bleeding are the most common presenting symptoms of gastric cancer. Unfortunately, tumors can grow to a large size before any symptoms develop.

BOX 16–3 PRESENTING SYMPTOMS OF GASTRIC CANCER

- Weight loss
- Abdominal pain
- Nausea and anorexia
- Melena
- Early satiety
- Ulcer-type pain

Upper endoscopy should be performed in patients with symptoms that are suspicious for carcinoma, including unexplained epigastric pain, postprandial discomfort, GI bleeding, or unexplained weight loss. Endoscopic biopsy should be performed on all gastric ulcers, except those that are clearly superficial, because it is difficult to differentiate benign and malignant ulcers accurately by gross endoscopic appearance alone. At a minimum, four-quadrant biopsies should be performed. Brush cytology complements biopsy and increases diagnostic accuracy. Endoscopy appears to be more sensitive than contrast radiography for the detection of small gastric carcinomas.

Because of the low incidence of gastric cancer in the United States, screening programs are not currently considered to be cost effective. An argument can be made for screening certain groups at higher risk in the United States, such as patients with chronic atrophic gastritis, pernicious anemia, Ménétrièr's disease, adenomatous polyps, or a prior history of partial gastrectomy.

No laboratory determination is specific for gastric cancer. Overall, the sensitivity of commonly used cancer markers, such as carcinoembryonic antigen, is less than 50%. A new marker, CA72-4, is elevated in 94% of patients with gastric cancer; however, further studies are needed to confirm these results and to assess this marker's practical usefulness as a screening tool for high-risk populations.

Gastric carcinoma can quickly invade adjacent organs, spread via lymphatics or throughout the peritoneal cavity, or metastasize via hematogenous dissemination. The most common mode is lymphatic metastases to lymph nodes along the greater and lesser curvature of the stomach. Occasionally, spread via the thoracic duct can lead to an involved, palpable supraclavicular node (Virchow's node). The liver is by far the most common site for hematogenous spread. Less commonly, gastric cancer can metastasize to the lungs, brain, or ovaries (Krukenberg's tumor). Peritoneal spread can involve many locations in the abdominal cavity; sometimes, this can be detected on physical examination by the detection of a rectal (Blumer's) shelf or a periumbilical (Sister Mary Joseph's) nodule.

After a diagnosis of gastric cancer has been made, staging should begin with a thorough history and a physical examination (Table 16-1 and Figures 16-1 and 16-2). Complete staging should include a computed tomography (CT) scan of the upper abdomen to look for direct local invasion of the pancreas or liver and to detect regional lymphadenopathy or liver metastasis, and it should also include a chest radiograph to detect pulmonary metastases. Although air-contrast barium radiography may help delineate gastric anatomy and provide a reference for the surgeon regarding the location of the tumor, radiologic contrast examination has, for the most part, been superseded by endoscopy. Endoscopic ultrasonography can provide accurate staging by assessing gastric wall invasion and determining the presence or absence of lymph-node metastases. This technique is likely to have special importance during the pretreatment staging evaluation of patients considered for preoperative (neoadjuvant) chemotherapy. However, an extensive preoperative evaluation is not always needed, because many of these patients may require exploration and resection for palliation of obstruction or bleeding.

Treatment

The standard approach to patients with gastric cancer remains surgical resection. After gastric cancer has been diagnosed and a staging workup has demonstrated the absence of metastatic disease, an exploratory laparotomy should be undertaken. This should begin with a thorough evaluation of the peritoneal cavity and liver for metastases that would preclude curative resection. After that, the surgeon should assess the nature and extent of the primary tumor, looking for invasion into the pancreas, colon, or liver. The surgeon should also document the status of the regional lymph nodes (Figure 16-3). Many surgeons begin with laparoscopic exploration to spare the patient the morbidity of an exploratory laparotomy if metastatic disease is identified. Despite a negative staging workup, many patients thought to have curable lesions

TABLE 16-1 • *American Joint Committee on Cancer Staging of Gastric Carcinoma*

Primary Tumor (T)			
Tx	Primary tumor cannot be assessed		
T0	No evidence of primary tumor		
Tis	Carcinoma in situ		
T1	Tumor invades lamina propria or submucosa		
T2	Tumor invades muscularis propria		
T3	Tumor invades adventitia		
T4	Tumor invades adjacent structures		
Regional Lymph Nodes (N)			
NX	Regional lymph node(s) cannot be assessed		
N0	No regional lymph node metastasis		
N1	Metastasis in 1 to 6 regional lymph nodes		
N2	Metastasis in 7 to 15 regional lymph nodes		
N3	Metastasis in more than 15 regional lymph nodes		
Distant Metastasis (M)			
MX	Distant metastasis cannot be assessed		
M0	No distant metastasis		
M1	Distant metastasis		
Stage			
0	Tis	N0	M0
IA	T1	N0	M0
IB	T1	N1	M0
	T2	N0	M0
II	T1	N2	M0
	T2	N1	M0
	T3	N0	M0
IIIA	T2	N0	M0
	T3	N1	M0
	T4	N2	M0
IIIB	T3	N2	M0
IV	T4	N1-2	M0
	T1-3	N3	M0
	Any T	Any N	M1

are found to have occult metastases at the time of abdominal exploration. However, these patients may benefit from a resection to avoid future bleeding or obstruction.

Gastrectomy

For patients without evidence of distant disease, a curative resection should be performed. The principle guiding the curative resection of gastric cancer is to remove both the primary tumor and associated involved lymph nodes. There is, however, controversy surrounding both the magnitude of the operation required to achieve local control and the role of radical lymphadenectomy. Although the gross margins of the tumor can usually be determined intraoperatively through careful inspection and bimanual palpation of the stomach, pathologic studies show that microscopic submucosal tumor extension is common in patients with gastric cancer. Therefore, the minimal requirements to ensure the complete microscopic resection of gastric carcinomas are gross margins of 4 cm to 6 cm around the primary tumor.

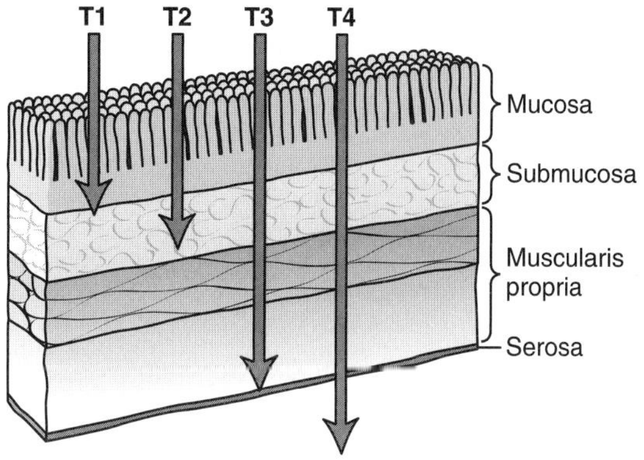

Figure 16-1. Penetration of gastric cancer through the gastric wall.

Some controversy exists regarding the use of subtotal and total gastrectomy for patients with gastric carcinoma. For tumors in the gastric antrum, randomized trials in France and Italy have demonstrated equivalent survival for total and subtotal gastrectomies. Reconstruction can be accomplished by either Billroth II or roux-en-Y reconstruction, both of which have similar long-term results for morbidity, 5-year survival, and functional results (Figure 16-4). All lesions in the mid body or fundus should undergo a total gastrectomy. Total gastrectomy is also indicated for linitis plastica (diffusely infiltrating gastric cancer causing a "leather-bottle" stomach), cancer in the face of Ménétrièr's disease, gastric remnant carcinoma, and cancer associated with multiple diffuse gastric polyps. Some surgeons opt to use total gastrectomy routinely, even for distal lesions. Supporters of this approach cite the benefit of wider excision of the primary tumor and potentially improved cure rates, although this claim has not been borne out in controlled trials. Moreover, quality of life is generally worse after total gastrectomy with standard reconstruction (a roux-en-Y esophagojejunostomy)

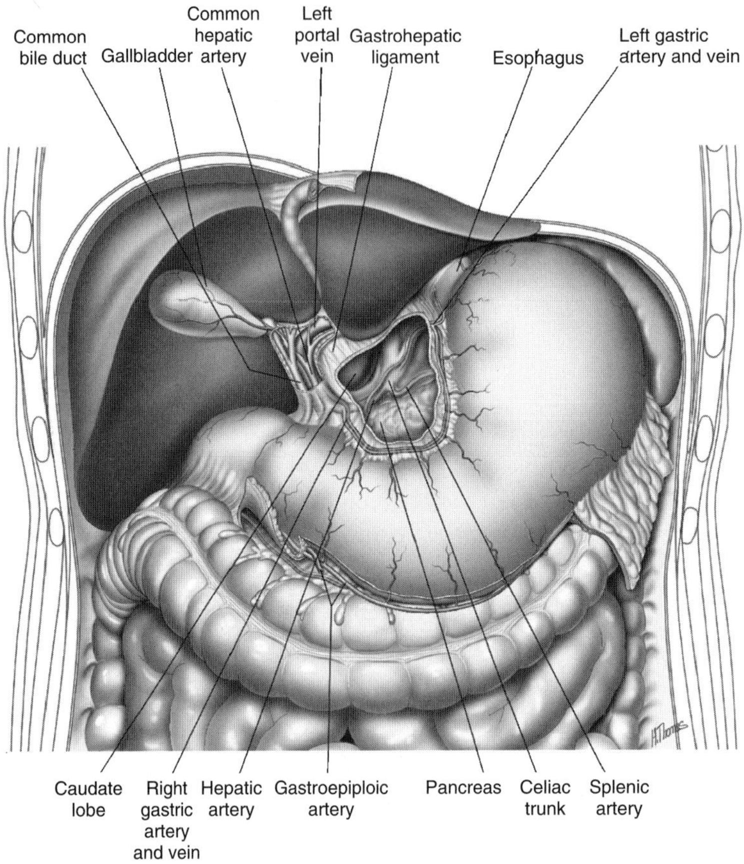

Figure 16–2. Anatomy of the upper abdomen. (From Bloom ND, Beattie EJ, Harvey JC. *Atlas of cancer surgery*. Philadelphia: WB Saunders, 2000.)

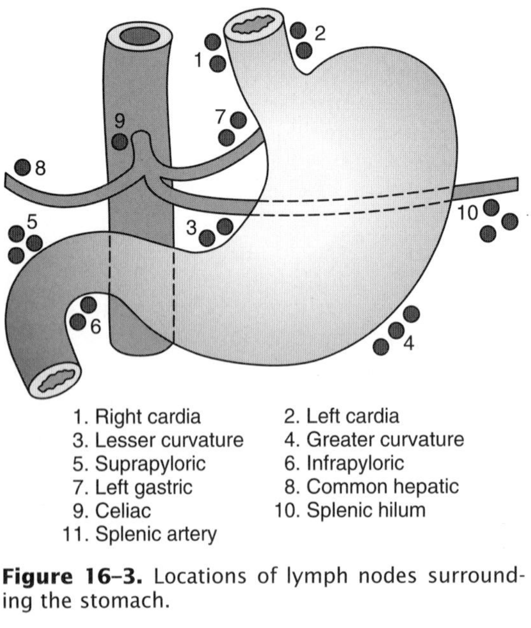

Figure 16–3. Locations of lymph nodes surrounding the stomach.

than after a more limited resection and gastrojejunostomy reconstruction. Newer reconstructive techniques for total gastrectomy patients, such as the Hunt-Lawrence pouch, attempt to reconstruct the gastric reservoir function, although there is little evidence to date that these improve quality of life (see Figure 16-4).

Lymph Node Dissection

Few topics in surgical oncology are as controversial as the necessary extent of lymph-node dissection in patients undergoing the curative resection of gastric cancer (see Figure 16-3). To provide uniformity of reporting in gastric cancer trials, the Japanese have developed standards for nodal dissection (Table 16-2). The nodal groups include N1 (perigastric along the greater and lesser curvatures), N2 (adjacent to the celiac axis and its major branches), N3 (hepatoduodenal ligament, retropancreatic region, celiac plexus, and superior mesenteric artery) and N4 (para-aortic).

A D0 resection thus includes a gastrectomy with the incomplete resection of N1 nodes, whereas a D1 gastric resection includes a complete dissection of N1 nodes. A D2 resection includes both the N1 and N2 nodes. A D3 resection includes the resection of N1 to N3 nodes, and a D4 resection is the most extensive and includes the removal of all nodal groups. It was once thought that routine splenectomy

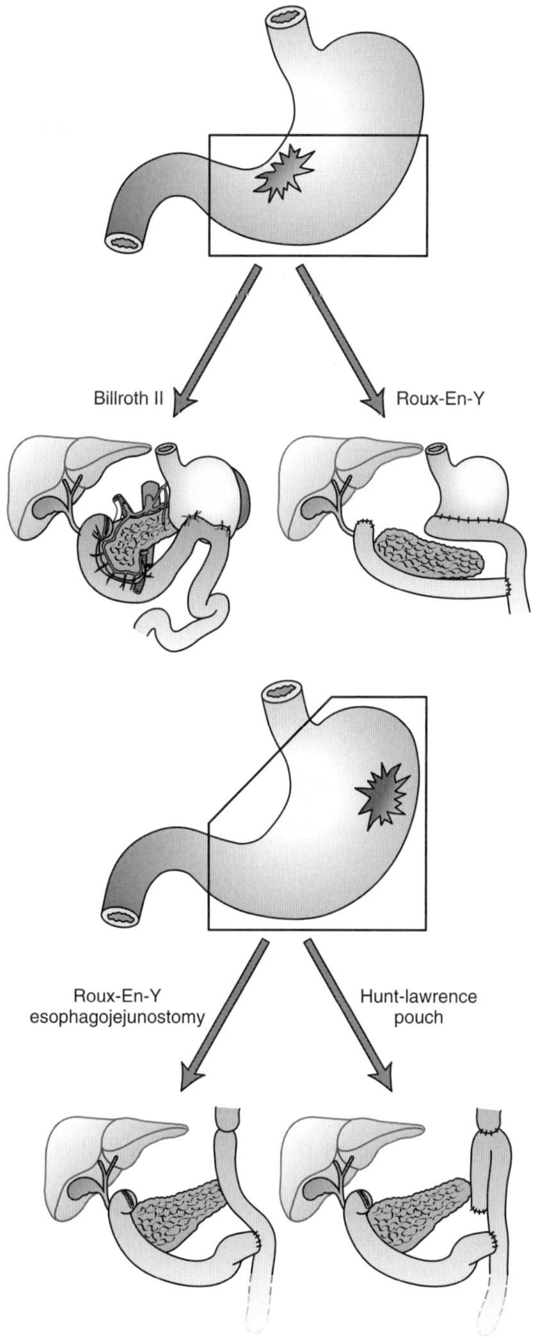

Figure 16–4. Figures of gastric resections and reconstructions.

was necessary for adequate tumor clearance; however, it results in increased morbidity without any clear survival benefit, and it is not recommended. Splenectomy may be necessary when the spleen is involved by direct extension from greater curvature lesions or when there is a proximal lesion of the greater curvature with macroscopic metastases to nodes in the splenic hilum. Distal pancreatectomy is also not recommended for the clearance of the level 2 nodes, but it may be necessary when there is direct invasion by the primary tumor.

Two major randomized trials from the Netherlands and the United Kingdom randomized patients between D1 and D2 dissections; there was no survival advantage but significantly more morbidity for D2 dissections (Table 16-3). The first study was by the Dutch Gastric Cancer Group. They found that the patients

TABLE 16–2 • *Upper Abdominal Lymph Node Stations, According to the Japanese Research Society for Gastric Cancer*

Level	Station	Location
Level 1	1	Right paracardial
	2	Left paracardial
	3	Lesser curvature
	4	Greater curvature
	5	Suprapyloric
	6	Infrapyloric
	7	Left gastric artery
Level 2	8	Common hepatic artery
	9	Celiac axis
	10	Splenic hilus
	11	Splenic artery
Level 3	12	Hepatic pedicle
	13	Retropancreatic
	14	Mesenteric root
	15	Middle colic artery
Level 4	16	Paraaortic

TABLE 16–3 • *Comparison of Two Large Prospective Randomized Trial of D1 Versus D2 Resection in Gastric Cancer*

	Medical Research Council Trial, United Kingdom	Dutch Gastric Cancer Trial, Netherlands
No. of patients	400	711
Operative mortality of D1 versus D2	6.5% versus 13%; $P < .04$	4% versus 10%; $P = .004$
Postoperative complications of D1 versus D2	28% versus 46%; $P < .001$	25% versus 43%; $P < .001$
5-year survival	35% versus 33%; P = NS	42% versus 47%; P = NS

with D2 dissections had significantly higher rates of complications (43% versus 25%; $P < .001$), postoperative deaths (10% versus 4%; $P = .004$), and longer hospital stays (median, 16 versus 14 days; $P < .001$) than patients with D1 dissections without a detectable survival advantage. The second trial was conducted by the Surgical Cooperative Group in the United Kingdom. They reported that the patients with D2 dissections had higher postoperative mortality (13% versus 6.5%; $P = .04$) and higher postoperative morbidity (46% versus 28%; $P < .001$) than patients with D1 dissections. Furthermore, 3-year overall survival was only 30% with D2 dissections as compared with 50% with D1 dissections. Thus, extensive lymphadenectomy is not the standard in Europe or the United States, and it remains unclear whether outcomes among Western patients can be improved by the more radical surgery. In Japan, more extensive nodal resections are still recommended. Survival for gastric cancer in Japan is superior to that seen in the United States (5-year survival rates of 50% versus 15–20%), and this has in part been attributed to a more widespread application of radical lymphadenectomy. However, differences in the biology of the gastric cancer between Western and Asian populations may explain some of the difference. Enthusiasm for radical lymphadenectomy among patients with gastric cancer should be tempered with the perspective that, for most other tumors, more radical surgery does not increase survival but does increase operative complication rates. Patients with potentially curable gastric cancer should have, at the very least, a complete D1 dissection.

Adjuvant Chemoradiation

Postoperative chemotherapy has been extensively evaluated, with generally equivocal results. In studies to date, adjuvant chemotherapy by itself has not made an impact on the long-term survival of patients undergoing the complete resection of gastric carcinoma. Based on the increased activity of combined chemotherapy and radiation therapy in the treatment of unresectable gastric cancer, several studies have examined adjuvant chemoradiation after potentially curative resection. The Southwest Oncology Group coordinated the Intergroup 0116 study (SWOG-9008), in which more than 600 patients with stages Ib to IV gastric cancer who had undergone curative resection were randomized to receive either observation or adjuvant therapy with 5-flourouracil and leucovorin plus 45 Gray of external-beam radiotherapy. Overall survival after 3 years was improved from 41% to 52%, and postoperative chemoradiation is now considered the standard of care by many clinicians. Critics of this study point out that more than half of the patients had a D0 lymphadenectomy. The survival rates in the treatment arm are similar to control arms in other studies, in which a more adequate lymph node dissection had been performed, thus suggesting that the chemoradiation may simply be compensating for inadequate surgery. The role of multimodality therapy for gastric cancer, however, is expanding. The recently completed MAGIC trial demonstrated that perioperative chemotheraphy (given before and after surgery) not only decreased tumor size and increased resectability rates, but also improved suvival. Other approaches being examined inculde alternate approaches to neoadjuvant therapy, intraperitoneal chemotherapy, and the use of biologic response modifiers (see Chapter 20: Multimodality Therapy for Select Gastro-intestinal Malignancies).

Small-Bowel Tumors

Incidence

Small-bowel tumors are rare, which is surprising when one considers that the total length of the duodenum, jejunum, and ileum is much greater than that of the remaining gastrointestinal tract. The most common benign lesions of the small bowel are leiomyomas and adenomas, whereas four histologic tumors make up most small-bowel malignancies: adenocarcinoma, carcinoid, lymphoma, and sarcoma Adenocarcinomas are more frequent in the duodenum, particularly in the vicinity of the ampulla. Carcinoids are more frequently distal in the small bowel, being predominantly ileal or jejunal.

There are approximately 5,300 new cases of small-bowel cancer per year in the United States. They comprise 1% to 3% of all gastrointestinal tumors, and they occur 30 to 60 times less frequently than malignancies of the colon. Several hypotheses have been introduced to explain the low incidence of small-bowel tumors. First, the transit time is more rapid in the small intestine than it is in the colon. Therefore, the effect of any carcinogen would be minimized. In addition, the proximal small bowel contains hydroxylases, which may detoxify carcinogens. There is also an alkaline environment as compared with the relatively acid environment of the stomach and large bowel, where carcinoma is more prevalent. The relative lack of bacteria in the small bowel may provide protection by minimizing exposure to bacteria-produced carcinogens. Finally, the distal ileum contains increased numbers of immunoglobulin-secreting B cells as well as T lymphocytes, which may contribute to a more effective local immune surveillance system.

Predisposing Factors for Small-Bowel Adenocarcinoma

Dietary fat intake has been correlated with the incidence of small-bowel tumors in various countries around the world. Weekly or more frequent consumption of red meat and monthly or more frequent consumption of salt-cured smoked foods have been associated with a two- to three-fold increased risk for the development of small-bowel adenocarcinoma. Tobacco and alcohol use have not been correlated with increased risk.

Several groups of individuals are at increased risk for the development of small-bowel tumors. Duodenal and small-intestinal neoplasms are associated with certain inherited disorders of the gastrointestinal tract, including von Recklinghausen's disease (neurofibromatosis), familial adenomatous polyposis, Gardner's syndrome, and Peutz-Jeghers syndrome. Along with increasing age and male sex, patients with chronic inflammation of the bowel (e.g., Crohn's disease) are at risk for small-bowel adenocarcinoma. Patients with longstanding celiac sprue are more likely to develop both lymphoma and adenocarcinoma of the small bowel.

Diagnosis

The presenting features of tumors of the small bowel are often vague, leading to a significant delay from the onset of symptoms to the time of diagnosis. Abdominal pain, nausea and vomiting, and abdominal distention may arise from a bowel obstruction or intussusception. Gastrointestinal hemorrhage as a result of ulceration may occur. Perforation and gross bleeding are rare. Physical examination is usually not helpful. Laboratory findings are usually nonspecific, but they may include mild anemia from chronic blood loss, elevated 5-hydroxyindolacetic acid levels from a carcinoid, or hyperbilirubinemia as a result of a periampullary lesion.

The diagnosis of small-bowel tumors remains largely the domain of the radiologist. Plain films may show an obstruction, but they are usually not helpful. Standard small-bowel follow through using orally administered barium is the traditional approach, but it is limited by the presence of multiple peristalsing intestinal loops overlapped in a limited area. This results in the lower sensitivity and specificity of barium studies in the small bowel as compared with the equivalent study of the stomach and colon. Enteroclysis is the preferred method for detecting resectable small-bowel tumors. This involves passing a balloon-tipped catheter under fluoroscopic control to the proximal jejunum. The catheter balloon is inflated before the infusion of contrast material to prevent reflux and maintain enough pressure in the small-bowel lumen to actively distend it, thereby resulting in superior detection rates for intraluminal lesions of the small bowel.

The use of CT scanning in the setting of nonspecific abdominal symptoms is increasing. Neoplastic disease should be suspected on CT if the thickness of the wall of the small bowel is greater than 1.5 cm or if there are discreet mesenteric masses larger than 1.5 cm. CT scans can also aid in the histologic diagnosis of small-bowel masses. Lipomas, leiomyomas, leiomyosarcomas, and carcinoid tumors are more easily recognized by their CT characteristics than adenocarcinomas and lymphomas, which are often mistaken for each other. Promising new techniques for examining the small bowel may eventually replace barium studies, which are currently the most sensitive modality for the early detection of small-bowel tumors. Both magnetic resonance imaging and CT enteroclysis have been reported in the literature for the investigation of partial small-bowel obstruction and inflammatory bowel disease.

Ultimately, endoscopy is the gold standard for evaluating small-bowel tumors. Three methods are used: push endoscopy, enteroscopy, and colonoscopy with intubation of the terminal ileum. Push endoscopy has the advantages of using standard endoscopic techniques to directly advance the scope along the small intestinal lumen and standard endoscopic instruments to biopsy or snare abnormal areas. Enteroscopy, which is a newer method, uses a 5-mm endoscope up to 9 feet in length, with dual 1-mm diameter internal channels. One channel is used to inflate a balloon along the side of the endoscope to permit peristalsis to carry the scope distally into the small intestine over time. The other channel is used to pass air into the small intestinal lumen during the examination, but it is too small to permit the use of standard endoscopic instruments, precluding biopsy of small-bowel tumors. Colonoscopy with intubation of the terminal ileum may allow for the diagnosis of distal small-bowel lesions. A promising new technique involves swallowing a tiny, capsule-sized endoscopy camera that records digital images as it travels through the intestines.

Management of Benign and Malignant Small-Bowel Neoplasms

All patients diagnosed with a small-bowel tumor should have a CT scan in an attempt to identify mesenteric infiltration, regional lymphadenopathy, and distant metastases. However, despite all of the studies available to detect, diagnose, and stage small-bowel tumors, the final diagnosis is typically not made until exploratory laparotomy. One third of these lesions will turn out to be benign, with the most common benign tumors (in descending order) being leiomyomas, adenomas, lipomas, and hemangiomas.

Leiomyomas

Leiomyomas of the small intestine account for 37% of all benign small-bowel tumors. They arise from smooth muscle cells and lack mitotic figures. These tumors may outgrow their blood supply and ulcerate, causing hemorrhage. Obstruction is also common, and perforation has been reported. On both gross inspection and frozen section analysis, it is sometimes difficult to distinguish these lesions from their malignant counterparts. Treatment should therefore consist of segmental resection, including adequate margins of normal tissue. Extensive lymphadenectomy is not required, because lymph-node metastasis is rare, even for leiomyosarcoma of the small bowel.

Adenomas

Adenomas are most commonly located in the duodenum, and the lesion that is most commonly noted is the villous adenoma. These lesions tend to involve the region of the ampulla of Vater. Simple local excision (endoscopically or via transduodenal excision) with negative surgical margins is feasible. A wide range of local recurrence rates have been reported, and there is concern about the risk of malignant degeneration in a significant proportion (up to 30%) of these tumors should they recur. Close endoscopic surveillance is thus mandated after this type of resection. If there is any suspicion of adenocarcinoma in the first or second part of the duodenum, the treatment of choice is a pancreaticoduodenectomy. For tumors that are more distal, in the third or fourth portion of the duodenum, or in the distal small bowel, treatment is wedge or segmental resection with the histologic control of margins.

Hamartomas

Hamartomas are small intestinal polyps that contain myoepithelial elements. Multiple hamartomas, along with melanin pigmentation in the buccal mucosa, lips, and face, constitutes the syndrome known as Peutz-Jeghers syndrome, which is inherited as a single, autosomal dominant gene. Patients with hamartomas usually present during the second decade of life with bleeding and obstruction as a consequence of intussusception. The incidence of carcinoma is less than 3%. The treatment is conservative unless obstruction or uncontrollable bleeding occurs.

Adenocarcinoma of the Small Bowel

Adenocarcinomas are most common in the duodenum, but when they arise in association with Crohn's disease, they tend to occur more often in the ileum. Segmental resection is the treatment of choice, and this is usually sufficient for patients with tumors in the third or fourth portions of the duodenum, jejunum, or ileum. Patients whose primary lesions arise in the first and second portion of the duodenum often require a pancreaticoduodenectomy, although there is no evidence of a superior outcome with the procedure as compared with a segmental resection when technically possible. Many patients with small bowel adenocarcinoma will have positive lymph nodes; therefore, curative resection should always include a regional lymphadenectomy. Prognostic factors include depth of penetration, lymph-node involvement, distant metastases, perineural invasion, grade, and resectability. The overall 5-year survival rate in most of the larger series is in the range of 20% to 35%, ranging from 45% to 70% among patients with negative lymph nodes to 12% to 14% among patients with histologically involved lymph nodes. There is no standard adjuvant chemotherapy or radiation therapy for small-bowel adenocarcinoma.

Ampullary Cancers

Periampullary cancers are defined as those cancers that arise within 2 cm of the ampulla of Vater in the duodenum. They account for only 5% of gastrointestinal tract cancers. Periampullary cancers can be divided into four categories: ampullary, biliary, pancreatic, and duodenal. Pancreatic is the most common, followed by ampullary. Although there are differences in the cells of origin, the anatomic location of these tumors and the difficulty in accurately classifying these tumors histologically dictate a common operative approach: a pancreaticoduodenectomy, with or without preservation of the pylorus. Although they are much less common than cancers of the head of the pancreas; periampullary cancers are overrepresented in series of pancreaticoduodenectomies because they are more often resectable. Cancers of the head of the pancreas account for 50% to 70% of pancreaticoduodenectomies, whereas ampullary cancer accounts for 15% to 20%. Biliary cancer and duodenal cancer account for 10% each.

BOX 16-4 PERIAMPULLARY CANCERS

- Ampullary (cancer of the ampulla of Vater)
- Biliary (intrapancreatic distal bile duct)
- Pancreatic (cancer of the head-uncinate process of the pancreas)
- Duodenal (second portion of the duodenum)

Although the operative approach is similar, the outcome varies with the type of periampullary cancer. The 5-year survival rate ranges from 32% to 67% for duodenal cancers and 33% to 48% for ampullary cancer. These are significantly better than the outcomes for cancer of the head of the pancreas or of the distal bile duct. Some of this is related to the timing of the onset of jaundice. Cancers of the ampulla almost always present with early jaundice, when the primary tumor is still small and before the onset of constitutional symptoms such as nausea and vomiting or abdominal pain. However, this is not the only factor, because distal bile-duct cancers, which also obstruct the bile duct early, have a worse prognosis. Other factors, such as growth pattern (intraluminal versus extraductal invasion), lymphatic and perineural invasion, and molecular factors, also play a role.

Surgical treatment for periampullary cancers remains pancreaticoduodenectomy (classic or pylorus-preserving); however, less-radical approaches have been investigated. With the advent of endoscopic ultrasound, it is possible to preoperatively determine the T stage of the tumor. It may be feasible to treat small (<1 cm) Tis or T1 ampullary or distal bile-duct cancers with transduodenal ampullectomy. Selected duodenal cancers may be treated by partial duodenectomy or transduodenal excision. These approaches are particularly attractive for patients who may not be good candidates for pancreaticoduodenectomy. However, for patients with invasive periampullary cancers, overall survival appears to be less for these limited approaches, with increased local recurrence rates described.

Other Malignant Tumors of the Stomach and Small Intestine

Carcinoid Tumors

Carcinoid tumors arise from enterochromaffin cells, and they are characterized by the ability to secrete many biologically active substances. They are the second most common malignancy of the small bowel; however, they are rare within the stomach. Gastric carcinoid tumor accounts for about 4% of all GI carcinoids.

Gastric carcinoids are the only carcinoid tumors with a well-documented hyperplasia-dysplasia-neoplasia sequence based on experimental and clinical observations. It was postulated that the lack of feedback inhibition by gastric acid (hypochlorhydria) is the common cause of G-cell hyperplasia resulting from various conditions, including atrophic gastritis with or without pernicious anemia, vagotomy, chronic administration of H^2 antagonists, or proton-pump inhibitors. Hypergastrinemia as a result of G-cell hyperplasia causes enterochromaffin-like (ECL)-cell hyperplasia in turn. ECL-cell hyperplasia leads to dysplasia and finally to microcarcinoids and invasive carcinoid. There are three clinical subtypes of gastric carcinoid (Table 16-4):

1. **Type I: carcinoid associated with type A chronic atrophic gastritis, with or without pernicious anemia.** This is presumably autoimmune in etiology, and it is caused by antibodies to parietal cells and intrinsic factor in the

patient's serum. This is the most common variant, and it often has a benign course. Conservative therapies, such as endoscopic removal or partial gastric resection, seem appropriate. Tumor regression has been reported after antrectomy, which removes the bulk of the G cells.

2. **Type II: carcinoid associated with Zollinger-Ellison syndrome.** These occur almost exclusively in patients with multiple endocrine neoplasia type 1 syndrome. Unlike the carcinoid tumors associated with chronic atrophic gastric, the hypergastrinemia comes not from G-cell hyperplasia in the antrum but rather from a gastrinoma. Treatment should center on the localization and excision of the gastrinoma (see Chapter 14: Tumors of the Endocrine Pancreas).
3. **Type III: carcinoid tumor of sporadic form or neuroendocrine carcinoma.** This is not associated with hypergastrinemia, and it has a worse prognosis than the other two subtypes. Patients usually have larger tumors and present at a more advanced stage of disease. Therapy should therefore be more aggressive, and, in addition to surgery, combined chemotherapy and radiation may be required.

After the appendix, the ileum is the second most common site of gastrointestinal carcinoids. Most intestinal carcinoid tumors are clinically silent and are discovered only during a laparotomy performed for other causes or at autopsy. Only 10% of patients with carcinoid tumors present with a carcinoid syndrome, which is usually associated with hepatic metastases. The carcinoid syndrome consists of such signs and symptoms as secretory diarrhea, telangiectasia, and bronchial constriction. Patients with mid gut carcinoids may have flushing that lasts only a few minutes after consuming alcohol, red wine, or foods that contain tyramine (e.g., blue cheese, chocolate). About 50% of patients will have elevated urinary levels of 5-hydroxyindolacetic acid.

Diagnostic Evaluation

For patients with a presumed carcinoid tumor, the diagnostic evaluation consists of (1) biochemical confirmation of elevated hormones and/or their metabolites and (2) localization studies. The localization and imaging studies follow a presumptive biochemical diagnosis. Contrast studies, such as small-bowel follow through and enteroclysis, may demonstrate mucosal abnormalities, although small lesions (<2 cm) may be missed. Standard CT scans also have limited ability to detect small tumors (<l cm), although they may be useful for evaluating retroperitoneal and mesenteric involvement and for detecting hepatic metastases. Newer multidetector scanners allow for thinner collimation and faster scanning, and they may allow for the visualization of even small submucosal masses.

Nuclear medicine studies can take advantage of the ability of carcinoid tumors to concentrate radioisotope complexed to somatostatin ana-

TABLE 16–4 • *Gastric Carcinoid Tumors*

	Type I Associated With Type A Atrophic Gastritis	Type II Associated With Zollinger-Ellison Syndrome/ Multiple Endocrine Neoplasia Type 1	Type III Sporadic
Location	Fundus	Fundus	Fundus or antrum
Size	<1-2 cm	<1-2 cm	2-5 cm
Growth	Slow growing	Slow growing	Aggressive
Metastases	Rare	Rare	Common
Plasma gastrin level	Elevated	Elevated	Normal
Gastric acid output	Low	High	Normal
Secretin test	Negative	Positive	Negative
Treatment	Endoscopic polypectomy; antrectomy for recurrence	Treatment of the gastrinoma, somatostatin analogs; possible local excision or antrectomy	En bloc resection with regional lymph nodes; possible chemotherapy or x-ray therapy

logues, such as indium-111 octreotide or iodine-123 MIBG, the former being more sensitive. In equivocal cases, mesenteric angiography may demonstrate a tumor "blush" that reflects the high vascularity of these lesions. Conventional angiography can be avoided if good-quality CT scanning or magnetic resonance angiography is available. These are less invasive, they use less intravenous contrast, and they can visualize vessels in an infinite number of planes.

Treatment

After the diagnosis is made, treatment consists of wide resection of the tumor, along with complete resection of the supporting mesentery. It is important to remember that a small subset of patients with carcinoid tumors may develop "carcinoid crisis," precipitated by anesthesia or surgery. Symptoms are intense in nature, and they are often refractory to treatment with intravenous fluids and vasopressors. Octreotide blockage preoperatively is therefore important, particularly for patients with a large tumor burden.

Nodal metastases are unusual with tumors smaller than 1 cm in diameter, but they occur with 33% to 67% of tumors 1 cm to 3 cm and with 75% to 90% of tumors larger than 3 cm. Approximately 30% of small-bowel carcinoids are multiple, and submucosal nodules may be present; therefore, a careful search of the remainder of the small bowel is mandatory. For these lesions that have metastasized, surgical debulking may still provide considerable palliation and prolonged symptomatic benefit. Because carcinoids tend to be slow growing and to metastasize late in their course, the prognosis for carcinoid tumors of the small intestine is considerably better than for adenocarcinomas arising from the same site. Patients who undergo complete resection of localized disease have a 5-year survival of 75% to 94%; those with positive regional lymph nodes have a 5-year survival rate of 45% to 90%; and the 5-year survival rate of patients with liver metastases is 19% to 54%.

For patients who cannot undergo complete resection of their disease, the management of carcinoid tumors consists of managing the complications of hormonal excess. The most active agent is the somatostatin analog octreotide acetate (SMS201-995). Because octreotide has a longer half-life (8 to 12 hours) than somatostatin (<2 minutes) and because it may be administered subcutaneously, it has been the preferred drug for the outpatient therapy of patients with carcinoid tumors. Octreotide is well tolerated, although long-term treatment may be associated with cholelithiasis, increased fecal fat excretion, fluid retention, nausea, and glucose intolerance. Other agents that have been used for symptomatic management include histamine H1 and H2 receptor antagonists, methoxamine, cyproheptadine, and diphenoxylate with atropine (Lomotil).

In addition to managing the symptoms of hormonal excess, octreotide may have the ability to affect the tumor biologically. Although objective responses occur in less than 20% of patients, disease stabilization is seen in approximately half of the patients treated, presumably to a cytostatic effect. Interferon-alfa has also been shown to be cytostatic in the management of carcinoid tumors, with response rates similar to those of octreotide. Carcinoid tumors tend to be resistant to most chemotherapeutic agents. Doxorubicin and 5-fluorouracil are considered the most active agents. When used in combination, these drugs may produce objective responses in 30% to 35% of patients; however, response durations are typically less than 9 months.

Lymphoproliferative Disease of the Stomach

Primary Gastric Lymphoma

Malignant lymphoma can affect the stomach either as a primary tumor or as part of more widespread disease. The GI tract is the most common site of primary extranodal non-Hodgkin's lymphoma, and more than 50% of all GI lymphomas arise from the stomach. There are approximately 3,000 new cases of primary gastric lymphoma each year. The diagnosis of primary gastric lymphoma requires histologic confirmation of lymphoma without any evidence of peripheral lymphadenopathy or hepatosplenomegaly. Secondary gastric lymphoma indicates the involvement of the stomach by a diffuse lymphoma that has developed elsewhere. Tertiary gastric lymphoma, which is quite rare, is a recurrence within the stomach after the treatment of lymphoma of the peripheral nodal basin.

Primary gastric lymphoma is best divided into two types: low grade (indolent) and high grade (aggressive). The low-grade lymphomas nearly always arise in the mucosa or submucosa, from the mucosa-associated lymphoid tissues (MALT). For this reason, low-grade primary gastric lymphomas are also referred to as *gastric MALT lymphoma*. Despite its penchant for being the most common site for extranodal lymphoma, the stomach is normally devoid of lymphoid tissue. However, MALT can arise within the stomach in response to certain inflammatory conditions. The most common is *H pylori* infection; however, MALT can also be seen with transplant-related immunosuppression, ulcer disease, inflammatory bowel disease, and human immunodeficiency virus infection.

MALT lymphomas are B-cell lymphomas, and they have many features in common with B-cell non-Hodgkin's lymphoma. The distinction of low-grade MALT lymphoma from gastritis is becoming increasingly important, because early treatment could prevent progression toward a high-grade malignancy.

Other forms of primary gastric lymphomas, particularly the high-grade lymphomas, are non-MALT type, although many of these may have initially been MALT lymphomas that progressed. One third of high-grade lesions have a visible low-grade MALT component. Such transformation may be mediated through increasing genetic instability and specific gene mutations. Inactivation of the *P53* tumor-suppressor gene, expression of the replication error repair phenotype, and mutation of the *c-myc* proto-oncogene have been demonstrated to occur with the development of high-grade lymphomas. Cytogenetics have also detected specific chromosomal abnormalities in primary gastric lymphoma. Trisomy of chromosome 3 has been associated with low-grade lymphomas, whereas trisomies of chromosomes 12 and 18 have been demonstrated in high-grade lymphomas.

Diagnosis and Staging

There is considerable overlap in the clinical presentation of gastric lymphoma as compared with adenocarcinoma. Gastric lymphoma can present with nonspecific upper GI symptoms such as abdominal pain, anorexia, nausea, vomiting, and weight loss. Gastric lymphoma presents more commonly with bleeding (7–33% of cases) rather than perforation (6–18% of cases). The presentation of gastric lymphoma is relatively nonspecific; therefore, the time between the onset of symptoms and diagnosis can be significantly prolonged.

In early studies, gastric lymphoma was diagnosed preoperatively in less than 50% of cases. Because of improvements in endoscopic tissue sampling, more recent series have shown a greater accuracy in diagnosis with that method, without need for formal surgery. Endoscopy, alone or in combination with barium radiography, approaches the highest diagnostic sensitivity. Endoscopic findings include gastritis with superficial ulcers, diffuse thickening of the mucosal folds, or a submucosal mass. Occasionally an exophytic mass might look like carcinoma. Whereas primary gastric lymphoma can involve any portion of the stomach, tumor location within the gastric fundus should raise the suspicion of secondary lymphoma. Multiple biopsies should be obtained, along with biopsies of the antrum to assess for *H pylori* infection.

After gastric lymphoma is diagnosed, a thorough history and physical should focus on identifying disease outside of the abdomen. One should palpate all lymph node basins and look for hepatosplenomegaly on abdominal examination. Laboratory examinations should include a complete blood count, a chemistry panel, an LDH level, and serum protein electrophoresis. A bone marrow biopsy and CT scan of the chest, abdomen, and pelvis should be obtained. If the clinical features are suggestive of gastric pathology and the disease is predominantly confined to the stomach, then this is diagnosed as primary gastric lymphoma. Typically, a modification of the Ann Arbor classification has been used for staging GI lymphomas (see Chapter 22: Leukemia and Lymphoma); however, a new staging system has been put forward by the International Workshop (Table 16-5).

TABLE 16-5 • *International Workshop Staging System for Gastrointestinal Non-Hodgkin's Lymphoma*

Stage	Definition
Stage I	Tumor confined to the gastrointestinal tract
	Single primary site or multiple noncontiguous lesions
Stage II	Tumor extending in abdomen from primary gastrointestinal site
	Nodal involvement:
	II_1 local (paragastric or paraintestinal)
	II_2 distant (mesenteric, para-aortic, paracaval, pelvic, inguinal)
Stage III	Penetration of serosa to involve adjacent organs or tissues
Stage IV	Disseminated extranodal involvement or a gastrointestinal tract lesion with supradiaphragmatic nodal involvement

Treatment

Low-Grade Gastric Lymphoma Low-grade or MALT lymphomas are caused by chronic infection with *H pylori,* and they are typically slow growing. Eradication of *H pylori* often causes the regression of gastric MALT lymphomas, and this represents the first line of therapy. *H pylori* eradication requires the suppression of gastric acid (by either proton pump inhibitors or H2 blockers) and antibiotics (Table 16-6). Eradication rates range between 80% and 95%. This results in a complete remission rate of the lymphoma of between 50% and 100%, with the largest study showing a complete remission rate of 81%.

Not all patients will respond to *H pylori* eradication. A second course of eradication treatment should be considered, because not all patients respond after one attempt. Patients with stage II disease are less likely to have a complete response rate than patients with stage I disease, as are patients with a t(11:18) chromosomal translocation in the tumor. For those patients, external beam radiation using relatively low doses (30 Gray) does an excellent job of controlling disease. With more extensive disease, chemotherapy should be combined with radiation. Patients who present with stage III or IV disease will require initial treatment with *H pylori* eradication, chemotherapy, and radiation. These patients then require endoscopic surveillance looking not only for lymphoma recurrence but also for recurrence of *H pylori,* which can lead to subsequent lymphoma recurrence. In addition, these patients are at risk for intestinal metaplasia and eventual adenocarcinoma development (Table 16-7 and Figure 16-5).

TABLE 16–6 • *Regimens for Eradicating* Helicobacter pylori

Regimen 1
Omeprazole (20 mg twice daily)
Amoxicillin (1 gm twice daily)
Clarithromycin (500 mg twice daily)
Regimen 2 (for those allergic to penicillin)
Omeprazole (20 mg twice daily)
Metronidazole (500 mg twice daily)
Clarithromycin (500 mg twice daily)
Regimen 3
Omeprazole (20 mg twice daily)
Tetracycline (500 mg three time a day)
Metronidazole (500 mg three time a day)
Bismuth (525 mg three time a day)

High-Grade Gastric Lymphoma The management of high-grade or non-MALT gastric lymphoma has changed significantly over the past two decades. In the past, surgery played a crucial role in the diagnosis, staging, and treatment of this disease. Surgery, with or without adjuvant radiation or chemoradiation, results in extremely high cure rates when the disease is confined to the operative specimen, but it is associated with significant morbidity. This has prompted a shift toward treating gastric lymphoma with chemotherapy and radiation therapy without resection. Several single-institution series reported excellent results without surgery. The German Multicenter Study group performed a prospective, nonrandomized study of 185 patients with stage I or II gastric lymphoma; 106 were treated by surgery followed by adjuvant radiation with or without chemotherapy, and 79 were treated by chemotherapy plus radiation. There was no significant difference in survival, with an 82% 5-year survival for surgery and an 84% 5-year survival for nonsurgical therapy. Much of the hesitancy to treat gastric lymphoma by chemotherapy and radiation was the concern for gastric perforation or bleeding; however, there was only one perforation and no GI bleeds in the nonsurgical arm of this trial. Primary treatment for early-stage, high-grade gastric lymphoma should be chemotherapy with or without radiation. Rituximab, which is a monoclonal antibody that targets CD20 on B cells, is often used in combination with chemotherapy.

Surgery for gastric lymphoma should be reserved for urgent situations, although these are rare. Gastric lymphomas are unlikely to present with severe hemorrhage requiring gastrectomy. Stable patients with chronic anemia can be treated without operation. For patients

TABLE 16–7 • *Success Rates for Treating Low-Grade Gastric MALT Lymphoma* With Helicobacter pylori *Eradication*

Report	Number of Patients Remissions	Complete
Fischbach et al (2000)	36	89%
Pinotti et al (1997)	49	67%
Neubauer et al (1997)	50	80%
Thiede et al (2000)	84	81%
Stolte et al (2002)	120	81%

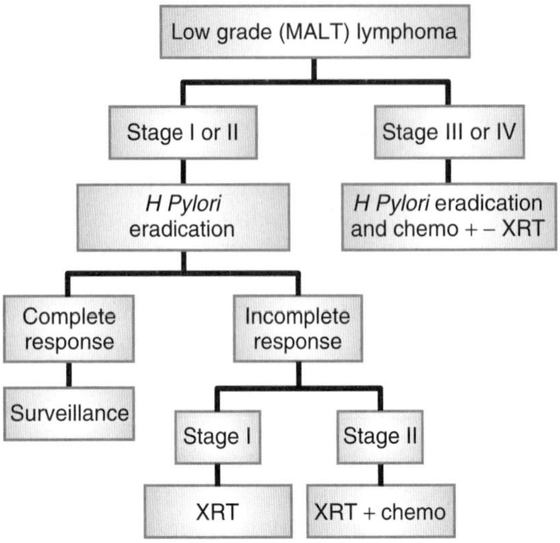

Figure 16-5. Management of MALT lymphoma.

with complete or near-complete obstruction, surgery is still not mandated. Treatment with high-dose steroids can lead to immediate palliation, thereby allowing for nonoperative management. Surgery for gastric lymphoma is reserved for acute hemorrhage, obstruction not relieved by steroids, or a failure of response to chemotherapy and radiation.

Lymphoproliferative Disease of the Small Intestine

Small-Bowel Lymphoma

Small-bowel lymphomas parallel the distribution of lymphoid follicles, resulting in the ileum being the most common site of involvement. In about 15% of patients, the disease may be multifocal. The disease may be primary or secondary (i.e., a manifestation of generalized involvement by disease originating outside of the small bowel). The development of this tumor is associated with immunodeficiency diseases (e.g., AIDS), rheumatoid arthritis, and immune disorders in transplant patients, as well as Crohn's disease and celiac sprue. Most lymphomas of the small bowel are diffuse, high-grade, non-Hodgkin's, B cell lymphomas. Bulky disease is characteristic at the time of diagnosis. Typical clinical presentations include malaise and fatigue, weight loss, ulceration and bleeding, an obstructing mass (with crampy abdominal pain), and perforation in up to 25% of cases. In contrast with other types of lymphomas (particularly Hodgkin's lymphomas), small-bowel lymphomas do not typically present with fever and night sweats. The most commonly used staging system is the Ann Arbor system (see Chapter 22: Lymphoma and Leukemia).

For low-grade localized tumors, resection alone suffices. For intermediate- and high-grade lesions, resection is combined with chemotherapy. The ideal chemotherapeutic regimen is the subject of intense debate. Most evidence indicates that the most efficacious regimen will be an intensive anthracycline-based regimen, such as CHOP (cyclophosphamide, doxorubicin, vincristine, prednisone, and bleomycin) or ProMACE (etoposide, cytarabine, bleomycin, vincristine, and methotrexate), which is used for nodal non-Hodgkin's lymphomas and other extranodal primary lymphomas.

The role of adjuvant radiation therapy for lymphoproliferative disorders of the small bowel is not well defined. Results have been equivocal. The doses of radiation used to treat intestinal lymphomas are low—usually 25 Gray to 35 Gray at 1.5 Gray per fraction—because these tumors are highly radioresponsive and because the treated area is usually relatively large.

Palliative radiation is highly effective for lymphoproliferative disease affecting the small bowel because of the low doses needed for this radioresponsive tumor. Symptom control is important for patients with advanced disease because, even with unresectable disease, an overall 5-year survival rate of 25% has been reported.

Immunoproliferative Small-Intestinal Disease

In developing countries, particularly among people living in substandard hygienic conditions, a chronic lymphoproliferative disorder known as immunoproliferative small intestinal disease (IPSID) is quite common. IPSID begins as a benign-appearing diffuse mucosal infiltration of plasma cells, and, in many cases, it may progress to large-cell immunoblastic lymphoma. IPSID has been reported predominately in patients from the Mediterranean basins, with most of the cases being noted in Arab and non-European Jews, Iranians, and South-African blacks.

In contrast with other lymphomas, which occur during the sixth decade of life, the peak incidence of IPSID is between the ages of 15 and 35 years. Most patients present with weight loss, anorexia, abdominal pain, and progressive diarrhea. On physical examination, most patients are profoundly emaciated, and they are noted to have dependent edema and digital clubbing. Fever, abdominal masses, peripheral lymphadenopathy, hepatosplenomegaly, and ascites are found late in this disease. Surgery plays little role in this disease other than for diagnosis and staging and for the treatment of rare abdominal catastrophes.

For the premalignant phase, most researchers have recommended tetracycline, although metronidazole with or without ampicillin, appears to be an effective alternative. If significant improvement has not been noted within 6 months, an underlying lymphoma should be ruled out. After the diagnosis of an IPSID lymphoma has been made, cytotoxic chemotherapy with an anthracycline-based regimen is warranted.

Enteropathy-Associated T Cell Lymphoma

Enteropathy-associated T cell lymphoma (EATCL) most often develops in patients with previously diagnosed, long-standing celiac sprue and/or dermatitis herpetiformis. Because patients with celiac sprue have a 50- to 100-fold greater-than-normal risk of developing lymphoma, some authors have suggested that celiac sprue is a premalignant state.

EATCL is usually a high-grade lesion, and, as such, it progresses rapidly, with a poor clinical outcome. Most patients present with exacerbation of celiac disease, such as a worsening of malabsorption syndrome and a loss of responsiveness to a gluten-restricted diet; nearly a quarter of patients will present with an intestinal perforation. The treatment of EATCL is difficult at best. Although the Epstein-Barr virus may play a role in the etiology of a subset of EATCL, this relationship is not certain, and antiviral therapy of Epstein-Barr virus infections is ineffective at present. Although the lymphoma tends to be localized in the jejunum, surgical resection for cure is precluded by the large area of gut involved, and it is reserved for the emergency treatment of abdominal catastrophes.

These tumors appear to be chemosensitive to many chemotherapy regimens. However, responses are usually brief, and therapy is poorly tolerated as a result of the malnourished state of most patients.

Key Selected Readings

Donohue JH. Malignant tumors of the small bowel. *Surg Oncol* 1994;3:61–68.

Roth AD. Curative treatment of gastric cancer: towards a multidisciplinary approach? *Crit Rev Oncol Hematol* 2003;46:59–100.

Selected Readings

Abu-Hamda EM, Hattab EM, Lynch PM. Small bowel tumors. *Curr Gastroenterol Rep* 2003;5:386–393.

Bonenkamp JJ, Hermans J, Sasako M, van de Velde CJ. Extended lymph node dissection for gastric cancer. Dutch Gastric Cancer Group. *N Engl J Med* 1999;340:908–914.

Cunningham D, Allum WH, Stenning SP, *et al.* Perioperative chemotheraipy versus surgery alone for resctable gastroesophagal cancer. *N Engl J Med* 2006;355:11–20.

Cuschieri A, Weeden S, Fielding J, *et al.* Patient survival after D1 and D2 resections for gastric cancer: long-term results of the MRC randomized surgical trial. Surgical Co-operative Group. *Br J Cancer* 1999;79:1522–1530.

Dicken BJ, Bigam DL, Cass C, *et al.* Gastric adenocarcinoma. Review and considerations for future directions. *Ann Surg* 2005;241:27–39.

Gold JS, DeMatteo RP. Combined surgical and molecular therapy: the gastrointestional stromal tumor model. *Ann Surg* 2006,244:176–184.

Gouzi JL, Huguier M, Fagniez PL, *et al.* Total versus subtotal gastrectomy for adenocarcinoma of the gastric antrum. A French prospective controlled study. *Ann Surg* 1989;209:162–166.

Jansen EP, Boot H, Verheji M, van de Velde CJ. Optimal locoregional treatment in gastric cancer. *J Clin Oncol* 2005;23:4509–4517.

Lim L, Michael M, Mann GB, Leong T. Adjuvant therapy in gastric cancer. *J Clin Oncol* 2005;23:6220–6232.

MacDonald JS, Smalley SR, Benedetii J, *et al.* Chemoradiotherapy after surgery compared with surgery alone for adenocarcinoma of the stomach or gastroesophageal junction. *N Engl J Med* 2001;345: 725–730.

McCulloch P, Eidi NM, Kazi H, Gama-Rodrigues JJ. Gastrectomy with extended Lymphadenectomy for primary treatment of gastric cancer. *Br J surg* 2005;92:5–13.

Minardi AJ Jr, Zibari GB, Aultman UF, *et al.* Small bowel tumors. *J Am Coll Surg* 1998;186:664–668.

Modlin IM, Lye KD, Kidd M. Carcinoid tumors of the stomach. *Surg Oncol* 2003;12:153–172.

Noguchi Y, Yoshikawa T, Tsuburaya A, *et al.* Is gastric carcinoma different between Japan and the United States? A comparison of patient survival among three institutions. *Cancer* 2000;89:2237–2246.

Roder JD, Bottcher K, Busch R, *et al.* Classification of regional lymph node metastasis from gastric carcinoma. *Cancer* 1998;82:621–631.

Yang C-S, Blaser MJ, Correa P, *et al.* Gastric dysplasia and gastric cancer: *Helicobacter pylori,* serum vitamin C, and other risk factors. *J Natl Cancer Inst* 2000;92:1607–1612.

17

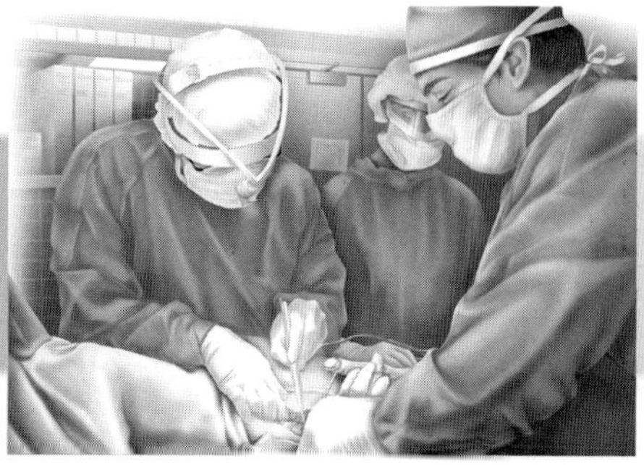

Tumors of the Exocrine Pancreas

Diane M. Simeone and Charles E. Binkley

Tumors of the Exocrine Pancreas: Key Points

- Relate the symptoms of pancreatic adenocarcinoma to its pathologic processes.
- Outline the steps taken to diagnose pancreatic cancer.
- Compare the various imaging methods with regard to their ability to assess pancreatic cancer.
- Describe the surgical treatment of pancreatic cancer and list the criteria for determining resectability.
- Identify the controversies associated with the Whipple operation.
- Describe the contraindications to surgical treatment and the palliation options for pancreatic cancer.
- Outline the characteristics of cystic pancreatic neoplasms.
- Discuss the procedures for diagnosing and differentiating cystic pancreatic neoplasms.

Epidemiology

Pancreatic adenocarcinoma is one of the deadliest known human malignancies, with an overall 5-year survival rate of 4.4%. Among gastrointestinal malignancies, pancreatic adenocarcinoma is second to colorectal cancer in terms of incidence, with 33,730 estimated new cases occurring in 2006. Pancreatic cancer is predicted to account for 32,300 deaths in the United States in 2006, making it the fourth most common cause of cancer related mortality, just behind breast cancer, which is responsible for an estimated 40,580 deaths. Delayed diagnosis, relative chemotherapy and radiation resistance, and an intrinsic biologic aggressiveness all contribute to the abysmal prognosis associated with pancreatic adenocarcinoma. The incidence of pancreatic adenocarcinoma is approximately the same among both men and women, although African and Japanese Americans have a higher incidence than other ethnic groups, which suggests some as-of-yet undetermined specific genetic or environmental association.

BOX 17-1 PANCREATIC CANCER STATISTICS

- Overall 5-year survival, 4.4%
- 5-year survival after resection with negative margins, 25%
- Fourth most common cause of cancer death
- 33,730 new cases in 2006
- 32,300 deaths in 2006
- 20% of tumors resectable at presentation
- Postoperative mortality, 1–4%

Many risk factors for pancreatic adenocarcinoma have been identified, with cigarette smoking having the strongest overall association; it is thought to account for one quarter of all patients diagnosed. The mechanism believed to be responsible for the association between cigarette smoking and pancreatic cancer involves the *N*-nitroso compounds present in cigarette smoke. Exposure to these agents leads to pancreatic ductal hyperplasia, which is a possible precursor to adenocarcinoma.

BOX 17-2 RISK FACTORS FOR PANCREATIC CANCER

- Cigarette smoking
- Increased age
- Chronic pancreatitis
- Increased saturated fat intake
- Exposure to nonchlorinated solvents

Other factors associated with an increased risk of pancreatic adenocarcinoma include saturated fat intake and exposure to nonchlorinated solvents and the pesticide DDT, although the overall contribution of these is likely small. The risk of pancreatic adenocarcinoma increases with age, with most patients diagnosed between the ages of 60 and 80 years. Studies examining the link between alcohol consumption and pancreatic adenocarcinoma are equivocal, except in the case of heavy alcohol use leading to chronic pancreatitis. Chronic pancreatitis clearly increases the risk of pancreatic adenocarcinoma, although the direct or indirect role of alcohol has not yet been defined.

Molecular Genetics

Genetic analysis has shown two distinct patterns of inherited risk for developing pancreatic adenocarcinoma: those inheriting mutations, specifically in the *PRSS1* gene, which leads to chronic familial relapsing pancreatitis, and those inheriting mutations in general cancer-susceptibility genes (Table 17-1). Chronic familial relapsing pancreatitis is an autosomal dominant trait, with complete penetrance. Individuals inheriting a mutated *PRSS1* gene, which is a serine protease also known as *cationic trypsinogen,* develop recurrent acute pancreatitis, frequently beginning in childhood. These individuals have a 40-fold increased risk of developing pancreatic adenocarcinoma as compared with the general population. The mechanism seems to involve recurrent bouts of acute pancreatitis, with increased pancreatic ductal cell turnover that leads to increased rates of DNA synthesis and accompanying random mutations. It is believed that the accumulation of random genetic mutations in key oncogenes and tumor-suppressor genes finally leads to the development of pancreatic adenocarcinoma.

An increased risk for developing pancreatic adenocarcinoma also occurs when individuals inherit germline mutations in cancer-susceptibility genes. A germline mutation in the *BRCA2* gene is present in approximately 5% to 10% of pancreatic adenocarcinomas, and it predisposes an individual to pancreatic as well as breast and ovarian cancer. The tumor-

TABLE 17-1 • *Inherited Risk Factors for Pancreatic Cancer*

Syndrome	Gene	Characteristics	Pancreatic Cancer Association
Chronic familial relapsing pancreatitis	*PRSS1* (cationic trypsinogen)	Relapsing acute pancreatitis beginning at a young age	20 to 40 times increased risk
Familial breast cancer	*BRCA2* (tumor suppressor)	Familial breast cancer	4–7% incidence of gene mutation
Peutz-Jeghers syndrome	*LKB1/STK11* (tumor suppressor)	Hamartomatous gastrointestinal polyps, gastrointestinal cancer, perioral pigmentation	5% incidence of gene mutation
Hereditary nonpolyposis colorectal cancer	*hMSH2, hMLH1, hPMS1, hPMS2, hMSH6/GTBP, hMSH3* (mismatch repair genes)	Lynch II syndrome: colorectal, ovarian, endometrial, and gastrointestinal cancers	4% incidence of gene mutation
Gardner's syndrome	*APC* (tumor suppressor)	Colorectal and upper gastrointestinal malignancy; ocular, cutaneous, and skeletal lesions; desmoid and thyroid tumors	Up to 50% incidence of gene mutation
Familial atypical mole and melanoma syndrome	*p16* (tumor suppressor)	Dysplastic nevi and melanomas	20 times increased risk

suppressor gene *p16* is mutated in more than 95% of the cases of pancreatic adenocarcinoma, usually by a somatic mutation; however, germline mutations have been described and are associated with an increased risk of both pancreatic malignancy and melanoma.

Inherited mutations in the *LKB1/STK11* gene lead to Peutz-Jeghers syndrome, and they are associated with the development of benign gastrointestinal polyps as well an increased risk of gastrointestinal cancers, including pancreatic adenocarcinoma. Other familial cancer syndromes involving an increased risk of pancreatic adenocarcinoma include hereditary nonpolyposis colorectal cancer (Lynch II), Gardner's syndrome, and familial and atypical multiple mole melanoma.

In contrast with inherited or germline gene mutations, several genes have been found to be commonly spontaneously mutated in pancreatic adenocarcinoma (Table 17-2). Mutations in the oncogene *K-ras* confer constitutive activation of the gene, and they are found in more than 90% of pancreatic cancers. Mutations in *K*-ras have also been detected in hyperplastic foci within the duct of patients with chronic pancreatitis, and they may predict which of these patients is at risk of developing pancreatic adenocarcinoma. As might be expected, mutations in tumor-suppressor genes—both spontaneously arising and inherited—are common among patients with pancreatic tumors, with more than 95% of cases harboring mutations in *p16*, 50% to 75% having p53 mutations, and approximately 55% having mutations of Smad4/DPC4 (deleted in pancreatic cancer, locus 4). Other, less-frequent mutations occur in tumor-suppressors *MKK4* (4%), transforming growth factor-β receptors I or II (<5%), and *RB1* (<5%).

TABLE 17-2 • *Sporadic Gene Mutations in Pancreatic Cancer*

Gene	Function	Incidence in Pancreatic Cancer
K-ras	Proto-oncogene	80–100%
p16	Tumor suppressor	95%
p53	Tumor suppressor	75%
Smad4/DPC4	Tumor suppressor	50%
MKK4	Tumor suppressor	4%
Transforming growth factor-β receptor	Signal transduction	<5%
RB1	Tumor suppressor	<5%

Pathology

The pancreas has both exocrine and endocrine cell types, so neoplasms can arise from multiple cellular structures. Approximately 90% of tumors of the exocrine pancreas have a ductal phenotype, whereas less than 1% have an acinar cell phenotype, with the balance being of uncertain histogenesis. Overall, 75% of pancreatic neoplasms are ductal adenocarcinoma: 65% of these arise from the head, neck, or uncinate process; 15% arise from the body or tail; and 20% are diffuse. Hallmarks of pancreatic adenocarcinoma include an intense desmoplastic reaction and perineural invasion (Figure 17-1).

Areas of focal ductal proliferation have been noted both adjacent to infiltrating pancreatic cancers and in the setting of chronic pancreatitis. Molecular analysis of these lesions, called *pancreatic intraepithelial neoplasia,* has shown the progressive accumulation of genetic changes with increasing severity of histologic atypia (Figure 17-2). In addition, the genetic alterations in pancreatic intraepithelial neoplasia lesions are similar to those seen in pancreatic adenocarcinomas, thus supporting the hypothesis that they are precursor lesions. There appears to be a stepwise accumulation of specific genetic alterations in the continuum from normal tissue to infiltrating carcinoma, with mutations in *K-ras* and Her-2/neu occurring in low-grade lesions, mutations in p16 being present in intermediate-grade lesions and p53, and DPC4 and BRCA2 mutations appearing in high-grade lesions. Although the progressive accumulation of genetic alterations have been initially identified, some controversy remains as to whether these lesions originate from fully differentiated duct cells or metaplastic conversion of either islet or acinar to ductal cell.

Clinical Presentation

The early symptoms associated with pancreatic adenocarcinoma are nonspecific, and therefore patients often delay seeking medical attention until the disease has advanced. A common presenting symptom, which is present in more than 90% of patients with pancreatic cancer, is cachexia, and it usually precedes a diagnosis of pancreatic adenocarcinoma by many months.

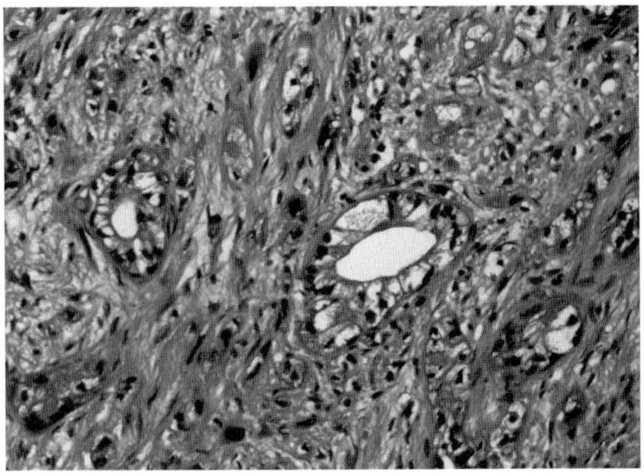

Figure 17-1. Histological section revealing the hallmarks of pancreatic adenocarcinoma, including an intense desmoplastic reaction and perineural invasion.

BOX 17-3 PRESENTING SYMPTOMS OF PANCREATIC CANCER

- Cachexia
- Nausea/vomiting
- Abdominal pain
- Jaundice
- Diabetes mellitus

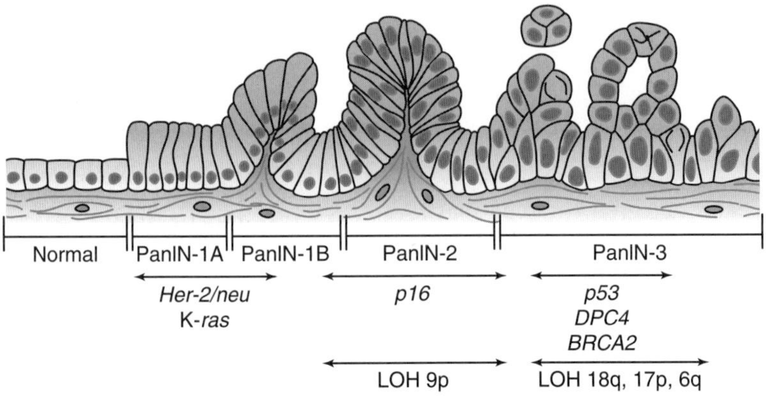

Figure 17-2. Pancreatic intraepithelial neoplasia (PanIn) progression model.

A major contributor to eventual mortality, cachexia is the result of both to weight loss from local obstructive factors causing nausea, vomiting, and anorexia as well as from the elaboration of tumor factors, such as tumor necrosis factor-α, and cytokines, such as interferon-α.

Abdominal pain is seen at presentation in 75% to 90% of patients with pancreatic cancer. The pain is believed to be caused by the compression of or the invasion into perineural and splanchnic neuronal structures as well as contiguous organs and the retroperitoneum. Because of the proximity of the common bile duct and the duodenum to the pancreas, tumors located in the head of the organ may grow and compress these structures. Bile-duct compression leads to obstructive jaundice in 70% to 85% of patients with pancreatic head lesions. Painless jaundice is more commonly associated with ampullary and distal bile-duct cancers, but it can accompany the presentation of pancreatic head or uncinate tumors, albeit less frequently than jaundice associated with abdominal pain. Compression of the duodenum leads to delayed gastric emptying and early satiety and contributes to nausea and vomiting, which is initially present in 35% to 45% of patients. In addition, up to 5% of patients present with advanced tumors that cause complete duodenal obstruction.

The onset of diabetes mellitus is also associated with pancreatic adenocarcinoma, with 10% to 15% of patients developing glucose intolerance 6 to 12 months before cancer diagnosis. The onset of diabetes appears to be the result of tumor elaboration of a yet undefined factor, which stimulates islet cells to secrete the prediabetic polypeptide amylin. Amylin levels are higher among patients with pancreatic adenocarcinoma as compared with patients with diabetes and other gastrointestinal malignancies, and both the serum level of amylin and insulin resistance abate after tumor resection. Pancreatic adenocarcinoma should be considered in any patient who develops severe diabetes with rapid progression to insulin dependence without either concomitant obesity or family history.

Diagnosis and Staging

Although the constellation of abdominal pain, weight loss, nausea, vomiting, and obstructive jaundice are highly suggestive of pancreatic malignancy, one must also consider other processes that can reproduce these symptoms. These symptoms can also be caused by benign processes, such as biliary strictures or choledocholithiasis, or other malignancies, such as cholangiocarcinoma and gallbladder cancer affecting the bile duct or ampullary and duodenal tumors. The possible diagnosis of pancreatic cancer is often raised during the evaluation of obstructive jaundice by transabdominal ultrasonographic imaging.

Because of multiple variables—including the skill of the examiner, patient habitus, and overlying loops of gas-filled bowel limiting complete imaging—the sensitivity of transabdominal ultrasound for diagnosing pancreatic cancer has ranged from 44% to 94% in different studies. Even with optimal results, transabdominal ultrasound is not able to stage patients or to determine resectability; thus, it must always be accompanied by another imaging modality.

When a diagnosis of pancreatic cancer is suspected, the modality of choice for confirmation is a helical CT scan of the abdomen with dual-phase scan acquisition (Figure 17-3). Dual-phase scans, which are acquired during both the arterial and portal phases, allow for pancreatic parenchymal and arterial enhancement during the former phase and for hepatic parenchymal as well as peripancreatic venous enhancement during the later phase (Figure 17-4). Enhancement of the pancreatic parenchyma allows for the detection of small, hypodense carcinomas as well as arterial involvement by the tumor, which directly affects resectability and possible cure. Tumor involvement of venous vessels and liver metastasis are delineated during the portal phase. The sensitivity of helical CT scanning to detect lesions greater than 2 cm in diameter is approximately 89%, and it is approximately 71% for lesions less than 2 cm in diameter,

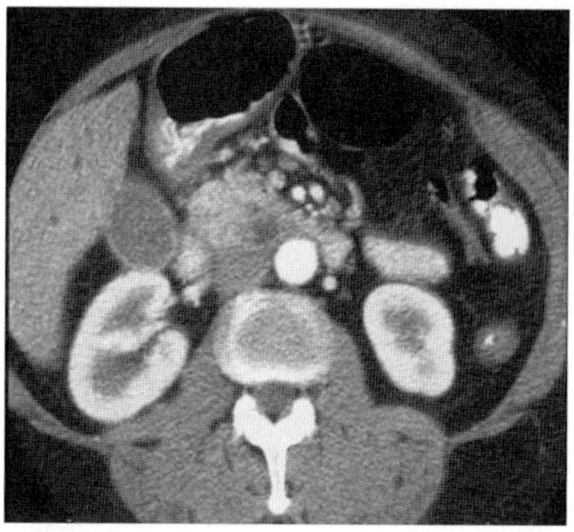

Figure 17-3. Dual-phase CT scan demonstrating a hypodense area in the pancreatic head that is consistent with pancreatic adenocarcinoma.

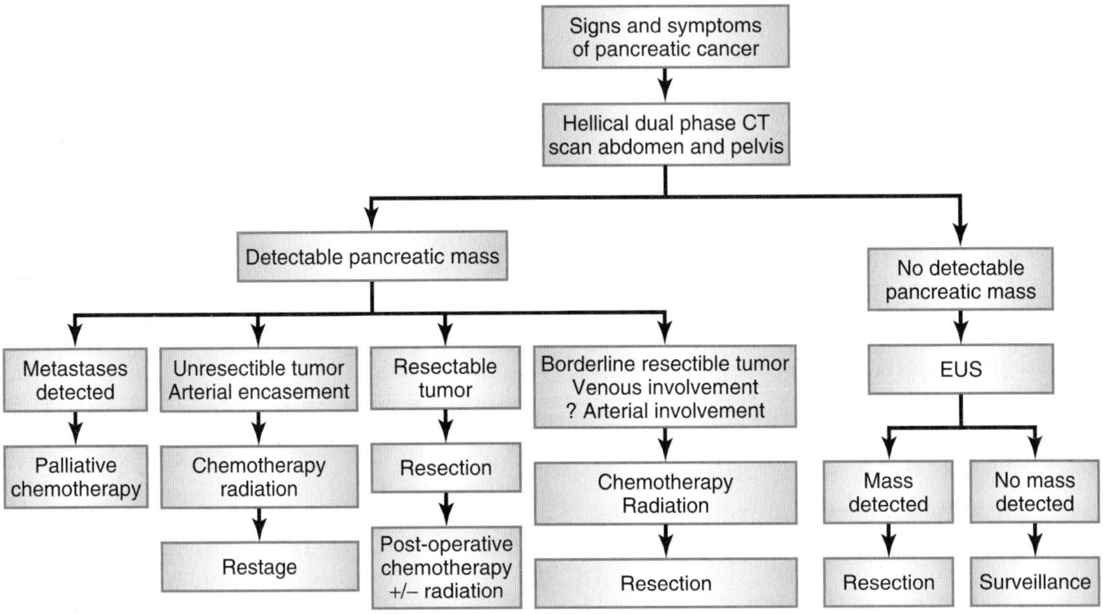

Figure 17–4. Management algorithm for pancreatic cancer.

with an overall diagnostic accuracy of 97% for pancreatic adenocarcinoma.

In addition to providing a diagnosis, CT scanning is useful for determining the resectability of the tumor. The criteria for resectability include the absence of extrapancreatic disease, the absence of tumor extension to the superior mesenteric artery and celiac axis, and a patent superior mesenteric–portal vein confluence. The accuracy of CT scanning for predicting unresectability approaches 100%; however, the accuracy for predicting resectability is only approximately 80% as a result of the limited ability to detect small metastases to the surface of the liver, the peritoneum, the lymph nodes, and the peripancreatic soft tissue.

Endoscopic ultrasonography (EUS) is highly sensitive for diagnosing pancreatic cancer, with an overall sensitivity of approximately 93% when combining data from various studies. EUS is particularly useful for detecting small (<2 cm) pancreatic tumors, which may not be well visualized by CT, as well as for the assessment of local vascular involvement. Combining EUS with fine-needle aspiration of the tumor increases the specificity over EUS alone for diagnosing pancreatic cancer.

Endoscopic retrograde cholangiopancreatography (ERCP) allows for the visualization of the biliary and pancreatic ductal structures, and it may be useful for diagnosing the cause of biliary obstruction when no mass is evident by CT scanning (e.g., ampullary tumors, cholangiocarcinoma) and for differentiating focal pancreatitis from neoplasm. Dilation of the distal pancreatic and common bile ducts with proximal stricturing of both structures—

BOX 17–4 DETERMINATION OF PANCREATIC CANCER RESECTABILITY

- Absence of extrapancreatic disease
- Absence of tumor extension to the superior mesenteric artery and celiac axis
- Patent superior mesenteric–portal vein confluence

BOX 17–5 DIAGNOSTIC MODALITIES

Dual-phase computed tomography scan
- 97% diagnostic accuracy
- 100% accuracy for predicting unresectability
- 80% accuracy for predicting resectability

Endoscopic ultrasonography
- 93% sensitivity
- Useful for lesions less than 2 cm and for assessing vascular involvement

Endoscopic retrograde cholangiopancreatography
- 92% sensitivity
- 96% specificity

Laparoscopy

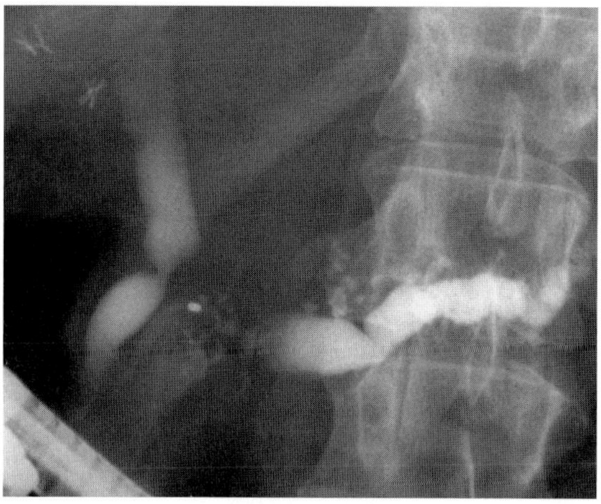

Figure 17-5. The "double-duct sign." Dilation of the distal pancreatic and common bile ducts is evident on endoscopic retrograde cholangiopancreatography; this is highly suggestive of adenocarcinoma affecting the head of the pancreas.

the "double-duct sign"—is highly suggestive of adenocarcinoma affecting the head of the pancreas (Figure 17-5). Data summarized from 16 studies suggest that ERCP has a sensitivity of 92% and a specificity of 96% for diagnosing pancreatic cancer. Bile aspiration for cytologic evaluation and tissue sampling by biopsy and ductal brushing can also be performed at the time of ERCP. Biliary decompression can also be achieved at ERCP if a tumor has been deemed unresectable or if a patient with symptomatic biliary obstruction will have a delay before resection. Multiple studies have failed to show a benefit from routine preoperative biliary decompression, and some studies have shown increased operative morbidity related to infectious complications.

In addition to radiographic and endoscopic assessment, laparoscopy has been proposed as an accurate means of evaluation for resectability before laparotomy. Evaluation begins with a thorough inspection of the abdomen, including the liver and the peritoneal surfaces. Any suspicious nodules should be biopsied for histological assessment. Metastatic disease not identified by spiral CT can be detected in as many as 30% of patients undergoing the laparoscopic staging of pancreatic cancer. The addition of laparoscopic ultrasonography to evaluate for intrahepatic and lymph-node metastasis, as well as for unrecognized vascular invasion, may further alter the management of additional patients.

Because of the limitations of detecting very early pancreatic cancers, the development of a biological marker that could detect these early lesions may translate into decreased mortality. Although many tumor markers have been investigated, currently none exists with acceptable specificity either for the confirmation of pancreatic adenocarcinoma in equivocal cases or for routine screening.

CA 19-9 is presently the most widely used serum marker for pancreatic cancer. CA 19-9 is a sialylated Lewis(a) antigen that is associated with circulating mucins, and it is expressed in normal pancreatic, biliary, and gastric epithelial cells. Although it is most frequently elevated in pancreatic adenocarcinoma, it may also be expressed in biliary, gastric, and colonic malignancies as well as acute and chronic pancreatitis, hepatitis, and biliary obstruction. Marked elevations are found in acute cholangitis and hepatic cirrhosis. The reported sensitivities and specificities of CA 19-9 for diagnosing pancreatic adenocarcinoma are related to the serum cutoff level selected. A cutoff of 15 U/mL produces a sensitivity of 92% and a specificity of 60%, whereas a cutoff of 1000 U/mL yields a sensitivity of 40% and a specificity of 99%. When using the usual cutoff of 37 U/mL, combined studies have shown a sensitivity of 81% to 85% and a specificity of 81% to 90%.Carcineoembryonic antigen (CEA) is commonly used as a serum marker for colon cancer, and it has been investigated as a marker for pancreatic adenocarcinoma; however, its sensitivity and specificity from combined studies is 58% and 75%, respectively. A higher diagnostic accuracy of 83% is observed when measuring CEA levels in pancreatic juice rather than serum. The oncogene *K-ras* is mutated in more than 90% of pancreatic adenocarcinomas, and it can be detected in the pancreatic juice from 55% to 77% of these patients. Several reports retrospectively examining pancreatic juice specimens from patients subsequently diagnosed with pancreatic adenocarcinoma have suggested that screening for *K-ras* mutations may be effective for the early detection of pancreatic cancer; however, its utility is limited by the finding that *K-ras* mutations are also present in some cases of chronic pancreatitis. Whether K-*ras* mutations in the setting of chronic pancreatitis predicts those who are at increased risk for developing pancreatic adenocarcinoma is currently unknown.

In some cases, even after multiple diagnostic modalities have been applied, it is still impossible to differentiate pancreatic adenocarcinoma from some other inflammatory process (often chronic pancreatitis) before laparotomy. In these instances—particularly when a pancreatic mass is identified in the setting of antecedent chronic pancreatitis—a tissue diagnosis is not necessary before resection. Although this approach risks overtreating a benign process, the greater concern is undertreating a potentially curable malignancy.

Management

Surgical Treatment

Approximately 20% of pancreatic tumors are resectable at the time of diagnosis, with 40% being unresectable because of local vascular invasion and 40% being unresectable because of metastatic disease. Currently, the only potential cure for pancreatic adenocarcinoma is surgical resection. Because lesions originating in the head and uncinate process of the pancreas obstruct the bile duct and cause jaundice, they tend to present at an earlier stage and to have a higher resectability rate than cancers in the tail and body. The uncommon lesion in the pancreatic body or tail that is resectable may be treated by distal or subtotal pancreatectomy and splenectomy, whereas pancreatic head and uncinate lesions are treated by pancreaticoduodenectomy. The survival rates for patients with body and tail cancers are similar to those with lesions located in the head or uncinate process when compared stage for stage.

Although survival rates after pancreaticoduodenectomy are approximately 25% at 5 years with negative margins of resection, given the low postoperative mortality of 1% to 4 % and the chance for cure, most patients with resectable disease and no prohibitive comorbidities undergo this operation. The procedure involves the division of either the distal stomach, in the classic Whipple operation, or the proximal duodenum 2 cm to 3 cm distal to the pylorus in the pylorus-preserving modification, with en bloc resection of the distal common bile duct and the involved portion of the pancreas, along with the duodenum to the ligament of Treitz (Figure 17-6). Reconstruction consists of pancreatic, biliary, and either gastroenteric or duodenoenteric anastomoses, usually in that anatomic order (see Figure 17-6). Typically, the proximal jejunum is used to reestablish pancreatic-enteric continuity, although the stomach is preferred by some surgeons, with roughly equivalent results.

Although this formidable operation involves many technical challenges, a few deserve emphasis. Although preoperative imaging may show a clear margin between the tumor and the underlying vasculature, because of the intense desmoplastic reaction characteristic of pancreatic adenocarcinoma, there may be dense adherence of the pancreas to these vessels, thereby making dissection difficult. In addition, among patients who have not developed biliary obstruction or who have been decompressed preoperatively, the distal common hepatic duct may be small, thereby making its anastomosis with the jejunum challenging. Also, in the

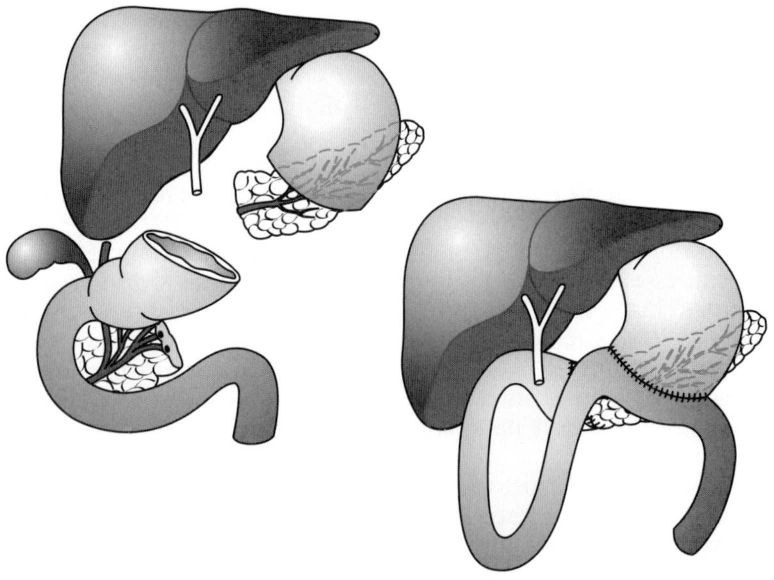

Figure 17-6. Resection specimen from Whipple procedure and reconstruction.

absence of significant pancreatic duct obstruction, this structure may be diminutive, thus posing a similar technical challenge.

Several important controversies surround the technical aspects of this operation. In Whipple's original description, the stomach was transected proximal to the antrum, whereas in the pylorus-preserving modification, the duodenum is transected 2 cm to 3 cm distal to the pylorus. The more extensive gastric resection was performed not only on oncologic grounds but also to reduce the acid burden and subsequent incidence of marginal ulceration. Pylorus preservation maintains normal gastrointestinal physiology, specifically in terms of acid production, the gastric reservoir, emptying functions, and hormone secretion. The rates of early postoperative delayed gastric emptying are similar for the two procedures, and pyloric preservation shortens operative time and is associated with no adverse early or late sequelae.

BOX 17-6 PANCREATICODUODENECTOMY CONTROVERSIES

- Pylorus-preserving versus pylorus-sparing approach
- Extent of retroperitoneal lymphadenectomy
- Superior mesenteric vein/portal vein resection for adherent tumor

The extent of peripancreatic lymph-node dissection is also the source of some controversy. The extended or radical pancreaticoduodenectomy entails en bloc wide retroperitoneal lymphadenectomy and often resection of the superior mesenteric vein–portal vein confluence, along with the tumor. Arguments that favor this approach claim improved resectability and cure rates; however, recent trials have failed to show a significant survival advantage for an extended pancreatic resection. In addition, any potential oncologic advantage associated with a radical pancreaticoduodenectomy would be negated by increased morbidity. Total pancreatectomy has been advocated by some as definitive therapy for pancreatic cancer based on the increased incidence of multicentric disease and complications resulting form the pancreatic-enteric anastomosis. However, neither of these factors justify the additional operative morbidity and lifelong insulin dependence that results from total pancreatectomy. Total pancreatectomy is only potentially justified if there is residual tumor at the pancreatic margin or if the pancreas is not suitable for anastomosis.

Tumor adherence to the lateral wall of the superior mesenteric vein (SMV) or the superior mesenteric-portal vein (SMPV) confluence has been accepted by many as a contraindication to resection with curative intent because of the presumption that a negative margin could not be achieved. However, this presumption has been challenged by those who advocate the resection of the SMV or SMPV confluence to achieve a negative margin. What is clear from studies in which patients underwent venous resection to achieve cure is that, although it is technically challenging, it is not associated with either greater perioperative morbidity or mortality or with a prognosis that is different than that of patients undergoing standard pancreaticoduodenectomy. In contrast with tumor invasion of the superior mesenteric artery, in which there is usually involvement of the mesenteric neural plexus (thereby making a negative retroperitoneal margin impossible to achieve), involvement of the SMV or SMPV confluence seems to be more a function of tumor location than innate biologic aggressiveness. Thus, the efficacy of venous resection is an increase in the number of patients who are candidates for a potentially curative resection, with outcomes similar to those patients without venous involvement.

Although operative mortality rates associated with pancreaticoduodenectomy are typically 1% to 4%, up to half of the patients undergoing this operation will experience a complication. Approximately 30% of patients undergoing a pancreaticoduodenectomy will experience delayed gastric emptying, which is thought to be related to decreased motilin levels, the removal of the duodenal pacemaker, and the disruption of gastroduodenal neural connections or to result from intra-abdominal complications, such as abscess or fistula development. Erythromycin, which is a motilin agonist, has been found to improve the gastric emptying of both solids and liquids when administered intravenously during the postoperative period.

BOX 17-7 COMMON MAJOR COMPLICATIONS OF PANCREATICODUODENECTOMY

- Delayed gastric emptying
- Pancreatic fistula
- Intra-abdominal abscess

Pancreatic fistula resulting from a failure of healing at the pancreatic–enteric anastomosis with subsequent intraperitoneal leakage of pancreatic secretions can usually be managed conservatively if there is no evidence of abdominal sepsis. Isolated fluid collections should be drained (percutaneously, if possible), and the patient should remain without oral intake, with nutrition provided parenterally. Intraoperatively, a drain is usually placed in the vicinity of the pancreatic-enteric anastomosis, and it should be maintained as the fistula is allowed to heal. The somatostatin analogue octreotide does not appear to shorten the duration of pancreatic fistulae nor does it appear to confer any benefit in terms of pancreatic fistula formation or overall morbidity or mortality when administered prophylactically.

Intra-abdominal abscesses can result from leakage at the pancreatic-enteric, gastroenteric or hepatoenteric anastomoses. Patients with evidence of systemic infection should be evaluated for an intra-abdominal abscess, and the collection drained, preferably percutaneously, with the initiation of appropriate antibiotics. In addition, hepatoenteric anastomotic leaks may require a transhepatic catheter to allow for external biliary drainage.

Palliation of Unresectable Pancreatic Adenocarcinoma

At the time of diagnosis, 80% of patients are not candidates for potentially curative resection. The majority of patients diagnosed with pancreatic adenocarcinoma will experience one or more of its complications, including biliary obstruction, gastric outlet obstruction, and severe abdominal pain. With improvements in determining preoperatively the resectability of pancreatic cancer, fewer patients undergo exploratory laparotomy, during which palliative procedures are performed. Palliation of the complications of pancreatic cancer may be achieved nonsurgically, in most cases.

Up to 70% of patients with pancreatic cancer will develop obstructive jaundice and accompanying pruritus, with an increased risk of cholangitis. In patients who are deemed unresectable intraoperatively, a biliary–enteric bypass may be performed for decompression. Hepatico- and choledochojejunostomy are the preferred procedures, because cholecystoenterostomy is associated with a rate of recurrent jaundice of 20%.

For patients who are deemed unresectable who do not undergo an operation, endoscopic or transhepatic radiographic placement of a biliary stent may be accomplished. The mortality and early morbidity rates after endoscopic biliary stent placement are similar or slightly less than those following surgical treatment, and the length of hospital stay is less with endoscopic palliation; however, surgical biliary decompression is associated with a longer rate of patency. Radiographically placed transhepatic catheters with exclusive external biliary drainage result in large fluid and electrolyte losses, and they are less desirable for the palliation of obstructive jaundice in patients with pancreatic cancer. This procedure is reserved for patients who fail internal endoscopic drainage. Biliary decompression before planned resection should be limited to cases with severe symptoms of obstructive jaundice in which surgery is delayed.

BOX 17–8 PALLIATIVE OPTIONS

Biliary obstruction
- Biliary-enteric bypass
- Endoscopic biliary stent placement
- Radiographic transhepatic stent placement

Gastric outlet obstruction
- Gastroenteric bypass
- Endoscopically placed duodenal stents

Abdominal pain
- Chemical splanchnicectomy

Chemoradiation

Gastric outlet obstruction from duodenal compression will affect up to 25% of patients with pancreatic cancer, and it may require surgical gastric bypass for palliation. Controversy exists regarding whether patients who are deemed unresectable at exploratory laparotomy should undergo a prophylactic gastroenteric bypass. Proponents cite the higher mortality rate, which approaches 25%, for patients requiring a second operation for the palliation of gastric outlet obstruction after exploratory laparotomy as well as no increase in mortality when gastric bypass is performed at the initial operation. Increased morbidity associated with gastric bypass (most notably delayed gastric emptying), increased hospital stay, and overestimation of the need for gastric bypass at the time of exploration are cited by its opponents. Clearly, any patient with radiographically confirmed gastric-outlet obstruction associated with pancreatic adenocarcinoma should undergo some form of palliation; currently, that is either gastroenterostomy using either an open or laparoscopic technique or endoscopically deployed duodenal stents. The experience with duodenal stents in this setting is increasing, and the data are promising; this suggests outcomes that are at least as good as—and potentially superior to—surgical gastroenterostomy, with a shorter postprocedure hospital stay and a decreased period of time before a regular diet can be resumed after the procedure.

Severe and debilitating abdominal and back pain are frequent complications of pancreatic adenocarcinoma, often requiring significant analgesia for adequate palliation. Chemical splanchnicectomy with 50% ethanol, performed either at the time of exploration or subsequently through the percutaneous route, has been shown to effectively palliate the pain associated with pancreatic adenocarcinoma, although its duration is limited. When performed intraoperatively, this procedure has not been accompanied by increases in morbidity, mortality, return to oral intake, or length of hospital stay.

For the 80% of patients deemed unresectable, palliative chemoradiation has been shown to increase survival and to possibly reduce the severity of pain as compared with untreated patients. In 1981, the Gastrointestinal Tumor Study Group published results of a trial in which patients who had been surgically staged to confirm unresectability and who had no evidence of peritoneal or liver metastases were randomized to receive either external beam radiation alone or external beam radiation with 5-fluorouracil (5-FU). Patients treated with chemoradiation fared better in terms of median survival (49 weeks) than those who received radiation alone (22 weeks).

A recent advance in the chemotherapeutic regimen to treat pancreatic adenocarcinoma is the use of gemcitabine, a potent radiosensitizer. Gemcitabine has been shown to improve survival as compared with 5-FU, with reported 1-year survival rates of 18% and 2%, respectively. In addition, gemcitabine appears to confer clinical benefit in terms of decreased pain intensity and analgesic consumption, with improvement in overall functional status.

Neoadjuvant Therapy

The observation that 25% to 30% of patients do not receive adjuvant therapy after pancreatic resection as a result of prolonged recovery, perioperative complications, or patient refusal has led to the investigation of preoperative chemoradiation. In addition to increasing the number of patients able to complete multimodality therapy, neoadjuvant therapy has been studied for its ability to convert locally unresectable pancreatic cancer to resectable disease. Other advantages of this modality include delivering radiation therapy to well-oxygenated cells not devascularized by surgery, reducing tumor dissemination during surgical manipulation, and targeting retroperitoneal margins of excision that may not be adequately treated surgically. Also, preoperative chemoradiation would allow an interval window for restaging before surgical resection so that previously occult metastatic disease could be detected, thus saving patients an unnecessary laparotomy. The utility of this approach is currently under intense investigation.

BOX 17-9 POTENTIAL ADVANTAGES OF NEOADJUVANT THERAPY

- Increased number of patients able to complete treatment regimen
- Decreased delay of treatment initiation
- Conversion of locally unresectable to resectable disease
- More effective radiation delivery to vascularized tissues
- Reduced tumor dissemination at the time of surgery
- Targeting retroperitoneal margins
- Provide a window of time to assess the biologic aggressiveness of the patient's individual cancer

Adjuvant Therapy for Resectable Pancreatic Adenocarcinoma

The basis for adjuvant therapy after surgical resection with negative margins comes from a Gastrointestinal Tumor Study Group study that showed a median survival of nearly twice as long for patients treated postoperatively with radiation and concurrent 5-FU as compared with those randomized to observation alone (20 versus 11 months, respectively). Single-institution studies investigating the benefit of postoperative chemoradiation as compared with observation have also shown a survival benefit. However, other studies, including the European Organization for Research and Treatment of

Cancer Trial, have shown no difference in survival after resection for those patients undergoing radiotherapy and 5-FU as compared with those receiving no further treatment. Although it is clear that a set of patients do benefit from combined-modality treatment after resection, the characteristics of those patients are yet to be defined. Given the abysmal prognosis for pancreatic cancer, even among those with a presumed curative resection, the trend has been to treat all patients who are candidates for chemoradiation with the intent of improving survival in at least some patients. Until either more efficacious agents are discovered or the select group of patients who will clearly benefit from the current regimen is defined, it is likely that postoperative adjuvant therapy will remain the recommendation for all patients who are candidates.

Cystic Pancreatic Neoplasms

In addition to the relatively more common solid pancreatic tumor, approximately 1% of pancreatic neoplasms are cystic, with the three most common being serous cystic neoplasms, mucinous cystic neoplasms, and intraductal papillary mucinous neoplasms (Table 17-3). Serous cystic neoplasms and mucinous cystic neoplasms have a mean age at presentation of 50 years, with a 4:1 female predominance. By contrast, patients with intraductal papillary mucinous neoplasms have a mean age of 65 years at presentation, with a slight male predominance. Additionally, most patients with serous cystic neoplasms and mucinous cystic neoplasms are asymptomatic, and the lesion is discovered incidentally, whereas most patients with intraductal papillary mucinous neoplasms present with symptoms similar to patients with adenocarcinoma, such as abdominal pain, jaundice, weight loss, and malaise, particularly if the tumor is invasive.

Differentiating between serous cystic neoplasms and mucinous cystic and intraductal papillary mucinous neoplasms can pose a clinical challenge, because the management of the former differs from the management of the latter two. Preoperatively, cystic neoplasms can be differentiated in many cases on the basis of radiographic, endoscopic, and ultrasonographic features. Serous cystic neoplasms occur most often in the body and tail of the pancreas, and they are composed of multiple small cysts less than 2 cm in diameter, 30% of which contain a pathognomonic central fibrous scar with a stellate pattern of calcification. Similarly, mucinous cystic neoplasms occur predominantly in the body and tail of the pancreas; however, in contrast with serous cystic neoplasms, they are macrocystic in 80% of cases, usually measuring 4 cm to 5 cm in diameter. Furthermore, mucinous cystic neoplasms have thick, irregular walls, and they are marked by a complex internal architecture

TABLE 17–3 • *Characteristics of Cystic Pancreatic Neoplasms*

	Serous Cystic Neoplasms	Mucinous Cystic Neoplasms	Intraductal Papillary Mucinous Neoplasms
Demographics	Mean age at presentation, 50 years; 4:1 female-to-male predominance	Mean age at presentation, 50 years; 4:1 female-to-male predominance	Mean age at presentation, 65 years; slight male predominance
Presentation	Commonly asymptomatic	Commonly asymptomatic	Commonly presents with abdominal pain, jaundice, weight loss, and malaise
Radiographic features	Microcystic or honeycomb appearance	Macrocystic, with thickened walls	Mixed macrocystic and microcystic; dilated pancreatic duct
Treatment	May be managed conservatively with serial imaging if asymptomatic; resect if symptomatic or if lesion cannot be differentiated from a potentially malignant cystic neoplasm	30–35% rate of invasive cancer; formal resection required	35–50% rate of invasive cancer; formal resection required
Prognosis	Essentially benign; resection is curative	Resection is curative if no invasive component; 15% to 30% 5-year survival for invasive lesions	Overall 5-year survival, 60% to 70%; less than 50% 5-year survival for invasive lesions

with papillary excrescences extending into the cysts; this is best appreciated ultrasonographically. This feature may allow for the differentiation of mucinous cystic neoplasms from serous cystic neoplasms. Calcifications, when present in mucinous cystic neoplasms, tend to be located within the peripheral cyst walls in an egg-shell distribution, and they are associated with an increased likelihood of invasive mucinous cystadenocarcinoma.

In contrast with serous cystic neoplasms and mucinous cystic neoplasms, which do not communicate directly with the pancreatic duct, intraductal papillary mucinous neoplasms communicate with and cause dilation of either the main pancreatic duct or a primary segmental side branch. As such, ERCP is the gold standard for the diagnosis of intraductal papillary mucinous neoplasms, demonstrating communication between the cystic tumor and the main pancreatic duct. Additionally, intraductal papillary mucinous neoplasms occur in the head of the pancreas in 60% to 75% of cases, although they may arise from the tail or show diffuse pancreatic involvement. Although tumors involving the main pancreatic duct and those with an intraductal tumor of more than 10 mm in diameter are often malignant, the reliable differentiation of malignant from benign intraductal papillary mucinous neoplasms is virtually impossible before histologic study.

Although endoscopic ultrasonography allows for the sampling of fluid from cystic neoplasms for cytological and biochemical analysis, the specificity of these evaluations is as of yet not great enough to make a definitive diagnosis in every case. However, a positive stain for mucin and a CEA concentration of more than 250 ng/mL can reliably differentiate mucinous cystic neoplasms from serous neoplasms. Furthermore, cystic fluid analysis can differentiate benign pancreatic pseudocysts from cystic neoplasms. In the setting of antecedent acute pancreatitis, a demarcated, unilocular cyst containing fluid with increased amylase or lipase activity is virtually diagnostic of a pancreatic pseudocyst.

The most reliable predictor of prognosis for cystic pancreatic neoplasms is the presence or absence of invasive adenocarcinoma. Whereas all mucinous cystic neoplasms and intraductal papillary mucinous neoplasms require resection based on a high incidence of invasiveness—30% to 35% for mucinous cystic neoplasms and 35% to 50% for intraductal papillary mucinous neoplasms—serous cystic neoplasms rarely contain an invasive component, and they can be managed expectantly with serial imaging. The indications for the resection of serous cystic neoplasms include an inability to distinguish them from mucinous cystic neoplasms and intraductal papillary mucinous neoplasms as well as gastrointestinal symptoms, such as jaundice and pain as a result of a mass effect. When indicated, the resection of serous cystic lesions should be limited, and it is curative. Mucinous cystic neoplasms and intraductal papillary mucinous neoplasms should be resected in a way similar to that of solid adenocarcinoma: pancreaticoduodenectomy for lesions involving the pancreatic head and distal pancreatectomy with splenectomy for body and tail lesions. Complete resection is curative for mucinous cystic neoplasms that do not have an invasive component. For invasive mucinous cystic neoplasms, the 5-year survival rate is approximately 15% to 30%. Because it is unclear whether intraductal papillary mucinous neoplasms represent a localized process or a field defect with the potential to affect all of the pancreatic ductal epithelium, the extent of resection is somewhat more controversial. What is clear is that, after localized resection, the distal margin should be analyzed by frozen section, and, if neoplastic cells are present, the resection should be extended, including total pancreatectomy if the patient is a suitable candidate. Overall 5-year survival rates for intraductal papillary mucinous neoplasms average 60% to 70%. In the presence of invasive cancer, even with negative margins of resection, the 5-year survival rate falls to less than 50%.

Key Selected Reading

Von Hoff D, Evans DB, Hruban RH, eds. *Pancreatic cancer.* Boston, MA: Jones & Bartlett Publishers, 2005.

Selected Readings

Barkin J, Goldstein J. Diagnostic approach to pancreatic cancer. *Gastroenterol Clin North Am* 1999;28:709–722.

Brugge WR, Lauwers GY, Sahani D, *et al.* Cystic neoplasms of the pancreas. *N Engl J Med* 2004;351: 1218–1226.

Chu QD, Khushalani N, Javle MM, *et al.* Should adjuvant therapy remain the standard of care for patients with resected adenocarcinoma of the pancreas? *Ann Surg Oncol* 2003;10:539–545.

Chua YJ, Cunningham D. Adjuvant treatment for resectable pancreatic cancer. *J Clin Oncol* 2005;23: 4532–4537.

Evans D. Preoperative chemoradiation for resectable and locally advanced adenocarcinoma of the pancreas. *J Gastrointest Surg* 2001;5:2–5.

Garofalo MC, Kwok Y, Regine WF. The evolving role of postoperative adjuvant radiation therapy for pancreatic cancer. *Surg Oncol Clin N Am* 2004;13:589–604.

Gold E. Epidemiology of and risk factors for pancreatic cancer. *Surg Clin North Am* 1995;75:819–843.

Hruban R, Iacobuzio-Donahue C, Wilentz R, *et al.* Molecular pathology of pancreatic cancer. *Cancer J* 2001;7:251–258.

Jimenez R, Warshaw A, Rattner D, *et al.* Impact of laparoscopic staging in the treatment of pancreatic cancer. *Arch Surg* 2000;135:409–415.

Kern S, Hruban R, Hollingsworth M, *et al.* A white paper: the product of a pancreas cancer think tank. *Cancer Res* 2001;61:4923–4932.

Kleef J, Michalski C, Friess H, Buchler MW. Pancreatic cancer: from bench to 5-year survival. *Pancreas* 2006;33:111–118.

Leach SD, Lee JE, Charnsangavej C, *et al.* Survival following pancreaticoduodenectomy with resection of the superior mesenteric-portal vein confluence for adenocarcinoma of the pancreatic head. *Br J Surg* 1998;85:611–617.

Li D, Xie K, Wolff R, Abbruzzese JL. Pancreatic cancer. *Lancet* 2004;363:1049–1057.

McGinn C, Zalupski M. Combined-modality therapy in pancreatic cancer: current status and future directions. *Cancer J* 2001;7:338–348.

Povoski S, Karpeh M, Conlon K, *et al.* Association of preoperative biliary drainage with postoperative outcome following pancreaticoduodenectomy. *Ann Surg* 1999;230:131–142.

Sener S, Fremgen A, Menck H, Winchester D. Pancreatic cancer: a report of treatment and survival trends for 100,313 patients diagnosed from 1985-1995, using the National Cancer Database. *J Am Coll Surg* 1999;189:1–7.

Siriwardana HPP, Siriwardena AK. Systematic review of outcome of synchronous portal-superior mesenteric vein resection during pancreatectomy for cancer. *Br J Surg* 2006;93:662–673.

Sohn T, Lillemoe K, Cameron J, *et al.* Surgical palliation of unresectable periampullary adenocar cinoma in the 1990s. *J Am Coll Surg* 1999; 188:658–666.

Spanknebel K, Conlon K. Advances in the surgical management of pancreatic cancer. *Cancer J* 2001;7: 312–323.

18

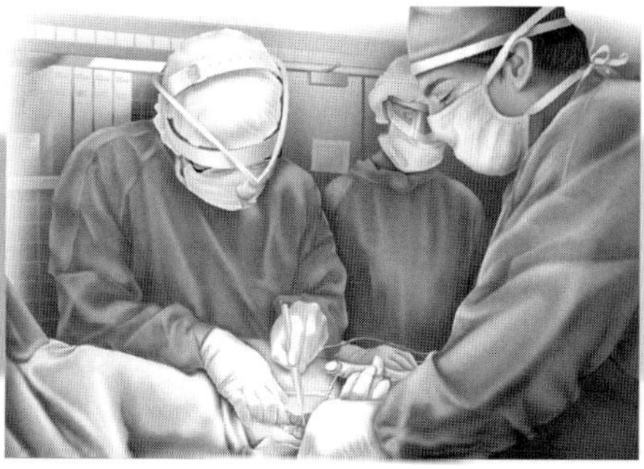

Hepatobiliary Cancer

Derek A. DuBay and Alfred E. Chang

Hepatobiliary Cancer: Key Points

- Describe the anatomic characteristics of the liver.
- List the risk factors for hepatocellular carcinoma (HCC).
- Outline the laboratory investigations used to diagnose and stage HCC.
- Compare the imaging options for HCC.
- Discuss the principal treatment options for HCC and how to determine which patients will benefit.
- Explain the alternative therapies possible for HCC patients.
- List the risk factors for cholangiocarcinoma.
- Discuss the laboratory investigations used to diagnose and stage cholangiocarcinoma.
- Compare the imaging modalities used to assess cholangiocarcinoma.
- Describe the treatment options for cholangiocarcinoma.

Surgical Anatomy of the Liver

The hepatic artery, the portal vein, and the bile duct maintain a close intrahepatic and extrahepatic anatomic relationship, and they are collectively referred to as a *portal pedicle*. The main portal pedicle divides into right and left lobar branches at the portal hepatis, and these then divide into segmental branches within the hepatic parenchyma. There are eight hepatic segments, each with distinct arterial, portal venous, and biliary supplies and segmental systemic venous drainage; these coalesce to form the main hepatic veins (Figure 18-1). A three-dimensional understanding of hepatic segmental anatomy is crucial for formal hepatic resections.

Grossly, the liver is divided into a right and left lobe by an imaginary line drawn between the gallbladder bed and the vena cava. The left lobe is further divided by the falciform ligament into the left medial and left lateral segments, whereas the right lobe is divided into anterior and posterior segments, although this boundary is not evident grossly (Figure 18-2). The hepatic veins run between the individual segments and separate the liver into four areas. The right hepatic vein divides segments six and seven (right posterior) from segments five and eight (right anterior). The middle hepatic vein divides segments five and eight from segment four (left medial). Finally, the left hepatic vein separates segment four from segments two and three (left lateral).

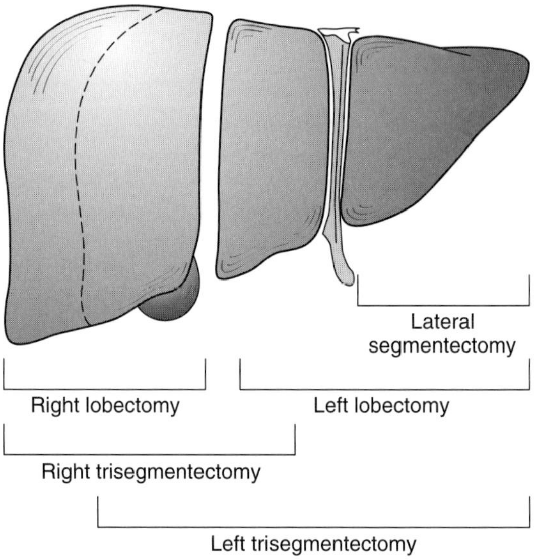

Figure 18-2. Gross hepatic anatomy illustrating the surgical hepatic lobes and formal margins of hepatic resections. The dotted line represents the boundary between the right anterior (segments V and VIII) and the right posterior (segments VI and VII) portions of the right lobe, corresponding with the position of the right hepatic vein.

There are several common hepatic arterial variations (Table 18-1). "Normal" anatomy is present 67% of the time. In about 12% of cases, there is a trifurcation of the gastroduodenal, right hepatic, and left hepatic arteries

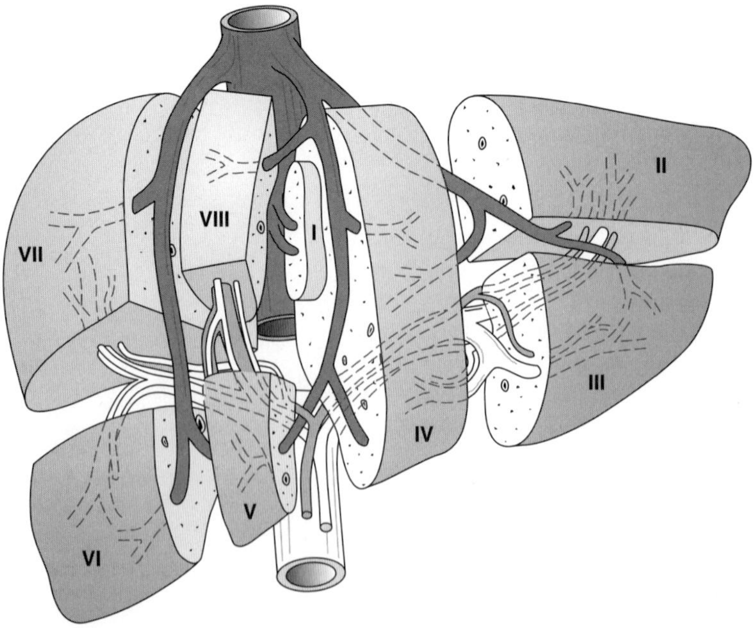

Figure 18-1. Schematic diagram of the hepatic segment anatomy based on the vasculobiliary structures that supply the liver parenchyma. (Reproduced with permission from Fan MH, Chang AE. Resection of liver tumors: technical aspects. *Surg Oncol* 2002;10: 139–152.)

TABLE 18-1 • *Hepatic Arterial Anatomy Variations*

Type	Percentage
1. Normal	66.5%
2. Replaced or accessory left hepatic artery	11.3%
3. Replaced or accessory right hepatic artery	14.9%
4. Combination of 2 and 3	1.7%
5. Common hepatic artery from superior mesenteric artery	1.9%
6. Other	3.8%

Adapted with permission from Skitzki JJ, Chang AE. Hepatic artery chemotherapy for colorectal liver metastases: technical considerations and review of clinical trials. *Surg Oncol* 2002;11:126. Table 1.

from a common point. The most common hepatic arterial anomalies include a replaced or accessory right hepatic artery arising from the superior mesenteric artery and a replaced or accessory left hepatic artery arising from the left gastric artery. Typical hepatic venous anatomy includes a single right vein, whereas the middle and left veins usually form a common trunk immediately before emptying into the vena cava. Hepatic venous variations are also common. An accessory right hepatic vein that drains segments six and/or seven as well as segmental veins that directly drain into the inferior vena cava are the most frequently encountered variations.

Hepatocellular Carcinoma

Epidemiology

Hepatocellular carcinoma (HCC) is the most frequent primary malignancy of the liver in adults. An estimated 350,000 new cases are diagnosed each year, making HCC one of the most common malignancies worldwide. More than two thirds of patients with HCC live in Asia. However, the incidence and mortality of hepatocellular carcinoma are rising sharply in Western cultures. Recent evidence suggests an 80% increase in the incidence of HCC in the United States, where approximately 15,000 new cases will occur each year. This increase has been attributed to the emergence of hepatitis C virus (HCV) infection as well as increased immigration from countries in which hepatitis B virus (HBV) infection is endemic.

Risk Factors

Male sex, age, cirrhosis, and certain metabolic diseases are the main epidemiological risk factors for the development of HCC. A 4:1 male-to-female ratio for HCC exists worldwide. With regard to age, there appears to be a lag period between the acquisition of risk factors and the subsequent development of cancer. HCC typically develops in elderly patients from Western countries as opposed to endemic Asian countries, where an earlier presentation is more common.

BOX 18-1 HEPATOCELLULAR CARCINOMA RISK FACTORS

- 4:1 male-to-female ratio
- Advanced age
- Cirrhosis
  - Chronic hepatitis B
  - Chronic hepatitis C
  - Alcoholic
- Metabolic diseases
  - Hemochromatosis
  - Tyrosinemia

The development of cirrhosis appears to be the most important risk factor associated with HCC. More than 80% of patients with HCC have cirrhosis, with the risk for HCC varying according to the etiology of the cirrhosis. Chronic infection with HBV is the most common cause of HCC worldwide. In the United States, however, more than half of HCC cases are the result of chronic HCV infection. Cirrhosis resulting from alcoholism is also a significant contributor to HCC, especially in the United States, where the incidence of chronic viral hepatitis is relatively low as compared with endemic Asian and African countries. Alcohol-related cirrhosis and HCV infection act synergistically, increasing the risk of HCC beyond what results from either risk factor alone.

Several metabolic diseases are also associated with an increased incidence of HCC, including hemochromatosis, Wilson's disease, glycogen storage disease, hereditary tyrosinemia, and α-1-antitrypsin disease.

Diagnosis and Staging

Patients with HCC usually have a history of HBV, HCV, alcoholic liver disease, or cirrhosis. Patients often present with advanced disease manifested clinically in right upper-quadrant pain referred to the right shoulder, abdominal fullness, early satiety, nausea, vomiting, jaundice, pruritus, or constitutional symptoms, such as weight loss and anorexia. On physical examination, scleral icterus, jaundice, firm nodular hepatomegaly, or palpable abdominal mass may be present. Signs of liver disease such as spider angioma, palmar erythema, gynecomastia, testicular atrophy, ascites, caput medusa, petechiae, or ecchymoses may also be detected.

The laboratory evaluation for patients with suspected HCC includes a complete blood cell count, a platelet count, basic chemistries, a liver panel, coagulation studies, hepatitis serologies, and the tumor marker α-fetoprotein. All patients should be staged with abdominal imaging and chest x-ray or CT scanning to evaluate for pulmonary metastases. Other imaging studies, such as a bone scan or a head CT, should only be obtained for related signs and symptoms.

Although a point of controversy, most hepatobiliary surgeons do not advocate preoperative biopsy when surgical resection is being contemplated. This is especially true when the clinical presentation makes the diagnosis of HCC likely. Biopsy may be obtained when the diagnosis is uncertain or to establish the diagnosis when unresectable disease is present. Alternatively, percutaneous biopsy of the unaffected liver may be obtained to evaluate for evidence of cirrhosis. Biopsy should be performed through a region of the liver that will be included in the planned resection. Existing coagulopathy must be corrected before biopsy.

HCC is staged according to the American Joint Committee on Cancer staging system (Table 18-2).

TABLE 18-2 • *American Joint Committee on Cancer TNM Staging System for Hepatocellular Carcinoma*

Tumor Size (T)			
T1	Solitary tumor without vascular invasion		
T2	Solitary tumor with vascular invasion or multiple tumors <5cm		
T3	Multiple tumors >5cm or tumor involving a major branch of the portal or hepatic vein		
T4	Tumor with direct invasion of adjacent organs other than the gallbladder or perforated tumor		
Regional Lymph Nodes (N)			
N0	No regional lymph node metastasis		
N1	Regional lymph node metastasis		
Distant Metastasis (M)			
N0	No distant metastasis		
N1	Distant metastasis		
Stage Grouping			
Stage	T	N	M
I	T1	N0	M0
II	T2	N0	M0
IIIA	T3	N0	M0
IIIB	T4	N0	M0
IIIC	Any T	N1	M0
IV	Any T	Any N	M1

Table adapted with the permission of the American Joint Committee on Cancer, Chicago. The original source for this material is the AJCC Cancer Staging Manual, 6th ed. New York: Springer-Verlag, 2002:133.

Screening

HCC is typically only curable if it is diagnosed and treated at an early stage. Most new cases of HCC develop within a defined population, thus prompting the development of diagnostic screening programs for patients with known chronic or active viral hepatitis in the setting of cirrhosis. Available screening strategies include periodic radiographic imaging or monitoring of HCC tumor-related serum proteins. The most popular screening protocol includes serial serum α-fetoprotein determination and hepatic ultrasonography at 3- to 12-month intervals. These screening programs

BOX 18-2 HEPATOCELLULAR CARCINOMA SCREENING PROTOCOL FOR HIGH-RISK PATIENTS

Rationale:

- Hepatocellular carcinoma is only curable if it is detected at an early stage. Aggressive screening programs detect the disease in up to 3–6% of patients with chronic active viral hepatitis and cirrhosis each year.

Screening Strategy:

- Serial sonographic studies every 6 months
- Serial serum α-fetoprotein levels

for HCC in Western cultures detect the development of HCC in about 3% to 6% of high-risk patients per year. Aggressive screening programs have been successful for detecting single, small HCCs, although this early detection surprisingly has not been accompanied by an increased overall resectability rate. Furthermore, it is unclear if screening improves patient survival, and the cost-effectiveness of these programs is in question.

Imaging Modalities

Aggressive surgical management of all liver lesions has paralleled the development of sensitive radiographic imaging. Historically, the main imaging modalities were radioisotope liver colloid scans and visceral angiography. Although occasionally used today to characterize a liver nodule, these modalities lack sensitivity for detecting small tumors; thus, they are not commonly employed for initial diagnostic purposes. Transcutaneous ultrasound examination has been used to detect the presence of liver tumors and to guide percutaneous biopsies or to direct percutaneous therapies. Ultrasound is also helpful when assessing for evidence of vascular invasion. This modality is readily available, low risk, and relatively inexpensive; thus, it is frequently employed as an initial diagnostic tool. Transcutaneous ultrasound is used almost universally in programs that screen high-risk patients for the development of HCC as outlined above. In this setting, serial ultrasound evaluations are more accurate for diagnosing the development of HCC than a single study in cirrhotic patients as a result of the overlapping sonographic appearance of benign nodules and small HCCs.

State-of-the-art abdominal CT scanning and magnetic resonance imaging (MRI) are the most sensitive diagnostic imaging procedures for HCC, especially tumors that are less than 2 cm in diameter. Refinements in CT scanning technique that facilitate rapid imaging after contrast administration and the development of protocols that take into account the increased vascularity of HCC have markedly improved tumor staging. HCC derives its blood supply predominately from the hepatic artery, whereas normal liver parenchyma and dysplastic nodules have mainly a portal venous supply. HCC lesions enhance 2 to 40 seconds after the administration of intravenous contrast material, during the "arterial phase" (Figure 18-3, *A*). By contrast, normal liver parenchyma and dysplastic nodules enhance 50 to 90 seconds after contrast administration, during the "portal venous phase" (Figure 18-3, *B*). Diagnostic hepatic CT imaging typically consists of a triphasic scan that includes imaging before the administration of contrast as well as during the arterial and portal venous phases. Triphasic imaging has significantly improved the sensitivity of the detection of small HCCs. A more-invasive CT protocol that is also based on the principle of hepatic arterial HCC blood supply is CT arterial portography. This involves hepatic imaging after the injection of contrast material directly into the celiac or hepatic arteries.

MRI is the most accurate imaging study to date for distinguishing between HCC, dysplastic nodules, and regenerative nodules (in contrast with CT scanning, which is considered more accurate for detecting hepatic colorectal

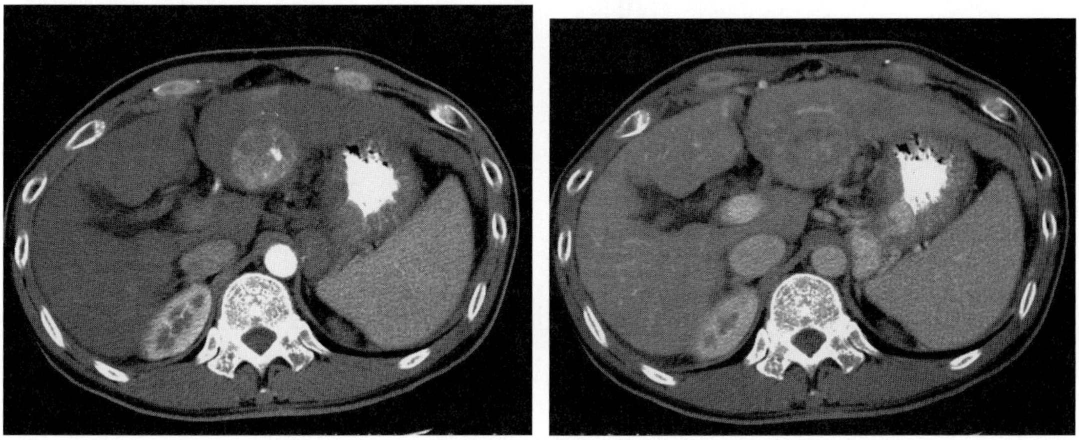

A B

Figure 18-3. Biphasic CT scan of hepatocellular carcinoma. **A,** Note the clear tumor demonstration during arterial phase enhancement. **B,** The tumor is relatively indistinct during the portal venous phase. (Courtesy of Dr. Isaac Francis, University of Michigan Department of Radiology, Ann Arbor, Mich.)

metastases). There appear to be unique signal characteristics for HCC, dysplastic nodules, and regenerative nodules. The typical appearance of HCC on MRI includes minimally hypointense signal as compared with normal parenchyma on T1-weighted imaging (Figure 18-4, *A*); hyperintense signal on T2-weighted imaging (Figure 18-4, *B*); brisk enhancement during the arterial phase (Figure 18-4, *C*); and hypointense signal with delayed imaging (Figure 18-4, *D*). By contrast, dysplastic nodules and regenerative nodules are isointense or hypointense on T2-weighted imaging. Additional MRI findings that are specific to HCC but that invariably present include the presence of intratumoral fat or a tumor capsule.

Management

Resection

Excluding hepatic transplantation, complete surgical extirpation offers the best 5-year survival rates for patients with HCC. Liver resection is the procedure of choice for all non-cirrhotic patients with technically resectable cancers without vascular invasion or extrahepatic disease. Many operative techniques have

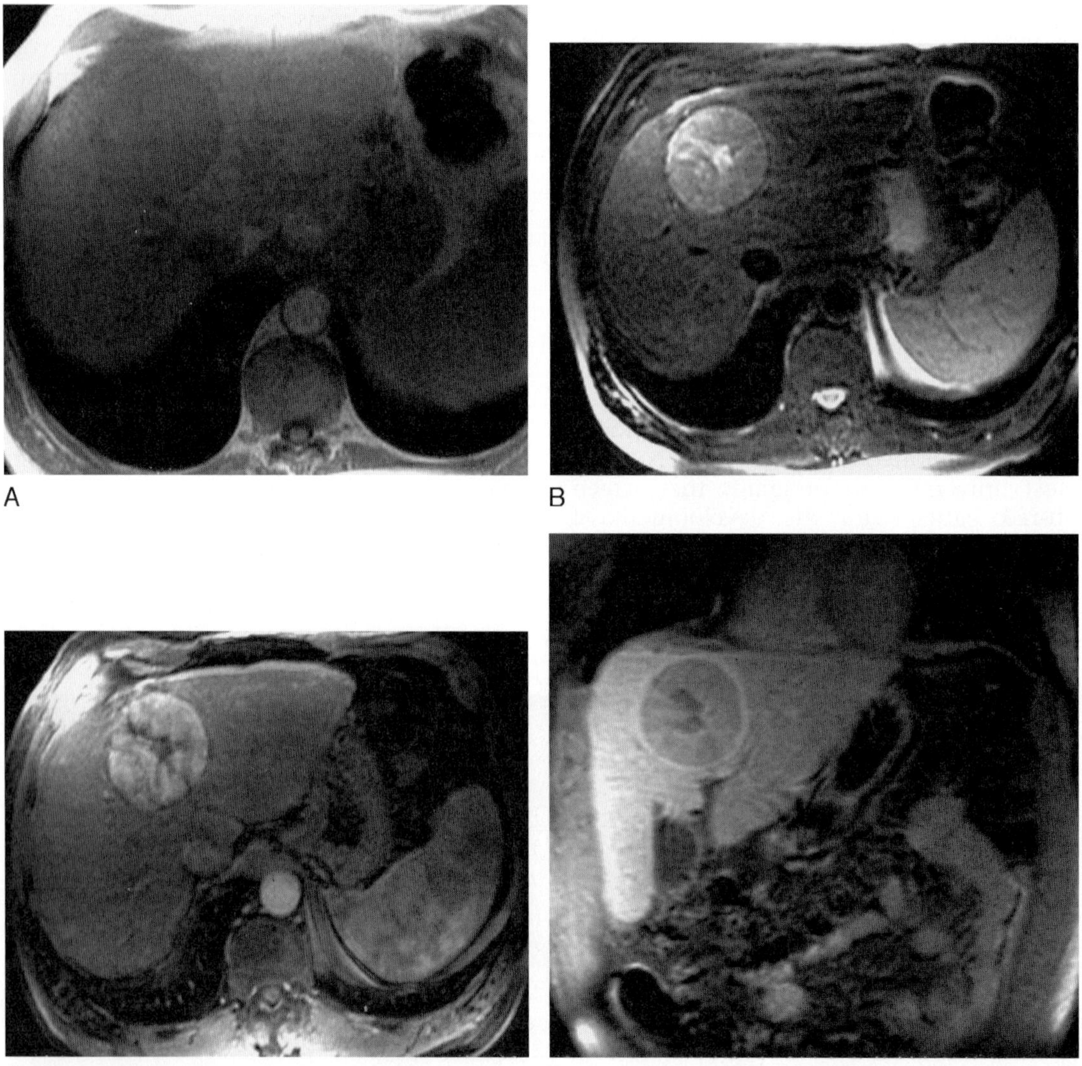

A B C D

Figure 18–4. Magnetic resonance imaging demonstrating the typical appearance of hepatocellular carcinoma. **A,** Minimally hypointense as compared with surrounding hepatic parenchyma on T1-weighted imaging. **B,** Hyperintense on T2-weighted imaging. **C,** Briskly enhances on arterial-phase imaging. **D,** Becomes hypointense on delayed-phase imaging. (Courtesy of Dr. Hero Hussain, University of Michigan Department of Radiology, Ann Arbor, Mich.)

been developed to facilitate safe tumor extirpation (Figure 18-5). However, more than 95% of all HCCs in patients in the Western world develop in the setting of cirrhosis, which limits the ability to perform major hepatic resection. Several studies have identified patient and tumor characteristics that predict successful outcomes after major hepatic resection. Only patients with well-compensated cirrhosis should be considered for major hepatectomy, because of the increased operative mortality and prohibitive postoperative fatal hepatic

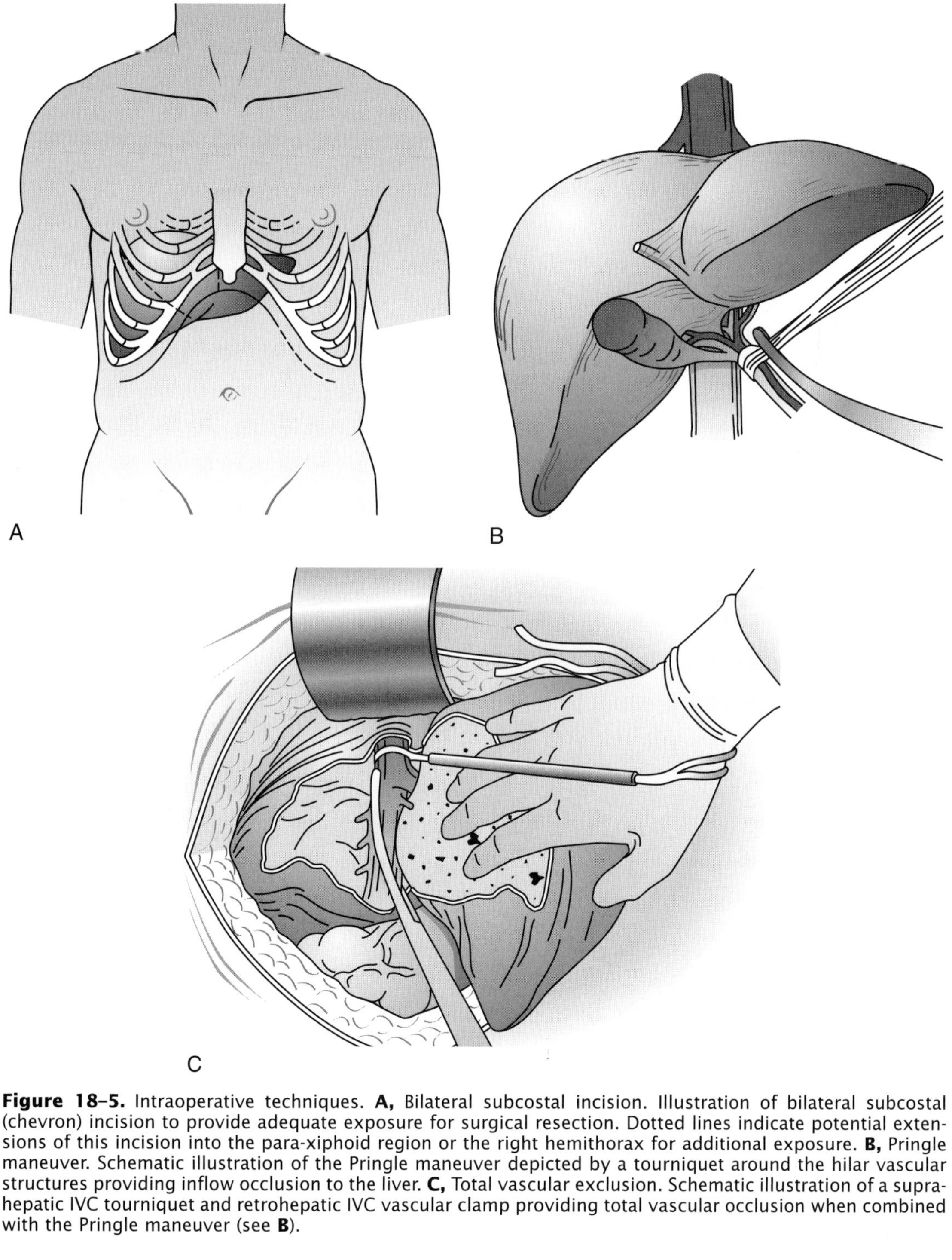

Figure 18-5. Intraoperative techniques. **A,** Bilateral subcostal incision. Illustration of bilateral subcostal (chevron) incision to provide adequate exposure for surgical resection. Dotted lines indicate potential extensions of this incision into the para-xiphoid region or the right hemithorax for additional exposure. **B,** Pringle maneuver. Schematic illustration of the Pringle maneuver depicted by a tourniquet around the hilar vascular structures providing inflow occlusion to the liver. **C,** Total vascular exclusion. Schematic illustration of a suprahepatic IVC tourniquet and retrohepatic IVC vascular clamp providing total vascular occlusion when combined with the Pringle maneuver (see **B**).

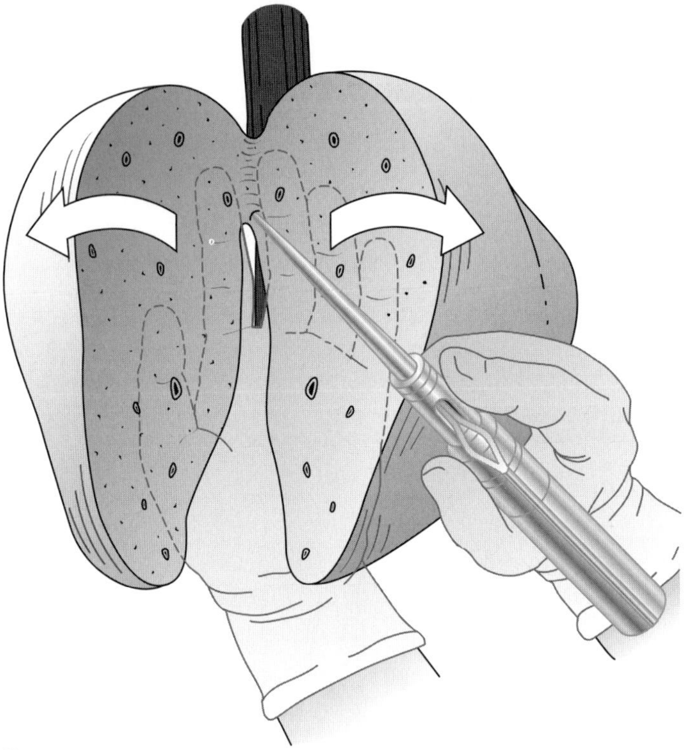

D

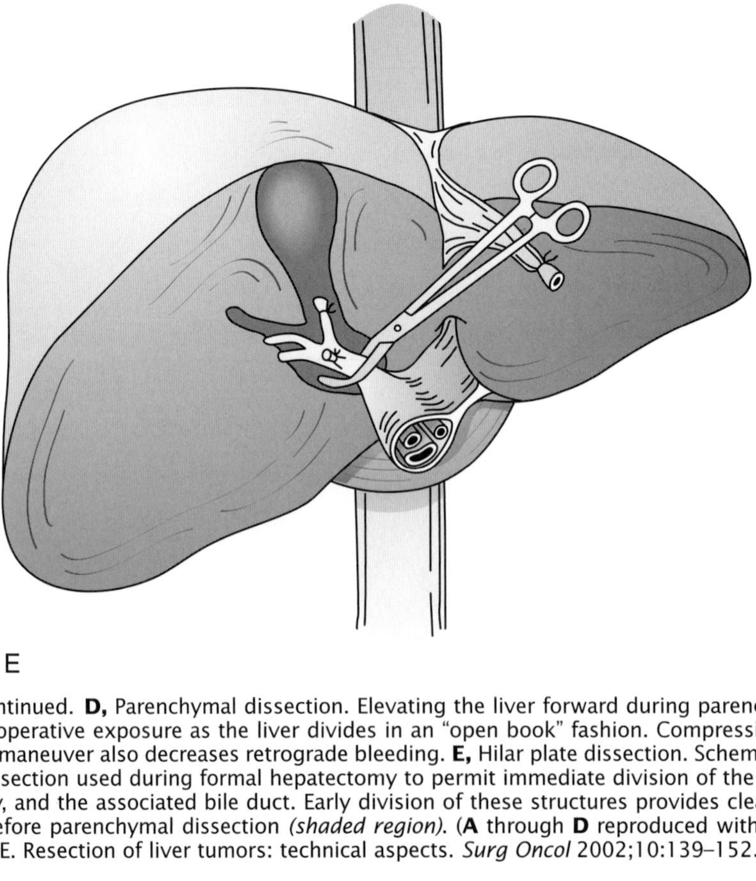

E

Figure 18–5 Continued. **D,** Parenchymal dissection. Elevating the liver forward during parenchymal dissection facilitates better operative exposure as the liver divides in an "open book" fashion. Compression of the hepatic veins during this maneuver also decreases retrograde bleeding. **E,** Hilar plate dissection. Schematic illustration of the hilar plate dissection used during formal hepatectomy to permit immediate division of the lobar portal vein, the hepatic artery, and the associated bile duct. Early division of these structures provides clear demarcation of lobar anatomy before parenchymal dissection *(shaded region)*. (**A** through **D** reproduced with permission from Fan MH, Chang AE. Resection of liver tumors: technical aspects. *Surg Oncol* 2002;10:139–152.)

decompensation associated with advanced cirrhosis (Figure 18-6). Functional tests have been described that specifically measure hepatic reserve (e.g., indocyanine green clearance, aminopyrine breath test, urea-nitrogen synthesis rate, galactose elimination capacity) in an attempt to define which patients are suitable for major hepatectomy. However, the most useful parameter is the Child-Turcotte-Pugh score, which considers several laboratory and clinical measurements of hepatic synthetic function, including serum albumin, coagulopathy, total bilirubin, and the presence of ascites and encephalopathy (Table 18-3). Child class A cirrhotic patients with solitary tumors of less than 5 cm and no evidence of vascular invasion or extrahepatic spread have 5-year survival rates in excess of 50%. Several recent series have further demonstrated that, with contemporary surgical technique and improved perioperative care, multiple tumors can be removed safely and large tumors approached with good surgical outcomes as long as complete tumor extirpation is achieved. Unfortunately, up to 8% of patients

BOX 18–3 RESECTION OF HEPATOCELLULAR CARCINOMA

Major hepatectomy is reserved for non-cirrhotic or Child class A cirrhotic patients. Patients with a single lesion of less than 5 cm who are completely resected have a 5-year survival rate of more than 50%. Portal and hepatic venous invasion, satellitosis, large tumor size, and advanced TNM stage are risk factors for local recurrence.

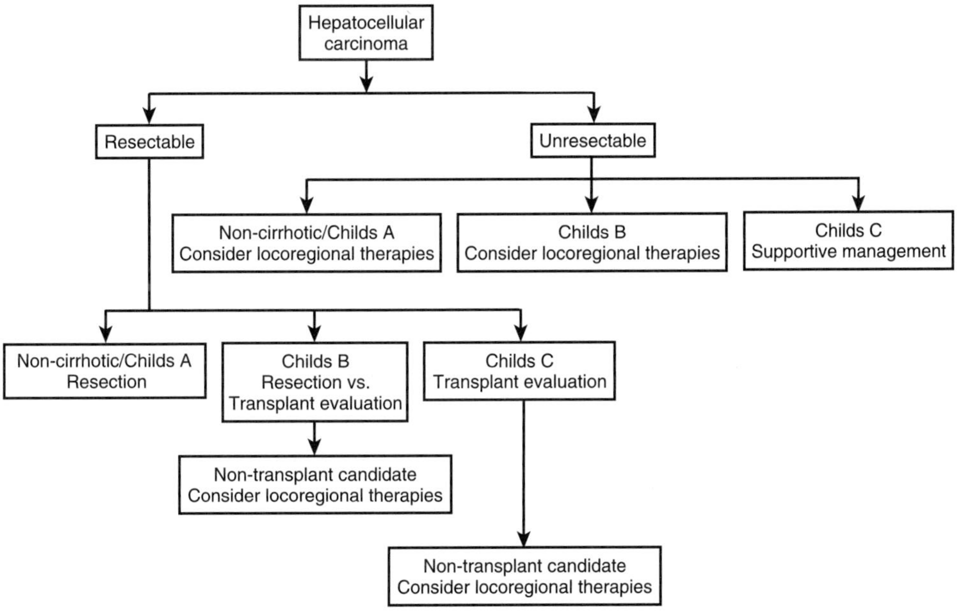

Figure 18–6. Hepatocellular carcinoma management algorithm incorporating hepatic resection, transplantation, and locoregional therapies.

TABLE 18–3 • *Child-Turcotte-Pugh Scoring System for Cirrhosis*

Parameter	1 Point	2 Points	3 Points
Albumin	>3.5	2.8–3.5	<2.8
Bilirubin	<2	2–3	>3
PT/INR	<1.7	1.7–2.3	>2.3
Ascites	None	Mild	Moderate to severe
Encephalopathy	None	Grade 1 or 2	Grade 3 or 4

Class A, 5 to 6 points; *Class B,* 7 to 9 points; *Class C,* 10 to 15 points.

with well-compensated Child class A cirrhosis may experience hepatic decompensation after major hepatic resection, despite favorable preoperative assessment. The presence of portal hypertension appears to be a major risk factor for the development of postoperative hepatic decompensation, which leads some hepatobiliary surgeons to not perform major hepatic resection in this setting. In clinical practice, less than a fourth of all patients with newly diagnosed HCC are candidates for surgical resection. The development of HCC in a cirrhotic liver is thought to be a field effect; thus, partial hepatectomy also has the negative attribute of leaving the remainder of the cirrhotic liver, which has a significant increased risk of subsequent HCC development. Risk factors for local recurrence after hepatic resection include portal or hepatic venous invasion, the presence of satellite nodules, large tumor size, and advanced TNM stage.

Hepatic Transplantation

The high incidence of recurrent HCC in the liver remnant after partial hepatectomy has prompted the practice of liver transplan tation for the primary treatment of HCC. Transplantation is particularly attractive for Child B or C cirrhotic patients, in whom partial hepatectomy is not a safe surgical option (see Figure 18-6). Clinical series have established tumor characteristics associated with HCC recurrence after hepatic transplantation, including size of more than 5 cm, vascular invasion, positive lymph nodes, and histologic grade. By contrast, those HCCs found incidentally in explanted livers and the fibrolamellar HCC variant have been associated with a better prognosis. These reports led to the integration of HCC size and stage into the United Network for Organ Sharing organ allocation guidelines. HCC cirrhotic patients can be listed at a higher status for transplant if they have a single tumor of less than 5 cm or no more than three tumors each of 3 cm or less. Historically, only a small portion of patients with known HCC were treated with liver transplant. With the revised United Network for Organ Sharing organ allocation guidelines and the more liberal use of liver donors, an increasing number of HCC patients are being treated with liver transplantation.

Local Ablation Therapies

More than 75% of all patients with HCC are not candidates for surgical resection, thus prompting the development of alternative treatments. Local ablative therapy is a minimally invasive technique that destroys HCC tumor tissue via chemical or thermal injury. Treatments can be administered percutaneously, laparoscopically, or during laparotomy. Ablation therapy can be used as an isolated treatment modality or as an adjunct to surgical resection. Patient populations ideally suited for local ablation therapies include those with technically resectable disease but poor hepatic function (Child class B or C), those with recurrent HCC in the liver remnant after partial hepatectomy, and possibly those needing a treatment bridge to liver transplant. Contraindications for local ablation therapy include gross ascites, coagulopathy that cannot be corrected, and obstructive jaundice. Tumors located on the surface of the liver are also hazardous to treat as a result of increased risks of bleeding and peritoneal tumor seeding. Finally, lesions positioned close to vital structures (e.g., central bile ducts, major blood vessels, adjacent abdominal viscera) pose distinct technical problems for this treatment modality.

Many forms of local ablative therapy for HCC have been introduced into the clinical arena (Table 18-4). The therapeutic potential of these modalities revolves around the ability to directly induce cytotoxic activity (e.g., chemicals, radioactive isotopes, chemotherapeutic drugs) or to produce thermal ablation (e.g., radiofrequency and microwave ablation, laser therapy, cryotherapy). There have been few head-to-head studies comparing the tumoricidal potential of the many available approaches; hence, it is difficult to determine the relative efficacy of the individual therapies. Of the available local ablative procedures, radiofrequency ablation is emerging in popularity in the United States. Complete tumor necrosis is possible in 80% to 100% of tumors of less than 3 cm with a single treatment. Long-term survival data—albeit limited—for the radiofrequency ablation of isolated HCC of less than 3 cm is reported to be as high as 40% at 5 years. Studies have demonstrated superior results of radiofrequency ablation as compared with ethanol injection as evidenced by a higher rate of necrosis with fewer treatment

TABLE 18-4 • *Local Ablation Options for Hepatocellular Carcinoma*

	Mechanism of Action	Pros	Cons
Percutaneous ethanol injection	Cellular dehydration; protein denaturation; thrombosis of small vessels	Relatively safe; performed as outpatient; effective for HCCs near large vessels	Multiple injections required; most effective for HCCs <3 cm; limited by tumor septa; cannot penetrate tumor capsule
Percutaneous acetic acid injection	Generation of acidic environment leading to lipolysis and protein dissociation	Relatively safe; performed as outpatient; effective for HCCs near large vessels; excellent tumor diffusion	Limited experience; multiple injections required; most effective for HCCs <3 cm
Radiofrequency ablation	Protein coagulation via thermoablation	Low complication rate; able to treat HCC lesions up to 7 cm; can be performed percutaneously	Not effective for HCCs near large vessels; unable to actively monitor tissue destruction accurately
Microwave coagulation therapy	Protein coagulation via thermoablation	Predictable area of tissue necrosis; able to penetrate the tumor capsule	High complication rate for HCCs >4 cm; open or laparoscopic approach required for HCCs >2–3 cm
Laser therapy	Protein coagulation via thermoablation	Able to actively monitor tissue destruction; can be performed percutaneously	Limited volume of tissue destruction; not effective for HCCs near large vessels; not safe for patients with severe liver dysfunction
Cryotherapy	Cellular necrosis via cell dehydration; destruction of cellular architecture	Able to actively monitor tissue destruction	Moderate complication rate; typically requires laparotomy; most effective for tumors <5 cm; difficult to treat HCCs near large vessels

HCC, Hepatocellular carcinoma.

sessions, a lower rate of tumor recurrence, and a higher patient survival benefit. However, radiofrequency ablation has significant limitations, including thermal injury to adjacent viscera, reduced effectiveness for lesions adjacent to the hepatic veins or vena cava (heat sinks), and significant tumor seeding. These largely percutaneous complications may be partially ameliorated with a laparoscopic or open surgical approach in which tumor destruction can be performed under direct vision and adjacent viscera retracted from the field of ablation.

Other Therapies

Systemic chemotherapy has provided disappointing results as the primary therapy for HCC or in an adjuvant setting, with a response rate of only 20% and no significant overall survival benefit. Other systemic therapies, such as tamoxifen and interferon, have likewise proved to be clinically ineffective. Given the poor response to systemic therapies, interest has grown in the locoregional administration of chemotherapy and radiation. Locoregional therapies are typically used in the setting of a clinical trial or as a palliative measure for the more than 75% of HCC patients with unresectable disease. HCC derives its blood supply from the arterial system; thus, the delivery of chemotherapy via a hepatic artery perfusion pump will directly bathe tumor cells in a much higher concentration of cytotoxic agents as compared with standard intravenous systemic delivery, and it will theoretically produce fewer systemic side effects as a result of first-pass hepatic metabolism (Figure 18-7). The most popular chemotherapy cocktail includes the coadministration of chemotherapeutic agents such as doxorubicin, cisplatin, and mitomycin C along with iodized poppyseed oil (Lipiodol) via the feeding artery. The Lipiodol drug vehicle is clinically advantageous, because HCC tumor selectively retains this agent via an unknown mechanism. Arterial embolization after chemotherapy administration improves survival as compared with intra-arterial chemotherapy alone. Retrospective studies report increased tumor necrosis and improved survival rate with this treatment modality. Prospective randomized studies have also documented marked antitumor effect, but they have failed to substantiate improved survival benefit. Potential benefits were balanced by the

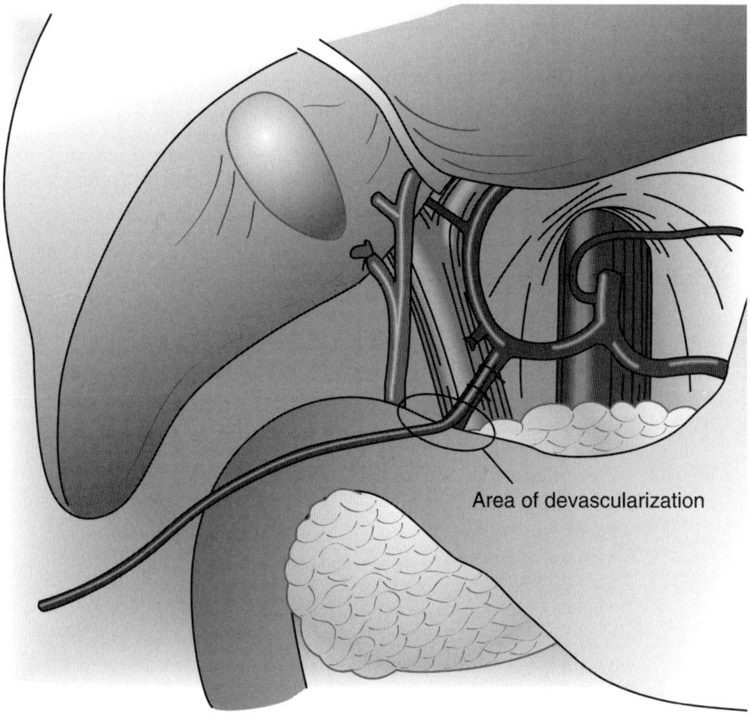

Figure 18–7. Placement of a hepatic arterial perfusion catheter into the gastroduodenal artery. Regional devascularization of the hepatoduodenal ligament is recommended to avoid chemotherapy-induced gastritis and duodenitis *(shaded area)*. (Reproduced with permission from Skitzki JJ, Chang AE. Hepatic artery chemotherapy for colorectal liver metastases: technical considerations and review of clinical trials. *Surg Oncol* 2002;11:123–135.)

deleterious effects of hepatic artery chemotherapy on liver function. Complications with hepatic arterial chemotherapy are frequent and include liver failure, liver abscess, tumor rupture, peptic ulcer formation, acute cholecystitis, acute pancreatitis, renal failure, and biliary sclerosis. In general, hepatic artery therapy is reserved for unresectable disease, and it is generally regarded as a palliative measure. Tumor chemoembolization has also been used to selectively induce hypertrophy of uninvolved liver to enhance the liver remnant mass before surgical resection.

One alternative locoregional approach that has shown promising results is focused chemoradiation. The concurrent administration of fluorodeoxyuridine (a radiosensitizer) and three-dimensional conformal irradiation directed only to the tumor burden (demonstrated on imaging studies) has been demonstrated to halt disease progression and to prolong survival in patients with unresectable HCC as compared with conventional radiation alone. In many centers across the United States, locoregional chemoembolization and chemoradiation therapies are reserved for patients with inoperable HCC and for those patients with recurrent HCC after standard hepatectomy.

Cholangiocarcinoma

Epidemiology

Cholangiocarcinoma is an uncommon tumor of the bile ducts. In the United States, approximately 2,500 new cases are diagnosed each year. Most patients are diagnosed between the ages of 50 and 70 years; men and women appear to be equally affected. This tumor may occur in the intrahepatic biliary ductal system or in the extrahepatic biliary tree at perihilar or distal ductal locations. Approximately two thirds of lesions are located in a perihilar position, and they are frequently referred to as *Klatskin tumors*.

Risk Factors

The pathogenesis of cholangiocarcinoma appears to be related to chronic inflammation, gallstones, and stasis in the biliary tree. Accordingly, this cancer has a strong association with ulcerative colitis, primary sclerosing cholangitis, biliary cystic disease, and choledochal cysts. Other, less-common risk factors include congenital hepatic fibrosis, hepatolithiasis, chronic typhoid carriers, *Clonorchis* parasitic infection, and certain chemicals used in the rubber industry.

BOX 18-4 CHOLANGIOCARCINOMA RISK FACTORS

- The pathogenesis of cholangiocarcinoma is associated with disease states characterized by chronic biliary inflammation and bile stasis:
  - Ulcerative colitis
  - Sclerosing cholangitis
  - Biliary cystic disease
  - Choledochal cysts

Diagnosis and Staging

Patients with cholangiocarcinoma present with obstructive jaundice. Associated symptoms may include pruritus, nausea, abdominal pain, fatigue, and weight loss. Patients may present acutely with cholangitis. Physical examination reveals scleral icterus, jaundice, and, with distal lesions, a palpable gallbladder.

The laboratory evaluation for patients with suspected cholangiocarcinoma includes a complete blood cell count, a platelet count, basic chemistries, a liver panel, coagulation studies, and evaluation for the presence of the tumor marker CA 19-9. All patients should be staged with abdominal imaging and chest x-ray or CT scanning to evaluate for pulmonary metastases. Other imaging studies should only be obtained for related signs and symptoms.

Cholangiocarcinomas are staged according to the TNM classification as either a perihilar or distal common bile-duct tumor (Table 18-5). Anatomic classification systems describe the extrahepatic biliary tree in thirds: the upper third (perihilar), the middle third, and the lower third (periampullary). Given the high incidence, perihilar cholangiocarcinomas are further divided into four types as described by Bismuth and Corlette (Figure 18-8) These anatomic classification systems have therapeutic relevance, because tumor position along the extrahepatic biliary tree governs the extent of surgical resection.

TABLE 18-5 • *American Joint Committee on Cancer TNM Staging System for Cancer of the Extrahepatic Bile Ducts*

Stage	Tumor	Node	Metastasis
IA	T1	N0	M0
IB	T2	N0	M0
IIA	T3	N0	M0
IIB	T1-3	N1	M0
III	T4	Any N	M0
IV	Any T	Any N	M1

T1, Tumor confined to the bile duct; *T2,* tumor invades beyond the wall of the bile duct; *T3,* tumor invades the liver, gallbladder, pancreas, or unilateral branches of the portal vein or hepatic artery; *T4,* tumor invades the main portal vein, the common hepatic artery, or adjacent structures; *N0,* no regional lymph node metastasis; *N1,* regional lymph node; *M0,* no distant metastasis; *M1,* distant metastasis.

Table adapted with the permission of the American Joint Committee on Cancer, Chicago. The original source for this material is the *AJCC Cancer Staging Manual,* 6th ed. New York: Springer-Verlag, 2002:147.

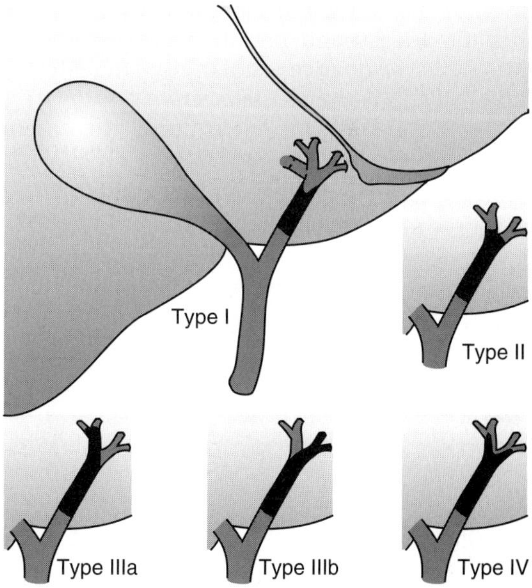

Figure 18-8. Perihilar cholangiocarcinoma, Bismuth classification.

Imaging Modalities

A variety of noninvasive and invasive imaging modalities are used during the workup for cholangiocarcinoma to do the following: (1) to delineate the biliary ductal anatomy; (2) to demonstrate local invasion into nonductal structures; and (3) to assess for distant metastasis. As with most patients presenting with painless jaundice, the diagnostic workup often begins with an abdominal ultrasound, which demonstrates evidence of biliary dilatation and establishes the level of obstruction. CT scanning or MRI is then used to assess for hepatic parenchymal invasion or portal vascular involvement. Hepatic CT protocols that include a portal venous phase facilitate lesion visualization, because tumor attenuation is noted to increase during the delayed portal venous images. However, the tumor frequently is not visualized, because it infiltrates along the wall of the bile duct rather than forming a discrete mass. Delayed imaging 15 to 20 minutes after contrast injection will demonstrate the lesions in up to 30% of cases (Figure 18-9, *A*). CT scanning is excellent for determining the level of biliary obstruction, and, thus, it indirectly demonstrates the position of the lesion (Figure 18-9, *B*).

MRI is the most sensitive imaging modality for visualizing cholangiocarcinoma and for determining parenchymal involvement. There typically is an ill-defined area of subtle enhancement with gadolinium contrast that is characteristic of cholangiocarcinoma MRI imaging (Figure 18-10, *A*). Magnetic resonance arteriography (MRA) provides additional information regarding the tumor involvement of hepatic arterial and portal venous structures. Magnetic resonance cholangiopancreatography (MRCP) is the most sensitive noninvasive imaging modality for determining the extent of bile-duct involvement (Figure 18-10, *B*). MRI/MRA/MRCP noninvasive imaging can be obtained at the same time, thereby providing a wealth of information regarding resectability. Ideally, MR imaging should be obtained before stenting the biliary tree, because the presence of stents can lead to imaging characteristics in the adjacent biliary wall, similar to tumor.

Most patients present with significant jaundice, and they will require biliary decompression either as a palliative procedure or to guide surgical intervention. Distal common bile-duct lesions are probably best approached with an endoscopic retrograde cholangiopancreatography-placed stent, whereas perihilar lesions are typically approached with a percutaneous transhepatic cholangiography stent. Bilateral percutaneous transhepatic cholangiography tubes are usually required for the adequate biliary decompression of perihilar lesions.

Management

Resection

The resection of cholangiocarcinoma is guided by the anatomic level of involvement. Intrahepatic cholangiocarcinomas are treated with standard hepatic resection of involved segments. Lower-third bile-duct lesions are typically treated in the same way as pancreatic cancer: with pancreaticoduodenectomy. Middle-third lesions are treated with cholecystectomy, common bile-duct excision, and perihilar lymphadenectomy. Reconstruction is achieved via roux-en-Y hepaticojejunostomy.

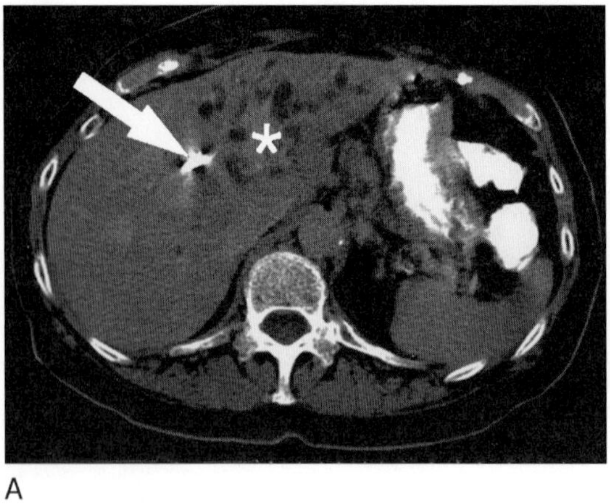

A

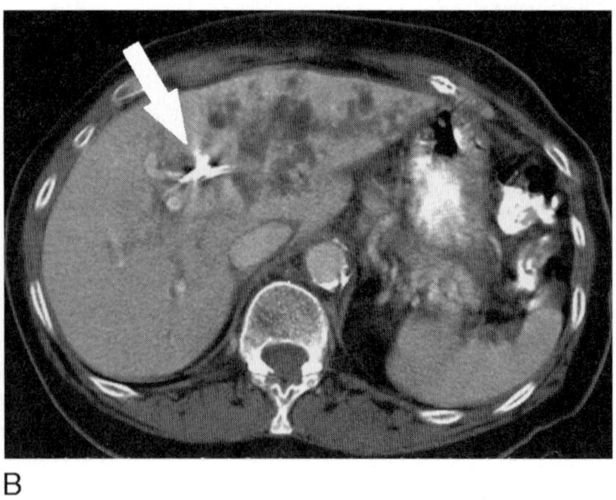

B

Figure 18-9. CT scan of cholangiocarcinoma. **A,** Delayed imaging 15 to 20 minutes after contrast administration will suggest the lesion *(asterisk)* in approximately 30% of cases. Arrow indicates percutaneous transhepatic cholangiography tube. **B,** CT scanning is excellent for demonstrating the level of biliary dilatation and thus indirectly suggests left main bile duct involvement in this case (same patient as in **A**). Arrow indicates percutaneous transhepatic cholangiography tube. (Courtesy of Dr. Isaac Francis, University of Michigan Department of Radiology, Ann Arbor, Mich.)

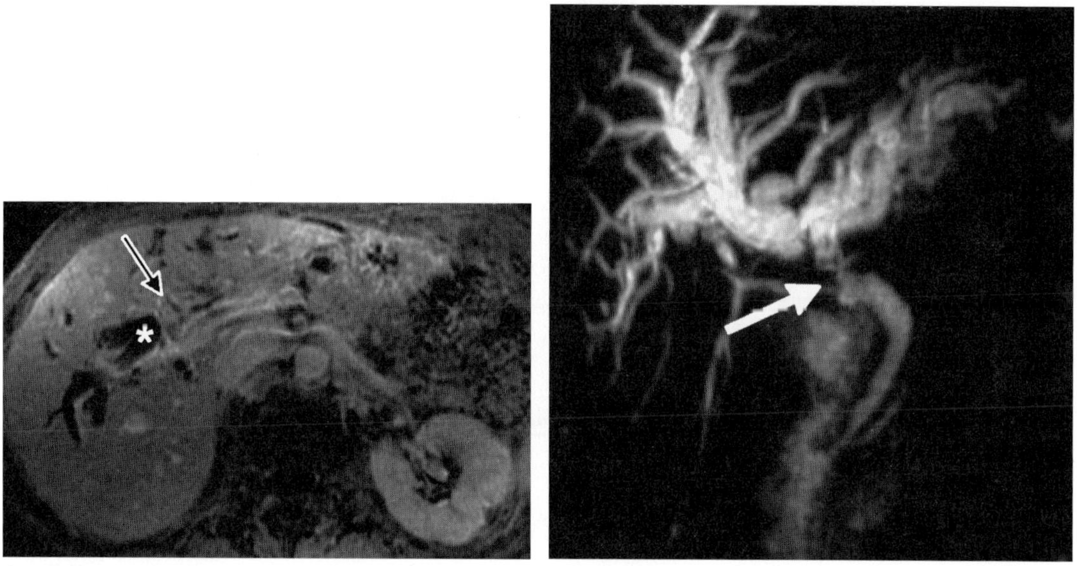

A B

Figure 18–10. Magnetic resonance imaging of cholangiocarcinoma. **A,** The central area of ill-defined subtle enhancement *(arrow)* corresponds with a hilar cholangiocarcinoma on this T1-weighted gadolinium-enhanced image. Dilated intrahepatic bile ducts *(asterisks)* appear as dark tubular structures. **B,** Magnetic resonance cholangiopancreatography sagittal view demonstrating perihilar cholangiocarcinoma *(arrow)* involving the proximal common hepatic, as well as right and left hepatic, bile ducts. (Courtesy of Dr. Hero Hussain, University of Michigan Department of Radiology, Ann Arbor, Mich.)

BOX 18–5 SURGICAL RESECTION OF CHOLANGIOCARCINOMA

Intrahepatic ducts: Hepatic resection of involved segments
Extrahepatic ducts:
1. **Proximal third:** Radical en bloc resection of extrahepatic biliary tree, hepatic lobectomy (± caudate resection), and perihilar lymphadenectomy
2. **Middle third:** Radical excision of extrahepatic biliary tree and perihilar lymphadenectomy
3. **Distal third:** Pancreaticoduodenectomy

Upper-third or perihilar lesions are treated with a radical extrahepatic bile-duct excision and perihilar lymphadenectomy, followed by biliary-enteric reconstruction with a roux-en-Y enteric limb. There is a growing body of evidence that suggests that combined liver resection along with extrahepatic bile-duct excision affords improved clinical outcomes for patients with perihilar lesions. This is especially true for Bismuth class III lesions, with which a right hepatic lobectomy would be included for IIIa lesions and a left hepatic lobectomy for IIIb lesions (Figure 18-11). The caudate lobe is frequently involved with perihilar lesions as a result of the proximity of the hepatic duct bifurcation; thus, caudate lobe resection is often included with major lobectomy. As expected, the frequency of curative resections decreases with more proximally located lesions. Approximately 60% of distal lesions, 33% of middle lesions, and 15% to 20% of perihilar lesions are amenable to surgical resection.

Complete surgical extirpation of proximally located cholangiocarcinomas is surgically challenging. Operative approaches that are helpful for identifying the hepatic duct bifurcation and assessing tumor involvement include early mobilization of the gallbladder and early division of the common bile duct. Preoperatively placed transhepatic biliary catheters in the right and left hepatic ducts also help in the identification of the extrahepatic biliary tree, and they greatly facilitate biliary-enteric reconstruction after radical extrahepatic biliary duct excision.

Other Therapies

There is limited experience with the administration of systemic chemotherapy as postoper-

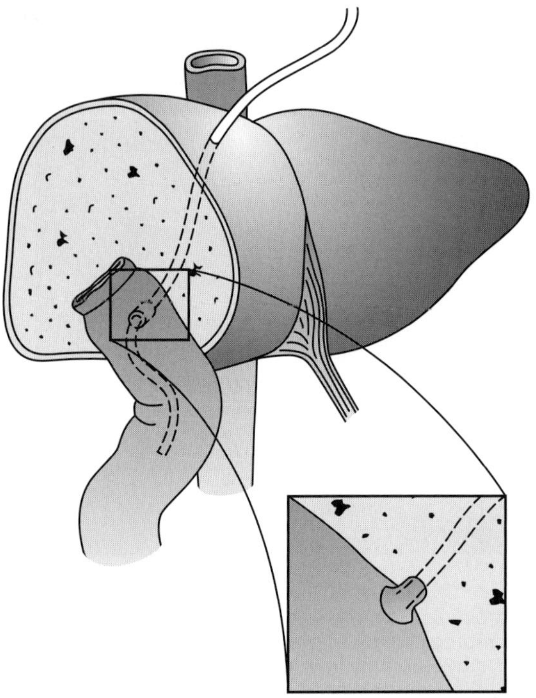

Figure 18–11. Surgical reconstruction after radical perihilar cholangiocarcinoma extirpation with en bloc right hepatic lobectomy. Reconstruction is performed via the anastomosis of a roux jejunal limb to the proximal left hepatic bile duct.

ative adjuvant therapy or to patients with unresectable cholangiocarcinoma. The most common agent used for bile-duct cancer is fluorouracil, but clinical results with this agent alone have been poor.

Most patients with cholangiocarcinoma receive radiation treatment. Conventional external beam or intraductal brachytherapy approaches can be used to deliver radiation doses. Radiation can be administered either as a primary therapy for unresectable disease or as an adjuvant therapy after complete surgical extirpation of the tumor. Unfortunately, the overall clinical results have been disappointing. Radiation-induced hepatotoxicity limits the ability to deliver large potentially curative doses with conventional external-beam radiation. Newer split-fraction approaches that direct the radiation field only at image-demonstrated disease facilitate a large dose delivery that often would be hepatotoxic if delivered to the entire liver parenchyma. Conformal irradiation administered jointly with fluorodeoxyuridine (a chemotherapy agent with radiosensitizing properties) has been demonstrated to produce long-term freedom from local disease progression and to significantly decrease radiation-induced complications as compared with conventional radiation alone.

Key Selected Reading

Schafer DF, Sorrell MF. Hepatocellular carcinoma. *Lancet* 1999;353:1253–1257.

Selected Readings

Akriviadis EA, Llovet JM, Efremidis SC, *et al.* Hepatocellular carcinoma. *Br J Surg* 1998;85: 1319–1331.

Brugge WR. Endoscopic techniques to diagnose and manage biliary tumors. *J Clin Oncol* 2005;23: 4561–4565.

Burke EC, Jarnagin WR, Hochwald SN, *et al.* Hilar cholangiocarcinoma: patterns of spread, the importance of hepatic resection for curative operation, and a presurgical clinical staging system. *Ann Surg* 1998;228:385–394.

Curley SA, Cusack JC Jr, Tanabe KK, Ellis LM. Advances in the treatment of liver tumors. *Curr Probl Surg* 2002;39:449–571.

El-Serag HB, Mason AC. Rising incidence of hepatocellular carcinoma in the United States. *N Engl J Med* 1999;340:745–750.

Fan MH, Chang AE. Resection of liver tumors: technical aspects. *Surg Oncol* 2002;10:139–152.

Kuvshinoff BW, Armstrong JG, Fong Y, *et al.* Palliation of irresectable hilar cholangiocarcinoma with biliary drainage and radiotherapy. *Br J Surg* 1995;82: 1522–1525.

McCormack L, Petrowsky H, Clavien P-A. Surgical therapy of hepatocellular carcinoma. *Eur J Gastroenterol Hepatol* 2005;17:497–503.

Misra MC, Guleria S. Management of cancer gallbladder found as a surprise on a resected gallbladder specimen. *J Surg Oncol* 2006;93:690–698.

Mulholland MW, Yahanda A, Yeo CJ. Multidisciplinary management of perihilar bile duct cancer. *J Am Coll Surg* 2001;193:440–447.

Pitt HA, Dooley WC, Yeo CJ, Cameron JL. Malignancies of the biliary tree. *Curr Probl Surg* 1995;32:1–90.

Poon RT, Fan ST, Tsang FH, Wong J. Locoregional therapies for hepatocellular carcinoma: a critical review from the surgeon's perspective. *Ann Surg* 2002;235: 466–486.

Sutherland LM, Williams JA, Padbury RT, *et al.* Radiofrequency ablation of liver tumors: a systematic review. *Arch Surg* 2006;141:181–190.

Washburn WK, Lewis WD, Jenkins RL. Aggressive surgical resection for cholangiocarcinoma. *Arch Surg* 1995;130:270–276.

19

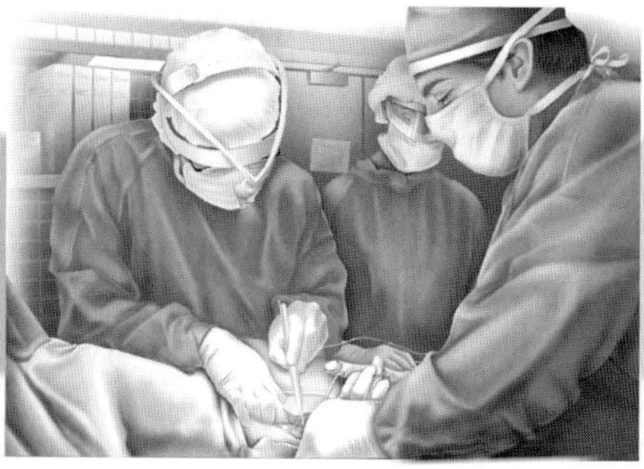

Colorectal Cancer

Susan Tsai and Emina H. Huang

Colorectal Cancer: Key Points

- List the risk factors for colorectal cancer.
- Outline the screening procedure for colorectal cancer for low-risk, normal-risk, and high-risk individuals.
- Describe the various clinical presentations of colorectal cancer.
- Explain the steps taken in a preoperative diagnostic evaluation for colorectal cancer.
- Outline the surgical management options of colon cancer.
- Discuss the use of adjuvant chemotherapy for colon cancer.
- Outline the surgical management options for rectal cancer.
- Outline the adjuvant and neoadjuvant therapies for rectal cancer.
- Outline the surveillance plan that should go into effect after the completion of colorectal cancer treatment.

Colorectal cancer is the third most common cancer in the United States in both men and women, with 106,680 new cases of colon cancer and 41,930 cases of rectal cancer being reported in 2006. Fortunately, both the overall incidence and the mortality rate for colon cancer are on the decline. This has largely been attributed to the improved detection and removal of premalignant adenomas as well as improved screening of high-risk patients. However, the disease remains the second leading cause of cancer-related deaths in the United States, with 55,170 deaths in 2006.

The average cumulative lifetime risk of colorectal cancer in Americans is 6%. The incidence greatly increases with increasing age, with 90% of colorectal cancers being diagnosed after the age of 50 years. In patients who present with colorectal cancer before the age of 50 years, the presence of a hereditary syndrome should be considered. Women have a lower incidence than men, possibly because of a beneficiary inhibitory role of female hormones.

As with many other cancers, the survival of patients with colorectal cancers depends on the stage of the disease. At the time of presentation, approximately 37% of patients will have localized disease; an additional 37% of patients will have regional disease. The remaining patients will present with metastatic disease. The 5-year survival rates of localized, regional, and metastatic disease are 91%, 66%, and 8.5%, respectively. Overall, approximately one in three patients who develop colorectal cancer will die of the disease.

BOX 19–1 RISK FACTORS FOR COLORECTAL CANCER

- Inherited syndromes
- Polyposis types
  - Familial adenomatous polyposis
  - Peutz-Jeghers syndrome
  - Turcot's syndrome
  - Juvenile polyposis
  - Nonpolyposis types
  - Lynch syndrome I
  - Lynch syndrome II
- Personal history of colorectal cancer
- Family history of colorectal cancer
- Inflammatory bowel disease
- Diabetes mellitus and insulin resistance
- Dietary factors
  - Obesity
  - Diet high in saturated fat from animal sources (red meat)
  - Diet low in fiber and vegetables
  - Alcohol
- Lack of physical activity
- Cigarette smoking

Risk Factors

Inherited Syndromes

Although the majority of colorectal cancers are sporadic, approximately 25% are attributable to heritable causes. Several inherited syndromes predispose a patient to colon cancer; these may be divided into the polyposis and the nonpolyposis types. The polyposis types include familial adenomatous polyposis (FAP) and Peutz-Jeghers syndrome. Hereditary nonpolyposis colorectal cancer (HNPCC) is not associated with multiple colonic polyps.

FAP results from a germline point mutation of the adenomatous polyposis coli (APC) gene on chromosome 5 (5q21 deletion). This mutation can be identified in 1 in 7,000 individuals, and it accounts for 1% of all colorectal cancer. Although most cases are familial, 15% of patients present with new mutations. FAP is an autosomal-dominant disease with 90% penetrance. Although polyps may develop anywhere within the gastrointestinal tract, they are predominantly found within the colon. Hundreds to thousands of polyps occur throughout the colon so that, on colonoscopy, it looks like the mucosa has been carpeted with multiple polyps. The first polyps appear by the mid teens. Without intervention, 100% of these patients will develop colon cancer by the fifth decade of life.

Other variants of APC mutations exist. An attenuated form of APC causes far fewer adenomas but a similarly high risk of colon cancer. An APC mutation found in approximately 6% of the Ashkenazi Jewish population is associated with a 20% to 30% risk of colon cancer.

Detailed studies of families with a high prevalence of colorectal cancer have identified a group of hereditary colon cancers not associated with polyposis. HNPCC is also known as *Lynch syndromes I and II*. HNPCC is an autosomal dominant disease with 30% to 70% penetrance that is associated with germ line defects of various mismatch repair genes. Overall, these patients have an 85% lifetime risk of developing colorectal cancer.

Ninety percent of the mutations are associated with the mismatch repair genes hMLH1 and hMLH2. These mutations result in microsatellite instability. Although HPNCC-related colorectal cancer may occur in any part of the bowel, it is more frequently right-sided. HNPCC patients not only have synchronous lesions, but they may also develop metachronous lesions. Although Lynch syndrome I is associated with only colorectal cancer, Lynch syndrome II is associated with endometrial, ovarian, gastric, and small bowel malignancies and cancers of the renal pelvis or ureter. Colorectal malignancies among Lynch syndrome patients tend to be biologically less aggressive, with improved stage-specific survival as compared with other patients. When screening for these patients, criteria that may direct the physician to the possibility of one of these familial syndromes include the modified Amsterdam criteria (Table 19-1).

In the absence of a defined syndrome, family history of colorectal cancer or advanced adenoma approximately doubles the risk of developing colorectal cancer to 11%. This group of individuals without a known genetic syndrome accounts for 15% to 20% of high-risk individuals. The risk is higher if more than one relative is affected or if the age at diagnosis is less than 45 years.

The Adenoma-Carcinoma Sequence

Sporadic colorectal cancers are thought to arise from a process of carcinogenesis involving a transition from normal colonic mucosa to adenomatous polyp to adenocarcinoma. This process probably takes at least 10 years in most people, and it results from an accumulation of genetic defects. Because polyps appear to be a precursor lesion for colorectal cancer, the endoscopic removal of those polyps (colonoscopic polypectomy) can significantly reduce the incidence of cancer. The National Polyp Study Work Group found that the incidence of colon cancer was 90% lower among patients who underwent colonoscopic screening and the removal of polyps than among a non-screened group of patients with a similar risk.

Although most colorectal cancers arise from polyps, not all polyps are cancerous. Polyps may be classified as neoplastic (adenomas that may be either benign or malignant) or non-neoplastic (i.e., hyperplastic, inflammatory, hamartomatous, mucosal). Adenomas may be further classified histologically as tubular, tubulovillous, or villous (Figure 19-1). The risk of an adenoma subsequently developing into a cancer is dependent on the histologic variant and size as well as the degree of dysplasia (Table 19-2).

BOX 19-2 THE ADENOMA-CARCINOMA SEQUENCE

- Normal colon
  ▼
- Small adenoma
  ▼
- Large adenoma
  ▼
- Large adenoma with high-grade dysplasia
  ▼
- Large adenoma with invasive carcinoma

TABLE 19-1 • *Modified Amsterdam Criteria*

- At least three relatives with a hereditary nonpolyposis colon-cancer–related cancer including cancer of any of the following:
  1. Colorectal cancer
  2. Endometrium
  3. Small bowel
  4. Ureter
  5. Renal pelvis
- One affected patient is a first-degree relative of the other two
- Two or more successive generations are affected
- One or more affected relative(s) received the colorectal cancer diagnosis at the age of less than 50 years
- Familial adenomatous polyposis excluded in any case of colorectal cancer
- Tumors verified by pathologic examination

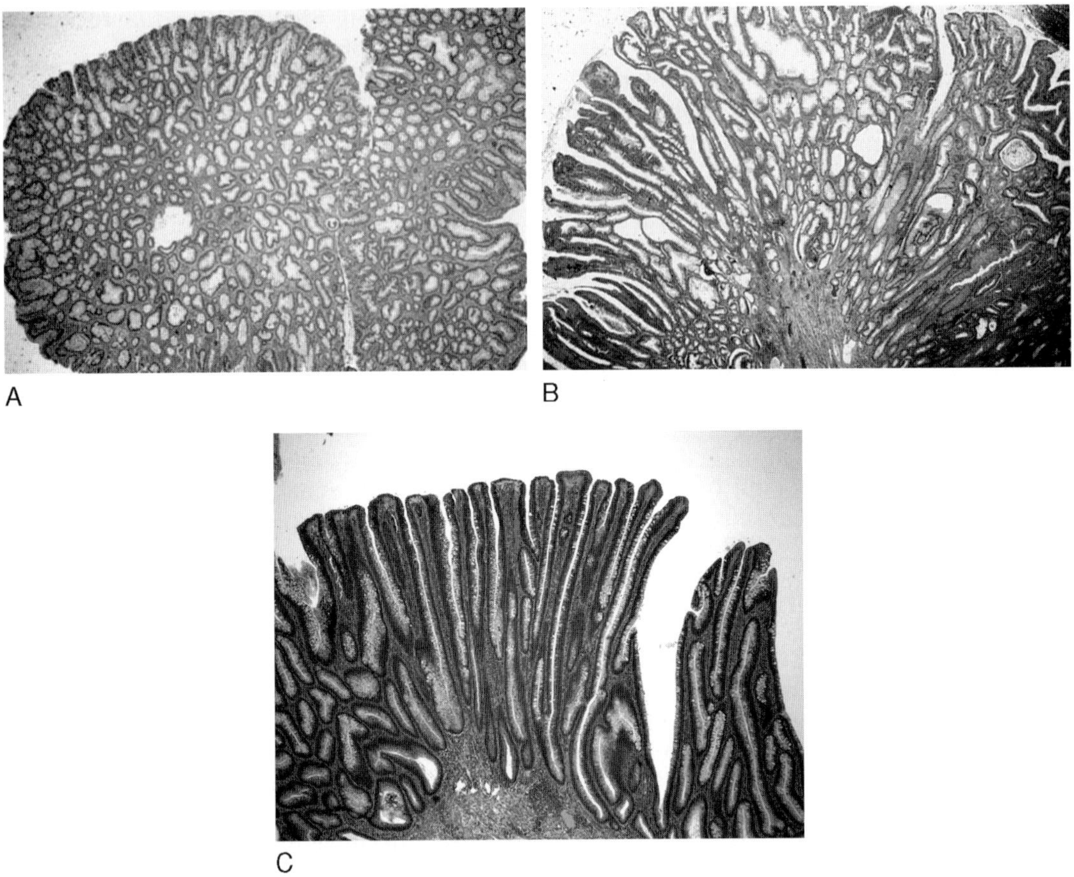

Figure 19–1. Adenomas may be classified histologically as tubular *(A)*, tubulovillous *(B)*, or villous *(C)*.

TABLE 19–2 • *Adenomatous Polyps*

Type	Incidence	Location	Cancer Risk
Tubular	75% of polyps	Throughout the large intestine	<5%
Tubulovillous	8–15%	Throughout the large intestine	25%
Villous	5–10%	Predominately in the rectum	40%

Tubular adenomas are found throughout the large bowel, and they account for 75% of polyps. Less than 5% of tubular adenomas are malignant. Tubulovillous polyps account for 8% to 15% of polyps, and they are also found with equal frequency throughout the large bowel; 25% of these polyps are malignant. Finally, villous adenomas are the least common polyp, accounting for 5% to 10% of all polyps. They are predominantly found in the rectum, and 40% are malignant. Size is also an important predictor of malignancy. Most lesions are less than 1 cm, and only 1.3% of polyps less than 1 cm are malignant. For polyps between 1 and 2 cm, 9.5% are malignant. Finally, 46% of polyps greater than 2 cm are malignant. The degree of dysplasia is a demonstration of the gradual transition from the benign to the malignant state. Polyps with mild, moderate, and severe dysplasia were found to have malignancy 6%, 18%, and 46% of the time, respectively.

Additional Risk and Protective Factors

An additional risk factor for developing colorectal cancer is a long history of active inflammatory bowel disease. Approximately 1% of all colorectal cancer develops in patients with inflammatory bowel disease. The risk of colorectal cancer in a patient with ulcerative colitis increases 1% per year after 8 to 10 years with active disease. Crohn's colitis associated with severe or chronic stricture is associated with an increased risk (7%) of colorectal dysplasia and carcinoma.

A personal history of colorectal cancer places patients at a threefold higher risk of developing a second primary colon cancer than the general population. Five to eight percent of these patients will develop metachronous lesions. Patients with a first-degree relative also have an increased risk of developing colorectal cancer; the risk is higher if more than one relative is affected and if the cancer developed at an age of less than 45 years. Alcohol consumption of more than two drinks per day doubles the risk of colorectal cancer. Cigarette smoking is associated with both an increased incidence and mortality. Several additional dietary factors can both increase and decrease the risk of colorectal cancer, although the links between diet and colorectal cancer risk are not as clear. An increased risk has been suggested for a diet high in saturated fats and low in fiber and vegetables. A protective effect has been described for folic acid, calcium, selenium, NSAIDS (particularly aspirin), and the cholesterol-lowering statins.

BOX 19-3 FACTORS POSSIBLY ASSOCIATED WITH A DECREASED RISK OF COLORECTAL CANCER

- Physical exercise
- Consumption of a high-fiber diet
- Consumption of fruits and vegetables
- Multivitamins with folic acid
- Postmenopausal hormone use
- Calcium supplementation
- Selenium
- Nonsteroidal anti-inflammatory drugs
- Statins

Screening

Given the improved prognosis associated with localized disease and the relative accessibility of the large intestine, screening asymptomatic patients for colorectal cancer plays a significant role in improving outcome. The recommendations for screening are based on the individual's risk of developing colorectal cancer and are generally divided into patients with no identifiable risk other than age, patients with increased risk (patients with adenomatous polyps or a personal or family history of colorectal cancer), and those with a high risk (patients with inflammatory bowel disease or a hereditary predisposition).

Screening Examinations

Fecal Occult Blood Testing

Fecal occult blood testing (FOBT) was one of the first tests used for colorectal cancer screening. Because of its availability, convenience, and affordability, it has been one of the most widely employed screening tools. As a test, it is limited by low sensitivity and specificity, which are affected by slide preparation techniques, exogenous peroxidase activity, and medications. In addition, many patients find testing stool samples displeasing. Despite this, at least five large controlled studies including more than 300,000 patients have demonstrated the detection of colorectal cancers in earlier stages with FOBT. A new type of FOBT is the fecal immunohistochemistry test (FIT), which may be more specific for lower gastrointestinal bleeding and better in sensitivity and specificity relative to guaic-based tests. A digital rectal examination and testing stool for occult blood should be a standard part of a health maintenance examination, and positive findings require appropriate evaluation.

Radiologic Examinations

Double-contrast barium enemas (DCBEs) have a sensitivity of 50% to 80% for polyps less than 1 cm and of 70% to 90% for polyps greater than 1 cm. Because it allows visualization of the remaining colon, it has been a useful adjunct to sigmoidoscopy. DCBEs and flexible sigmoidoscopy have been demonstrated to have a 98% sensitivity for carcinomas. The drawback of radiologic examination is that it does not allow for tissue diagnosis via biopsy or therapy as with an endoscopic polypectomy. If an abnormality is detected in the right colon on barium enema, a colonoscopy is still necessary. Therefore, the role of the DCBE is as an adjunctive tool in patients for those patients for whom colonoscopy is inaccessible, incomplete, refused, or intolerable.

A newer technique is "virtual colonoscopy," in which helical computed tomographic (CT) scanning followed by three-dimensional reconstruction can produce high-resolution colonic imaging. At the moment, bowel preparation is still needed, as with colonoscopy, although techniques using special markers to differentiate stool from mucosal abnormalities are in evolution so that bowel preparation may not be necessary. This technique is quite sensitive for lesions greater than 1 cm, with advancing discrimination of smaller lesions on the horizon. Although it is associated with few risks, this technique has the disadvantages of limited accessibility, radiation exposure, lack of tissue diagnosis or therapeutic possibilities, and few practitioners having the expertise necessary to interpret the results. Cost is also a concern because any patient with an abnormality still requires a colonoscopy. However, the greatest advantage may be for screening, because current health care providers are overwhelmed with the screening of patients with few risk factors. As technology improves, virtual colonoscopy may be used to screen low-risk individuals, thereby reserving colonoscopies only for those who have suspicious findings.

Endoscopy

Because 60% of colorectal cancers arise distal to the splenic flexure, flexible sigmoidoscopy has been a useful screening modality. A 60-cm flexible sigmoidoscope allows the clinician to reach the descending colon or even the splenic flexure. As compared with rigid proctoscopy, flexible sigmoidoscopy demonstrates improved patient comfort and additional proximal visualization. Advantages over colonoscopy include fewer complications and the ability to perform the procedure without sedation. Three case-controlled trials have demonstrated flexible sigmoidoscopy to be effective for reducing mortality from sigmoid and rectal cancers. However, an obvious limitation of sigmoidoscopy is that the entire colon is not visualized. Recent literature documents that nonvisualization of the proximal colon is associated with decreased detection of 30% to 50%. If flexible sigmoidoscopy is to be used, it should be performed every 5 years for screening patients with average risk.

Patients who have a positive FOBT, sigmoidoscopy, or DCBE will all require a colonoscopy. As a screening examination, colonoscopy rarely misses lesions greater than 1 cm in size, and it has been shown to be equivalent or better than DCBE for detecting larger lesions. Disadvantages include the risks associated with colonoscopy and the cost. The risk of perforation is 0.1%, the risk of hemorrhage is 0.3%, and the risk of mortality is 0.01%. The cecum is visualized in up to 98% of patients. If polyps are detected, colonoscopy should be performed every 2 to 3 years until the colon is cleared.

BOX 19–4 AMERICAN CANCER SOCIETY RECOMMENDATIONS FOR COLORECTAL CANCER EARLY DETECTION

- Beginning at age 50, men and women who are at average risk for developing colorectal cancer should have 1 of the 5 screening options below:
  - A fecal occult blood test (FOBT) or fecal immunochemical test (FIT) every year, OR
  - Flexible sigmoidoscopy every 5 years, OR
  - An FOBT or FIT every year plus flexible sigmoidoscopy every 5 years, OR
  - Double-contrast barium enema every 5 years, OR
  - Colonoscopy every 10 years
- Of the first 3 options, the combination of FOBT or FIT every year plus flexible sigmoidoscopy every 5 years is preferable.

There are several recommendations for the colorectal cancer screening of average-risk patients that include the combination of FOBT, flexible sigmoidoscopy, DCBE, and/or colonoscopy. FOBT should be performed annually. The American College of Gastroenterology recommends screening colonoscopy over the other options, and this is gaining in popularity over flexible sigmoidoscopy. If sigmoidoscopy is chosen, these examinations should be obtained every 5 years, as opposed to colonoscopy, which is recommended every 10 years. If polyps are found, a full colonoscopy is necessary. The various approaches differ with regard to cost, safety, and feasibility, so patients and their clinicians must decide which is the most appropriate for them (Table 19-3).

Screening of High-Risk Individuals (Table 19-4)

Patients with Prior Colon Cancer or Adenomatous Polyps

An increased risk of metachronous lesions exist in patients who have already had colorectal cancer. Approximately half of patients will develop a premalignant polyp in the 5 to 10 years after resection. American Cancer Society surveillance recommendations for patients with a prior adenoma or colon cancer resection are given in Table 19-4.

Patients with Family History of Colorectal Cancer

Individuals with first-degree relatives who have colorectal cancer are at a significantly greater risk of developing cancer than the general

TABLE 19-3 • *Comparisons of the Screening Tests for Colorectal Cancer*

Screening Test	Complexity	Risks	Advantages	Disadvantages
Fecal occult blood test	Minimal	Low	Easy to perform on an annual basis; strong level of evidence for its effectiveness	Low specificity and sensitivity; displeasing to some patients
Flexible sigmoidoscopy	Medium	Medium	Easy to perform; strong level of evidence for its effectiveness; does not require sedation or full bowel preparation	Does not examine entire length of colon; follow-up colonoscopy needed for abnormalities
Double-contrast barium enema	High	Low to medium	Does not require sedation; minimal risk	Bowel preparation required; follow-up colonoscopy needed for abnormalities
Colonoscopy	High	High	Examines entire colon; both diagnostic and therapeutic without follow-up examination	Bowel prep and intravenous sedation needed; risk of perforation; limited accessibility

TABLE 19-4 • *American Cancer Society Guidelines on Screening and Surveillance for the Early Detection of Colorectal Adenomas and Cancer—Womem and Men at Increased Risk or High Risk*

Risk Category	Screening Recommendations
Increased Risk	
Small (<1 cm) adenoma	Repeat colonoscopy 3–6 years after the polypectomy; if the examination is normal, the patient can return to screening every 10 years
One large adenoma; multiple adenomas; high-grade dysplasia or villous change	Colonoscopy 3 years after polypectomy; if normal, repeat examination in 3 years; if normal then, the patient can return to screening every 10 years
Personal history of curative-intent resection of colorectal cancer	Colonoscopy 1 year after resection (6 months if entire colon was not visualized preoperatively); if normal, repeat examination in 3 years; if normal then, repeat examination every 5 years
Colorectal cancer in any first-degree relative before the age of 60 years or in two or more first-degree relatives at any age	Colonoscopy beginning at age 40 or 10 years before the youngest case in the immediate family, then every 5–10 years
High Risk	
Family history of familial adenomatous polyposis	Endoscopy should begin during puberty; encourage genetic testing; if the genetic test is positive, colectomy is indicated
Family history of hereditary nonpolyposis colon cancer	Consider genetic testing; if the genetic test is positive or if the patient has not had genetic testing, colonoscopy every 1–2 years until age 40, and then annually
Inflammatory bowel disease; chronic ulcerative colitis; Crohn's disease	Begin screening 8 years after the onset of disease; consider proctocolectomy for ulcerative colitis; otherwise, colonoscopy with biopsies for dysplasia every 1–2 years

population, particularly if the relative was less than 60 years old. Patients with a first-degree relative with colorectal cancer who is less than 60 years old or with two or more first-degree relatives with colorectal cancer should begin their screening at the age of 40 years or 10 years earlier than the youngest occurrence. Those with a history of adenomatous polyps should have a repeat colonoscopy in 3 to 5 years.

If there is a significant family history, the patient may be part of an HNPCC family, and he or she may benefit from a more aggressive screening. Patients with HNPCC are recommended to undergo a full colonoscopy every 1 to 2 years starting between the ages of 20 and 30 years or at an age 10 years younger than that at which the youngest family member had colon cancer.

Familial Adenomatous Polyposis

Relatives of patients with FAP should undergo genetic testing. Prophylactic colectomy should be a strong consideration in individuals who bear the FAP mutation. It is important to remember that a negative genetic test only rules out FAP if an affected family member has an identified mutation. For patients who cannot be ruled out for FAP or for those who refuse prophylactic colectomy, colonoscopic screening should occur during or just after adolescence, when the phenotype is first expressed. The latency between the diagnosis of polyposis and the development of cancer is variable, averaging 10 to 15 years.

Inflammatory Bowel Disease

Patients with ulcerative colitis are known to be at increased risk of colorectal cancer. Endoscopic surveillance is mandated, and the presence of severe dysplasia on biopsy is an indication to remove the large bowel before cancer develops. Colonoscopy should be performed every 1 to 2 years beginning after 8 years of disease. However, 50% of patients with more than 10 years of active ulcerative colitis will develop bowel cancer, and endoscopic surveillance and eventual treatment are hampered by the diseased colon. Therefore, the recommendation is to consider proctocolectomy after 10 years of active ulcerative colitis. Patients with Crohn's disease also fall into the high-risk category. However, the disease is not limited to the large intestine, and removal of the colon does not prevent recurrence in the small intestine.

BOX 19–5 CLINICAL PRESENTATION OF COLORECTAL CANCER

- Anemia without other symptoms
- Hematochezia or melena
- Abdominal pain
- Change in bowel habits (left sided cancers)
- Tenesmus (rectal cancer)
- Weight loss
- Bowel obstruction
- Acute abdomen associated with perforation

Clinical Presentation

Colorectal cancer commonly presents in one of three ways: the slow onset of chronic symptoms (80–90%), acute obstruction (6–16%), or acute perforation (2–7%). When patients present with large bowel obstruction, colorectal malignancy should always be considered, because carcinoma is the most common cause of large bowel obstruction, contributing to 60% of cases in the elderly. Often the history and physical examination suggest the diagnosis, which may be confirmed with imaging studies or endoscopy. With acute presentations after a plain film of the abdomen, a contrast enema to confirm the obstruction and to determine the level of obstruction may be diagnostic. The majority of obstructing lesions occur at the splenic flexure and the left colon (60–70%), whereas 23% are right colonic lesions and 7% are rectal lesions. Not surprisingly (and likely related to stage), patients presenting with obstruction have a 1.4-fold greater mortality.

Acute perforation may present as peritonitis, or, if localized, it may present with obstruction or with a new fistula. Concurrent obstruction with perforation occurs in 12% to 19% of patients with obstruction. Perforation increases the mortality of colorectal cancer threefold.

The majority of patients will present with more chronic symptoms, most often bleeding. Although this usually presents as occult bleeding, melena or hematochezia may also be seen depending on the location. Iron-deficiency anemia or fatigue may be associated with bleeding as a result of colorectal neoplasms.

Changing bowel habits and abdominal pain are also common symptoms. Patients may complain of either diarrhea or constipation. Constipation is more often noted with left-sided lesions, with a gradual change in the caliber of stool. Left-sided lesions may also present with cramping abdominal pain associated with nausea and vomiting that are relieved by bowel movements. Rectal lesions may present with tenesmus (the constant feeling of the need to empty the bowel) or, in more advanced cases, pelvic pain. Advanced metastatic disease is suggested by symptoms of right upper quadrant discomfort, fever, hepatomegaly, ascites, or supraclavicular adenopathy.

Colonoscopy with biopsy of the suspicious lesion is the appropriate first step in patients with symptoms that are suggestive of colorectal cancer or abnormal findings on radiologic studies. Not only does colonoscopy allow for the assessment of tumor size, location, and histologic diagnosis, but it also allows for the detection of synchronous lesions. Synchronous carcinomas can occur in up to 7% of patients, whereas synchronous polyps may occur in up to 30% of patients. Clearly, the discovery of additional lesions may change the planned treatment.

After diagnosis, a staging evaluation should be performed. In 1932, Dukes related the stage (and corresponding mortality) of rectal cancer to the depth of tumor invasion. Currently, TNM staging is used for both colon and rectal cancer (Table 19-5). The workup should include routine laboratory blood work, including a complete blood count, liver function tests, and a baseline carcinoembryonic antigen (CEA) level. However, elevated liver-function tests are present in only 15% of patients with metastases. The false-positive rate for elevated liver-function tests is close to 40%. Metastatic disease to the liver is often associated with an elevated CEA. CEA levels exceeding 10 to 20 mg/dL (baseline, <3 mg/dL) have been associated with increased disease failure both in node-negative and node-positive patients.

Further radiographic imaging studies include the chest radiograph, seeking the presence of metastatic disease, and, possibly, CT scanning of the abdomen. The use of the abdominal CT scan is widely debated in the preoperative workup for colon cancer. CT scanning is recommended for patients in whom metastatic disease is suspected or if there is a suspicion of primary invasion into adjacent organs. Because the majority of patients with colon cancer will require an operative procedure, a preoperative CT scan is helpful for planning operative strategies for liver metastasis or contiguous organ involvement. In general, it does not alter the operative plan of patients with local or regional disease. However, discovering the presence of occult metastatic disease may obviate surgical treatment if the patient is neither obstructed or bleeding sufficiently to cause symptomatic anemia. If a preoperative CT scan is not obtained, intraoperative ultrasound of the liver is recommended.

Preoperative staging is critical with rectal cancers, because the staging may have an impact on decision making with regard to neoadjuvant therapies and strategies for sphincter-sparing procedures. In addition to the laboratory studies and chest x-ray obtained for colon cancer, the preoperative workup for rectal cancer should include a CT scan of the abdomen and pelvis as well as an endoscopic ultrasound. Transrectal ultrasound is the most accurate tool for determining tumor stage. Tumor infiltration into the rectal wall can be identified with 67% to 93% accuracy (Figure 19-2). Transrectal ultrasound is superior to CT and MRI for the evaluation of tumor penetration as well as lymph-node staging. Lymph nodes that are more than 3 mm in size and that are hypoechoic are more likely to contain metastases. Currently, low-lying rectal

BOX 19-6 PREOPERATIVE WORKUP OF COLON CANCER

- Full history and physical examination
- If not already performed, a complete colonoscopy (to the cecum) to rule out synchronous lesions
- Double-contrast barium enema if a complete colonoscopy cannot be performed
- Chest x-ray
- Carcinoembryonic antigen level
- Complete blood cell count, comprehensive metabolic profile with liver function tests (ALT, AST, alkaline phosphatase)
- CT scan of abdomen and pelvis (optional)
- If preoperative CT is not performed, intraoperative hepatic ultrasound may be used to assess the liver

TABLE 19–5 • *TNM Classification of Colon and Rectal Tumors*

Primary Tumor (T)			
Tx	Primary tumor cannot be assessed		
T0	No evidence of primary tumor		
Tis	Carcinoma in situ; intraepithelial or invasion of lamina propria		
T1	Tumor invades submucosa		
T2	Tumor invades muscularis propria		
T3	Tumor invades through muscularis propria into subserosa or into nonperitonealized pericolic or perirectal tissues		
T4	Tumor directly invades other organs or structures and/or perforates visceral peritoneum		
Regional Lymph Nodes (N)			
Nx	Regional lymph nodes cannot be assessed		
N0	No regional lymph node metastasis		
N1	Metastasis in one to three regional lymph nodes		
N2	Metastases in four or more regional lymph nodes		
Distant Metastasis (M)			
Mx	Distant metastasis cannot be assessed		
M0	No distant metastasis		
M1	Distant metastasis		
Staging			
Stage	T	N	M
0	Tis	N0	M0
I	T1/T2	N0	M0
II	T3/T4	N0	M0
III	Any T	N1/N2	M0
IV	Any T	Any N	M1

BOX 19–7 PREOPERATIVE WORKUP OF RECTAL CANCER

- Full history and physical examination
- If not already performed, a complete colonoscopy (to the cecum) to rule out synchronous lesions
- Double-contrast barium enema if a complete colonoscopy cannot be performed
- Chest x-ray
- Carcinoembryonic antigen level
- Complete blood cell count, comprehensive metabolic profile with liver-function tests (ALT, AST, alkaline phosphatase)
- CT scan of abdomen and pelvis
- Endoscopic ultrasound (especially if neoadjuvant treatment is considered)

cancers that are T3 or T4 on ultrasound or that demonstrate the possibility of nodal disease are eligible for preoperative chemoradiation therapy. Preoperative therapy often downstages these lesions, which facilitates sphincter-sparing techniques.

Surgical Management of Colon Cancer

Surgery remains the cornerstone of colorectal cancer management. A curative resection is possible in up to 50% of patients. Even in those patients who have disseminated disease at the time of operation, a resection prevents the tumor-related complications of bleeding or obstruction.

The essentials of an adequate oncologic operation involve two principles: (1) excision of the tumor and (2) a wide resection of its

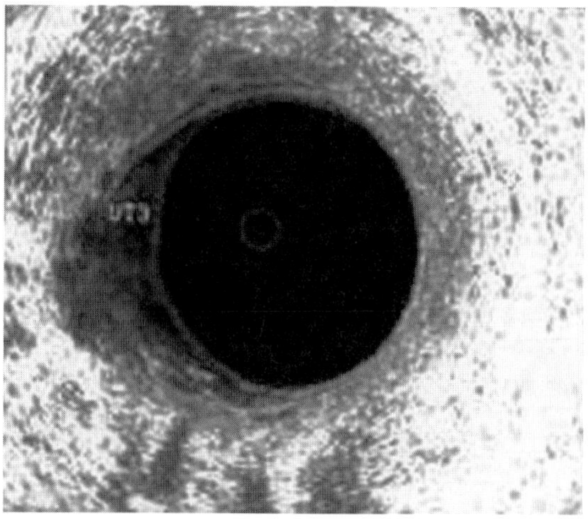

Figure 19–2. Transrectal ultrasound of a rectal cancer.

BOX 19–8 SURGICAL MANAGEMENT OF COLON CANCER

- Thorough exploration of peritoneal cavity to rule out extracolonic spread
- Bimanual palpation of liver to rule out hepatic metastases
- Intraoperative hepatic ultrasound may be considered
- Examination of the entire length of the colon to rule out synchronous lesions
- Complete resection of the involved bowel segment with negative proximal, distal, and radial margins
- Incorporation of all draining lymph nodes for the involved bowel segment

draining lymphatic bed. Because colorectal carcinoma spreads through the lymphatics, adequate lengths of bowel proximal and distal to the cancer must be resected in addition to its major lymphatic drainage within the mesentery. Currently, a minimum of a 5-cm margin is recommended to achieve this end for colon cancers, whereas a 2-cm margin is recommended for rectal cancers. The anatomically defined vascular region dictates the resection for colon cancer (Figure 19-3). Traditionally, the "no-touch" technique has been recommended; however, there has been no survival advantage demonstrated by this technique. This technique entails controlling the lymphovascular bundle proximal and distal to the tumor before manipulation of the tumor.

The cecum, the ascending colon, and the proximal transverse colon are derived from the embryonic midgut, and they are supplied by branches of the superior mesenteric antigen (SMA), including the ileocolic, the right colic, and the middle colic vessels (Figure 19-4). Branches of the inferior mesenteric artery (IMA), including the left colic, the sigmoid, and the superior rectal arteries, supply the descending colon, the sigmoid colon, and the rectum. The distal rectum is supplied by the middle and inferior rectal arteries, which are branches of the hypogastric and pudendal arteries. The marginal artery of Drummond provides the blood supply to the watershed region that connects the IMA and SMA over the distal transverse colon. The venous drainage accompanies the respective arteries. The superior and inferior mesenteric veins drain into the portal circulation, whereas the middle and inferior rectal veins drain into the internal iliac vein and the systemic circulation. The lymphatic drainage of the colon parallels the vascular anatomy. The lymphatic drainage of the upper third of the rectum follows the inferior mesenteric vein (IMV), whereas the lower two thirds are drained in the hypogastric nodes, which in turn drain to the paraaortic nodes or via the pudendal nodes, which drain to the inguinal nodes.

A right hemicolectomy is indicated for lesions involving the cecum, the ascending colon, or the hepatic flexure (Figure 19-3, *A* and *B*). Five to eight centimeters of terminal ileum are included in the bowel resection, which extends just proximal to or may include the right branch of the middle colic artery. Care is taken to not injure retroperitoneal structures such as the ureter, the gonadal vessels, the vena cava, and the duodenum.

Hepatic flexure lesions may be included in a right hemicolectomy, and, similarly, splenic flexure lesions may be addressed with a left hemicolectomy (Figure 19-3, *B* and *D*). Mid-transverse lesions may be amenable to a transverse colectomy or to an extended right hemicolectomy (Figure 19-3, *B* and *C*). An extended right hemicolectomy incorporates resection of the middle colic artery.

For cancers of the splenic flexure, the distal half of the transverse colon and the descending colon are removed in a left hemicolectomy (Figure 19-3, *D* and *E*). The left colic artery is resected with preservation of the left branch of the middle colic artery to supply the watershed

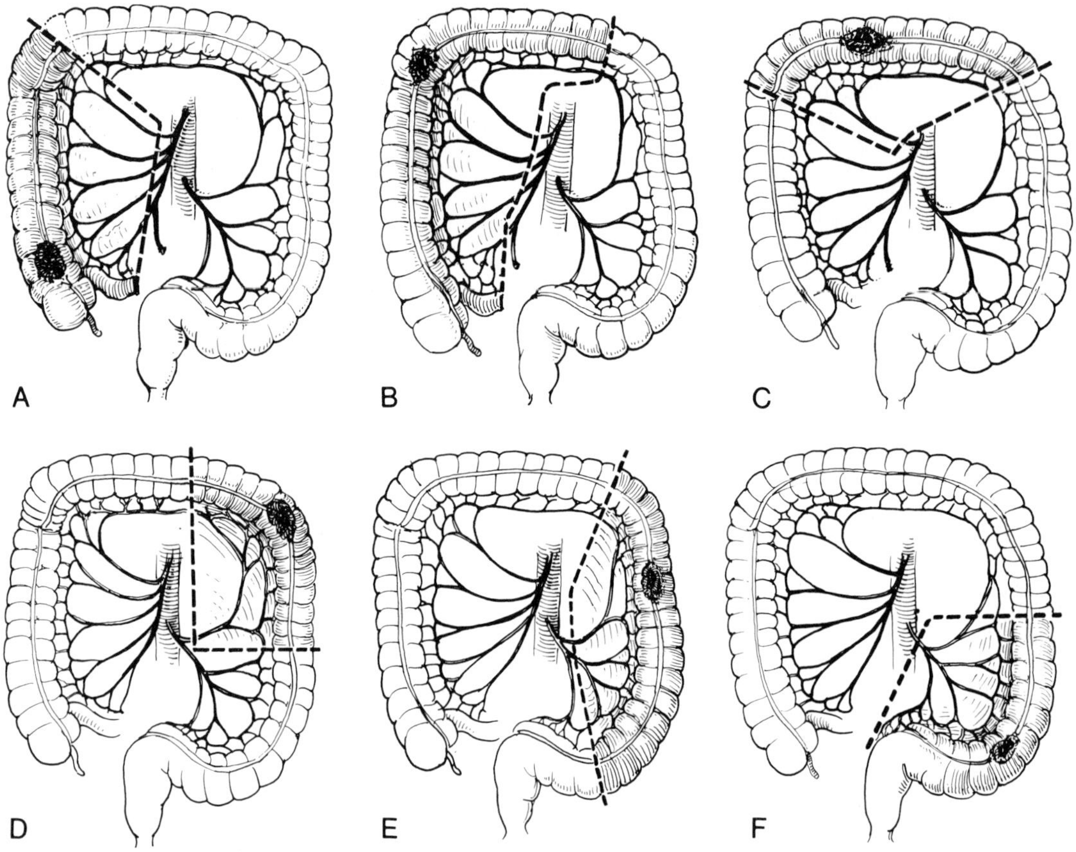

Figure 19–3. Standard operative approaches for cancers of the colon. (From Bland KI, Karakousis CP, Copeland EM. *Atlas of surgical oncology*. Philadelphia: WB Saunders, 1995.)

region. As with a right hemicolectomy, retroperitoneal structures are at risk, including the splenic vein, the duodenum, the pancreas, and the ureter.

Cancers of the sigmoid colon are managed by a sigmoid colectomy (Figure 19-3, *F*). This resection includes the distal descending colon to the proximal rectum. The IMA is ligated just distal to the origin of the left colic artery.

There are several instances in which a total abdominal colectomy may be warranted. These include the presence of synchronous lesions, obstruction, associated symptomatic sigmoid diverticulosis, a young patient age with a worrisome family history, and adherence of the sigmoid colon to a cecal carcinoma. The procedure entails the removal of the entire colon from the cecum to the level of the rectum with an ileorectal anastomosis.

Minimally invasive colon resection is a newer approach to the resection of selected colon cancers. The laparoscopic approach does not change the indication for the procedure and should not compromise the extent of the resection. Although this approach may offer decreased discomfort and convalescence, initial series reported an alarming rate of trocar-site tumors. This finding forced the vigorous examination of this technique via several small, randomized, controlled, clinical trials as well as in the basic science laboratory. The United States trial, sponsored by the National Cancer Institute and called the NCI-COST study (National Cancer Institute's Clinical Outcomes of Surgical Therapies), completed accrual in August 2001. Early reports do not reveal an increased incidence of trocar-associated tumors as compared with the traditional open technique among the more than 20 centers that contributed to the study. These operations, although technically demanding, are feasible and safe, and they yield a similar number of resected lymph nodes and comparable specimen length as do open procedures.

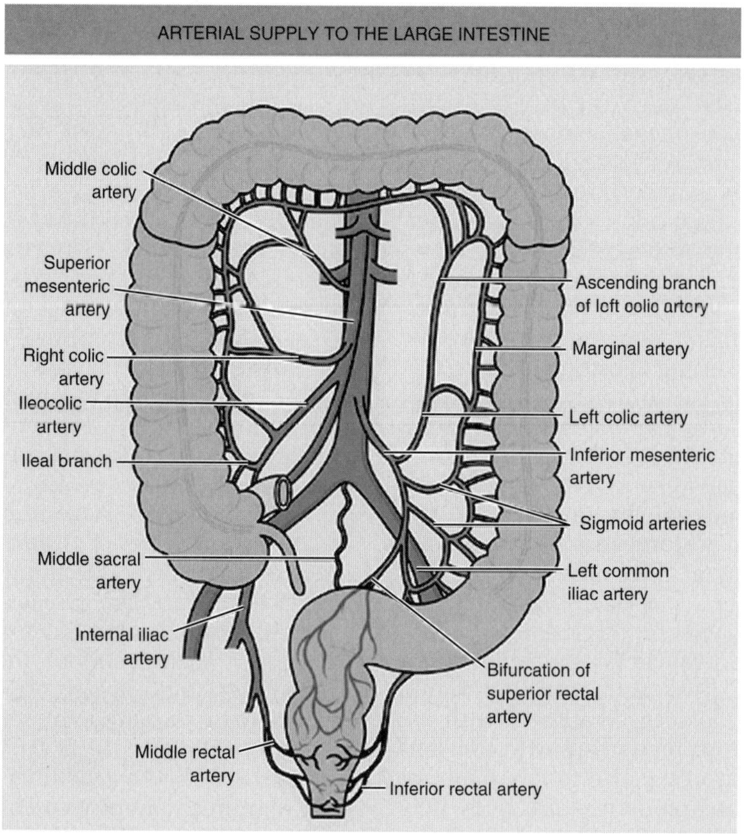

A

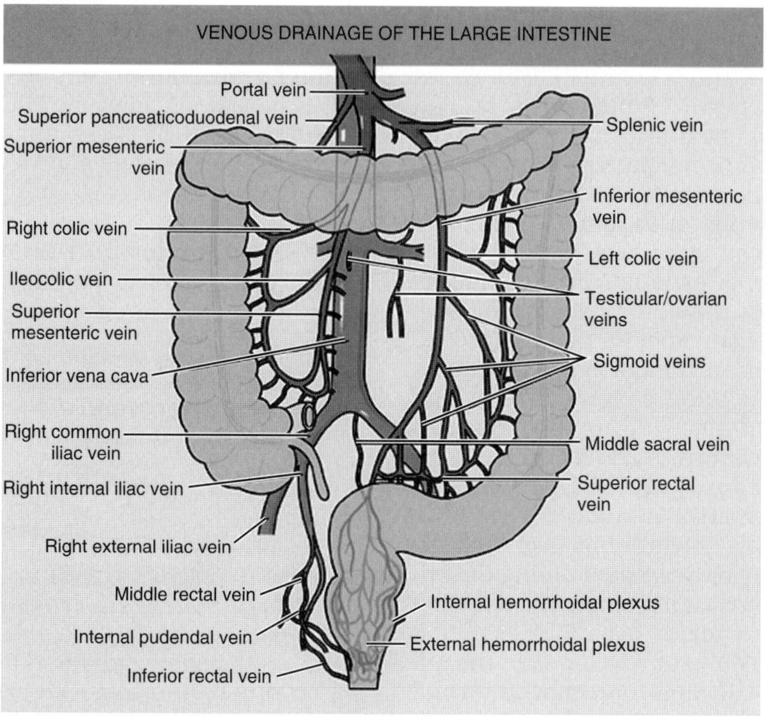

B

Figure 19–4. Arterial and venous supply of the large bowel. (From Bloom ND, Beattie ED, Harvey JC. *Atlas of cancer surgery*. Philadelphia: WB Saunders, 2000.)

Colon cancer is the most common cause of large-bowel obstructions. These are more often associated with larger cancers, and they are more frequently left sided. In general, right-sided lesions may be amenable to resection and primary anastomosis. For left-sided lesions, primary anastomosis may be possible if on-table lavage of the proximal colon can be safely performed or if a preoperative colonic stent allows for decompression before the resection. In circumstances in which the anastomosis is questionable, a primary anastomosis may be protected by a diverting ileostomy. An alternative is resection of the tumor with a proximal colostomy and Hartman's pouch. In addition, the historical option of a three-stage procedure consisting of a transverse colostomy followed by a resection and primary anastomosis and takedown of the colostomy may also be considered. Finally, subtotal colectomy with primary anastomosis offers a one-stage operation that may also address synchronous lesions.

Perforated colon cancer is associated with a poor prognosis. Two thirds of perforated lesions present as a localized abscess, with the remaining one third presenting with free perforation and peritonitis. The tumor may not always be the site of perforation that may often involve more proximal bowel. Both the tumor and the site of perforation should be included in the resection. If a primary anastomosis is performed, consideration should be given to a diverting proximal ostomy. In patients with generalized peritonitis, an end colostomy should be considered, with either a Hartman's pouch or mucus fistula formation. In the case of perforation that has occurred remote from the site of the primary tumor, a subtotal colectomy should be considered.

In the absence of metastatic disease, locally advanced tumors should be resected en bloc. The affected organ should be resected to include a margin of normal tissue. Although locally advanced colon cancers have a high rate of local recurrence (up to 50%), patients with negative margins on resection have the same survival as those with similar stage and no local involvement.

In patients with synchronous liver metastasis, resection may be attempted during the primary operation unless major hepatic resection is indicated. If a major hepatic resection is indicated, a delay of 6 to 8 weeks after the primary resection will allow for recuperation and for restaging of the hepatic burden. The goals of hepatic resection should be a pathologic margin of more than 1 cm and a resection of no more than 70% of liver parenchyma (see Chapter 26: Surgery for Advanced Disease).

Adjuvant Therapy of Colon Cancer

The cornerstone of adjuvant therapy for colon cancer has been 5-fluorouracil (5-FU). Although early trials with 5-FU alone showed no survival advantage, this changed when 5-FU was used in combination with other chemotherapeutic agents (MOF; methyl CCNU, vincristine [Oncovin], and 5-FU) or with modulators of 5-FU activity (leucovorin and levamisole). Subsequently, the combination of 5-FU and leucovorin were shown to be superior to MOF for stage III disease. In 1990, a National Institutes of Health consensus conference established 5-FU and leucovorin as the standard of care for resected node-positive (stage III) colon cancer. Since that time, newer drugs have demonstrated increased activity against metastatic disease, and they have been evaluated in the adjuvant setting. The addition of oxaliplatin to 5-FU and leucovorin (known as FOLFOX4) demonstrated a statistically significant improvement in disease-free survival for stage III colorectal cancer, and many consider this the new standard of care. Other drugs, such as irinotecan, capecitabine, and targeted therapies are still under investigation in the adjuvant setting.

The benefit of adjuvant chemotherapy for stage II colon cancer is less clear. Many of the trials that demonstrated a benefit of adjuvant

BOX 19–9 CHEMOTHERAPY REGIMENS FOR THE ADJUVANT THERAPY OF STAGE III COLON CANCER

- *The Roswell Park regimen:* bolus 5-fluorouracil (500 mg/m²) plus high-dose leucovorin (500 mg/m²) weekly for 6 of each 8 weeks for a total of four cycles
- *The Mayo regimen:* bolus 5-fluorouracil (425 mg/m²) daily for 5 days every 4 to 5 weeks, plus low-dose leucovorin (20 mg/m²) on days 1 to 5, for 6 cycles
- *The FOLFOX4 regimen:* infusional 5-fluorouracil (400 mg/m² then 600 mg/m² over 22 hours) on days 1 and 2 plus leucovorin (200 mg/m²) over 2 hours on days 1 and 2 plus oxaliplatin (85 mg/m²) on day 1, every 2 weeks for 12 cycles

chemotherapy in stage III disease also included stage II patients, and they failed to show a similar benefit. However, some showed a trend toward improved survival with adjuvant chemotherapy, but most were underpowered to detect small differences. Three trials that were designed solely to look at chemotherapy for stage II disease—INT 0035, QUASAR, and IMPACT B2—failed to demonstrate a statistically significant improvement in overall survival.

Several meta-analyses have been performed to help shed light on this question. The Intergroup Pooled Analysis looked at 3,302 patients in seven randomized trials and found that adjuvant 5-FU–based therapy was associated with a disease-free survival benefit but not with an overall survival benefit. The Cancer Care Ontario Program in Evidence-Based Care looked at 4,187 patients in 12 randomized trials and again failed to identify a statistically significant improvement in overall survival. Therefore, the routine use of adjuvant chemotherapy for stage II colon cancer is not recommended. However, it may be considered for patients with higher-risk disease (e.g., T4 lesion, inadequate nodal sampling, poorly differentiated histology). The benefits of therapy (at best a 2–3% survival advantage at 5 years) must be weighed against its toxicity.

Surgical Management of Rectal Cancer

Historically, rectal cancers were treated with an abdominoperineal resection (APR), which involves the removal of the entire rectum and anus. With the advent of neoadjuvant chemoradiotherapy, the management of rectal cancers has come to incorporate methods that provide the patient with sphincter preservation while providing 5-year survival rates equivalent to those of patients who have undergone an APR. Therefore, preoperative staging is critical for patient selection.

The length of the rectum is divided into three areas according to the distance from the anal verge. The upper third begins approximately 10 cm from the anal verge. Lesions in this region have similar vascular and lymphatic drainage as would a sigmoid colon cancer. The middle rectum is 6 to 10 cm from the anal verge, and the distal rectum 0 to 5 cm from the anal verge. These cancers can invade the internal or external sphincter and the levator muscles. The blood supply to the rectum, as previously discussed, arises from superior, middle, and inferior hemorrhoidal arteries, which drain either to the portal or the systemic circulation.

Multiple factors are considered when planning the surgical management of rectal cancer, including the depth of tumor invasion, lymph-node involvement, histologic grade, and location. T1 lesions have lymph-node metastasis in up to 10% of cases. T2 and T3 lesions have 20% and up to 70% lymph-node involvement, respectively. The criteria for transanal excision are the following: T1 or T2 lesions within 10 cm of the anal verge that are less than 4 cm or a fourth of the circumference, that are mobile, that are without evidence of lymph-node metastasis, and that are of low histologic grade. Excision should be full thickness and should incorporate 1 cm of grossly normal mucosa. Patients who are unfit for radical surgical excision may also benefit from transanal excision. Those with T2 lesions will most likely be advised to receive adjuvant therapy.

Those patients who have large or local tumor burden and who are not candidates for local excision should undergo transabdominal resection. As with colon cancer, an adequate lymphadenectomy should be performed. For resection of rectal cancer, a total mesorectal excision is increasingly recognized to be an important component of the multimodality approach (see Chapter 20: Multimodal Therapy for Select Gastrointestinal Malignancies).

A low anterior resection (LAR) may be performed in patients with middle to low rectal cancers for which a 2-cm margin may be obtained. Survival has been found to be dependent on the distance of the tumor from the anal verge, the presence of lymph-node metastasis, and the lateral extent of dissection. Retrospective studies have demonstrated no difference in local recurrence or survival between an APR and LAR for low to middle rectal cancers.

For low rectal cancers, an alternative to the LAR is a proctectomy with coloanal anastomosis. The cancer should be a minimum of 2 cm above the dentate line. Functionally, patients with anastomosis this close to the sphincter muscles may benefit from either a coloplasty or a colonic J pouch, especially during the first year or two after resection. A proximal diverting ileostomy may be indicated for those anastomoses less than 7 cm from the anal verge or if the anastomosis has been completed with some tension or performed in a patient with preoperative radiation or steroid use.

Adjuvant Therapy of Rectal Cancer

As opposed to colon cancer, adjuvant therapy for rectal cancer includes both radiation and chemotherapy. Whereas colon cancer recurrences are almost always distant, patients with rectal cancer are as likely to have local recurrences within the pelvis as they are to have distant recurrences. Another difference in adjuvant therapy between colon and rectal cancer is that, whereas adjuvant therapy for stage II colon cancer is controversial, it is clearly indicated for stage II rectal cancer. The Gastrointestinal Tumor Study Group trial 7175 randomly assigned 227 patients with stages II and III rectal cancer to either observation, postoperative radiation therapy, postoperative chemotherapy, or postoperative chemoradiation. The trial found a decrease in local recurrence from 24% to 11%, with a survival advantage at 7 years for chemoradiation. The researchers used a combination of 5-FU and methyl-CCNU, but subsequent trials have demonstrated no additional benefit to methyl-CCNU, and so it is no longer used for the adjuvant treatment of rectal cancer. The optimum dosing (bolus versus infusional versus prolonged venous infusion) and timing of 5-FU with respect to radiation (prior to, following, and/or during) have not been established conclusively, and practices vary among institutions.

Neoadjuvant Treatment of Rectal Cancer

An alternate approach is the delivery of chemoradiation before surgery. Neoadjuvant chemoradiation potentially downsizes tumors to increase the potential for sphincter-sparing operations. It may also decrease the potential of radiation enteritis because the absence of adhesions will limit exposure of the small bowel to radiation. Therefore, any patient with an ultrasound stage of T3 or greater or with suspicious mesorectal lymph-node involvement should be considered for preoperative chemoradiation. The full pelvis is treated to at least 4,500 cGy, with a boost to the tumor site for a total dose of at least 5,040 cGy. Chemotherapy is given to enhance the radiosensitivity of the tumors. The operation is then scheduled for 5 to 6 weeks after completion of the radiation therapy.

Surveillance for Colorectal Cancer Recurrence

Unfortunately, 50% of patients who undergo resection for colorectal cancer will have tumor recurrence. More than 80% of recurrences occur within the first 2.5 years. After the completion of therapy, patients require close surveillance. Surveillance practices are variable based on institution, although almost universally early and aggressive surveillance is performed for the first 2 to 3 years after resection. Aggressive postoperative surveillance may include a history and a physical examination every 3 months and laboratory testing, including a complete blood cell count, liver function tests, and CEA level. If it was elevated preoperatively, a postoperative CEA level should be obtained at 6 weeks. An elevated CEA level that fails to return to baseline suggests incomplete resection or metastatic disease. An elevated CEA level has been noted in up to 80% to 90% of patients with hepatic metastases. If the colon was able to be examined preoperatively, then colonoscopy 1 year after resection (6 months if entire colon was not visualized preoperatively) should be performed. If this is normal, repeat examination is done in 3 years and every 5 years unless an abnormality is noted. Anastomotic recurrence is rare; if it is present, it usually represents locally recurrent disease invading though the bowel wall. A chest radiograph is obtained every 6 months during the first 2 to 3 years and then yearly thereafter. Other imaging modalities, such as transrectal ultrasound, CT scans, and positron emission tomography (PET) scanning, are more controversial.

Key Selected Readings

Fazio VW, Church JM, Delaney CP. *Current therapy in colon and rectal surgery,* 2nd ed. St. Louis: Elsevier-Mosby, 2003.

Gordon PH, Nivotvongs S, eds. Malignant neoplasms of the colon and rectum. In: *Principles and practice of surgery for the colon, rectum and anus.* St. Louis: Quality Medical Publishing, Inc., 1999.

Selected Readings

Andre T, Boni C, Mounedji-Boudiaf L, *et al.* Oxaliplatin, fluorouracil, and leucovorin as adjuvant treatment for colon cancer. *N Engl J Med* 2004;350:2343–2351.

Arnoletti JP, Bland KI. Neoadjuvant and adjuvant therapy for rectal cancer. *Surg Oncol Clin N Am* 2006;15:147–157.

Barabouti DG, Wong WD. Current management of rectal cancer: total mesorectal excision (nerve sparing) technique and clinical outcome. *Surg Oncol Clin N Am* 2005;14:137–155.

Benson AB 3rd, Schrag D, Somerfield MR, *et al.* American Society of Clinical Oncology recommendations on adjuvant chemotherapy for stage II colon cancer. *J Clin Oncol* 2004;22:3408–3419.

Clevers H. Colon cancer—understanding how NSAIDs work. *N Engl J Med* 2006;354:761–763.

Corman ML, ed. *Colon and rectal surgery,* 4th ed. New York: Lippincott-Raven Publishers, 1998.

Deans G, Krukowski Z, Irwin S. Malignant obstruction of the left colon. *Br J Surg* 1994;81:1270–1276.

Fearon ER, Vogelstein B. A genetic model for colorectal tumorigenesis. *Cell* 1990;61:155–157.

Finlayson E, Nelson H. Laparoscopic colectomy for cancer. *Am J Clin Oncol* 2005;28:521–525.

Gastrointestinal Tumor Study Group. Prolongation of the disease-free interval in surgically treated rectal carcinoma. *N Engl J Med* 1985;312:1465–1472.

Jeong SY, Chessin DB, Guillem JG. Surgical treatment of rectal cancer: radical resection. *Surg Oncol Clin N Am* 2006;15:95–107.

Khatri VP, Petrelli NJ, Belghiti J. Extending the frontiers of surgical therapy for hepatic colorectal metastases: is there a limit? *J Clin Oncol* 2005;23:8490–8499.

McCormick JT, Gregorcyk SG. Preoperative evaluation of colorectal cancer. *Surg Oncol Clin N Am* 2006;15:39–49.

Meyerhardt JA, Mayer RJ. Systemic therapy for colorectal cancer. *N Engl J Med* 2005;352:476–487.

Moertel C, Fleming T, Macdonald J, *et al.* Fluorouracil plus levamisole as effective adjuvant therapy after resection of stage II colon carcinoma: a final report. *Ann Internal Med* 1995;122:321–326.

O'Connell M, Martenson J, Wieand H, *et al.* Improving adjuvant therapy for rectal cancer by combining protracted infusion fluorouracil with radiation therapy after curative surgery. *N Engl J Med* 1994;331: 502–557.

Perretta S, Guerrero V, Garcia-Aguilar J. Surgical treatment of rectal cancer: local resection. *Surg Oncol Clin N Am* 2006;15:67–93.

Pfister DG, Benson AB, Somerfield MR. Surveillance strategies after curative treatment of colorectal cancer. *N Engl J Med* 2004;350:2375–2382.

Poynter JN, Gruber SB, Higgins PDR, *et al.* Statins and the risk of colorectal cancer. *N Engl J Med* 2005;352:2184–2192.

Rossi H, Rothenberger DA. Surgical treatment of colon cancer. *Surg Oncol Clin N Am* 2006;15:109–127.

Sauer R, Becker H, Hohenberger W, *et al.* Preoperative versus postoperative chemoradiotherapy for rectal cancer. *N Engl J Med* 2004;351:1731–1740.

Stryker S, Wolff B, Culp C, *et al.* Natural history of untreated colonic polyps. *Gastroenterology* 1987;93: 1009–1013.

Twelves C, Wong A, Nowack MP, *et al.* Capecitabine as adjuvant treatment for stage III colon cancer. *N Engl J Med* 2005;352:2696–2704.

Van Cutsem E, Hoff PM, Harper P, *et al.* Oral capecitabine vs intravenous 5-flourouracil and leucovorin: integrated efficacy data and novel analyses from two large, randomized, phase III trials. *Br J Cancer* 2004;90:1190–1197.

Weitz J, Koch M, Debus J, *et al.* Colorectal cancer. *Lancet* 2005;365:153–165.

Winawer S, Fletcher R, Rex D, *et al.* Colorectal cancer screening and surveillance: clinical guidelines and rationale—update based on new evidence. *Gastroenterology* 2003;124:544–560.

Wolmark N, Rockette H, Fisher B, *et al.* The benefit of leucovorin-modulated fluorouracil as postoperative adjuvant therapy for primary colon cancer: results from National Surgical Adjuvant Breast and Bowel Project protocol C-03. *J Clin Oncol* 1993; 11: 1879–1887.

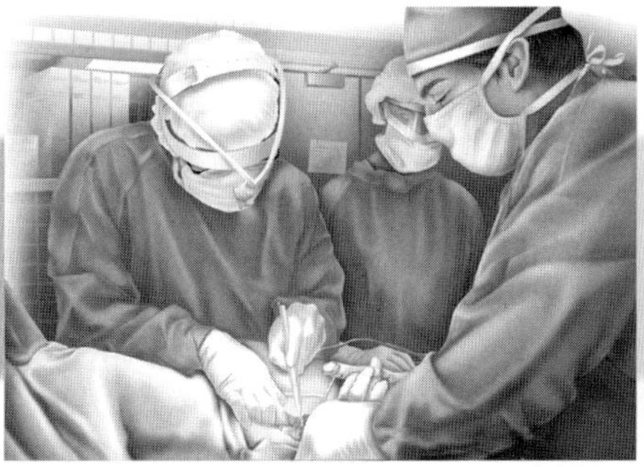

20

Multimodal Therapy for Select Gastrointestinal Malignancies

Joseph Kim and Syed A. Ahmad

Multimodal Therapy for Select Gastrointestinal Malignancies: Key Points

- Describe the clinical presentation, diagnosis, and treatment of anal cancer.
- Discuss treatment approaches specific to cancers of the upper anal canal.
- Outline the clinical assessment and treatment of rectal carcinoma.
- Discuss the incidence, diagnosis, and treatment approaches to gastric carcinoma.
- List the steps taken in the preoperative evaluation of pancreatic cancer.
- Compare the outcomes achieved with surgery versus multimodal strategies for pancreatic cancer.

Surgery alone is not enough to completely eliminate many gastrointestinal (GI) tract cancers. Therefore, for many patients, methods of management in addition to surgery will be necessary for cure, palliation, or prolongation of survival. In select patients, surgery may not even be warranted, and chemotherapy and/or radiation may be sufficient for cure.

The current treatment of many GI malignancies reflects these varied methods of treatment. Surgery, radiation, and chemotherapy all have roles in the treatment of GI malignancies, and the details of their use, sequencing, and combination have emerged as a major topic of research over the past several years. Although an overall discussion of the pathophysiology and surgical treatment is specifically covered in other chapters, this chapter will focus on the important aspects of multimodal therapy with respect to cancers of the anal canal, the rectum, the stomach, and the pancreas.

The importance of communication between the physicians of the treating specialties cannot be overstated. This minimizes patient confusion and allows for the proper coordination and planning of treatments. Communication may be enhanced through group tumor board or multidisciplinary conferences or through the repetitive close working relationships of the specialists.

Anal Cancer

Carcinoma of the anal canal is a rare disease, comprising approximately 1.6% of digestive tract cancers. Although the anal canal's definition has varied, it is best defined as extending proximally from the anorectal junction (where the rectum begins to pass through the levator ani muscles) to the anal verge distally. The lower anal canal, therefore, is lined by squamous epithelium up to the dentate line, where a transition occurs over approximately the next 1 cm until the mucosa becomes uniformly lined by columnar epithelium in the upper anal canal (Figure 20-1). Cancers arising within 5 cm distal to the anal verge in keratinized skin are referred to as *anal margin cancers;* they are considered skin cancers and treated accordingly.

Clinical Presentation

Anal cancer was once believed to be the result of chronic inflammation of the perianal area. Inflammatory bowel disease was even believed to be a risk factor. Recent epidemiologic surveys have discounted these notions, implicating genital viral infections, the human papilloma virus (predominately serotypes 16 and 18), chronic immunosuppression, human immunodeficiency virus infection, and smoking as risk factors. Among patients who have squamous cell carcinoma of the anus, rectal bleeding remains the most

BOX 20-1 RISK FACTORS FOR ANAL CANAL CANCER

- Human papilloma virus
- Immunosuppression
- Human immunodeficiency virus
- Tobacco use

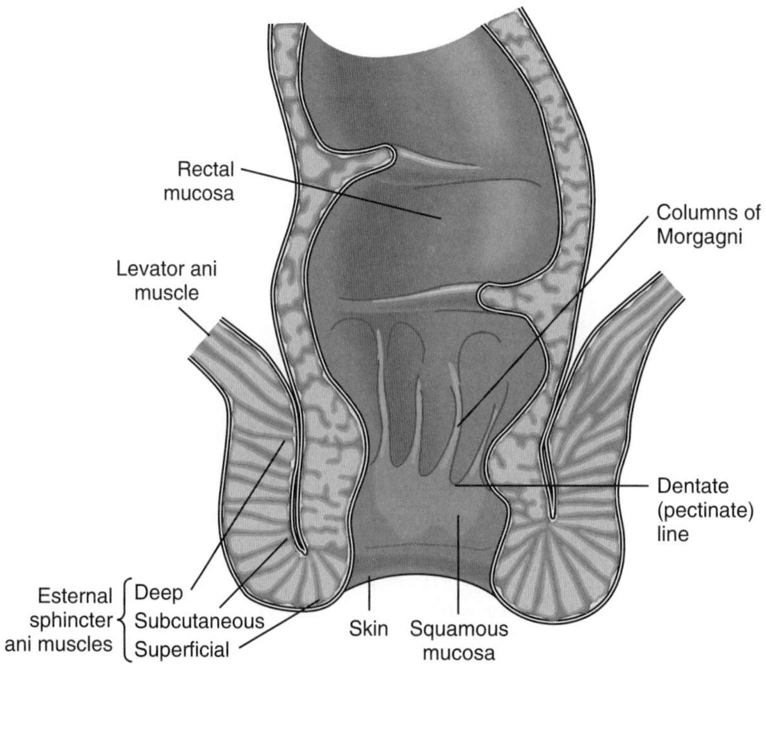

Figure 20-1. Diagram of the anatomic landmarks of the anal canal.

common initial presentation. Another 30% of patients will present with either pain or the sensation of a rectal mass.

Diagnostic Evaluation

In addition to a digital rectal examination, the patient with a suspicious anal lesion warrants an anoscopic visual examination and biopsy of such lesions. A thorough examination should include an evaluation for palpable lymphadenopathy in the inguinal regions, because lymph-node metastases can be present in up to 30% to 45% of patients. Suspicious regional lymph nodes should be evaluated by fine-needle aspiration. Lymph node involvement is directly related to primary tumor size and degree of invasion. Tumors of less than 2 cm rarely metastasize to lymph nodes.

For further evaluation, endoanal ultrasound or magnetic resonance imaging (MRI) may assist with the delineation of the depth and extent of invasion and with the detection of recurrences. Abdominal and pelvic computed tomography (CT) and chest radiography are helpful for assessing local disease and distant spread. Colonoscopy is warranted to survey the entire colon to evaluate for synchronous colonic lesions.

Treatment

Historically, an abdominoperineal resection (APR) with permanent colostomy was the treatment of choice for tumors in the anal canal, with 5-year survival rates ranging from 40% to 60%. In the early 1970s, Nigro and colleagues, on the basis of studies exploiting the potentiating effects of chemotherapy on radiation, investigated and reported on the multimodality treatment of anal canal cancers to improve survival. In their initial report, three patients were successfully treated with radiation therapy and concurrent chemotherapy, including fluorouracil and mitomycin. More recent studies have validated their initial conclusions, documenting 70% to 90% survival in select patients with chemoradiation regimens. Thus, radical surgery was used selectively only for patients who failed to completely respond to chemoradiation or for those whose disease recurred.

Several studies have examined the additive effect of chemotherapy to the radiation treatments (Table 20-1). The first of two large multicenter trials in Europe was conducted by the United Kingdom Coordinating Committee for Cancer. They demonstrated that, for the nonsurgical management of anal cancer, the addition of a regimen of 5-fluorouracil (5-FU) to 45 Gy of radiotherapy increased local control from 41% to 64% ($P < .0001$). However, there was no overall survival advantage ($P = .25$).

The second large multicenter trial in Europe was conducted by the European Organization for Research and Treatment of Cancer. Their study similarly demonstrated an improvement in local control with the addition of 5-FU to radiotherapy. The complete response improved from 54% to 80%, and local control improved from 55% to 73% for the combined regimen after surgical resection ($P = .02$). Again, however, there was no statistical difference in overall 5-year survival rates between the two groups.

In the United States, the Radiation Therapy Oncology Group and Eastern Cooperative Oncology Group trial confirmed the superiority of combination therapies over radiation alone while also addressing the contribution of mitomycin. Patients who were assigned to mitomycin and 5-FU treatment with radiation therapy as compared with radiation and 5-FU alone had improved disease-free survival at

TABLE 20-1 • *Randomized Studies of Radiation Therapy Versus Combined Therapy for Anal Cancer*

Study	Local Control with Radiation Therapy Alone	Local Control with Chemotherapy/ Radiation Therapy	Survival with Radiation Therapy Alone	Survival with Chemotherapy/ Radiation Therapy
United Kingdom Coordinating Committee for Cancer	41%	64%	58% (4 years)	65% (4 years)
European Organization for Research and Treatment of Cancer	55%	73%	52% (5 years)	57% (5 years)

4 years (73% versus 51%; $P = .0003$). However, a significant difference in overall survival was not observed at 4 years. Patients who initially fail the standard regimen of chemoradiation are eligible for additional nonoperative management. In the Radiation Therapy Oncology Group and Eastern Cooperative Oncology Group trial, salvage chemotherapy with 5-FU and cisplatin combined with a radiation boost avoided a permanent colostomy in selected patients with small amounts of residual tumor. Of 24 patients undergoing salvage chemoradiation, 12 (50%) were rendered disease-free using this regimen.

Surgery

The surgical indications for anal canal carcinoma are summarized in Table 20-2. When the anal sphincter is not involved, local excision is appropriate for carcinoma in situ and some T1 lesions. The presence of metastatic disease within the inguinal basins (unilateral or bilateral) designates stage III disease. Failure of these nodes to respond to standard chemoradiation therapy or recurrence in these nodes mandates surgical treatment, which may include unilateral or bilateral superficial and deep inguinal node dissections. Patients with stage IV or distant metastatic disease are candidates for palliative surgery, as are patients with severely symptomatic disease (e.g., perineal sepsis, fistulae, intolerable incontinence). Finally, radical resection is reserved for residual or recurrent cancer in the anal canal after nonoperative therapy.

Upper Anal Canal

Cancers of the upper anal canal are typically adenocarcinomas in origin. They should be considered as low rectal cancers and treated accordingly. Because they are by definition at the level of the anal sphincter, they will require an APR unless they are well-differentiated T1 lesions that are amenable to complete local excision.

Rectal Carcinoma

There were approximately 42,000 new cases of rectal carcinoma in the United States in 2006, making it the second most common GI tract malignancy, after colon cancer. Historically, APR had been the gold-standard resection for rectal carcinoma at all levels; however, local recurrence rates of 36% to 67% demanded additional measures for cure and/or palliation. Over the last 20 years, adjuvant therapies have been actively investigated, allowing for the performance of less radical surgery while improving the overall prognosis of rectal carcinoma.

Clinical Evaluation

Patients are commonly diagnosed with rectal carcinoma after screening or evaluation for bleeding. When carcinoma is discovered, full evaluation of the patient, including digital rectal examination, must be performed. The entire colon and rectum should be inspected endoscopically or radiographically, and all suspicious lesions should be biopsied. Where available, endorectal ultrasound or MRI can more accurately determine the depth of invasion, because both can identify discrete layers of the rectal wall. Their major limitation is the inability to adequately predict lymph-node involvement. CT scanning is useful for the evaluation of metastatic disease. Additionally, chest radiography should be employed to exclude metastatic pulmonary disease.

Treatment

As previously stated, APR has been the surgical treatment of choice for rectal carcinoma. Today, although complete surgical extirpation

TABLE 20-2 • *Possible Surgical Treatment Options for Anal Canal Cancer*

Treatment	Most Applicable Situation
Local excision	In situ or T1 disease
Biopsy only for diagnosis	Most situations in which chemoradiation is the primary treatment
Radical excision	Recurrent or persistent disease; fistula; incontinence; perineal sepsis
Inguinal/iliac-node dissection	Involvement of nodal basins; unresponsive to chemotherapy/radiation therapy

BOX 20–2 INDICATIONS FOR LOCAL EXCISION FOR RECTAL CANCER

- Tumor <3 cm
- Tumor <30% of the circumference of the rectum
- Only submucosa or superficial muscularis invasion
- No lymphatic or vascular invasion or evidence of lymph-node involvement
- Well-differentiated to moderately differentiated histology
- Can be visualized through the transanal approach

remains the mainstay of treatment, there are options that offer sphincter preservation in many instances. For example, early small distal lesions may be amenable to local excision. Ideal patients are those who have small, well-differentiated distal lesions amenable to a full-thickness excision and who have a low risk of harboring occult lymph node metastases. Fragmentation, piecemeal excision, and poor visualization all increase local recurrence rates. Appropriate imaging is also important, because the T stage will have an impact on the recurrence rate. Endoscopic ultrasound or specialized MRI evaluation can often distinguish T1, T2, and T3 lesions. Local recurrence after surgery alone is approximately 5% for T1 lesions, but it is an excessive risk for all but the most fragile patients, with T2 lesions recurring in approximately 8% to 27% of cases. Failure rates can be reduced by approximately half by adding postoperative radiotherapy with or without chemotherapy, which makes this a reasonable approach for selected patients to avoid more radical surgery. Occasionally, sphincter-preserving trans-sacral and posterior-approach local resections are useful, because they avoid an abdominal incision; however, these procedures have their own set of complications.

Most patients have more advanced lesions at presentation and are not good candidates for local excisional approaches. Low rectal lesions may be resected in a combined APR that includes the removal of the anal sphincter or transabdominally with a low colo-anal anastomosis. For lesions in the middle to upper rectum, a low anterior resection and anastomosis is the treatment of choice today. These resections should encompass a wide anatomic dissection of the rectum with surrounding fat-containing lymph nodes (mesorectum). This surgical strategy is referred to as a *total mesorectal excision* (TME), and it has led to a significant decrease in the rate of local recurrence (Figure 20-2). Local recurrence rates between 4% and 10% have been reported with this operative approach alone; however, not all surgeons are trained in proper sharp TME techniques and thus may not achieve these results. A local recurrence can cause difficult-to-control symptoms such as severe pelvic pain and tenesmus. Bowel obstruction and/or fistulas to the bladder or vagina can occur. These complications may be impossible to correct or even to adequately palliate, and they can lead to death. Therefore, despite optimal surgical therapy, patterns of locoregional recurrence over the years have indicated a need for adjuvant regional therapy in most patients with resected tumors of the rectum.

Most studies of adjuvant radiation have shown a reduction in the local recurrence rate of rectal cancer as compared with surgery alone (Table 20-3). This is particularly true when TME surgery is not rigorously performed and the control group's recurrence rate is high. When the surgery-alone group's recurrence

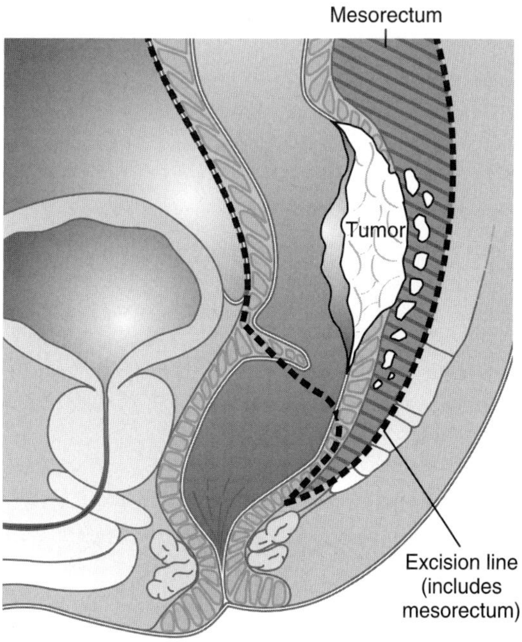

Figure 20–2. Surgical margins of total mesorectal excision. (From Nelson, H, Sargent, DJ. Refining multimodal therapy for rectal cancer. *N Engl J Med* 2001;345:691.)

rate is low, some studies were underpowered statistically to demonstrate a small benefit of radiation; however, in general, radiation appears to reduce the local recurrence rate by one third to one half as compared with surgery alone. The absolute benefit varies with how high the recurrence rate is in the surgery-alone control group. In one Dutch trial, there was a survival difference seen in favor of patients treated with radiation therapy. Although radiation may produce undefined systemic effects, it is presumed that radiation's effects result from one of two circumstances: (1) decreasing intraoperative tumor shedding; or (2) decreasing local recurrences, leading to fewer fatal complications from local recurrences in a few patients and the elimination of metastatic disease spread from recurrences in others.

Similarly, combining chemotherapy (as a radiation sensitizer) with radiation therapy further reduces the rate of local recurrence (Table 20-4). Combined chemoradiation use is more controversial, because the absolute amount of additive benefit attributable to chemotherapy on top of the radiation's effects alone for improving the recurrence rate may be small, and the toxicity is greater. However, there is a higher complete pathologic response

TABLE 20–3 • *Multimodality Therapy Versus Surgery Alone for Rectal Cancer*

Trial	Year	Treatment	Local Recurrence Rate
European Organization for Research and Treatment of Cancer	1998	Surgery alone	30%
		Surgery + preoperative RT	15%
National Surgical Adjuvant Breast and Bowel Project	1988	Surgery alone	25%
		Surgery + postoperative RT	16%
Imperial Cancer Research Fund	1994	Surgery alone	24%
		Surgery + preoperative RT	17%
Stockholm I	1995	Surgery alone	28%
		Surgery + preoperative RT	14%
MRC3	1995	Surgery alone	34%
		Surgery + postoperative RT	21%
Swedish RCT	1997	Surgery alone	27%
		Surgery + preoperative RT	11%
Dutch RCT	2001	Surgery alone (TME)	8%
		Surgery (TME) + preoperative RT	2%

MRC3, Medical Research Council 3; *RCT,* Randomized Controlled Trial; *RT,* radiation therapy; *TME,* total mesorectal excision.

TABLE 20–4 • *Single Modality Therapy Versus Combination Radiation Therapy/Chemotherapy for Rectal Cancer*

Randomized Trial	Year	Treatment	Local Recurrence Rate
European Organization for Research and Treatment of Cancer	1984	Preoperative RT	15%
		Preoperative RT + chemotherapy	15%
GITSG	1985	Postoperative RT	20%
		Postoperative RT + chemotherapy	11%
North Central Cancer Treatment Group	1991	Postoperative RT	23%
		Postoperative RT + chemotherapy	14%
GITSG	1992	Postoperative RT	15%
		Postoperative RT + chemotherapy	11%
National Surgical Adjuvant Breast and Bowel Project	1996	Chemotherapy	14%
		Chemotherapy + RT	9%

GITSG, Gastrointestinal Tumor Study Group; *RT,* radiation therapy.

rate when chemotherapy is combined with radiation therapy. In addition, overall survival is improved among patients with rectal cancer when chemotherapy is administered. One major trial that has recently underscored these conclusions is the Norwegian Adjuvant Rectal Cancer Project Group study, which analyzed the outcomes after surgery alone as compared with surgery with combined chemoradiation. The local recurrence rate was 12% in the adjuvant arm as compared with 30% in the surgery-alone arm (P = .01). Five-year overall survival was improved in the combined modality adjuvant arm, from 50% to 64% (P = .05).

There is also controversy surrounding how and when to administer the adjuvant chemotherapy and radiation therapy. Advantages and disadvantages are seen with both preoperative and postoperative administration. The dosing of the radiation and the specifics of chemotherapy agents and dosing are also not standardized.

Attempts at further defining best practices have met with difficulty because of strong clinician biases. Nonetheless, on the basis of many of the early studies, the National Institutes of Health Consensus Conference concluded in 1990 that combined modality therapy was the standard adjuvant treatment for patients with T3, N1, or N2 disease.

BOX 20–3 PREOPERATIVE TREATMENT OF RECTAL CANCER

Advantages:

1. Decrease in tumor size, thereby allowing for improved operative exposure, resectability, and improved sphincter preservation
2. Decreased risk of spread of cancer cells as a result of tumor manipulation
3. Increase in tissue-plane edema improving ease of resectability
4. Improved radiation tumoricidal effects, because tumor is well oxygenated

Disadvantages:

1. Loss of accurate pathologic staging as a result of the downstaging of T and N stage
2. Delay in performing operative procedure
3. Possibility of treating some patients with early-stage disease who do not need adjuvant treatment at all

BOX 20–4 POSTOPERATIVE TREATMENT OF RECTAL CANCER

Advantages:

1. Accurate pathologic staging
2. Avoidance of overtreating some patients mistakenly thought to have more advanced cancers than what is present
3. Decrease in complications related to tissue healing
4. No delay in operation

Disadvantages:

1. Cells that are still viable may be shed during the operation
2. Residual cancer is rendered hypoxic by surgery and thus more resistant to radiation therapy
3. Long delay in initiating adjuvant therapy if postoperative complications occur

Gastric Carcinoma

Although the overall incidence of gastric adenocarcinoma is declining, it remains an important cause of cancer deaths worldwide. In 2006, approximately 22,280 new cases of gastric adenocarcinoma were diagnosed in the United States, and an estimated 11,430 deaths occurred, making it the eighth leading cause of cancer deaths in the United States. In the West, proximal gastric tumors are occurring more frequently along the proximal lesser curvature, in the cardia, and at the gastroesophageal junction.

The curative treatment of gastric carcinoma requires resection, although the survival rates are dismal for patients who are diagnosed at advanced stages. A review from the National Cancer Data Base reported the 10-year survival for patients with stage IA disease who had undergone resection to be only 65%.

Local or regional recurrence has been found to occur in 40% to 65% of patients with curative gastric operations. This high rate of relapse and low survival even for IA disease makes adjuvant treatment important for patients with gastric adenocarcinoma. An area of controversy in the field of gastric carcinoma has been the higher rates of survival after more extended gastric resections reported by surgeons in Japan as compared with those in the West.

Diagnosis and Evaluation

Gastric cancer is difficult to diagnose early because of the lack of identifying symptoms and signs during the initial stage. Instead, patient's complaints are nonspecific and are commonly evaluated and treated, including vague indigestion, early satiety, postprandial fullness, eructation, and occasional nausea and vomiting. One study found that the most common presenting symptom of gastric cancer was weight loss, followed by abdominal pain and nausea. Physical examination signs when present are usually indicative of advanced disease. These include massive ascites, a palpable supraclavicular node (Virchow's node), a periumbilical node (Sister Mary Joseph node), palpable metastasis on rectal examination (a Blumer's shelf), and a palpable ovarian mass (a Krukenberg tumor).

Historically, contrast upper GI radiography was used to identify mucosal abnormalities. Today, the suspicion for gastric pathology mandates endoscopic examination using flexible fiberoptic endoscopy. Gastric ulcers, masses, and any suspicious lesions warrant biopsy. After the diagnosis of carcinoma is made, CT scanning of the abdomen and pelvis should be obtained for staging. For patients undergoing neoadjuvant therapy, endoscopic ultrasound has been reported to have the highest sensitivity and specificity for correct T and N staging. Laparoscopy may also play an important role as a staging tool, often identifying patients who have occult subradiographic disease.

Surgery

As has been already mentioned, the reported improved survival rates by Japanese surgeons have been attributed to the extended lymph-node dissections that are commonly performed in Japan during the gastric resectional surgery. In the West, D1 dissections are traditionally performed, which entail the resection of the involved portion of the stomach and the greater and lesser omentum. The D2 dissection, which is advocated by Japanese surgeons, adds to the D1 dissection the resection of the anterior leaf of the transverse mesocolon, a splenectomy, a distal pancreatectomy, and the nodal clearance of the hepatic portal, splenic, and celiac arteries.

Two major randomized controlled trials compared the outcomes of patients with D1 versus D2 dissections. The first study was by the Dutch Gastric Cancer Group. They found that the patients with D2 dissections had significantly higher rates of complications (43% versus 25%; $P < .001$), higher rates of postoperative death (10% versus 4%; $P = .004$), and longer hospital stays (median, 16 versus 14 days; $P < .001$), and that there was no survival advantage over the results for patients who underwent the D1 dissections. The second trial was conducted by the Surgical Cooperative Group in the United Kingdom. They reported that the patients with D2 dissections had higher postoperative mortality (13% versus 6.5%; $P = .04$) and higher postoperative morbidity (46% versus 28%; $P < .001$) than patients with D1 dissections. Furthermore, 3-year overall survival was 30% with D2 dissections as compared with 50% with D1 dissections. Although debate continues regarding the trial details, general recommendations for extended gastric resections cannot be made in this country. Experienced centers able to perform improved nodal clearing resections safely still advocate this approach. The better results seen in Japan may in part result from better surgery, but they also have been largely attributed to improved staging with the extended dissection technique, thereby eliciting a stage migration effect (the Will Rogers phenomenon).

Adjuvant Therapy

The frequency of local or regional recurrence has made regional radiation an attractive possibility for adjuvant therapy. Although initial studies showed no benefit for the administration of radiation alone, a Japanese phase III trial comparing neoadjuvant radiation with surgery versus surgery alone was conducted. The investigators reported clinically limited but significant improvement in survival (30% versus 20%; $P = .009$) after preoperative regional radiotherapy among patients with gastric cancer.

Most trials have examined the combined uses of radiotherapy and chemotherapy for the adjuvant treatment of gastric carcinoma. The first important study by Moertel and colleagues demonstrated a statistically significant survival advantage for patients receiving combined chemoradiation (40 Gy radiation with 5-FU), in addition to surgery, as compared with surgery alone. These results were bolstered by the Gastrointestinal Tumor Study

Group trial, which found improved survival among patients with combined therapy versus single radiation therapy alone.

Recently, the Intergroup trial INT 0116 published a landmark study of the use of adjuvant therapy for gastric carcinoma. They assigned patients to one of two arms: surgery alone or surgery plus postoperative chemoradiotherapy. Adjuvant treatment consisted of 4,500 cGy of radiation along with a regimen of 5-FU and leucovorin. They demonstrated that the addition of adjuvant chemoradiotherapy improved the median length of survival from 27 to 36 months (P = .005) and that it improved 3-year overall survival to 50% from 41%. Additionally, the investigators found a significant decrease in local failure (19% versus 29%). This has led to a new standard of care in this country regarding the use of multimodality therapy for gastric cancer. However, there is a concern that more than half of the patients in this trial did not have a D1 lymphadenectomy and that the chemoradiotherapy may be "cleaning up" suboptimal surgery. It is still not clear if adjuvant chemoradiotherapy would improve the survival of patients who undergo a complete lymph-node dissection or an extended Japanese-type resection. Moreover, the adjuvant chemoradiotherapy is toxic, and attention to detail regarding radiation ports and chemotherapy side effects is critical.

Preliminary results of the European MAGIC trial have also suggested the benefits of systemic therapy for patients with resectable gastric cancer. A total of 503 patients were randomized to surgery alone or to a combination of preoperative and postoperative epirubicin, cisplatin, and infusional 5-FU therapy without radiation. Survival at 5 years was improved from 23% to 36% in the chemotherapy arm. Formal publication of these results is still pending.

Gastric cancer also tends to spread to peritoneal surfaces, even without nodal and distant metastatic disease being present. Randomized trials in Japan have demonstrated improved survival for high-risk patients (T3 primaries) who receive intraperitoneal heated chemotherapy immediately after the gastric resection, while the abdomen is still open. This has been correlated with positive peritoneal cytology samples converting to negative with the topical chemotherapy. This form of multimodality therapy is being explored by several centers in the United States, usually in the setting of macroscopic peritoneal disease, but it theoretically does have more appeal to treat microscopically based peritoneal disease if those patients can be clearly identified.

Pancreatic Cancer

Despite current treatment modalities, pancreatic cancer remains a highly aggressive disease with an overall dismal prognosis. Of the estimated 33,730 cases in 2006, 80% to 90% presented with clinically apparent metastatic disease or radiographic evidence of unresectability. For those who are diagnosed early, surgery remains the only option for cure. Unfortunately, even surgery for cure confers patients a median survival of less than 20 months. Such results have increased the interest in using adjuvant multimodality therapy to improve survival.

Preoperative Evaluation

Accurate clinical staging is obtained by high-quality CT scanning. The relationship of the mass to the superior mesenteric artery and the celiac axis is the main focus of preoperative imaging studies (Figure 20-3). When there is an absence of distant extrapancreatic disease, the absence of tumor extension to the superior mesenteric artery or the celiac axis, and a patent superior-mesenteric–portal-vein confluence, the cancer is potentially resectable. The aim is to obtain a negative retroperitoneal margin of resection and to safely remove the involved pancreas and the associated duodenum and nodal tissue. Patients with positive margins have a median survival of 8 to 12 months, which is the same as that for patients with locally advanced cancer who are treated with chemoradiation alone.

Surgery

Surgical resection should only be undertaken with an intent to cure, because a survival benefit is gained only among those patients who undergo a negative-margin resection. Current data indicate that the surgical resection for cancer of the head of the pancreas can be performed in a standard or pylorus-preserving fashion without statistically significant differences in outcomes. Furthermore, involvement of the superior mesenteric vein or the superior-mesenteric–portal-vein confluence does not preclude resection, and it can be treated with

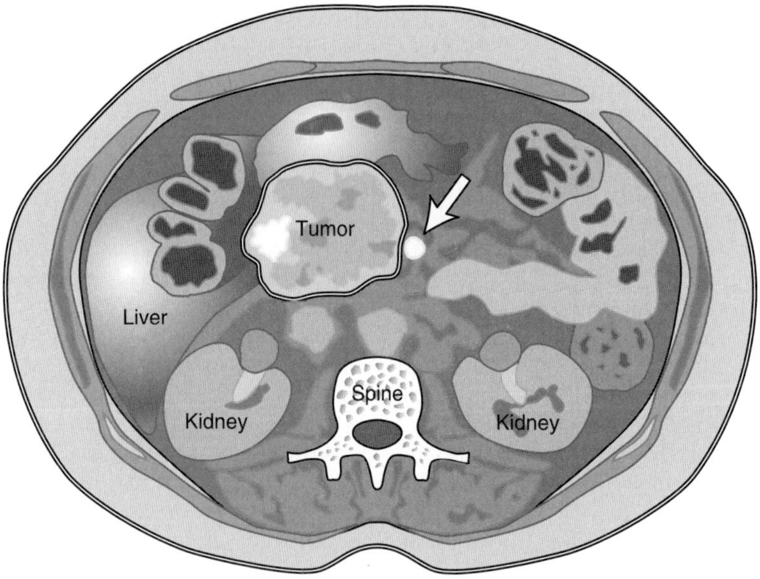

Figure 20–3. CT scan of pancreatic cancer demonstrating fat plane between tumor and superior mesenteric artery.

venous resection and reconstruction without alteration in survival outcomes.

Multimodal Strategies

The dismal outcomes with surgery alone have prompted searches for adjuvant therapies. The first study of significance to show a benefit of additional therapy involved a regimen of postoperative external-beam radiation therapy and concomitant chemotherapy with 5-FU for unresectable pancreatic cancer; this was designed by the Gastrointestinal Tumor Study Group. Researchers in this trial demonstrated that the addition of 5-FU to 4,000 or 6,000 cGy of external-beam irradiation significantly increased the median survival from 20 weeks in the radiation treatment group alone to 36 weeks and 40 weeks in the two combined chemoradiation groups, respectively. There was no significant difference between the 4,000 cGy plus 5-FU and the 6,000 cGy plus 5-FU groups. A survival advantage was also seen from chemoradiation among patients undergoing curative resections in a follow-up study by the Gastrointestinal Tumor Study Group as compared with resection alone.

With some controversy, two large European trials have demonstrated no survival advantage for chemoradiation in the adjuvant setting. The first study was conducted by the European Organization for Treatment and Research of Cancer Trials. They demonstrated no differences in survival between the surgery-alone arm versus the surgery plus adjuvant chemoradiation arm; there was a median duration of survival of 19 months and 24.5 months and a 2-year survival of 41% and 51%, respectively ($P = .2$). However, this trial had major flaws and limitations. First, the researchers did not make a distinction between pancreatic and periampullary tumors. Second, 20% of their patients assigned to receive chemoradiation did not receive this treatment as a result of a prolonged recovery, refusal, or comorbidity. Third, there was no assessment of a retroperitoneal margin, thereby not validating the number of complete resections. Finally, there exists the possibility of a missed clinically significant difference as a result of a small sample size.

The second major trial conducted in Europe was organized by the European Study Group for Pancreatic Cancer. In this multicenter trial, patients were randomized to a two-by-two factorial study, randomizing patients between chemoradiation and no chemoradiation, and chemotherapy and no chemotherapy. The combined study results demonstrated no benefit for the use of adjuvant chemoradiotherapy as compared with surgery alone. Median survival was 15.5 months with chemoradiotherapy versus 16.1 months in the control arm ($P = .24$). There was, however, evidence of benefit for surgery plus chemotherapy as compared with surgery alone. Median survival in this treatment group was 19.7 months versus 14.0 months ($P = .0005$). There has been much skepticism regarding the findings of this trial, because clinicians were allowed to choose which randomization schema the patient enrolled in; the statistical analyses incorporated different randomized subsets; the data regarding radiotherapy quality assurance were not clear, with more-than-usually-seen toxicity in the radiation-containing arms; there were no data about background chemotherapy for a significant portion of patients; and there was a 9% protocol violation, with patients not receiving their assigned treatments.

Chemoradiation in the neoadjuvant setting has been explored as a result of the outcomes of adjuvant trials. Neoadjuvant chemoradiation has several advantages, including the better performance status of the patients at the time of chemotherapy; no delays or omissions as a result of prolonged surgical recovery; increased efficacy of treating well-vascularized tissues; downstaging the primary to potentially make the surgery easier or to make it more likely to be margin negative; and the identification of patients with rapidly progressive disease to avoid operating on those individuals. In addition, chemoresponsive or radiosensitive tumors can be identified for selection of those patients who might benefit from additional postoperative adjuvant therapies. To date, there are no controlled studies showing survival benefits from the employment of neoadjuvant treatments.

New radiation-sensitizing agents, such as paclitaxel and gemcitabine, have been used with some limited success. A recent randomized study found gemcitabine to be more effective than 5-FU for locally advanced pancreatic cancer. A new promising adjuvant chemoradiation treatment that adds interferon has been popular recently. The researchers initially reported 2-year overall survival rates of 84% in the interferon group versus 54% in the traditional 5-FU group. The follow-up study later reported 5-year survival rates of 55% using this treatment regimen. These results await confirmation from large multicenter studies.

BOX 20–5 POTENTIAL ADVANTAGES OF NEOADJUVANT THERAPY FOR PANCREATIC CANCER

1. More patients can actually receive the adjuvant therapy, because recovery from surgery often delays or prevents the patient from receiving the therapy postoperatively.
2. Systemic therapy is received promptly to eradicate the micrometastases that are most often the life-limiting problem.
3. If patients develop obvious metastases during neoadjuvant therapy and before surgery, then surgery can be avoided.
4. Response to chemotherapy is evaluated because the tumor is left in situ. If this is favorable, then, postoperative adjuvant therapy may prove useful.
5. Downstaging of the tumor can occur, thereby making surgery technically easier and potentially converting an unresectable patient to a resectable one.
6. Tumor response may lower the risk of tumor spread through manipulation and spillage during surgery.
7. Preoperative irradiation may lower the risk of pancreaticojejunal anastomotic complications by causing the pancreas to become more fibrotic.
8. Preoperative therapy may be more effective for killing tumor cells when they are better vascularized preoperatively.

Key Selected Readings

Evans DB, Abbruzzese JL, Willett CG. Cancer of the pancreas. In: DeVita VT, Hellman S, Rosenberg SA, eds. *Cancer principles and practice of oncology,* 6th ed. Philadelphia: Lippincott, 2001.

Gordon PH. Malignant neoplasms of the rectum. In: *Principles and practice of surgery for the colon, rectum, and anus,* 2nd ed. New York: Quality Medical Publishing, Inc, 1999.

Karpeh MS, Kelsen DP, Tepper JE. Cancer of the stomach. In: DeVita VT, Hellman S, Rosenberg SA, eds. *Cancer principles and practice of oncology,* 6th ed. Philadelphia: Lippincott, 2001.

Nivatvongs S. Perianal and anal canal neoplasms. In: *Principles and practice of surgery for the colon, rectum, and anus,* 2nd ed. St. Louis: Quality Medical Publishing, Inc, 1999.

Selected Readings

Arnaud JP, Norlinger B, Bosset JF, *et al.* Radical surgery and postoperative radiotherapy as combined treatment in rectal cancer. Final results of a phase III study of the European Organization for Research and Treatment of Cancer. *Br J Surg* 1997;84:352–357.

Balslev I, Pedersen M, Teglbjaerg PS, *et al.* Postoperative radiotherapy in Dukes' B and C carcinoma of the rectum and rectosigmoid. A randomized multicenter study. *Cancer* 1986;58:22–28.

Barrett MW. Chemoradiation for rectal cancer: current methods. *Semin Surg Oncol* 1998;15:114–119.

Bartelink H, Roelofsen F, Eschwege F, *et al.* Concomitant radiotherapy and chemotherapy is superior to radiotherapy alone in the treatment of locally advanced anal cancer: results of a phase III randomized trial of the European Organization for Research and Treatment of Cancer Radiotherapy and Gastrointestinal Cooperative Groups. *J Clin Oncol* 1997;15:2040–2049.

Bonadeo FA, Vaccaro CA, Benati ML, *et al.* Rectal cancer: local recurrence after surgery without radiotherapy. *Dis Colon Rectum* 2001;44:374–379.

Bonenkamp JJ, Hermans J, Sasako M, van de Velde CJ. Extended lymph-node dissection for gastric cancer. Dutch Gastric Cancer Group. *N Engl J Med* 1999;340:908–914.

Bonenkamp JJ, Songun I, Hermans J, *et al.* Randomised comparison of morbidity after D1 and D2 dissection for gastric cancer in 996 Dutch patients. *Lancet* 1995;345:745–748.

Burris HA III, Moore MH, Andersen J, *et al.* Improvements in survival and clinical benefit with gemcitabine as first-line therapy for patients with advanced pancreas cancer: a randomized trial. *J Clin Oncol* 1997;15:2403–2413.

Conlon KC, Klimstra DS, Brennan MF. Long-term survival after curative resection for pancreatic ductal adenocarcinoma. Clinicopathologic analysis of 5-year survivors. *Ann Surg* 1996;223:273–279.

Cuschieri A, Fayers P, Fielding J, *et al.* Postoperative morbidity and mortality after D1 and D2 resections for gastric cancer: preliminary results of the MRC randomised controlled surgical trial. The Surgical Cooperative Group. *Lancet* 1996;347:995–999.

de Manzoni G, Verlato G, Roviello F, *et al.* The new TNM classification of lymph node metastasis minimises stage migration problems in gastric cancer patients. *Br J Cancer* 2002;87:171–174.

Fisher B, Wolmark N, Rockette H, *et al.* Postoperative adjuvant chemotherapy or radiation therapy for rectal cancer: results from NSABP protocol R-01. *J Natl Cancer Inst* 1988;80:21–29.

Flam M, John M, Pajak TF, *et al.* Role of mitomycin in combination with fluorouracil and radiotherapy, and of salvage chemoradiation in the definitive nonsurgical treatment of epidermoid carcinoma of the anal canal: results of a phase III randomized intergroup study. *J Clin Oncol* 1996;14:2527–2539.

Frisch M, Olsen JH, Bautz A, Melbye M. Benign anal lesions and the risk of anal cancer. *N Engl J Med* 1994;331:300–302.

Fuchshuber PR, Rodriguez-Bigas M, Weber T, Petrelli NJ. Anal canal and perianal epidermoid cancers. *J Am Coll Surg* 1997;185:494–505.

Fuhrman G, Leach S, Staley C, *et al.* Rationale for en bloc vein resection in the treatment of pancreatic adenocarcinoma adherent to the superior mesenteric-portal vein confluence. *Ann Surg* 1996;223:154–162.

Gamliel Z, Krasna MJ. Multimodality treatment of esophageal cancer. *Surg Clin North Am* 2005;85: 621–630.

Gastrointestinal Tumor Study Group. A multi-institutional comparative trial of radiation therapy alone and in combination with 5-fluorouracil for locally unresectable pancreatic carcinoma. *Ann Surg* 1979;189:205–208.

Gastrointestinal Tumor Study Group. Prolongation of the disease-free interval in surgically treated rectal carcinoma. *N Engl J Med* 1985;312:1465–1472.

Gastrointestinal Tumor Study Group. Further evidence of effective adjuvant combined radiation and chemotherapy following curative resection of pancreatic cancer. *Cancer* 1987;59:2006–2010.

Gastrointestinal Tumor Study Group. The concept of locally advanced gastric cancer: effect of treatment on outcome. *Cancer* 1990;66:2324–2330.

Gerard A, Buyse M, Nordlinger B, *et al.* Preoperative radiotherapy as adjuvant treatment of rectal cancer. *Ann Surg* 1988;208:606–614.

Goldberg PA, Nicholls RJ, Porter NH, *et al.* Long-term results of a randomised trial of short-course low-dose adjuvant preoperative radiotherapy for rectal cancer: reduction in local treatment failure. *Eur J Cancer* 1994;30A:1602–1606.

Heald RJ, Ryall RD. Recurrence and survival after total mesorectal excision for rectal cancer. *Lancet* 1986;1:1479–1482.

Hundahl SA, Phillips JL, Menck HR. The National Cancer Data Base report on poor survival of US gastric carcinoma patients treated with gastrectomy: fifth edition American Joint Committee on Cancer staging, proximal disease, and the "different disease" hypothesis. *Cancer* 2000;88:921–932.

Kapiteijn E, Marijnen CAM, Nagtegaal ID, *et al.* Preoperative radiotherapy combined with total mesorectal excision for resectable rectal cancer. *N Engl J Med* 2001;345:638–646.

Klinkenbijl JH, Jeekel J, Sahmoud T, *et al.* Adjuvant radiotherapy and 5-fluorouracil after curative resection of cancer of the pancreas and periampullary region: phase III trial of the EORTC gastrointestinal tract cancer cooperative group. *Ann Surg* 1999;230:776–782.

Ko CY, Stamos MJ, Zimmerman A, Yang HC. Adjuvant therapy for rectal cancer. *Clinics in Colon and Rectal Surgery* 2002;15:55–62.

Kockerling F, Reymond MA, Altendor-Hofmann A, *et al.* Influence of surgery on metachronous distant metastases and survival in rectal cancer. *J Clin Oncol* 1998;16:324–329.

Krook JE, Moertel CG, Gunderson LL, *et al.* Effective surgical adjuvant therapy for high-risk rectal carcinoma. *N Engl J Med* 1991;324:709–715.

Landry J, Tepper JE, Wood WC, *et al.* Patterns of failure following curative resection of gastric cancer. *Int J Radiat Oncol Biol Phys* 1990;191:1357–1362.

MacDonald JS, Smalley SR, Benedetti J, *et al.* Chemoradiotherapy after surgery compared with surgery alone for adenocarcinoma of the stomach or gastroesophageal junction. *N Engl J Med* 2001;345:725–730.

Marsh PJ, James RD, Schofield PF. Adjuvant preoperative radiotherapy for locally advanced rectal carcinoma. Results of a prospective, randomized trial. *Dis Colon Rectum* 1994;37:1205–1214.

Medical Research Council Rectal Cancer Working Party. Randomised trial of surgery alone versus surgery followed by radiotherapy for mobile cancer of the rectum. *Lancet* 1996;348:1610–1614.

Moertel CG, Childs DS, O'Fallon JR, *et al.* Combined 5-fluorouracil and supervoltage radiation therapy for locally unresectable gastrointestinal cancer. *Lancet* 1969;2:865–867.

Neoptolemos JP, Dunn JA, Stocken DD, *et al,* and the European Study Group for Pancreatic Cancer. Adjuvant chemoradiotherapy and chemotherapy in respectable pancreatic cancer: a randomized controlled trial. *Lancet* 2001;358:1576–1585.

Nigro ND, Vaitkevicius VK, Considine B. Combined therapy for cancer of the anal canal. *Dis Colon Rectum* 1974;17:354–356.

National Institutes of Health Consensus Conference. Adjuvant therapy for patients with colon and rectal cancer. *JAMA* 1990;264:1444–1450.

Nitecki S, Sarr M, Colby T, van Heerden J. Long-term survival after resection for ductal adenocarcinoma of the pancreas. Is it really improving? *Ann Surg* 1995;221:59–66.

Nukui Y, Picozzi VJ, Traverso LW. Interferon-based adjuvant chemoradiation therapy improves survival after pancreaticoduodenectomy for pancreatic adenocarcinoma. *Am J Surg* 2000;179:367–371.

Picozzi VJ, Kozarek RA, Traverso LW. Interferon-based adjuvant chemoradiation therapy after pancreaticoduodenectomy for pancreatic adenocarcinoma. *Am J Surg* 2003;185:476–480.

Reis Neto JA, Quilici FA, Reis JA Jr. A comparison of nonoperative vs preoperative radiotherapy in rectal carcinoma. A 10-year randomized trial. *Dis Colon Rectum* 1989;32:702–710.

Rousseau DL Jr, Thomas CR Jr, Petrelli NJ, Kahlenberg MS. Squamous cell carcinoma of the anal canal. *Surg Oncol* 2005;14:121–132.

Rousseau DL Jr, Petrelli NJ, Kahlenberg MS. Overview of anal cancer for the surgeon. *Surg Oncol Clin N Am* 2004;13:249–262.

Ryan DP, Compton CC, Mayer RJ. Medical progress: carcinoma of the anal canal. *N Engl J Med* 2000;342:792–800.

Spitz FR, Abbruzzese JL, Lee JE, *et al.* Preoperative and postoperative chemoradiation strategies in patients treated with pancreaticoduodenectomy for adenocarcinoma of the pancreas. *J Clin Oncol* 1997;15:928–937.

Stockholm Colorectal Cancer Study Group. Randomized study on preoperative radiotherapy in rectal carcinoma. *Ann Surg Oncol* 1996;3:423–430.

Stockholm Rectal Cancer Study Group. Preoperative short-term radiation therapy in operable rectal carcinoma. A prospective randomized trial. Stockholm Rectal Cancer Study Group. *Cancer* 1990;66:49–55.

Swedish Rectal Cancer Trial. Improved survival with preoperative radiotherapy in resectable rectal cancer. *N Engl J Med* 1997;336:980–987.

Tocchi A, Mazzoni G, Lepre L, *et al.* Total mesorectal excision and low rectal anastomosis for the treatment of rectal cancer and prevention of pelvic recurrences. *Arch Surg* 2001;136:216–220.

Touboul E, Schlienger M, Buffat L, *et al.* Epidermoid carcinoma of the anal canal: results of curative-intent radiation therapy in a series of 270 patients. *Cancer* 1994;73:1569–1579.

Treurniet-Donker AD, van Putten WL, Wereldsma JC, *et al.* Postoperative radiation therapy for rectal cancer. An interim analysis of a prospective, randomized multicenter trial in the Netherlands. *Cancer* 1991;67:2042–2048.

Tveit KM, Guldvog I, Hagen S, *et al.* Randomized controlled trial of postoperative radiotherapy and short-term time-scheduled 5-fluorouracil against surgery alone in the treatment of Dukes' B and C rectal cancer. Norwegian Adjuvant Rectal Cancer Project Group. *Br J Surg* 1997;84:1130–1135.

United Kingdom Coordinating Committee for Cancer: Anal Cancer Trial Working Party. Epidermoid anal cancer: results from the UKCCCR randomized trial of radiotherapy alone versus radiotherapy, 5-fluorouracil, and mitomycin. *Lancet* 1996; 348: 1049–1054.

Wanebo HJ, Kennedy BJ, Chmiel J, *et al.* Cancer of the stomach: a patient care study by the American College of Surgeons. *Ann Surg* 1993;218:583–592.

Willett C, Lewandrowski K, Warshaw A. Resection margins in carcinoma of the head of the pancreas. Implications for radiation therapy. *Ann Surg* 1993;217:144–148.

Wolmark N, Wieand HS, Hyams DM, *et al.* Randomized trial of postoperative adjuvant chemotherapy with or without radiotherapy for carcinoma of the rectum: National Surgical Adjuvant Breast and Bowel Project Protocol R-02. *J Natl Cancer Inst* 2000;92: 388–396.

Yeo CJ, Cameron JL, Sohn TA, *et al.* Six hundred fifty consecutive pancreaticoduodenectomies in the 1990s: pathology, complications, and outcomes. *Ann Surg* 1997;226:248–257.

Zhang ZX, Gu XZ, Yin WB, *et al.* Randomized clinical trial on the combination of preoperative irradiation and surgery in the treatment of adenocarcinoma of gastric cardia (AGC)—report on 370 patients. *Int J Radiat Oncol Biol Phys* 1998;42:929–934.

21

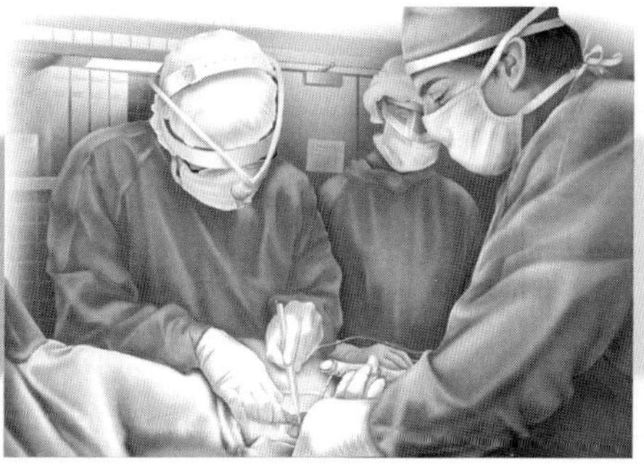

Head and Neck Cancer

Michael J. Wolfe and Keith Wilson

Head and Neck Cancer: Key Points

- List the risk factors for head and neck malignancies.
- Discuss the imaging performed for the diagnosis of head and neck cancer.
- Describe the general treatment options to consider for head and neck cancers.
- Outline the pattern of spread and staging considerations of head and neck cancers.
- Walk through the procedures for radical neck dissection, modified radical neck dissection, and selective neck dissection.
- List the diagnostic steps to take when evaluating an unknown primary.
- Describe the anatomy, treatment, and reconstruction pertinent to cancer of the oral cavity.
- Outline the treatment, reconstruction, and outcomes for nasopharyngeal, oropharyngeal, and hypopharyngeal carcinomas.
- Describe the anatomy, staging, and treatment of laryngeal cancers.
- Detail the workup, treatment, and complications associated with cancer of the major salivary glands.

Head and neck cancer (HNCa) is composed of malignancies that stem from the upper aerodigestive tract, the major salivary glands, and the thyroid gland. Excluding the thyroid gland, HNCa accounts for nearly 5% of all cancers diagnosed in the United States. Prevalence varies widely around the world, and it is one of the main cancers diagnosed in many parts of Africa and Asia. The focus of this chapter will be the diagnosis and treatment of malignancies of the oral cavity, the pharynx, the larynx, and the salivary glands.

Head and neck oncologists rely on many techniques to diagnosis cancer. After malignancy is diagnosed, treatment options are considered. Even with the advancement of medical technology, the overall survival of patients with HNCa has not greatly changed over the past 30 years. Newer strategies are focusing on organ preservation and the avoidance of total laryngectomy, glossectomy, and other disfiguring procedures. This is very important given that derangements of the upper aerodigestive tract alter the normal functions of eating, swallowing, speech, and breathing. Changes in such basic life functions can lead to a significant decrease in the quality of life of the patient. Many patients will become dependent on tracheostomies or gastric feeding tubes, and vocal communication can become nearly impossible. Treatment success can no longer be measured solely in terms of cancer cure rates; it must include the ability to preserve or resume function and to return to normal life without the stigmata of sometimes deforming treatments.

Risk Factors

By far the most prevalent type of HNCa is squamous cell carcinoma (SCCa). The list of risk factors for this condition is exceedingly broad. (Table 21-1). The most common factors are tobacco use and alcohol intake. Both are inde-

BOX 21–1 RISK FACTORS FOR SQUAMOUS CELL CARCINOMA OF THE HEAD AND NECK

- Tobacco use
- Alcohol consumption
- Nutritional deficiencies
- Immunosuppression
- Viruses (human papilloma virus, Epstein-Barr virus)
- Occupational exposures (wood dust, nickel dust, paint fumes, metal work ing, gasoline, plastics production, radiation, textiles, asbestos, benzenes)
- Older age
- Male gender
- Low socioeconomic status

BOX 21–2 DIFFERENTIAL DIAGNOSIS OF HEAD AND NECK CANCER

- Squamous cell carcinoma
- Minor salivary gland tumors
    - Mucoepidermoid carcinoma
    - Adenoid cystic carcinoma
    - Acinic-cell carcinoma
    - Pleomorphic adenoma
- Adenocarcinoma
- Sarcoma
- Lymphoma
- Mucosal melanoma
- Granular-cell tumor (benign)
- Plasmacytoma
- Metastasis from distant primary
    - Renal cell carcinoma most common
- Necrotizing sialometaplasia (benign)
- Pseudoepitheliomatous hyperplasia (benign)

TABLE 21–1 • *Syndromes Associated with Increased Cancer Risk*

Plummer-Vinson syndrome	Women with esophageal webs, iron-deficiency anemia, and postcricoid squamous cell carcinoma
Bloom's syndrome	Chromosome breaks cause cancer at young age; 18% of patients with this syndrome have head and neck cancer
Fanconi's anemia	Dysfunctional marrow, leukemia, soft-tissue tumors, oral tumors
Xeroderma pigmentosum	Unable to repair DNA; leads to sensitivity to ultraviolet light and skin cancers
Li-Fraumeni syndrome	Predisposition for cancer at a young age; breast, brain, and adrenal carcinoma; leukemia, sarcoma

pendent elements, but, when taken together, their effects are synergistic. As exposure increases over time, the relative risk also increases. Differences in the method of consumption also increase risks, such as smokeless tobacco, reverse smoking (with the lit end of the cigarette in the mouth, as practiced in southeast Asia), and betel-nut chewing (as practiced in India).

Other risk factors include older age, male gender, and low socioeconomic status. Certain medical conditions can predispose an individual to the development of cancer: immune compromise, malnutrition, chronic inflammation, and premalignant lesions, such as leukoplakia, erythroplakia, and lichen planus. Laryngopharyngeal reflux, which involves the spilling of gastric secretions proximal to the upper esophageal sphincter and into the pharynx and larynx, can also increase the risk of laryngeal cancer. Epstein-Barr virus plays a major role in the carcinogenesis of nasopharyngeal carcinoma, and human papilloma virus increases the risk of laryngeal carcinoma in the presence of laryngeal papillomatosis. Several syndromes can also lead to HNCa.

Evaluation

The workup of the patient with a suspected HNCa begins with a full history and physical examination. Imaging is very important for both staging and treatment planning. Laboratory data is needed to assess the patient's overall health status and to identify abnormal values that may need correction to help in the success of treatment.

BOX 21-3 DIFFERENTIAL DIAGNOSIS OF A NECK MASS

Metastatic Cancer

- Squamous cell carcinoma
- Salivary gland
- Skin (squamous cell carcinoma, melanoma)
- Thyroid
- Distant primary
- Unknown primary
- Lymphoma

Benign Masses

- Inflammatory lymphadenopathy
    - Viral, bacterial
- Congenital
- Branchial cleft cyst, thyroglossal duct cyst, dermoid cyst
- Lymphangioma/hemangioma
- Paraganglioma (carotid body tumor, glomus tumors)
- Schwannoma
- Neurofibroma

History and Physical Examination

Symptoms usually are centered on the anatomic areas affected by the tumor. Sixty percent of patients will complain of otalgia (ear pain). Complete questioning about airway status will help the physician decide if concern is needed for an emergent airway (i.e., is the patient complaining of dyspnea, increasing snoring, or overt sleep apnea?).

BOX 21-4 FIVE "T's" OF OTALGIA

- Patients complaining of ear pain but no ear pathology noted on examination warrant evaluation of these areas:
    1. Temporomandibular joint (most common site of referred pain to the ear)
    2. Teeth
    3. Tongue
    4. Tonsil
    5. Throat

The examination not only centers on the areas of concern but also on the entire aerodigestive tract; this is because of a 5% to 7% risk of a second primary. A headlight or head mirror allows for the use of both hands. Bimanual examination of the oral cavity, the oropharynx, and the neck increase the likelihood of finding masses (Figures 21-1 and 21-2). The pharynx and the larynx can be examined with a laryngeal mirror (indirect laryngoscopy) or by transnasal flexible laryngoscopy.

Imaging

The mainstay of imaging for HNCa is CT scanning with contrast. It shows good soft-tissue resolution as well as the involvement of bone. The size, location, and extent of the primary tumor are assessed. The neck is examined for the presence of metastases.

Magnetic resonance imaging (MRI) is excellent for the evaluation of soft tissue. Extension into surrounding areas is easily Extension into surrounding areas is easil seen. Bony invasion can be seen if the marrow

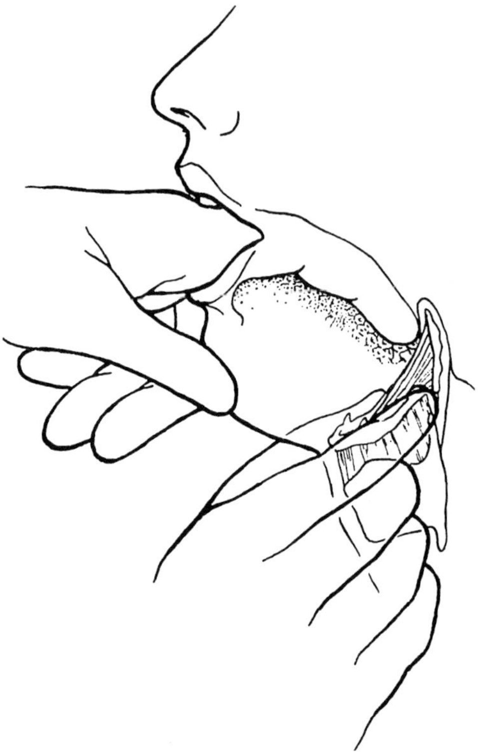

Figure 21–1. Bimanual (intraoral and cervical) palpation of the oral cavity and the oropharynx. (From Close LG, Larson DL, Shah JP. *Essentials of head and neck oncology.* New York: Thieme Medical Publishers, Inc., 1998. Figure 5-3.)

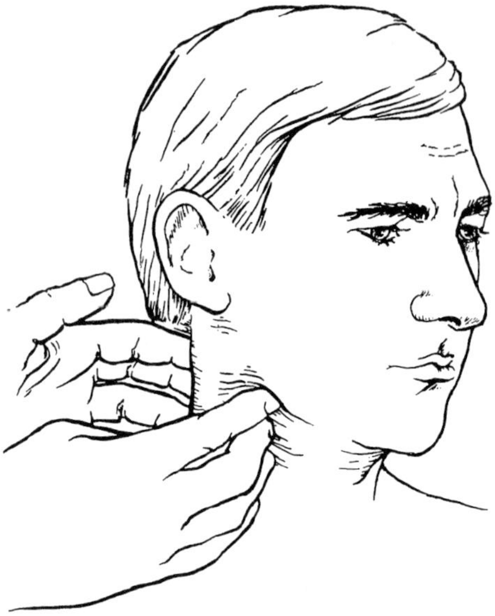

Figure 21–2. Technique for the bimanual palpation of cervical lymph nodes. (From Close LG, Larson DL, Shah JP. *Essentials of head and neck oncology.* New York: Thieme Medical Publishers, Inc., 1998. Figure 5-2.)

space is replaced by tumor. The multiplanar images are also advantageous for the better assessment of areas of infiltration.

Chest x-rays can diagnose lung and mediastinal metastases. Any suspicious findings should be further examined with chest CT. Large primary tumor masses and extensive neck disease warrant evaluation for distant metastases with multiple CT scans (chest, abdomen, pelvis), a bone scan, or a positron emission tomography scan.

Angiography can be used if a vascular tumor is suspected (usually paraganglioma), and it can be both diagnostic and therapeutic if embolization is needed. Involvement of the carotid artery can also be assessed. Balloon occlusion can help with the decision to resect the carotid artery.

Head and neck ultrasound is increasing in its usefulness. The information derived depends on the expertise of the technologist performing the scan. It is mostly used to assess for the presence of neck metastases: number, size, attachment to carotid, and so on. Thyroid nodules and parathyroid adenomas can be examined. The ultrasound can also be used to guide the needle in a fine-needle aspiration (FNA) biopsy.

BOX 21–5 PHYSICAL EXAMINATION OF THE PATIENT WITH SUSPECTED HEAD AND NECK CANCER

- Vital signs/performance status
- Ears
- Nose
- Oral cavity
  - Trismus
  - Dental status
  - Tongue movement, protrusion
- Palpation
  - Bimanual examination of the floor of the mouth
- Neck
- Nasopharynx
- Oropharynx
  - Symmetry, displacement
  - Palpation of the base of the tongue and the pharynx
- Hypopharynx (mirror or endoscopic examination)
  - Pooling
  - Pyriform sinus opening
- Larynx (indirect mirror examination or flexible transnasal laryngoscopy)
  - Voice quality
  - Symmetry
  - Movement

Modified from Close LG, Larson DL, Shah JP. *Essentials of head and neck oncology.* New York: Thieme Medical Publishers, Inc., 1998. Table 5-3.

Biopsy

Definitive diagnosis by biopsy is crucial before treatment can start. Tumors of the oral cavity can be biopsied with cup forceps, punch biopsy, or scalpel. Accessible oral pharyngeal lesions should also be sampled. Laryngeal masses are difficult to biopsy in the clinic without appropriate instruments and proper anesthesia. Neck nodes can be biopsied using FNA techniques (Figure 21-3). If FNA is not possible or is indeterminate and there is no obvious primary lesion, then the patient can be taken to the operating room for excision or incisional biopsy. The surgeon must be prepared to proceed with a formal neck dissection, depending on the frozen pathologic section results. "Node plucking" is discouraged because of the risk of seeding the soft tissues of the neck.

BOX 21-6 COMPUTED TOMOGRAPHY CRITERIA FOR METASTATIC CERVICAL LYMPH NODES

- Size: >1.5 cm in level I, >1.0 cm in other levels
- Shape: oval is normal, round is suspicious
- Necrotic center
- Border: fuzziness indicative of extra capsu-lar spread
- Loss of the fatty hilum

Panendoscopy

Virtually all HNCa patients will require a trip to the operating room for full evaluation of the mass by panendoscopy or quadruple endoscopy. This latter procedure entails direct

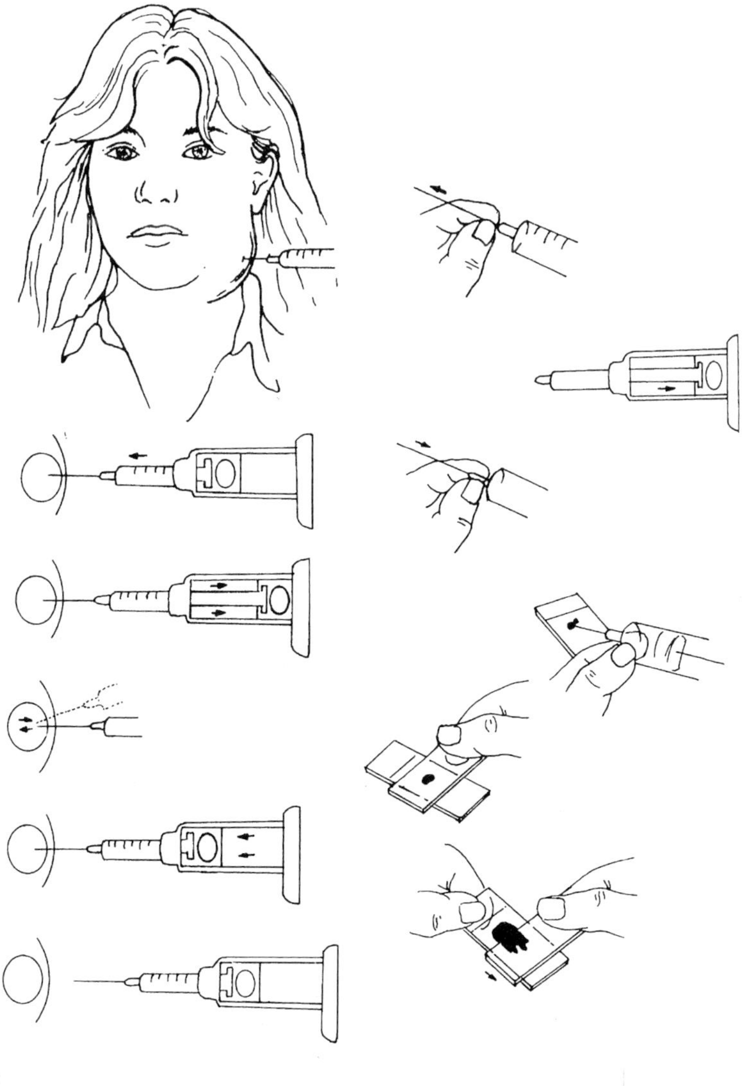

Figure 21-3. Steps of a fine-needle aspiration biopsy of a neck mass. With a small amount of air in the chamber of the syringe, the needle is placed into the tumor. Negative pressure is then applied to the syringe as the needle is passed to and fro in the specimen. Negative pressure is then released, and the needle is withdrawn. The needle is removed, the syringe is filled with air, the needle is replaced, and a gentle positive pressure is applied to displace tumor cells from the needle onto a glass slide. A second slide is applied to create a smear of the aspiration. (From Close LG, Larson DL, Shah JP. *Essentials of head and neck oncology.* New York: Thieme Medical Publishers, Inc., 1998. Figure 22-3.)

laryngoscopy, bronchoscopy, esophagoscopy, and nasopharyngoscopy. Another crucial part of the operation is palpation of the mass and neck. The utility of these procedures is threefold: full assessment of the mass for staging, biopsy for diagnosis, and full evaluation of the upper aerodigestive tract for second primaries.

It is essential that the patient is under general anesthesia and fully paralyzed. This aids in easier placement of the rigid scopes as well as deep palpation. Location of the mass in the aerodigestive tract prohibits a full examination in the clinic as a result of patient discomfort. Pharmacologic paralysis allows for palpation in the deep pharynx and for firm palpation of the neck that would not otherwise be possible as a result of gagging, pain, and muscular splinting.

Treatment

General Principles of Therapy

There are general principles regarding the treatment of HNCa that pertain to most anatomic sites and diagnoses. Intuitively, the earlier a cancer is diagnosed, the higher the chance of cure and survival. T1 and T2 tumors are considered early. Late tumors are T3 and T4, with T4a being still operable and T4b being inoperable.

In most sites, early cancers are equally curable using surgery or radiation. Later stages require a combination approach that involves the use of both modalities. Recent advancements in the addition of chemotherapy can increase treatment response rates, and they will be discussed in more detail later. Surgery first ensures an easier procedure and better wound healing, but it creates a relatively hypoxic environment that decreases the efficacy of the radiation and chemotherapy. However, radiation can be reserved for recurrent tumor or for a second primary malignancy. Radiation first makes surgery more difficult, and healing is prolonged. After the full dose of radiation is given, the patient generally is not eligible for further courses in the same area.

HNCa spreads in a somewhat predictable fashion. The malignancy usually spreads through the lymphatics first to predictable regional lymph-node beds (first-echelon nodes), depending on the anatomic site of the primary tumor before it spreads to other nodal levels. After excessive growth of the primary or extensive lymphatic spread, one must worry about distant metastases, and the workup needs to be appropriately tailored. Distant spread portends a dismal prognosis, and local and regional therapies will not improve the outcome. Typically, distant metastases from HNCa go to the lungs most frequently, followed by the bones and the liver.

Regional Metastases

The main predictor of the success of treatment is the presence of regional metastases. Spread to the cervical lymph nodes halves the survival rate. A positive node upstages the cancer to stage III, and more extensive nodal involvement increases it to stage IV. HNCa staging uses the TNM classification, with the letter *N* pertaining to the extent of nodal disease (Table 21-2).

The neck has been divided into several anatomic levels (Figure 21-4):

Level I: This level contains the submental and submandibular triangles, and it is bounded by the anterior and posterior bellies of the digastric muscle, the hyoid bone inferiorly, and the body of the mandible superiorly.

Level II: This level contains the upper jugular lymph nodes, and it extends from the level of the skull base superiorly to the hyoid bone inferiorly.

BOX 21-7 HISTORY TO BE TAKEN FROM THE PATIENT WITH SUSPECTED HEAD AND NECK CANCER

- Present illness
  - Time course
  - Pain, otalgia, dysphagia, dyspnea, voice change, weight loss, diet
- Past medical and surgical history
- Medications
- Social history/risk factors
  - Tobacco: age of initiation, quantity
  - Alcohol
  - Dental problems
  - Reflux
  - Occupation
- Other physicians
- Family history
  - Cancer, diabetes, heart disease
- Family support

TABLE 21-2 • *Nodal Staging*

NX	Regional lymph nodes cannot be assessed
N0	No regional lymph-node metastasis
N1	Metastasis in a single ipsilateral lymph node, 3 cm or less in greatest dimension
N2a	Metastasis in a single ipsilateral lymph node, more than 3 cm but not more than 6 cm in greatest dimension
N2b	Metastasis in multiple ipsilateral lymph nodes, none more than 6 cm in greatest dimension
N2c	Metastases in bilateral or contralateral lymph nodes, none more than 6 cm in greatest dimension
N3	Metastasis in a lymph node more than 6 cm in greatest dimension

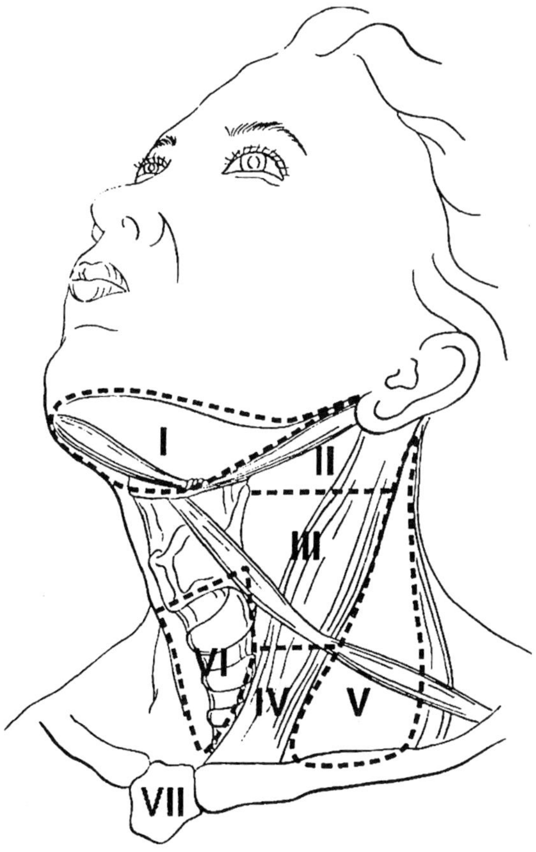

Figure 21-4. Schematic diagram indicating the location of the lymph-node levels in the neck, as described in the text. (From Greene FL, Page DL, Fleming ID, *et al. AJCC cancer staging handbook*, 6th ed. New York: American Joint Commission on Cancer, 2002. Figure 2.1.)

Level III: This level contains the middle jugular lymph nodes from the hyoid bone superiorly to the level of the lower border of the cricoid cartilage inferiorly.

Level IV: This level contains the lower jugular lymph nodes from the level of the cricoid cartilage superiorly to the clavicle inferiorly.

Level V: This level contains the lymph nodes in the posterior triangle, and it is bounded by the anterior border of the trapezius muscle posteriorly, the posterior border of the sternocleidomastoid muscle anteriorly, and the clavicle inferiorly.

Neck Dissections

In 1906, Crile described the first removal of regional neck nodes for the treatment of metastatic spread. Since that time, neck dissection in some form has been incorporated into the complete treatment of HNCa. The gold standard for the treatment of neck disease is the *radical neck dissection* (RND). By definition, it includes the removal of the lymph nodes from levels I through V, the sternocleidomastoid muscle (SCM), the internal jugular vein (IJ), and the spinal accessory/eleventh cranial nerve (CN11).

In an attempt to decrease the morbidity involved with the removal of some of the structures, the *modified radical neck dissection* (MRND) was developed (Table 21-3). The SCM, the IJ, and/or the CN11 are variably left in place, depending on the location of the metastatic nodes. Lymph nodes on levels I through V are still removed. Further reductions in morbidity have lead to various *selective neck dissections* (SNDs). In their various forms, these procedures preserve whole nodal levels. The proper dissection is selected on the basis of the site of the primary tumor.

External Beam Radiation

External beam radiation can also be used to treat neck disease. Indications for postoperative radiation include multiple nodes, nodes larger than 2 cm, extracapsular spread, and nodes in levels beyond those thought to be in the first echelon for the primary tumor. If a neck dissection is not performed, pathologic findings of the primary tumor may indicate that neck radiation is needed. These are deep infiltration of more than 2 mm (oral cavity, palate), angiolymphatic invasion, and neuroinvasion.

TABLE 21-3 • *Types of Neck Dissection*

Name	Levels	Preserved
Radical neck dissection	I-V	None
Modified radical neck dissection type 1	I-V	Eleventh cranial nerve
Modified radical neck dissection type 2	I-V	Eleventh cranial nerve, internal jugular vein
Modified radical neck dissection type 3	I-V	Eleventh cranial nerve, internal jugular vein, sternocleidomastoid muscle
Supraomohyoid	I-III	All
Lateral	II-IV	All
Anterolateral	I-IV	All
Posterolateral	II-V	All

Indications for Treatment of the Neck

The decision to treat the positive neck (N^+) is an easy one. There is an element of controversy with regard to choosing the modality, and it may depend on the modality chosen for the treatment of the primary. With regard to radiation of the neck, the N1 neck can also be successfully treated. As the bulk of disease increases, the risk of regional failure also rises. The N2 neck status after neoadjuvant radiation may need subsequent neck dissection. The N3 neck will likely need preoperative radiation to shrink the tumor mass and to hopefully reduce adherence to vital structures such as the carotid artery and prevertebral fascia; such involvement precludes successful extirpation.

The RND is used for extensive neck disease: multiple nodes, large tumor mass (single large or matted nodes), after incision biopsy of a positive node, after radiation failure in the neck, and after radiation of the N3 neck.

MRND can be used in the N^+ neck if the CN11 is clearly not involved. Neck disease staged at N2 can be treated with MRND after radiation therapy.

Some feel that in certain, carefully chosen cases, an SND can be therapeutic during the earliest of stages of regional metastasis (N1). This should, however, be followed by radiation therapy.

The treatment of the neck without obvious metastasis (N0)—*elective neck dissection*—is more controversial. Some primary tumors have a high propensity for early metastases, such as the tongue, the floor of the mouth (FOM), the supraglottis, the hypopharynx, and the oropharynx. In these situations, elective treatment is warranted. It is accepted that, if the chance of occult disease (metastases present but too small for detection clinically or radiographically) is greater than 20%, then the neck should be treated electively. If the primary tumor is to be radiated, then that is sufficient for the neck. The appropriate form of SND can also be used.

Indications for adjuvant radiation therapy to the neck after neck dissection include multiple nodes, large nodes (N2 or greater), extracapsular spread, and nodes in levels beyond the first echelon.

Surgical Techniques for Neck Dissection

Incisions for the various dissections vary (Figure 21-5). One should choose the variation that allows for the best access to the nodal levels to be removed and to the primary tumor if it is to be excised through the neck.

Prior radiation, prior neck incisions, the need for trifurcating incisions, and the need for possible subsequent surgery should all be considered. The incisions can be modified depending on the tumor, skin creases, and patient factors (e.g., neck length, obesity). The trifurcation should never be placed over the carotid artery. Wound breakdown after a neck dissection can leave the carotid exposed. Reconstruction with a pedicled flap is then an urgent matter before the carotid ruptures, which carries an 80% mortality.

Radical Neck Dissection

Skin incisions are made and carried out through the platysma muscle. The skin flaps are elevated in this subplatysmal plane (Figure 21-6, *A*). Keeping the platysma in view (directly on the undersurface of the thin muscle belly) will avoid the anterior veins, the external jugular

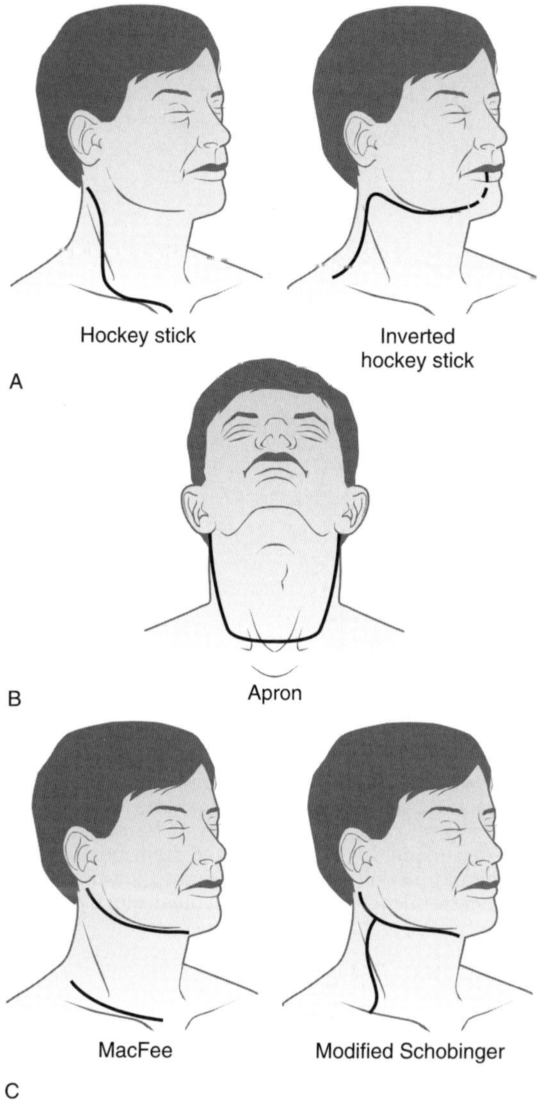

Figure 21-5. Common incisions used for neck dissections. (From Cummings CW, Fredrickson JM, Harker LA, *et al. Otolaryngology head and neck surgery*, 3rd ed. St. Louis: Mosby, 1998.)

vein, the greater auricular nerve (it is saved in an SND), and the marginal mandibular nerve. A Hayes-Martin flap will raise the marginal mandibular nerve (Figure 21-6, *B*). It lies within the submandibular fascia and superficial to the facial vein. The facial vein is ligated and raised with the flap, thus protecting the nerve.

Level I of the neck can now be dissected. The fibrofatty tissue of the submental triangle is excised from the contralateral anterior belly of the digastric muscle and removed from the deeper mylohyoid muscle. It is kept intact with the contents of the submandibular triangle. The mylohyoid is once again located posterior to the ipsilateral anterior belly of the digastric. It is retracted anteriorly, and the lingual nerve is located and preserved. The contents of the submandibular triangle are then dissected from the deep tissue in an anterior-to-posterior direction. The hypoglossal nerve is located and preserved. The nodes contained in the fat and the submandibular gland are removed from the body of the mandible and included in the specimen. The facial artery both superior and inferior to the gland, the duct of the gland, and the submandibular ganglion from the lingual nerve are located and ligated. The contents of level I are then left attached posteriorly.

Next, the boundaries around levels II, III, and V are defined. The SCM is divided at its attachments to the mastoid process, the sternum, and the clavicle. Care is taken to not damage the IJ, the carotid artery, or the vagus nerve, which lie deep to the muscle. The omohyoid muscle is divided in level V. Inferiorly, the internal jugular vein is isolated and divided between 0-silk ties and 2-0 silk suture ligatures. The carotid artery and the vagus nerve are located and protected during this maneuver. The phrenic nerve is located just lateral to the IJ. The tissue comprising levels IV and V is separated from the superior mediastinal fat, parallel to the clavicle at the depth of the deep cervical fascia. This tissue must be ligated with ties or with a stapler to avoid large lymphatic leaks, especially on the left side, where the thoracic duct is located. The posterior border is dissected along the trapezius muscle to the skull base (Figure 21-6, *C*).

Now, up at the skull base, the IJ is located, ligated, and divided. It is ensured that the hypoglossal nerve is preserved. The CN11 is cut at the skull base. The contents of level II are then removed from the skull base. The occipital artery may require ligation.

The fibrofatty contents of level V are now dissected from the deep layer of the deep cervical fascia in a posterior-to-anterior direction (Figure 21-6, *D*). The brachial plexus and the phrenic nerve must be avoided by remaining superficial to this fascial layer. Cervical nerve roots are encountered and cut about 1 cm from the phrenic nerve. The IJ is removed from the rest of the carotid sheath components as it is lifted with the rest of the specimen. The tissue is dissected from the strap muscles medially (Figure 21-6, *E*). Depending on how the primary tumor is removed, the neck dissection specimen can be left attached to it for an en bloc resection. Active drains are placed to avoid fluid collections.

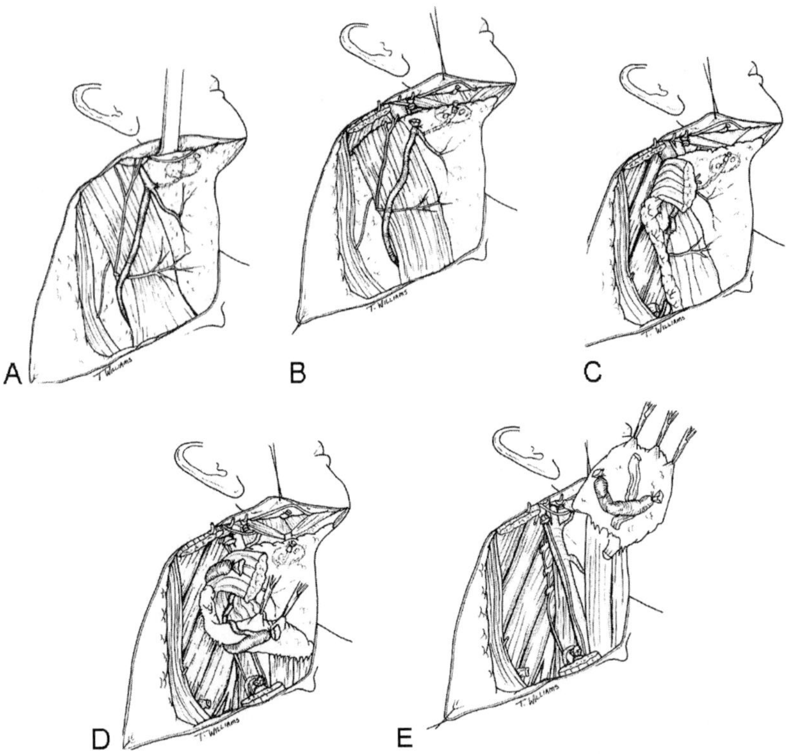

Figure 21-6. Steps in a radical neck dissection. **A,** Skin flaps are raised. The sternocleidomastoid muscle is exposed, along with cranial nerve 11. **B,** A Hayes-Martin flap is raised to protect the marginal mandibular nerve. **C,** The sternocleidomastoid muscle is detached from the mastoid, and the posterior border is delineated. **D,** The internal jugular vein is ligated, and the neck-dissection specimen is raised from posterior to anterior. **E,** The specimen is removed from the carotid sheath and medial attachment. (From Cummings CW, Fredrickson JM, Harker LA, *et al. Otolaryngology head and neck surgery,* 3rd ed. St. Louis: Mosby, 1998. Figure 95-4.)

Modified Radical Neck Dissection

Many of the steps of the MRND are the same as those of the RND. Some steps vary, depending on which structures are being removed (Figure 21-7, *A–F*). The CN11 must be located at the anterior or posterior border of the SCM; it is then carefully dissected and isolated from surrounding tissue from the skull base to the junction of the trapezius muscle and the clavicle. The course of the nerve is followed through the SCM, noting that it may lie deep to the entire muscle. If the SCM is to be taken, it is divided superiorly and inferiorly, as it is during the RND.

If the SCM is to be preserved, the fascia surrounding the muscle must be removed circumferentially and left with the specimen. Level I is dissected as it is in the RND. The boundaries of level V are then delineated, avoiding the CN11 next to the trapezius. The fibrofatty contents of level V are then dissected in an inferior-to-superior direction. As the tissue is freed, it can be passed under the CN11and SCM. At the skull base, the proximal end of the CN11 must be lightly retracted and protected in level II.

If the IJ is to be preserved, the dissection of the specimen is carried to its posterior border. The fascia is removed from the wall of the vein, keeping it attached to the specimen. Several branches of the vein need to be properly ligated. The carotid artery and the vagus nerve are protected, and the specimen is removed from the strap muscles medially.

Selective Neck Dissections

The sternocleidomastoid muscle, the spinal accessory nerve, and the internal jugular veins are always preserved. The *supraomohyoid neck dissection* requires the dissection of level I. The fascia is taken off of the anterior border of the SCM, around to the deep aspect of the muscle, to the posterior border. The CN11 is located anteriorly and followed to the skull base.

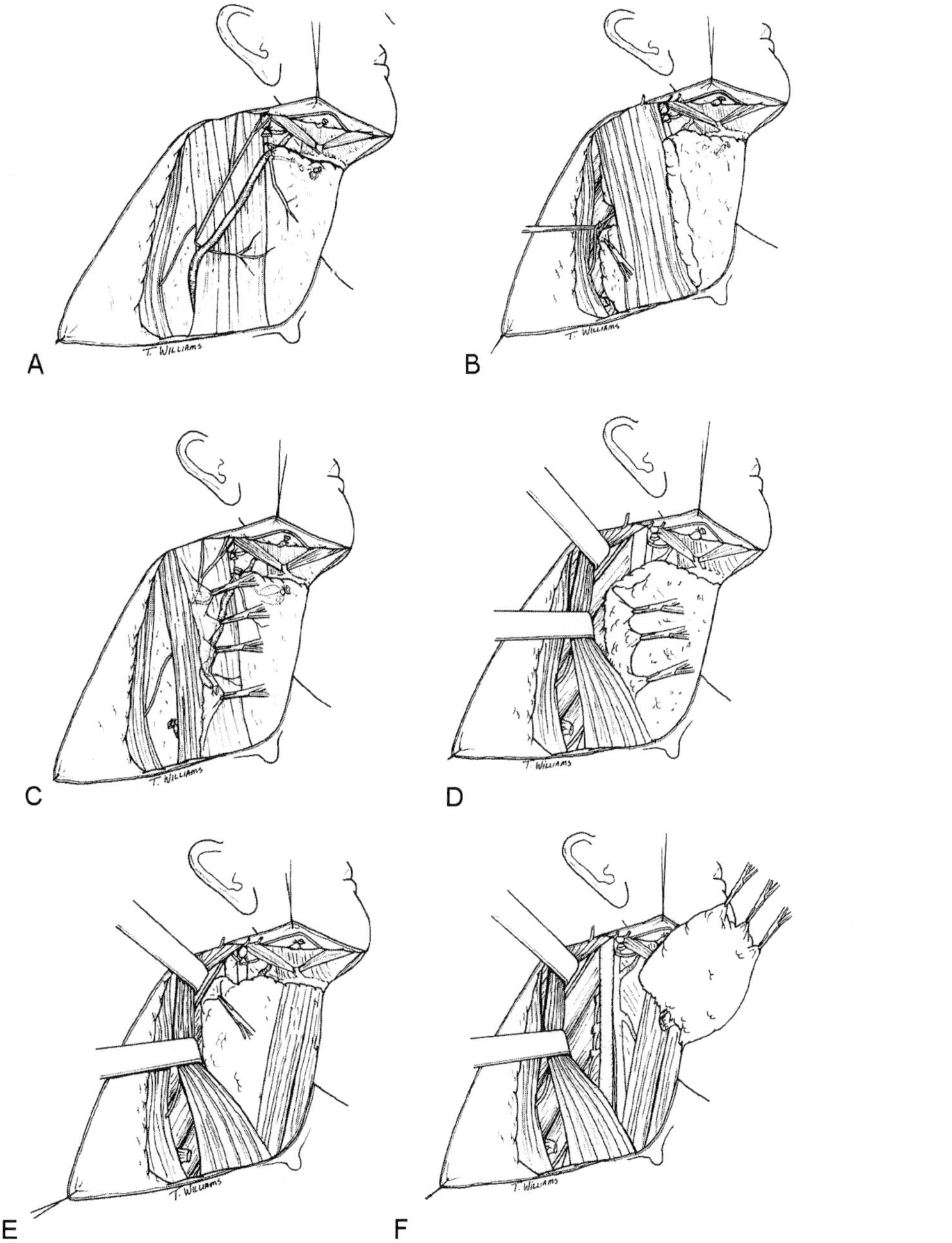

Figure 21–7. Steps in a modified radical neck dissection. **A,** Skin flaps are raised, and level I is dissected. **B,** The level V tissue is passed under cranial nerve 11. **C,** Removal of the sternocleidomastoid muscle fascia. **D,** The sternocleidomastoid muscle is retracted laterally and level V tissue is passed under toward the carotid sheath. **E,** The sternocleidomastoid muscle is retracted, cranial nerve 11 is seen, and level II is removed from the skull base. **F,** Levels I through V are removed; sternocleidomastoid muscle, internal jugular vein, and cranial nerve 11 are intact. (From Cummings CW, Fredrickson JM, Harker LA, *et al. Otolaryngology head and neck surgery,* 3rd ed. St. Louis: Mosby, 1998. Figure 95-6.)

Great care is needed to avoid damaging the CN11 as it exits the posterior SCM. The muscle is retracted posteriorly. The omohyoid is located and the fascia is removed, but the muscle is preserved.

At the junction of the omohyoid and the SCM, a dissection plane is created down to the deep layer of the deep cervical fascia. The phrenic nerve is once again avoided. This plane is then brought superiorly. As it is made, the contents of levels II through IV are retracted anteriorly. Avoid pulling the contents of level V into the surgical plane; this makes the dissection more difficult and puts CN11 in danger.

The cervical nerve roots are preserved. The specimen is removed from the IJ in the same manner as it is in the MRND types 2 and 3.

Knowing how to approach each level of the neck in a dissection will allow for other selective neck dissection procedures. If level I is to be left, as it is in the lateral neck dissection and the posterolateral neck dissection, the anterior border of level II is the posterior belly of the digastric muscle. The array of SNDs was developed to decrease the morbidity of the neck dissection. As such, efforts should be made to preserve muscles, nerves, and blood vessels that should not be part of the specimen.

Complications of Neck Dissection

The complications of neck dissection are the result of the removal of structures with the specimen or of damage to neighboring anatomy. Meticulous dissection and gentle tissue handling techniques are required. A thorough knowledge of the normal anatomy and its variations is important. The surgeon must be aware of how normal landmarks can be distorted by tumor mass and scarring from prior treatment.

BOX 21-8 COMPLICATIONS OF NECK DISSECTION

- Bleeding
- Infection
- Nerve damage: hypoglossal, vagus, spinal accessory, phrenic, brachial plexus, lingual, marginal mandibular
- Shoulder syndrome: severe shoulder pain and dysfunction from damage to eleventh cranial nerve
- Neck and ear numbness: damage of the greater auricular and cervical nerves
- Skin-flap necrosis: may leave carotid artery exposed, thus requiring flap reconstruction
- Chyle leak: may lead to dehydration, malnutrition, and immunocompromised state
- Horner's syndrome: damaged sympathetic trunk
- Loss of bilateral internal jugular vein (removal and/or thrombosis): severe facial edema, increased intracranial pressure, blindness, syndrome of inappropriate secretion of antidiuretic hormone

The Unknown Primary

A neck mass in an adult is presumed to be neoplastic until proven otherwise. A patient with a neck mass but no symptoms of an upper aerodigestive tract pathology can be a diagnostic dilemma. The patient needs a full head and neck examination. Cancers in various areas of the aerodigestive tract metastasize to predictable nodal levels. Supraclavicular nodes may be indicative of a lymphoma or a primary site below the clavicles. An FNA biopsy can aid in tailoring the investigation.

The mass will most likely be a metastatic node from a squamous cell primary. If the clinic examination and imaging are still negative (which is less common with advancements in imaging with high-resolution CT scanning, MRI, and positron emission tomography scanning), then a panendoscopy in the operating room is warranted. Biopsies of suspicious areas are performed. The main areas of concern are the nasopharynx, the base of the tongue (BOT), the piriform sinus, and the tonsil. If no primary is found, then treatment is centered around the neck and these areas. Radiation therapy is started with the field encompassing a region from the nasopharynx to the piriform sinus and the neck. Morbidity is high because of the large surface being irradiated. Treatment of the neck may include neck dissection; this is dependent on the extent of nodal involvement.

Cancer of the Oral Cavity

Anatomy

The oral cavity is made up of many different parts. Anteriorly, the border is the vermilion border of the lips. Posteriorly, the boundaries are the bilateral ascending rami of the mandible (retromolar trigone), the junction of the hard and soft palate, and the circumvallate papillae of the tongue. This area also contains the mobile tongue, the upper and lower alveolar ridges, the buccal mucosa, the FOM, and the hard palate (Figure 21-8). Cancers in each area of the oral cavity spreads in a predictable pattern. The risk of regional metastases is related to T stage, depth of invasion, and anatomic location (Table 21-4).

Treatment

Choices of treatment are dependent on the anatomic site as well as the extent of disease (Table 21-5). Radiation and surgery have equal

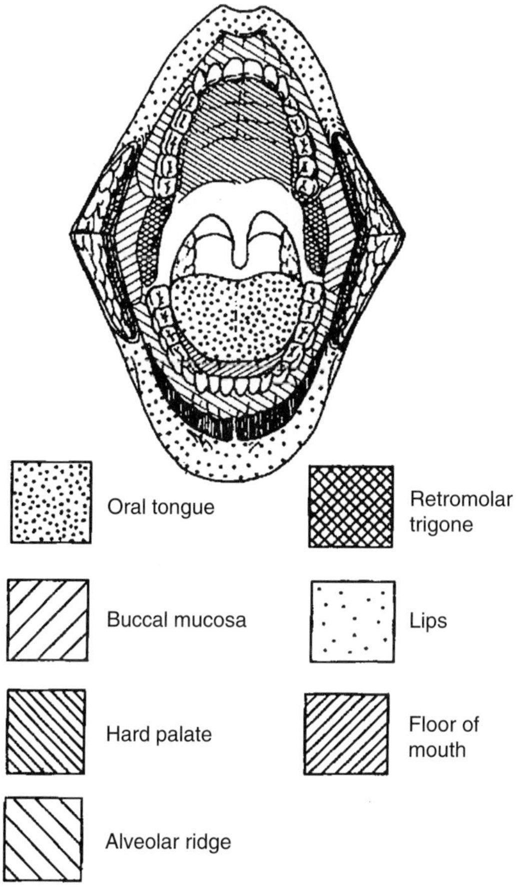

Figure 21–8. The oral cavity and its constituents. (From Close LG, Larson DL, Shah JP. *Essentials of head and neck oncology*. New York: Thieme Medical Publishers, Inc., 1998. Figure 7-1.)

survival rates for early lesions (i.e., T1, T2). Radiation may cause less functional morbidity, and there is no external scar. However, it is not without its complications. Disadvantages include the time commitment (up to 7 weeks), poor coverage of tumors that have infiltrated bone, full dental extractions if poor dental hygiene is present, and loss of radiation as an option for subsequent HNCa primary tumors.

There are several surgical approaches to tumors of the oral cavity:

Peroral excision is for small, easily accessible lesions.

Upper or lower cheek flaps allow access to larger peripheral lesions. An incision is made in the upper or lower gingivobuccal sulcus and deepened to allow the cheek to be further retracted.

The *visor flap* allows access to anterior, inferior areas (mandible, FOM). After the neck incision is made bilaterally, the skin and deep tissue are dissected from the mandible, and full-length lower gingivobuccal incisions are made. The lower face can then be retracted superiorly while the mandible and lower oral cavity are retracted inferiorly. A significant morbidity is caused by the loss of both of the mental nerves, which leaves both the lower lip and the chin insensate.

BOX 21–9 COMPLICATIONS OF EXTERNAL-BEAM RADIATION THERAPY

- Xerostomia
- Loss of taste and smell
- Mucositis
- Skin desquamation
- Pigmentation changes
- Fibrosis
- Tissue necrosis
- Pain
- Trismus
- Edema
- Osteoradionecrosis
- Dental caries
- Poor healing
- Neuropathies
- Vascular thrombosis

TABLE 21–4 • *Lymphatic Spread by Primary Site*

Site	Risk	Primary Lymph Node Groups
Lip	Low	I to II
Hard palate	Low	I to II/retropharyngeal
Alveolar ridge	Low	I to II/retropharyngeal
Retromolar trigone	Med	II to III
Tongue	High	See 1 and 2
Floor of mouth	High	See 2

(1) Posterior mobile tongue spreads to the higher levels. Tip of the tongue cancers are more likely to go to the middle to low neck. (2) The closer to the midline the primary is, the more likely bilateral necks can be involved.

TABLE 21-5 • *American Joint Committee on Cancer Staging of Oral Cavity Cancer*

Primary Tumor (T)			
TX	Primary tumor cannot be assessed		
T0	No evidence of primary tumor		
Tis	Carcinoma in situ		
T1	Tumor 2 cm or less in greatest dimension		
T2	Tumor more than 2 cm but not more than 4 cm in greatest dimension		
T3	Tumor more than 4 cm in greatest dimension		
T4 (lip)	Tumor invades through cortical bone, inferior alveolar nerve, floor of mouth, or skin of face (i.e., chin or nose)		
T4a (oral cavity)	Tumor invades adjacent structures (e.g., through cortical bone, into deep [extrinsic] muscle of tongue [genioglossus, hyoglossus, palatoglossus, and styloglossus], maxillary sinus, skin of face)		
T4b	Tumor invades masticator space, pterygoid plates, or skull base and/or encases internal carotid artery		
Regional Lymph Nodes (N)			
NX	Regional lymph nodes cannot be assessed		
N0	No regional lymph-node metastasis		
N1	Metastasis in a single ipsilateral lymph node, 3 cm or less in greatest dimension		
N2a	Metastasis in single ipsilateral lymph node more than 3 cm but not more than 6 cm in greatest dimension		
N2b	Metastasis in multiple ipsilateral lymph nodes, none more than 6 cm in greatest dimension		
N2c	Metastases in bilateral or contralateral lymph nodes, none more than 6 cm in greatest dimension		
N3	Metastasis in a lymph node more than 6 cm in greatest dimension		
Distant Metastases (M)			
MX	Distant metastases not assessed		
M0	No distant metastases		
M1	Distant metastases located		
Stage Groupings			
Stage	T	N	M
0	Tis	N0	M0
I	T1	N0	M0
II	T2	N0	M0
III	T3	N0	M0
	T1	N1	M0
	T2	N1	M0
	T3	N1	M0
IVA	T4a	N0	MO
	T4a	N1	M0
	T1	N2	M0
	T2	N2	M0
	T3	N2	M0
	T4a	N2	M0
IVB	Any T	N3	M0
	T4b	Any N	M0
IVC	Any T	Any N	M1

The *mandibulotomy* and the *mandibular swing* give wide access to the posterior oral cavity and the oropharynx. The neck incision is extended around the mentum and through the midline of the lower lip. The periosteum of the mandible is incised and raised a short distance bilaterally. A titanium reconstruction plate is fashioned before the mandibulotomy and saved for use during closure. A midline vertical, full-thickness cut through the bone is made, avoiding the tooth roots. The incision is then extended lateral to the FOM paralleling the lower alveolar ridge. This allows the ipsilateral mandible to be rotated (swung) laterally to gain access posteriorly.

The *pull-through* is performed by gaining access to the oral cavity from the neck through the floor of mouth. The primary tumor is excised, with exposure from the mouth and the neck, and it is removed through the neck. It gives excellent access to large tumors of the FOM and the tongue. The primary and neck specimens are removed en bloc.

If the periosteum of the mandible is involved, a *marginal mandibulectomy* may need to be performed (Figure 21-9). The involved bony cortex and adjacent teeth are removed with the specimen. The other cortex is left intact to maintain the integrity of the mandibular arch.

If the bone is grossly eroded, a *segmental mandibulectomy* is required; the full-thickness section of the mandible is removed (Figure 21-10). If the marrow space is infiltrated, the resection must extend from distal to the mental foramen to the angle of the mandible.

Reconstruction

Small defects can be left to close by secondary intention or by primary closure. A split-thickness skin graft with a bolster can be used on small to intermediate sites. Large defects and those that connect the oral cavity to the neck cavity (after concurrent neck dissection) need more elaborate flap reconstruction.

The most commonly used regional flap is the pectoralis myocutaneous (PMC) flap. The muscle, subcutaneous fat, and a chest skin paddle are removed from the anterior chest wall and rotated into the neck on a muscle pedicle containing the thoracoacromial artery. The skin paddle is used to patch the defect in the oral cavity, and it is sewn in with 3-0 polyglactic acid sutures. If the flap adds too much bulk, the skin and fat can be removed and a split-thickness skin graft sewn directly to the muscle. Other regional flaps include the deltopectoral flap, the sternocleidomastoid myocutaneous flap, the latissimus dorsi flap, and the platysma flap (Table 21-6).

The last two decades have seen the introduction and advancement of free tissue transfer. A piece of tissue is removed from a distant area of the body, along with the vascular pedicle (i.e., the artery and veins). The tissue is used to patch the defect, and microvascular techniques are used to anastomose the vessels to the blood supply in the neck.

Mandibular reconstruction after segmental mandibulectomy of the anterior mandible is

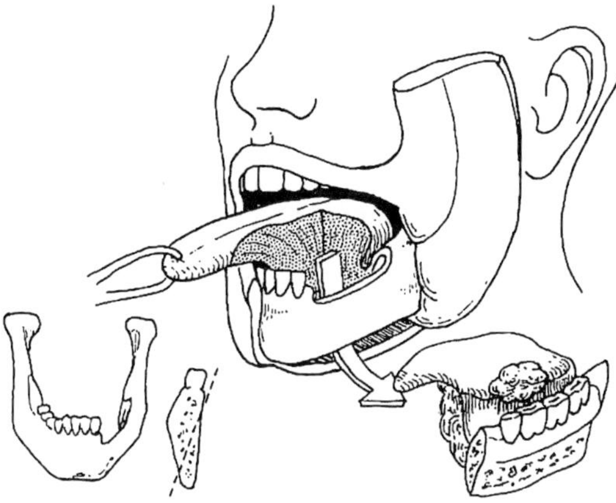

Figure 21-9. Marginal resection of the mandible. (From Close LG, Larson DL, Shah JP. *Essentials of head and neck oncology*. New York: Thieme Medical Publishers, Inc., 1998. Figure 17-2.)

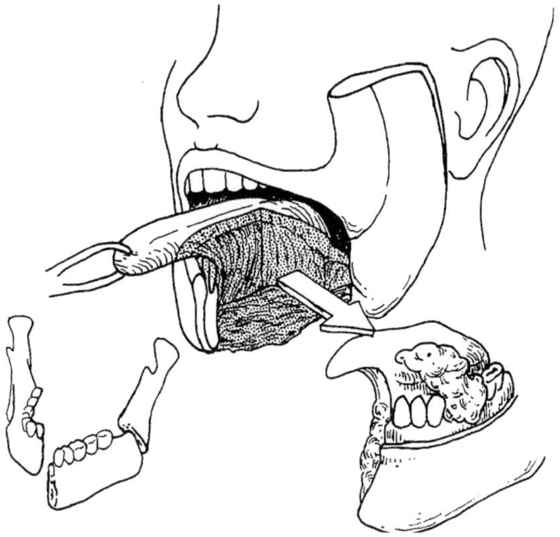

Figure 21-10. Segmental resection of the mandible. (From Close LG, Larson DL, Shah JP. *Essentials of head and neck oncology*. New York: Thieme Medical Publishers, Inc., 1998. Figure 17-1.)

TABLE 21-6 • *Common Free Flaps Used for Head and Neck Reconstruction*

Radial forearm	Fasciocutaneous, thin and pliable patch
Fibular free flap	Osteocutaneous, longest bone stock for mandibular defects
Anterolateral	Fasciocutaneous, fat thigh adds bulk to large defects
Rectus	Myocutaneous, fat and muscle add bulk
Iliac crest	Osteocutaneous
Jejunal graft	Conduit for total pharyngeal/esophageal defects

required to recreate support for the tongue. Bare reconstruction plate filling the defect with or without a PMC flap is wrought with wound complications and should be avoided. The best method for this reconstruction is an osteocutaneous free flap. Lateral mandible defects in edentulous patients need not be reconstructed, because dental occlusion is not a factor.

Cancer of the Pharynx

The pharynx is divided into three distinct areas: the nasopharynx, the oropharynx, and the hypopharynx (Figure 21-11). With regard to neoplastic involvement, treatment, reconstruction, and outcomes vary greatly among regions.

Nasopharyngeal Carcinoma

The nasopharynx is the area of the airway that starts at the posterior choana of the nose and ends at the plane created by the free edge of the soft palate. This can be broken into regions: the lateral walls, which contain the Eustachian tube orifices and the fossae of Rosenmueller; the posterior wall, which holds the adenoid; and the floor, which is the nasal surface of the soft palate.

Risk Factors

Genetic and environmental factors play a large role in the etiology of nasopharyngeal carcinoma (NPC). People of Asian decent are at highest risk. First-generation Asian Americans born in the United States to Asian immigrants have a lower risk, but it does not reach the normal baseline. It is felt that eating salted fish at a young age is a risk factor, as are smoking and exposure to quarry dust, wood/grass smoke, and formalin.

An interesting and important fact is the association of NPC with Epstein-Barr virus. Titers for immunoglobulin A to viral capsid antigen and early antigen are high among patients with NPC. Pretreatment titers can be compared to post-treatment measurements. A persistently high level is indicative of persistent or recurrent disease and a poor prognosis. Titers have also been used as a screening test, with some success in high-risk populations.

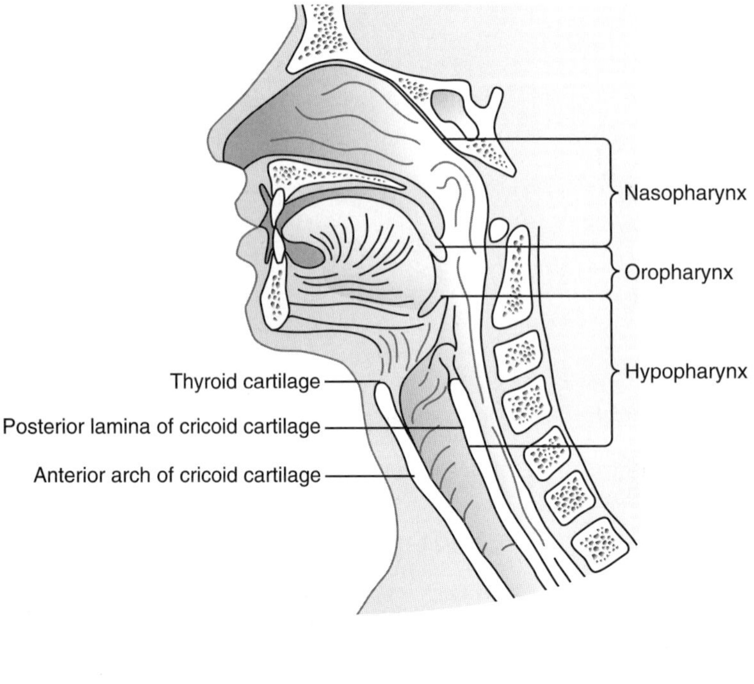

Figure 21-11. Sagittal view of the face and neck depicting the subdivisions of the pharynx. (From Greene FL, Page DL, Fleming ID, *et al. AJCC cancer staging handbook*, 6th ed. New York: American Joint Commission on Cancer, 2002. Figure 4.1.)

Presentation

Nasopharyngeal carcinoma presents with a classic triad: neck mass, ear fullness/hearing loss, and nasal obstruction. Other symptoms include epistaxis, headache, otalgia, neck pain, weight loss, diplopia, and other cranial nerve deficits.

Workup

The history should include ethnic origin and environmental exposures. The examination requires a careful evaluation of the neck. A zero-degree 4-mm rigid endoscope or a nasopharyngeal mirror examination will allow for visualization of the mass. The biopsy of a nasal or a nasopharyngeal mass in the clinic can be dangerous as a result of excessive bleeding that is difficult to control. An FNA of a neck mass can be helpful. The patient is taken to the operating room for full evaluation of tumor extent for staging, biopsy for diagnosis, and evaluation for second primaries. MRI is the scan of choice for its better definition of soft-tissue planes to evaluate deep extension.

The differential diagnosis for masses in the nasopharynx is limited. NPC has been divided into three histologic patterns by the World Health Organization (WHO):

WHO I	Keratinizing SCCa
WHO II	Non-keratinizing SCCa
WHO III	Undifferentiated carcinoma

Differentiation is important, because it can aid with the treatment plan and with predicting prognosis. WHO II and III are more prevalent (especially in Asia), and they are more strongly associated with Epstein-Barr virus. They are more responsive to chemotherapy, and they have a better prognosis.

BOX 21-10 DIFFERENTIAL FOR NASOPHARYNGEAL MASSES

Benign
- Adenoid hyperplasia
- Thornwaldt's cyst 1
- Inclusion cyst

Malignant
- Nasopharyngeal carcinoma
- Lymphoma
- Minor salivary gland tumor
- Sarcoma
- Chordoma

The staging of NPC differs from other HNCa (Table 21-7). Lymphatic spread from a primary NPC goes to the retropharyngeal, upper jugular, and spinal accessory nodes (level V). A solitary nodal mass in level V warrants careful inspection of the nasopharynx.

The distribution and the prognostic impact of regional lymph-node spread from NPC—particularly of the undifferentiated type—are different from those of other head and neck mucosal cancers and justify the use of a different N classification scheme. The supraclavicular zone or fossa is relevant to the staging of nasopharyngeal carcinoma, and it is the triangular region originally described by Ho. It is defined by three points: (1) the superior margin of the sternal end of the clavicle; (2) the superior margin of the lateral end of the clavicle; and (3) the point at which the neck meets the shoulder (Figure 21-12). Note that this would include caudal portions of levels IV and V. All cases with lymph nodes (whole or part) in the fossa are considered N3b.

Treatment

Difficult access and the involvement of critical structures (i.e., the internal carotid artery, multiple cranial nerves, the cavernous sinus, the skull base, and intracranial extent) preclude surgery as a realistic option for NPC. External-beam radiation is the mainstay of therapy. Some controversy exists regarding the role of chemotherapy. Late-stage disease warrants either neoadjuvant or concurrent chemotherapy with platinum-based agents. 5-Fluorouracil can be added, but there is then increased toxicity. Surgery is reserved for salvage therapy, and patients must be chosen carefully. Exposure of the nasopharynx includes transpalatal, transmaxillary, and transcervical approaches.

Oropharyngeal Cancer

Anatomy

The oropharynx starts superiorly at the junction of the hard and soft palate and at the plane created by the free edge of the soft palate. The anterior border of the base of the tongue is the circumvallate papillae. It extends inferiorly to the level of the plane created by the hyoid bone. It includes the anterior tonsillar pillars and the soft palate, the tonsillar fossae, the lateral and posterior pharyngeal walls, and the BOT. It extends into the vallecula and ends where the vallecular mucosa reflects superiorly onto the

TABLE 21–7 • *American Joint Committee on Cancer Staging of Nasopharyngeal Cancer*

Primary Tumor (T)	
TX	Primary tumor cannot be assessed
T0	No evidence of primary tumor
Tis	Carcinoma in situ
T1	Tumor confined to the nasopharynx
T2	Tumor extends to soft tissues
T2a	Tumor extends to the oropharynx and/or nasal cavity without parapharyngeal extension*
T2b	Any tumor with parapharyngeal extension*
T3	Tumor involves bony structures and/or paranasal sinuses
T4	Tumor with intracranial extension and/or involvement of cranial nerves, infratemporal fossa, hypopharynx, orbit, or masticator space
Regional Lymph Nodes (N)	
Nx	Regional lymph nodes cannot be assessed
N0	No regional lymph node metastasis
N1	Unilateral metastasis in lymph node(s), 6 cm or less in greatest dimension, above the supraclavicular fossa*
N2	Bilateral metastasis in lymph node(s), 6 cm or less in greatest dimension, above the supraclavicular fossa*
N3a	Lymph node metastasis greater than 6 cm in dimension
N3b	Lymph node metastases greater than 6 cm in dimension
Distant Metastases (M)	
MX	Distant metastases not assessed
M0	No distant metastases
M1	Distant metastases located

Stage Groupings

Stage	T	N	M
0	Tis	N0	M0
I	T1	N0	M0
IIA	T2a	N0	M0
IIB	T1	N1	M0
	T2	N1	M0
	T2a	N1	M0
	T2b	N0	M0
	T2b	N1	M0
III	T1	N2	M0
	T2a	N2	M0
	T2b	N2	M0
	T3	N0	M0
	T3	N1	M0
	T3	N2	M0
IVA	T4	N0	M0
	T4	N1	M0
	T4	N2	M0
IVB	Any T	N3	M0
IVC	Any T	Any N	M1

*Parapharynged extension denotes posterolateral infiltration of tumor beyond the pharyngobasilar fascia.
**Midline nodes are considered ipsilateral nodes.
Modified from Close LG, Larson DL, Shah JP. *Essentials of head and neck oncology*. New York: Thieme Medical Publishers, Inc., 1998.

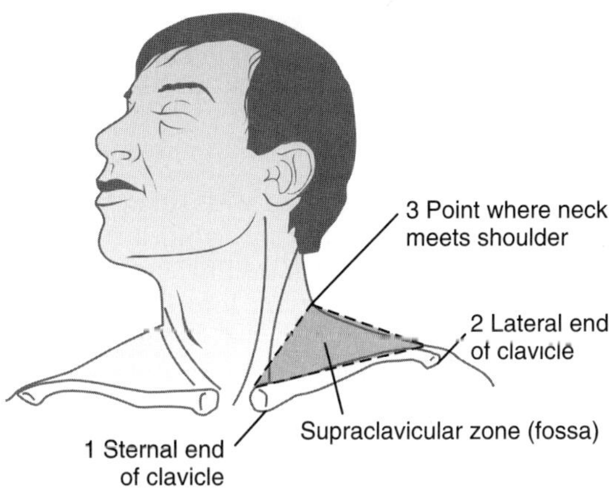

Figure 21-12. The supraclavicular fossa as defined by Ho. (From Greene FL, Page DL, Fleming ID, *et al. AJCC cancer staging handbook*, 6th ed. New York: American Joint Commission on Cancer, 2002. Figure 4.2.)

lingual surface of the epiglottis. Lymphatic spread is usually to the upper and mid-jugular nodes. Midline lesions have a higher propensity for bilateral spread. Nodal staging is the same as for the oral cavity.

Treatment

As there are for oral cavity cancer, there are several options for treatment. Both surgery and radiation therapy are equally effective for early lesions. Large resections can lead to functional deficits, and they require complicated reconstruction. If small lesions can be removed with surgery, it can leave radiation available for recurrence or any second primaries.

SCCa of the BOT usually presents in late stages. Multimodality therapy is the norm. The mainstay of therapy has been surgical resection followed by radiation or vice versa. Large tumors often involve the deep tongue musculature and the neurovascular pedicles to the tongue, thereby necessitating wide resection (i.e., the tumor and an additional 1.5- to 2-cm margin of normal tissue). A total glossectomy may require a concomitant total laryngectomy, because, without the tongue, a patient can no longer protect the airway. This leads to uncontrolled aspiration and chronic lung problems. Up to 80% of patients have neck involvement, and a quarter of these have bilateral disease. Neck dissection is indicated for anything larger than a T1 tumor.

Surgical approaches include many of those seen for the oral cavity: peroral, cheek flap, and mandibulotomy/mandibular swing. Others include the midline tongue split (Figure 21-13), the transhyoid (Figure 21-14), and the transcervical pharyngotomy. Small tongue base and posterior pharyngeal wall tumors can be removed using endoscopic techniques with a CO_2 laser. Various degrees of mandibulectomy may also be indicated if the bone is involved.

Several radiation therapy schemes can be used; preoperative and postoperative are the most common. Radiation alone is used for patients with unresectable disease and for those who cannot tolerate a large resection or the morbidity of chemotherapy. Deep infiltration of bone decreases the success of radiation. Brachytherapy, or the placement of radioactive seeds directly into the tumor bed, gives extra boosts of radiation in a very localized area and spares surrounding structures.

In more recent years, later-stage disease has been treated with chemoradiation regimens: either neoadjuvant chemotherapy followed by radiation or concurrent chemotherapy and radiation. In the former scheme, if there is no or limited response after two courses of chemotherapy, then this may predict a poor response to radiation, and the patient should undergo surgical resection. In the concurrent chemotherapy and radiation scheme, large tumors that may not be susceptible to radiation alone are thought to be sensitized to the radiation, thereby increasing the likelihood of a favorable response. This is often called *organ preservation therapy,* and the hope is to avoid debilitating surgery.

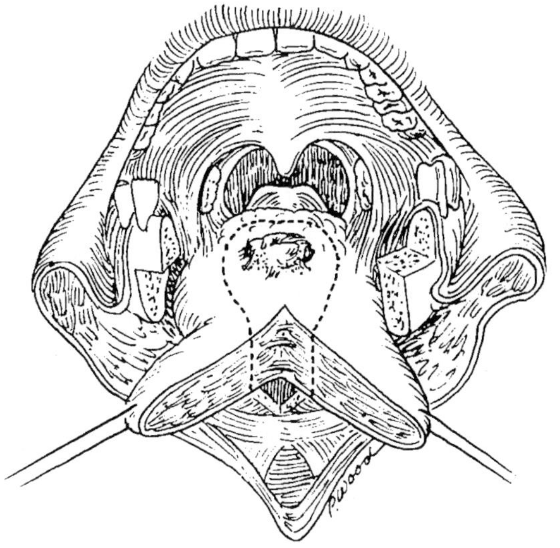

Figure 21-13. For midline base-of-the-tongue lesions, the anterior midline glossotomy approach may be indicated. (From Cummings CW, Fredrickson JM, Harker LA, *et al. Otolaryngology head and neck surgery,* 3rd ed. St. Louis: Mosby, 1998. Figure 78-52.)

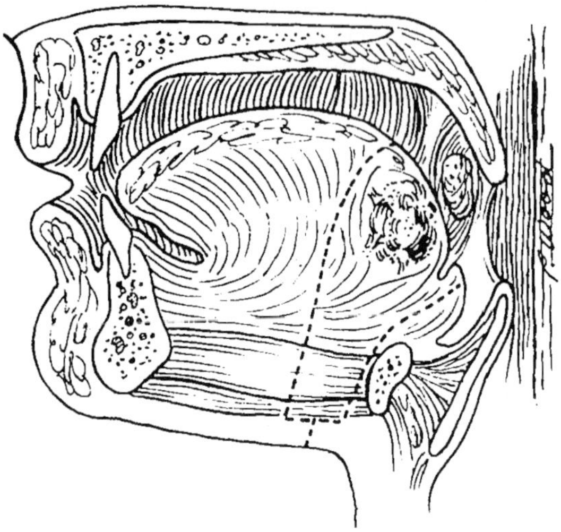

Figure 21–14. The transhyoid or suprahyoid approach allows for access of the tongue from the neck area. (From Cummings CW, Fredrickson JM, Harker LA, *et al. Otolaryngology head and neck surgery,* 3rd ed. St. Louis: Mosby, 1998. Figure 78-54.)

Chemotherapy is not curative when it is used alone. It is used for the palliation of those with unresectable tumors who have already had their full dose of radiation.

Tonsil

Many of the principles of BOT treatment also apply to other areas of the oropharynx. Tonsillar SCCa is thought to be more responsive to radiation, especially when it involves undifferentiated tumors or lymphoepithelioma. Tumors can spread to the BOT, the palate, the pharyngeal wall, and the larynx. Small tumors respond equally well to surgery and radiation. They can be removed perorally by way of a radical tonsillectomy. Larger tumors have been treated with combined-modality therapy, with surgery and preoperative or postoperative radiation. Chemoradiation protocols for organ preservation are gaining in popularity.

Soft Palate

Early lesions can be treated with surgery or radiation. Large resections create significant morbidity with velopharyngeal insufficiency (i.e., the opening of the oropharynx into the nasopharynx, thus causing the reflux of air and liquids/food during swallow and speech). Oropharyngeal obturators decrease this problem.

Hypopharyngeal Carcinoma

Anatomy

The cone-shaped hypopharynx extends from the hyoid bone inferiorly to the lower border of the cricoid cartilage. It is separated into regions called the piriform (pyriform) sinuses, the posterior wall, and the postcricoid mucosa. The piriform sinuses are at the lateral aspects of the hypopharynx, from the pharyngoepiglottic ligament tapering to an apex that is roughly at the level of the true vocal folds. Medially they are closely associated with the aryepiglottic folds and the arytenoid cartilages of the larynx. The postcricoid area contains the mucosa from the posterior surfaces of the arytenoids cartilages and the intervening space, and it extends inferiorly to the inferior edge of the cricoid. The posterior wall lies between the piriform sinuses, overlying the prevertebral fascia. The cervical esophagus starts at the inferior edge of the cricoid and is involved when tumor extends inferiorly past the borders of the hypopharynx.

Staging

Table 21-8 outlines the staging of hypopharyngeal carcinomas. A rich lymphatic plexus

TABLE 21–8 • *T Staging of Hypopharyngeal Carcinoma*

TX	Primary tumor cannot be assessed
T0	No evidence of primary tumor
Tis	Carcinoma in situ
T1	Tumor limited to one subsite of hypopharynx and 2 cm or less in greatest dimension
T2	Tumor invades more than one subsite of hypopharynx or an adjacent site or measures more than 2 cm but not more than 4 cm in greatest diameter without fixation of hemilarynx
T3	Tumor more than 4 cm in greatest dimension or with fixation of hemilarynx
T4a	Tumor invades thyroid/cricoid cartilage, hyoid bone, thyroid gland, esophagus, or central compartment soft tissue*
T4b	Tumor invades prevertebral fascia, encases carotid artery, or involves mediastinal structures

*Central compartment soft tissue includes prelaryngeal strap muscles.

leads to early spread to the neck nodes and a high incidence of bilateral involvement. Nodal staging is consistent with the oral cavity and the oropharynx.

Treatment

These tumors present at late stages with extensive local disease and nodal spread. The proximity to the larynx often requires that it is included in the treatment. SCCa has a tendency to spread in the submucosal plane, so wide margins are needed to increase the risk of success. Inferior spread leads to the involvement of the cervical esophagus. Sometimes the inferior extent cannot be safely evaluated with endoscopy. Barium esophagram can be used to assess the inferior extent.

Multimodality therapy is usually used. Radiation with or without chemotherapy can be used as neoadjuvant treatment. In this setting, surgery is reserved for salvage after treatment failure. Surgery with preoperative-or postoperative radiation is the norm, with increasing use of chemotherapy for larger tumors in organ-preservation protocols. To achieve adequate margins, portions or all of the laryngeal structures may need to be addressed.

Partial pharyngectomy. This approach is suited for early, superficial lesions. Posterior-wall tumors are usually exophytic, and they infiltrate the prevertebral fascia late. Before excision is started, the surgeon must assess mobility of the tumor on the prevertebral fascia. Fixation precludes a successful resection. Early tumors can be reached using endoscopic techniques and excised with the CO_2 laser or transcervically with a transhyoid or lateral pharyngotomy approach. Piriform sinus tumors are more difficult to remove this way as a result of submucosal spread.

An *extended supraglottic laryngectomy* allows for a partial pharyngectomy and removal of an affected supraglottic larynx. The portion of the larynx that is removed is the epiglottis, the ipsilateral aryepiglottic (AE) fold, the false vocal fold, and the upper half of the thyroid cartilage. This is not possible if the arytenoid, the true vocal fold, or the paraglottic space are involved in tumor. This procedure is best for small- to moderate-sized masses of the piriform sinus.

The *total laryngectomy with partial pharyngectomy* is probably the most used procedure. Involvement of the larynx is usually extensive enough (to the true vocal fold, the paraglottic space, and the arytenoids) to make preservation impossible. If too much is taken, the remaining portion may not be functional, leaving the patient dependent on feeding and tracheostomy tubes and unable to form a voice. A total laryngectomy is generally more desirable than this. The pharyngeal defect should be able to be closed primarily. Tumors involving the postcricoid region or the apex of the piriform sinus are indications for total laryngectomy.

If the pharyngeal tumor is circumferential or the remnant is too small to close primarily, then a *total laryngopharyngectomy* is needed. Extension to the cervical esophagus requires inferior margins of 4 cm as a result of submucosal spread. If an adequate margin inferiorly is not attainable, the patient will require a *total laryngopharyngoesophagectomy.*

Concurrent neck dissections are performed as needed (i.e., RND versus MRND for known neck metastases). Necks staged as N0 have a high likelihood of occult disease and should be treated with elective neck dissection or with external-beam radiation. Level I is rarely involved and can be retained if an elective neck dissection is performed (posterolateral neck dissection).

Reconstruction

Small defects can be closed primarily. Those created with endoscopic resection can be left to be closed by secondary intention, as long as the neck is not entered, which can then cause a pharyngocutaneous fistula. Other partial pharyngectomies coupled with partial or total laryngectomies can be closed primarily. If the mucosal remnant is too small, primary closure may cause pharyngeal stenosis. The pharynx can then be reconstructed with a PMC flap, with the lateral edges of the skin sewn to the mucosal edges. The upper end of the skin is then sewn to the upper pharyngeal remnant, and the inferior edge is sewn to the lower remnant.

Total pharyngectomy defects are more complicated. A new conduit must be placed that will allow food to move from the pharynx into the esophagus. The PMC flap can be used in the same fashion except that the exposed prevertebral fascia needs a split-thickness skin graft cover (Figure 21-15). The lateral skin edges of the flap must be sewn to the fascia. A radial forearm free flap can be rolled into a tube and placed into the defect; a free jejunal graft can also be used. A separate laparotomy must be made for harvest, and the re-anastomosis of the gut is another area of concern during the postoperative period. After the total laryngopharyngoesophagectomy, a gastric pull-up is the mode of reconstruction that is most preferred.

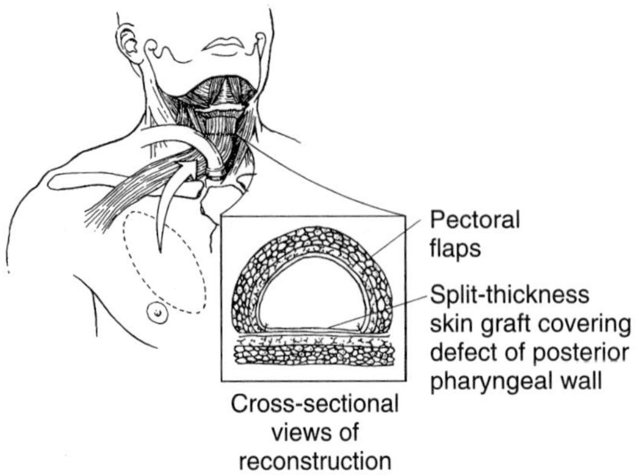

Figure 21–15. Pectoralis myocutaneous flap reconstruction after total laryngopharyngectomy. (From Close LG, Larson DL, Shah JP. *Essentials of head and neck oncology*. New York: Thieme Medical Publishers, Inc., 1998. Figure 20-2.)

Cancer of the Larynx

The larynx is a complex structure made up of a cartilage and membranous framework with muscular attachments covered by mucosa. These structures provide pathways that lead to predictable patterns of spread of carcinoma. This subject is beyond the scope of this work, but more in-depth reading is available. The functions of the larynx are to provide an inlet to the trachea, to protect the airway from foreign matter, and to form a voice. Tumors in this sensitive area and/or their treatment cause disruption of all of these functions.

Anatomy

The larynx is divided into three main regions: the supraglottis, the glottis/true vocal folds (cords), and the subglottis. The supraglottis contains the epiglottis, the AE folds, the arytenoids, and the false vocal folds. The ventricle is the mucosa-lined "pocket" between the false and true vocal folds. The border between the glottis and the supraglottis is the reflection of the ventricle onto the upper surface of the true vocal fold. The glottis extends from the ventricle, it contains the upper and lower surfaces of the true fold, and it ends at a line 1-cm inferior to the free edge of the fold. The subglottis extends from this line to the inferior border of the cricoid cartilage.

The main cartilages of the larynx are the epiglottis, the thyroid cartilage, the cricoid cartilage, and the arytenoids. The hyoid bone is an integral component that is attached to the larynx by the strap muscles and the thyrohyoid membrane (Figure 21-16). Another membrane is the quadrangular membrane, which stretches from the free edge of the epiglottis to the arytenoid cartilages. The upper edge of this membrane forms the AE folds, and the lower edge forms the false vocal folds. The conus elasticus is a condensation of fibrous tissue from the upper border of the cricoid to the arytenoids and the thyroid cartilage. The free edge of this membrane forms the true vocal folds (Figure 21-17). Various adductor and abductor muscles attach to the thyroid and cricoid cartilages and to the arytenoids to provide the movements to open and close the airway and to produce vocalization.

Two spaces within the larynx are the pre-epiglottic space and the paraglottic space. The pre-epiglottic space is filled with fat and is bounded by the epiglottic cartilage posteriorly and anteriorly by the thyroid cartilage and the thyrohyoid membrane. The paraglottic space is inside the thyroid cartilage, the cricothyroid membrane, and the cricoid cartilage. The inner boundary is the quadrangular membrane superiorly, the ventricular mucosa, and the conus elasticus inferiorly; it contains the muscles of the true vocal fold.

Lymphatic drainage is dependent on the region of the larynx. Cancers of the supraglottis spread to the upper and mid-jugular nodes first. The subglottic primary is rare, and direct extension from neighboring regions is more common. The lymphatics flow to the paratracheal, pretracheal, paralaryngeal, and prela-

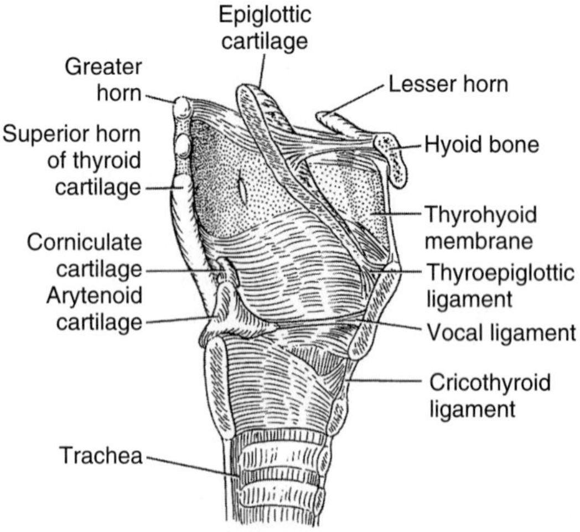

Figure 21–16. Sagittal section of the larynx. (From Cummings CW, Fredrickson JM, Harker LA, *et al. Otolaryngology head and neck surgery,* 3rd ed. st. Louis: Mosby, 1998. Figure 97-3.)

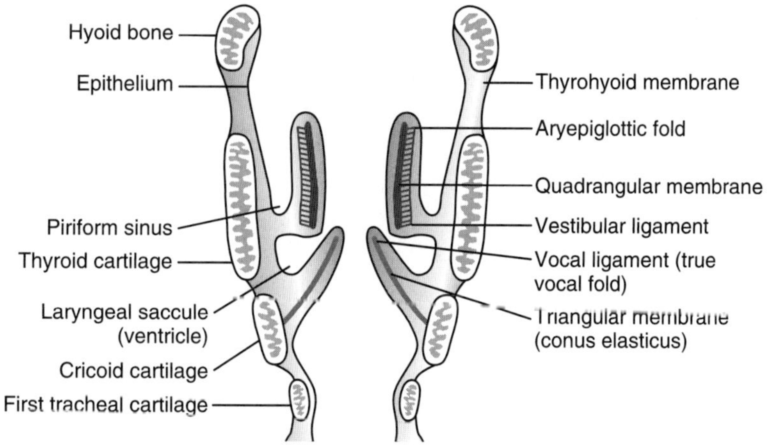

Figure 21-17. Coronal diagram of the larynx. (From Cummings CW, Fredrickson JM, Harker LA, *et al. Otolaryngology head and neck surgery,* 3rd ed. St. Louis: Mosby, 1998. Figure 97-6.)

ryngeal (Delphian) nodes; these groups make up level VI. The glottis is nearly free of lymphatics, and nodal spread is rare. As cancers spread from the glottis to adjacent areas, nodal metastases are more common.

Staging

Table 21-9 outlines the staging of laryngeal cancer.

Treatment

During the evaluation of the patient before treatment, it is imperative to assess the stability of the airway. Tumor bulk or fixation of the vocal folds can compromise breathing. Many patients present with stridor, but patients in distress must have the airway secured. The use of tracheostomy is somewhat controversial, because many feel that it increases the risk of stomal recurrence after treatment. If a surgical airway is needed, it is placed high so as to put it into the surgical field to be excised with the primary. Treatment should then begin within 3 days. Another option would be to do an emergent laryngectomy if that is to be the treatment of choice for the primary.

As with other areas of the aerodigestive tract, early lesions are equally amenable to surgery and radiation. Carcinoma in situ is removed endoscopically with microlaryngeal instruments. The boundaries of the lesions are difficult to identify, and patients must be brought back at regular intervals (3 months) for re-evaluation in the operating room and biopsy and re-excision until no more carcinoma in situ can be found.

Surgery for small T1 lesions of the glottis can include endoscopic laser resection or laryngofissure with cordectomy (Figure 21-18). By definition, there can be no invasion of the paraglottic space or vocal fold fixation. The main disadvantage is the poor voice result. The voice returns after several months, when scar fills the defect and the other vocal fold can vibrate against it. The main advantage is the reservation of radiation therapy for recurrence or later primaries.

Partial laryngectomies are reserved for larger T1 and some T2 and T3 lesions; they are performed in conjunction with a tracheostomy. The *vertical partial laryngectomy* entails thyrotomy and excision of the ipsilateral thyroid cartilage ala, the true vocal fold, the paraglottic space, and the false vocal fold (Figure 21-19). If the anterior commissure must be taken, the contralateral thyroid ala is entered, and the anterior aspect is removed with the specimen; this is called the *frontolateral partial laryngectomy* (Figure 21-20, *A*). If the arytenoid mucosa is involved, it can also be removed with the arytenoid cartilage (Figure 21-20, *B*). This requires reconstruction with cartilage, mucosal, or strap muscle flaps to aid in swallowing and in the prevention of aspiration. If the cricoarytenoid joint is involved, a total laryngectomy is performed. Some T3 carcinomas can also be resected using these techniques, if chosen wisely.

Supraglottic carcinoma staged at T1 and T2 may be amenable to a *supraglottic/horizontal laryngectomy* (Figure 21-21). A transverse thyrotomy on the ipsilateral side is made just above the level of the true vocal folds; this is estimated to be halfway between the thyroid notch and the lower border of the thyroid cartilage. The true vocal fold must be avoided. The thyrotomy is continued onto the contralateral side, angling superiorly from the midline to

TABLE 21–9 • *T Staging of Laryngeal Cancer*

Primary Tumor (T)	
TX	Primary tumor cannot be assessed
T0	No evidence of primary tumor
Tis	Carcinoma in situ
Supraglottis	
T1	Tumor limited to one subsite of supraglottis, with normal vocal cord mobility
T2	Tumor invades mucosa of more than one adjacent subsite of supraglottis or glottis or region outside of the supraglottis (e.g., mucosa of base of tongue, vallecula, medial wall of pyriform sinus) without fixation of the larynx
T3	Tumor limited to larynx with vocal cord fixation and/or invades any of the following: postcricoid area, pre-epiglottic tissues, paraglottic space, and/or minor thyroid cartilage erosion (e.g., inner cortex)
T4a	Tumor invades through the thyroid cartilage and/or invades tissues beyond the larynx (e.g., trachea, soft tissues of neck including deep extrinsic muscle of the tongue, strap muscles, thyroid, or esophagus)
T4b	Tumor invades prevertebral space, encases carotid artery, or invades mediastinal structures
Glottis	
T1	Tumor limited to the vocal cord(s) (may involve anterior or posterior commissure), with normal mobility
T1a	Tumor limited to one vocal cord
T1b	Tumor involves both vocal cords
T2	Tumor extends to supraglottis and/or subglottis and/or with impaired vocal cord mobility
T3	Tumor limited to the larynx with vocal cord fixation and/or invades paraglottic space and/or minor thyroid cartilage erosion (e.g., inner cortex)
T4a	Tumor invades through the thyroid cartilage and/or invades tissues beyond the larynx (e.g., trachea, soft tissues of neck including deep extrinsic muscle of the tongue, strap muscles, thyroid, or esophagus)
T4b	Tumor invades prevertebral space, encases carotid artery, or invades mediastinal structures
Subglottis	
T1	Tumor limited to the subglottis
T2	Tumor extends to vocal cord(s) with normal or impaired mobility
T3	Tumor limited to larynx, with vocal cord fixation
T4a	Tumor invades cricoid or thyroid cartilage and/or invades tissues beyond the larynx (e.g., trachea, soft tissues of neck including deep extrinsic muscles of the tongue, strap muscles, thyroid, or esophagus)
T4b	Tumor invades prevertebral space, encases carotid artery, or invades mediastinal structures

the superior cornu of the thyroid cartilage. Calcified cartilages will require a sagittal saw for the thyrotomies. The pharynx is then entered in the vallecula, and the tip of the epiglottis is grasped and retracted out of the wound. Now, with a headlight, the surgeon must look directly at the tumor and guide the cuts to remove the tumor with adequate margin but leave all needed mucosa to aid in healing. The epiglottis, the false vocal fold, the AE fold, the hyoid bone, and pre-epiglottic space are taken; the true vocal fold and the arytenoid are left. Any arytenoid fixation or paraglottic involvement precludes this as a viable procedure. The remaining thyroid cartilage is suspended from the BOT to aid in swallow rehabilitation. Postoperative assessment and treatment by trained speech pathologists is crucial.

The *supracricoid laryngectomy* is a procedure that is indicated in some T2 and T3 lesions of the supraglottis or glottis. It involves the removal of the supraglottic larynx with the vocal folds and the thyroid cartilage. One or both arytenoids must be left, along with the cricoid cartilage and the hyoid bone. The crux of the procedure is the suspension of the cricoid from the hyoid bone, also called the *cricohyoidopexy*. If the lesion is of the glottis,

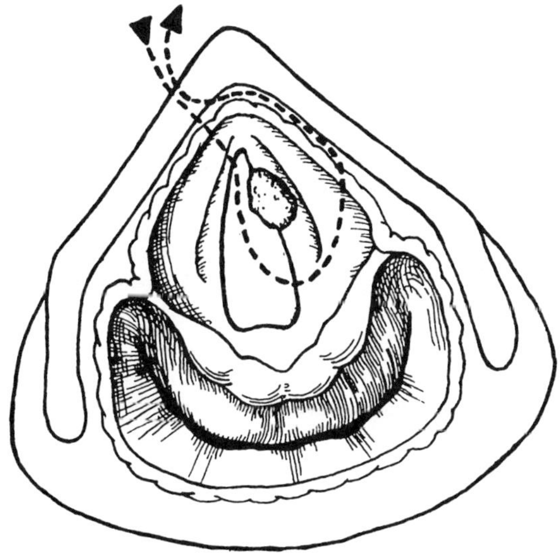

Figure 21–18. Laryngofissure and cordectomy. (From Close LG, Larson DL, Shah JP. *Essentials of head and neck oncology*. New York: Thieme Medical Publishers, Inc., 1998. Figure 21-5.)

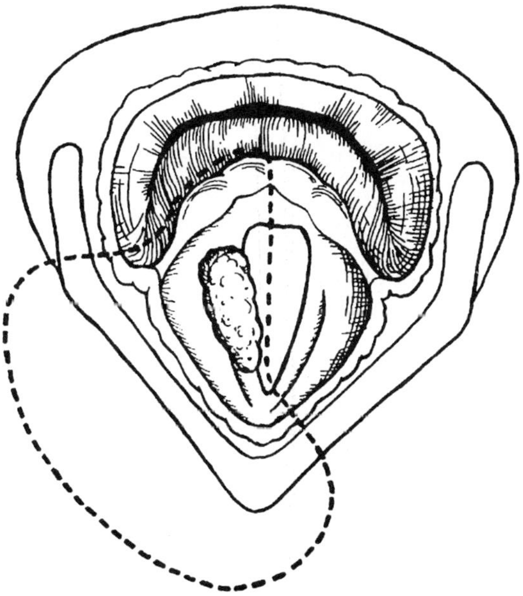

Figure 21–19. Vertical hemilaryngectomy. (From Close LG, Larson DL, Shah JP. *Essentials of head and neck oncology*. New York: Thieme Medical Publishers, Inc., 1998. Figure 21-6.)

the epiglottis can be left, and the suspension is called a *cricohyoidoepiglottopexy*. Contraindications are the involvement of the subglottis, the arytenoids, the cricoid cartilage, the cricoarytenoid joints, the hyoid bone, or the surrounding pharynx. Once again, extensive speech and swallowing rehabilitation is needed. Some patients may not be able to regain any function of the larynx.

The *total laryngectomy* entails the removal of the entire larynx and the formation of a permanent tracheostoma. Exposure is from the hyoid bone to the sternal notch, and it is indicated for most T3 and T4 lesions. The strap muscles are left attached anteriorly; they are then excised from their sternal attachments. The thyroid isthmus is incised and ligated. The ipsilateral thyroid lobe is removed with the larynx if there is cartilage invasion or subglottic extension. The parathyroid glands are

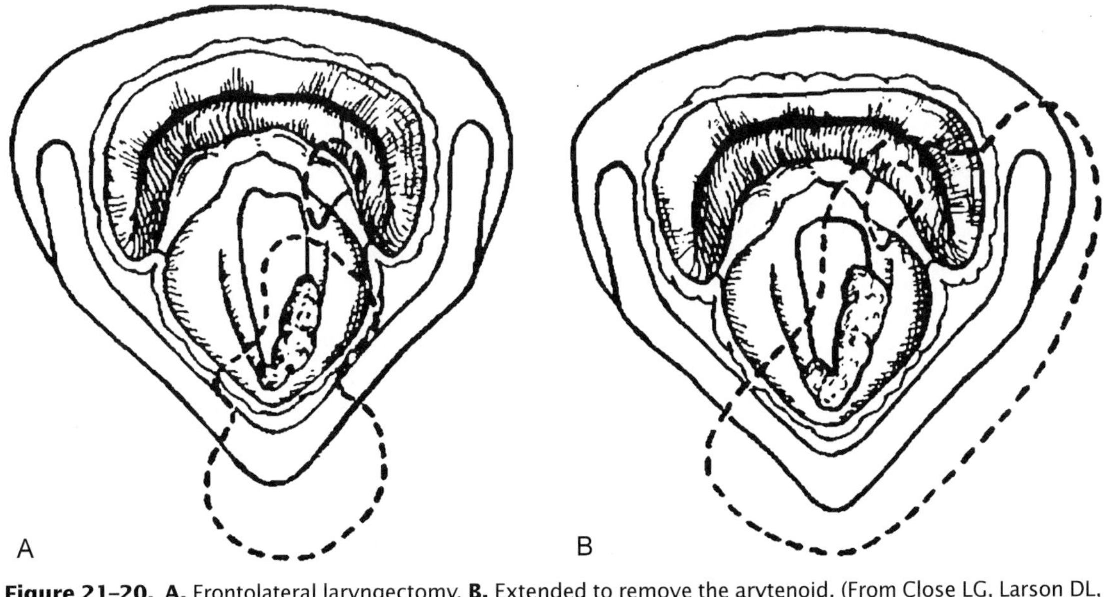

Figure 21–20. A, Frontolateral laryngectomy. **B,** Extended to remove the arytenoid. (From Close LG, Larson DL, Shah JP. *Essentials of head and neck oncology*. New York: Thieme Medical Publishers, Inc., 1998. Figure 21-7.)

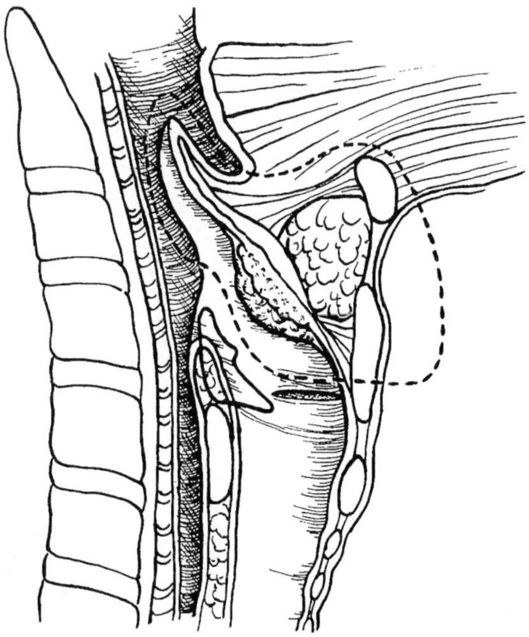

Figure 21–21. Supraglottic laryngectomy. (From Close LG, Larson DL, Shah JP. *Essentials of head and neck oncology*. New York: Thieme Medical Publishers, Inc., 1998. Figure 21-9.)

located and preserved along with their vasculature. The suprahyoid muscles are removed from the hyoid bone. The resection must stay directly on the bone to avoid the hypoglossal nerves. Bilateral carotid sheathes are dissected away from the central compartment (neck-dissection specimens can be left attached at the thyrohyoid membrane). The inferior constrictor muscles are now incised at the posterior border of each side of the thyroid cartilage. Next, the tracheal incision is made at about the third or fourth ring, depending on the subglottic extent. The posterior tracheal wall is incised, with care taken to not to enter the esophagus. The plane between the trachea and the esophagus is followed superiorly until the arytenoids are reached. Thus, the boundaries of the resection have been defined.

The pharynx is now entered either at the vallecula or the piriform. At this point, the surgeon can look into the larynx with a headlight and guide the rest of the resection. As much mucosa as possible is left without sacrificing oncologic principles. The incisions are brought down along the medial piriform sinuses, and they are connected with the inferior incisions in the postcricoid area. If this area is involved with tumor, then the excision must be tailored appropriately. The specimen can then be removed.

A cricopharyngeal myotomy or a pharyngeal neurectomy is now performed to aid in postoperative healing. If a primary tracheoesophageal puncture is planned, it is performed now. This will allow for the placement of a speech prosthesis after healing that will allow the patient to vocalize as air is forced into the pharynx through a one-way valve. The pharyngeal defect is closed primarily or reconstructed as described earlier.

As with other head and neck SCCa, radiation is also frequently used. Early cancers have a good chance of being cured. Later lesions are treated neoadjuvantly, and surgery can then be used for salvage. Most late lesions will require multimodality therapy.

The larynx has been the subject of several large studies evaluating chemoradiation for organ preservation. The survival is nearly equal, but many undergoing the chemoradiation regimen are able to keep their larynges. The functional outcome is in question, and not much is known about how many of these patients have functional larynges or how many are tracheostomy- and/or feeding-tube dependent and unable to phonate.

Outcome

Stage I and II tumors have excellent control rates. Stage I survival is greater than 90%, and stage II survival is greater than 75%. Stage III disease reduces survival to 60%, and stage IV reduces it to 40% to 50%. The presence of nodal spread reduces survival by 50%.

Cancer of the Major Salivary Glands

There are three sets of major salivary glands: the parotid glands, the submandibular glands, (SMG), and the sublingual glands. There are also 600 to 800 minor salivary glands throughout the mucosal lining of the upper aerodigestive tract. These are treated like other cancers of the specific region, and they are staged and treated according to the region in which they arise. The differential diagnosis of salivary gland tumors is large and contains both benign and malignant tumors. The larger the gland, the more likely the mass is benign: roughly 80% of parotid tumors, 50% of SMG tumors, and 20% of sublingual tumors (rare) are benign.

BOX 21-11 PAROTID TUMORS

Benign
- Pleomorphic adenoma (benign pleomorphic adenoma)
- Warthin's tumor
- Monomorphic adenoma
- Oncocytoma

Malignant
- Mucoepidermoid carcinoma
- Carcinoma ex-pleomorphic adenoma
- Acinic-cell carcinoma
- Adenocarcinoma
- Adenoid cystic carcinoma
- Metastasis to intraparotid node
- Squamous cell carcinoma

The benign pleomorphic adenoma or the benign mixed tumor is the most common salivary gland neoplasm. There is a real risk of untreated benign pleomorphic adenomas degenerating into a carcinoma ex-pleomorphic adenoma, which is a high-grade malignancy. Warthin's tumor can be bilateral or multifocal.

The most common malignant tumor is the mucoepidermoid carcinoma. These are graded histologically into low, intermediate, and high grades. Adenoid cystic carcinoma is an indolent malignancy that has a propensity for neural invasion; this increases the risk of local recurrence, which can occur after many years. It usually spreads to the lungs. Acinic-cell carcinoma can be bilateral. One must always rule out that the parotid malignancy is not a metastasis to an intraparotid lymph node from another primary, usually a skin cancer (i.e., SCCa or melanoma).

Workup

The evaluation of the patient with a parotid or SMG mass requires an examination of all major salivary glands, the ipsilateral facial nerve, the lingual nerve (SMG), and the ipsilateral neck. A deep lobe tumor may cause oropharyngeal asymmetry or bulging of the tonsil and deviation of the uvula to the contralateral side. Deep invasion can cause trismus and suggests a poor prognosis. The mainstay of imaging is the CT scan. Ultrasound can be helpful, and it can be used to guide the needle in an FNA biopsy. Deep invasion can be evaluated with an MRI.

BOX 21-12 SUBMANDIBULAR TUMORS

Benign
- Pleomorphic adenoma
- Oncocytoma

Malignant
- Adenoid cystic carcinoma
- Mucoepidermoid carcinoma
- Adenocarcinoma
- Acinic-cell carcinoma

Treatment

The decision must be made whether to perform a superficial or total parotidectomy. The parotid gland is artificially divided into a superficial lobe and a deep lobe by the course of the facial nerve. The excision of benign and most low-grade malignant tumors is dependent on the location of the mass within the parotid. A CT scan can show if the mass is intraparotid or adjacent to it and, if it is within the parenchyma of the gland, the lobe in which it is in. Masses in the superficial lobe can be excised with a superficial parotidectomy with facial nerve dissection and preservation. Deep-lobe lesions require total parotidectomy with facial nerve preservation. New advances in nerve monitoring help in the identification and preservation of the nerve.

The parotidectomy incision is made in the preauricular crease and curved into the neck (Figure 21-22, *A*). The skin and the subcutaneous fat are then raised off of the parotid fascia. The creation of the skin flap is stopped at the anterior extent of the parotid to avoid the separate branches of the facial nerve as they exit the gland. The anterior border of the SCM is found in the neck, and the tail of the parotid is removed from it. A deeper dissection locates the posterior belly of the digastric muscle; this is at about the level of the depth of the facial nerve as it exits the stylomastoid foramen. Next, the parotid gland is dissected from the auricular cartilage in a wide plane in a superficial-to-deep direction. As the depth of the nerve is reached, great care is taken to get meticulous hemostasis and to not create a confining "hole" with minimized exposure (Figure 21-22, *B*). The main nerve trunk is then located by using several landmarks. Its identification is confirmed with a nerve stimulator.

The trunk of the nerve is then followed to the *pes anserinus*, the area where it separates

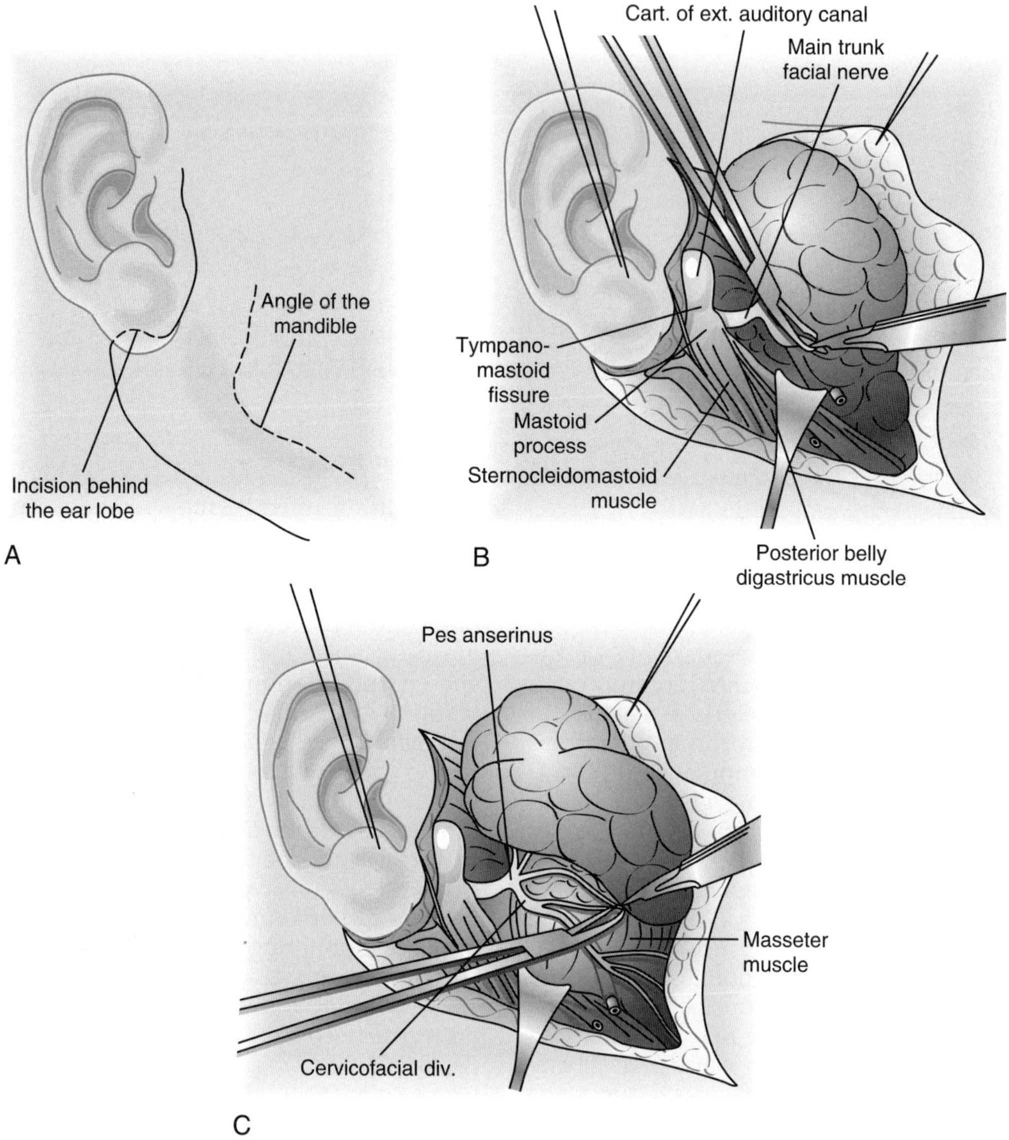

Figure 21-22. A, Incision for a parotidectomy. **B,** The main trunk of the facial nerve is found deep to the tympanomastoid suture line. **C,** Each branch is dissected, and the intervening parenchyma is excised. The gland is being retracted superiorly here. (From Lore JM, Medina JE. *An atlas of head and neck surgery,* 4th ed. New York: Elsevier, 2005. Figure 17-1.)

into the five main branches. The branches are then each followed out to the distal margin of the gland in successive order. The gland parenchyma between the branches is incised, and the specimen is retracted superiorly or inferiorly (Figure 21-22, *C*). Care is taken to not violate the capsule of the mass. Tumor seeding may increase the chance of multifocal recurrence, which is difficult to treat.

Deep-lobe masses are carefully dissected from deep to the nerve branches off of the masseter muscle. Risk to the nerve is increased with these tumors. An active drain is placed, and the skin is meticulously closed.

High-grade or late-stage tumors of the parotid require more extensive resections. A cuff of normal tissue is needed for a margin. Skin and masseter muscle are commonly excised. If the facial nerve is intact, the fate of the nerve is somewhat controversial. Some would remove the nerve if it comes in contact with the cancer, whereas others would leave the nerve and rely on postoperative radiation to eradicate any residual microscopic disease.

BOX 21-13 ANATOMIC LANDMARKS FOR FACIAL NERVE IDENTIFICATION

- Tragal pointer (nerve is approxi mately 1-cm medial and ante roinferior to the tip of the pointer)
- Tympanomastoid suture (nerve is approximately 6-mm to 8-mm medial to suture)
- Digastric muscle attachment to digastric groove (nerve just superior to and on same plane as muscle attachment)
- Nerve within mastoid bone
- Retrograde dissection from distal nerve branch

From Eisele, Table 22-2.

This latter approach is justified by the high morbidity of a dense total facial palsy (i.e., oral incompetence, nasal obstruction, xerophthalmia, severe cosmetic deformity).

High-grade tumors also require a neck dissection. Overtly positive necks must receive an RND or an MRND. If the necks appear negative, then an SND may be substituted (supraomohyoid heck dissection and arterolateral neck dissection). Low-grade tumors rarely metastasize, but vigilance is needed.

Benign and low-grade SMG tumors can be removed with simple SMG excision. High-grade tumors need excision of the contents of the submandibular triangle with or without excision of the hypoglossal and lingual nerves, as appropriate for oncologic resection.

Radiation is used for high-grade malignancies, for recurrent tumors, and for neck involvement, usually postoperatively.

Complications

There are a number of complications that are unique to parotid or SMG surgery (Table 21-10). Facial nerve injury as a result of nerve traction is usually transient, unless the branches are severed. A thin facial skin flap increases the risk of flap necrosis. Sialoceles and salivary fistulas are caused by remnants of viable salivary tissue. Saliva is secreted into the wound. Repeat needle aspiration of fluid collections, compression dressings, and botulinum toxin injections may stop the drainage. Frey's syndrome or gustatory sweating is caused by reinnervation of the cutaneous sweat glands by the parasympathetic nerves that once innervated the parotid gland. Smelling, seeing, or tasting food can cause a profuse facial sweating from the area overlying the parotidectomy site. Diagnosis is by history or the Minor's starch-iodine test. Treatment is with topical antiperspirants, barriers placed under the skin flap (AlloDerm, fascia lata), or botulinum toxin injections.

TABLE 21-10 • *Early and Late Complications of Parotidectomy*

Early Complications	Late Complications
Facial nerve injury	Frey's syndrome
Hemorrhage, hematoma	Trismus
Infection	Amputation neuroma (greater auricular nerve)
External otitis	Tumor recurrence
Sialocele, seroma	Cosmetic deformity
Salivary fistula	Hypertrophic scar, keloid
Flap necrosis	Earlobe malposition, "crosshatch" scars

From Eisele, Table 22-1.

Key Reading

Close LG, Larson DL, Shah JP. *Essentials of head and neck oncology*. New York: Thieme Medical Publishers, Inc., 1998.

Selected Readings

Cummings CW, Fredrickson JM, Harker LA, *et al. Otolaryngology head and neck surgery,* 3rd ed. St. Louis: Mosby, 1998.

Lore JM, Medina JE. *An atlas of head and neck surgery,* 4th ed. New York: Elsevier, Inc., 2005.

Perez-Ordonez B, Beauchemin M, Jordon RCK. Molecular biology of squamous cell carcinoma of the head and neck. *J Clin Pathol* 2006;59:445–453.

Schwarz JK, Giese W. Organ preservation in patients with squamous cancers of the head and neck. *Surg Oncol Clin N Am* 2004;13:187–199.

Thawley SE, Panje WR, Batsakis JG, Lindberg RD. *Comprehensive management of head and neck tumors,* 2nd ed. Philadelphia: WB Saunders Company, 1999.

22

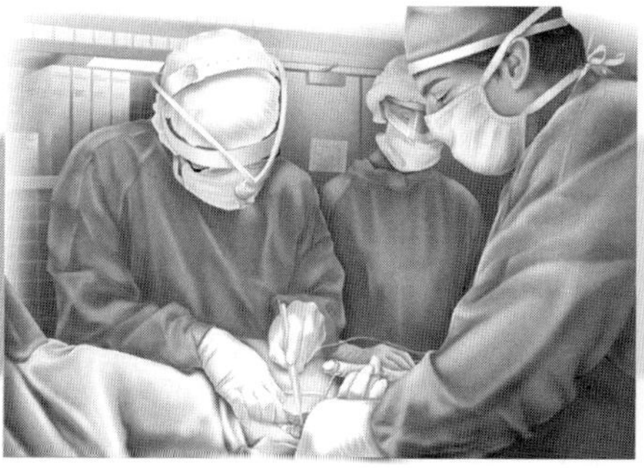

Leukemia and Lymphoma

Scott D. Gitlin

Leukemia and Lymphoma: Key Points

- Describe the presenting symptoms of acute leukemia and the diagnostic and staging tests required to identify the acute leukemias.
- Outline the treatment of patients with acute leukemia.
- Compare chronic lymphocytic and chronic myelogenous leukemia.
- Discuss the treatment of chronic myelogenous leukemia.
- Compare Hodgkin's disease and non-Hodgkin lymphoma.
- Discuss the evaluation process and treatment options for lymphoma.

Leukemias and lymphomas comprise a widely heterogeneous group of malignancies of the hematopoietic and lymphatic systems. The different leukemias and lymphomas have vastly different pathogenic, epidemiologic, diagnostic, staging, therapeutic, and prognostic characteristics. As a result of these differences, it is crucial to establish a histopathologic diagnosis at the time of presentation. Although there have been a variety of pathologic classification systems used over time, the World Health Organization (WHO) Classification of Tumours of Haematopoietic and Lymphoid Tissues is the system that is currently being used for leukemias and lymphomas (Table 22-1).

Leukemias

The leukemias consist of diseases that result from the dysregulated growth and proliferation of hematopoietic cells.

BOX 22–1 LEUKEMIA AND LYMPHOMA IN THE UNITED STATES IN 2006

Leukemia

- 35,070 new cases of leukemia
- Eighth most common form of new cancer diagnosis
- 22,280 deaths from leukemia
- Sixth most common cause of cancer deaths

Lymphoma

- 66,670 new cases of lymphoma
- Sixth most common form of new cancer diagnosis
- 20,330 deaths from lymphoma
- Seventh most common cause of cancer deaths

Acute Leukemias

Those diseases that arise from the malignant transformation of hematopoietic progenitor cells are known as *acute leukemias*. These diseases are characterized by the accumulation of blast cells that retain the ability of self-renewal but that have lost the potential for terminal differentiation. Pathologic evaluation allows for classifying the acute leukemias as either *acute myelocytic leukemia* (AML) or *acute lymphocytic leukemia* (ALL).

The incidence of AML increases with age. The median age at the time of diagnosis of AML is approximately 65 years. AML accounts for 80% of acute leukemia in adults but only 15% to 20% of acute leukemia in children. ALL typically occurs in a younger patient, with a peak incidence at the age of 3 to 5 years. Although a specific predisposing cause of a patient's acute leukemia is usually not identifiable, there are a number of genetic, environmental, and clinical factors associated with acute leukemia.

The clinical presentation of a patient with an acute leukemia is typically the result of the infiltration of leukemic blasts into the bone-marrow space and, occasionally, into other tissues. The replacement of the marrow space with leukemia results in bone marrow failure with cytopenias of one or more lineage of hematopoietic cell. As a result, patients can present with symptoms and signs of anemia, infection, and/or bleeding. When the leukemic blast count exceeds 50,000 per μL, there is a risk of stasis of blood flow in the cerebral and pulmonary vasculature. The risk of leukostasis depends on the size of the blasts (more common in AML than ALL due to larger blasts in AML), the blast count, and the type of leukemia. Symptoms and signs associated with leukostasis may include headache, change in mentation, neurologic dysfunction (e.g., visual disturbances), dyspnea at rest, and respiratory distress. Some patients with acute leukemia will develop coagulation defects, including disseminated intravascular coagulation (DIC) or primary fibrinolysis. The infiltration of leukemic cells into extramedullary organs and tissues may result in hepatomegaly, splenomegaly, lymphadenopathy, skin involvement, gingival hypertrophy, or leukemic meningitis. Solid masses of leukemic cells (called *chloromas*) may be seen in various extramedullary locations in patients with AML. Metabolic abnormalities may be present either before or after the initiation of therapy. These include hyperuricemia, tumor lysis syndrome, and renal and/or hepatic dysfunction.

BOX 22–2 SYMPTOMS ASSOCIATED WITH ACUTE LEUKEMIA

Symptoms Associated with Marrow Replacement

- Anemia
- Infection
- Bleeding

Symptoms Associated with Leukostasis

- Headache
- Mental status changes
- Changes in vision
- Neurologic dysfunction
- Dyspnea and respiratory distress

As a result of the progressive proliferation of leukemic cells and the presence of potentially life-threatening conditions, acute leukemias should be approached as medical emergencies. Patients typically should be admitted to the hospital to facilitate the diagnosis and initiation of therapy. In addition, intervention for significant clinical sequelae should be aggressively pursued.

The diagnosis of acute leukemia requires morphologic, immunohistopathologic, flow cytometric, and cytogenetic evaluations of the leukemic cells. The traditional French-American-British (FAB) classification system defines acute leukemia as being present when

TABLE 22–1 • *World Health Organization (WHO) Classification of Tumours of Haematopoietic and Lymphoid Tissues*

Acute Myeloid Leukemias (AMLs)
AML with recurrent cytogenetic abnormalities
AML with t(8;21)(q22;q22), (*AML1/ETO*)
AML with inv(16)(p13q22) or t(16;16)(p13;q22), (*CBFbeta/MYH11*)
AML with t(15;17)(q22;12), (*PML/RARalpha*) and variants
AML with 11q23 (*MLL*) abnormalities
AML with multilineage dysplasia
AML with prior myelodysplastic syndrome
AML without prior myelodysplastic syndrome
AML and myelodysplastic syndrome, therapy related
Alkylating-agent related
Topoisomerase-II–inhibitor related
AML not otherwise categorized
AML minimally differentiated
AML without maturation
AML with maturation
Acute myelomonocytic leukemia
Acute monoblastic and monocytic leukemia
Acute erythroid leukemia
Acute megakaryoblastic leukemia
Acute basophilic leukemia
Acute panmyelosis with myelofibrosis
Myeloid sarcoma
Acute leukemia of ambiguous lineage
Myelodysplastic Syndromes
Refractory anemia
Refractory anemia with ringed sideroblasts
Refractory anemia with excess blasts
Refractory cytopenia with multilineage dysplasia
Myelodysplastic syndrome associated with isolated del(5q) chromosome abnormality
Myelodysplastic syndrome, unclassifiable
Chronic Myeloproliferative Diseases
Chronic myelogenous leukemia with t(9;22)(q34;q11), (*BCR/ABL*)
Chronic neutrophilic leukemia
Chronic eosinophilic leukemia/hypereosinophilic syndrome
Polycythemia vera
Chronic idiopathic myelofibrosis
Essential thrombocythemia
Chronic myeloproliferative disease, unclassifiable
Myelodysplastic/Myeloproliferative Diseases
Chronic myelomonocytic leukemia
Atypical chronic myeloid leukemia
Juvenile myelomonocytic leukemia
Myelodysplastic/myeloproliferative diseases, unclassifiable

(Continued)

TABLE 22–1 • *World Health Organization (WHO) Classification of Tumours of Haematopoietic and Lymphoid Tissues*—Cont'd

B Cell Neoplasms
Precursor B cell neoplasm
Precursor B lymphoblastic lymphoma/leukemia
Mature B cell neoplasms
Chronic lymphocytic leukemia/small lymphocytic lymphoma
B cell prolymphocytic leukemia
Lymphoplasmacytic lymphoma
Splenic marginal zone lymphoma
Hairy-cell leukemia
Plasma-cell myeloma
Solitary plasmacytoma of bone
Extraosseous plasmacytoma
Primary amyloidoisis
Heavy chain disease
Extranodal marginal zone B cell lymphoma of mucosa-associated lymphoid tissue
Nodal marginal zone B cell lymphoma
Follicular lymphoma
Mantle cell lymphoma
Diffuse large B cell lymphoma
Mediastinal (thymic) large B cell lymphoma
Intravascular large B cell lymphoma
Primary effusion lymphoma
Burkitt's lymphoma/leukemia
B cell proliferations of uncertain malignant potential
Lymphomatoid granulomatosis
Post-transplant lymphoproliferative disorder, polymorphic
T Cell and Natural Killer (NK) Cell Neoplasms
Precursor T cell neoplasms
Precursor T lymphoblastic leukemia/lymphoma
Blastic NK cell lymphoma
Mature T cell and NK cell neoplasms
T cell prolymphocytic leukemia
T cell large granular lymphocytic leukemia
Aggressive NK cell leukemia
Adult T cell leukemia/lymphoma
Extranodal NK/T cell lymphoma, nasal type
Enteropathy-type T cell lymphoma
Hepatosplenic T cell lymphoma
Subcutaneous panniculitis-like T cell lymphoma
Mycosis fungoides
Sézary syndrome
Primary cutaneous anaplastic large-cell lymphoma
Peripheral T cell lymphoma, unspecified
Angioimmunoblastic T cell lymphoma
Anaplastic large-cell lymphoma
T cell proliferations of uncertain malignant potential
Lymphomatoid papulosis

TABLE 22-1 • *World Health Organization (WHO) Classification of Tumours of Haematopoietic and Lymphoid Tissues*

Hodgkin Lymphoma
Nodular lymphocyte predominant Hodgkin lymphoma
Classical Hodgkin lymphoma
Nodular sclerosis classical Hodgkin lymphoma
Lymphocyte-rich classical Hodgkin lymphoma
Mixed-cellularity classical Hodgkin lymphoma
Lymphocyte-depleted classical Hodgkin lymphoma
Histiocytic and Dendritic Cell Neoplasms
Macrophage/histiocytic neoplasm
Histiocytic sarcoma
Dendritic cell neoplasms
Langerhans cell histiocytosis
Langerhans cell sarcoma
Interdigitating dendritic cell sarcoma/tumor
Follicular dendritic-cell sarcoma/tumor
Dendritic cell sarcoma, not otherwise specified
Mastocytosis
Cutaneous mastocytosis
Indolent systemic mastocytosis
Systemic mastocytosis with associated clonal, hematological, non–mast-cell lineage disease
Aggressive systemic mastocytosis
Mast-cell leukemia
Mast-cell sarcoma
Extracutaneous mastocytoma

LGL, Large granular lymphocytic; *MDS,* myelodysplastic syndrome.

more than 30% of the nucleated cells in the peripheral blood or bone marrow aspirate are leukemic blasts. The WHO classification system proposes that a diagnosis of acute leukemia can be made when there are at least 20% blasts. A lumbar puncture to evaluate the cerebral spinal fluid for the presence of leukemic blasts by morphologic evaluation and flow cytometry or to evaluate for the presence of infection might be necessary. Occasionally an excisional biopsy of a chloroma or a core-needle biopsy of an infiltrated organ is necessary to confirm the presence of leukemia at that site. Punch skin biopsies are sometimes useful to differentiate leukemic skin involvement (i.e., leukemia cutis) from other causes of skin changes.

There are eight morphologic subtypes of AML and three morphologic subtypes of ALL, according to the French-American-British classification system (Table 22-2). Some of the acute leukemias have characteristic cytogenetic and molecular genetic abnormalities associated with them. These often play a useful role in diagnosis, classification, and the determining treatment. For example, the translocation t(15;17)(q22;q21) is found only in acute promyelocytic leukemia, and it is the result of a fusion of the *PML* gene on chromosome 15 with the retinoic acid receptor-α gene on chromosome 17. This leukemia can be treated with retinoic acid analogues and other agents that other AMLs cannot. Translocations t(8;14) and t(8;22) are found only in mature B cell ALL and Burkitt's lymphoma, and they result in dysregulation of the *c-myc* gene on chromosome 8. Other cytogenetic abnormalities provide prognostic information about the leukemia.

The initial management of patients with acute leukemia involves supportive measures, which may include red blood cell and/or platelet transfusions. Transfusions of blood products will be necessary throughout the management of a patient who is receiving potentially curative therapy for acute leukemia.

TABLE 22-2 • *French-American-British Classification of Acute Leukemias*

Acute Myelogenous Leukemia	
M0	Myeloblastic without cytologic maturation
M1	Myeloblastic with minimal cytologic maturation
M2	Myeloblastic with significant cytologic maturation
M3	Acute promyelocytic leukemia (usual form)
M3 variant	Acute promyelocytic leukemia, unusual hypogranular form
M4	Acute myelomonocytic leukemia
M4eo	M4 with eosinophilic maturation
M4baso	M4 with basophilic maturation
M5a	Acute monoblastic leukemia (poorly differentiated)
M5b	Acute monoblastic leukemia (more differentiated)
M6	Acute erythroid leukemia
M7	Acute megakaryoblastic leukemia
Acute Lymphocytic Leukemia	
L1	Predominantly small lymphocytes
L2	Heterogeneous large lymphocytes
L3	Homogeneous large lymphocytes

Blood products should be depleted of leukocytes to prevent the transmission of cytomegalovirus, alloimmunization, and febrile transfusion reactions. Irradiated blood products are often used to decrease the risk of transfusion-associated graft-versus-host disease and for patients who may be expected to undergo a bone-marrow transplantation procedure. Leukostasis, if present, should be immediately treated with intravenous hydration and leukapheresis. This should be followed by initiating hydroxyurea or appropriate induction chemotherapy to decrease the leukemic blast count. DIC should be managed by providing the replacement of severely deficient plasma coagulation factors and/or platelets. Cryoprecipitate (especially as a source of fibrinogen), fresh-frozen plasma, and platelets are typically used to manage DIC. Unless contraindicated, patients should be started on intravenous hydration with brisk saline diuresis, alkalinization of the urine, and allopurinol in anticipation of hyperuricemia that may occur upon beginning induction chemotherapy. Patients will also typically require an assessment of their cardiac function (e.g., radionuclide ventriculogram) in anticipation of anthracycline use and the placement of an indwelling central venous catheter as well as the human leukocyte antigen–typing of peripheral blood for possible allogeneic hematopoietic stem-cell transplant.

Curative treatment of acute leukemia is divided into induction and postremission phases. Induction chemotherapy is intended to obtain a complete remission, which is defined as fewer than 5% blasts in a bone marrow sample, no peripheral blood blasts, transfusion independence, normal hematopoiesis of all cell lines, and the resolution of any extramedullary leukemic infiltrates.

Induction chemotherapy is very toxic, and this is primarily the result of temporary severe marrow hypoplasia. This results in the need for intensive supportive care, with transfusions of blood products, the treatment of mucositis, and the administration of antimicrobials for bacteria, fungus, and viruses. Use of leukocyte-poor, irradiated blood products is important if hematopoietic stem-cell transplantation may be a future therapeutic option. Despite aggressive supportive care, 10% to 25% of patients undergoing induction chemotherapy will die from treatment-associated toxicities. Postremission therapy ("consolidation therapy") consists of additional chemotherapy or hematopoietic stem-cell transplantation. Patients who fail to achieve a complete remission with induction chemotherapy for AML have a poor prognosis. However, 10% to 20% can be salvaged with allogeneic hematopoietic stem-cell transplantation.

Treatment of acute promyelocytic leukemia (APL) is different from that used for the other forms of AML. Because of the molecular characteristics of this malignancy, the treatment of APL includes the use of all-*trans*-retinoic acid with chemotherapy. Arsenic trioxide also has a role in the treatment of APL. The complete remission rate for the treatment of APL is at least 90%.

The treatment of ALL usually requires the administration of chemotherapy over a 2- to 3-year period. Despite the very good cure rate for children with ALL, adults do not do as well. Remission induction therapy usually includes the use of four or five chemotherapy drugs. Postremission chemotherapy includes the prophylactic treatment of the central nervous system with the intrathecal administration of chemotherapy with or without cranial irradiation. If the patient continues in complete remission, this is followed by a prolonged administration of "maintenance" chemotherapy. Allogeneic hematopoietic stem-cell transplantation plays a useful role for those patients who fail to obtain a complete remission, for those who relapse after complete remission, or for those who are at high risk for relapse.

Chronic Leukemias

The so-called chronic leukemias are characterized as presenting with a clonal proliferation of cells that are more mature and differentiated than the blasts seen in the "acute" leukemias. Although the progression and course of disease may be less aggressive than that of the acute leukemias, the chronic leukemias do progress, and they can shorten patients' lives. The two most common chronic leukemias are chronic lymphocytic leukemia and chronic myelogenous leukemia.

Chronic Lymphocytic Leukemia

Chronic lymphocytic leukemia (CLL) is a clonal expansion of lymphocytes with a low proliferative index but prolonged cell survival. B lineage cells are responsible for 95% of CLL. CLL is the most common adult leukemia in the United States, and its incidence increases with age.

The prognosis of CLL depends on the stage of disease (Table 22-3). Median survival ranges from 10 or more years for stage 0 to 2 years for stage IV. Patients are usually asymptomatic at the time of discovery of lymphocytosis on routine blood screening. Diagnosis of CLL is made by the demonstration of a monoclonal lymphocytosis in the blood, with characteristic phenotypic features of the malignant lymphocytes.

Treatment of this incurable malignancy varies, depending on the rate of disease progression and the presence of clinical sequelae. Because the aggressiveness of this disease is variable, some patients can be observed without treatment. When treatment is necessary, a variety of chemotherapy and biologic agents (e.g., monoclonal antibodies), either alone or in combination, are effective choices. Autologous and allogeneic hematopoietic stem-cell transplantation have demonstrated utility for some patients, but they should be considered investigational.

Chronic Myelogenous Leukemia

Chronic myelogenous leukemia (CML) is a clonal myeloid stem-cell disorder that accounts for 15% to 20% of all leukemias. Although CML can occur at any age, the median age at presentation is between 50 and 60 years. Because this is a stem-cell disorder, all myeloid elements (except possibly T lymphocytes) are involved. Ionizing radiation exposure increases the risk of developing CML.

CML is characteristically associated (i.e., in 90% to 95% of patients) with the presence of the Philadelphia (Ph) chromosome in the patient's white blood cells. This represents a translocation of the *BCR* and *ABL* genes located

TABLE 22-3 • *Clinical Staging Systems for Chronic Lymphocytic Leukemia*

Rai Staging System		
Stage	**Clinical Features**	**Median Survival (years)**
0	Lymphocytosis only (blood and bone marrow)	>10
I	Lymphocytosis + lymphadenopathy	>8
II	Lymphocytosis + splenomegaly and/or hepatomegaly ± lymphadenopathy	6
III	Lymphocytosis + anemia (hemoglobin <110 g/L) ± lymphadenopathy ± splenomegaly ± hepatomegaly	2
IV	Lymphocytosis + thrombocytopenia (platelets $<100 \times 10^9$/L) ± anemia ± lymphadenopathy ± splenomegaly ± hepatomegaly	2
Binet Staging System		
Stage	**Clinical Features**	**Median Survival (years)**
A	<3 node-bearing areas	>10
B	>3 node-bearing areas	7
C	Anemia and/or thrombocytopenia	2

on chromosomes 9 and 22 [t(9;22)(q34;q11)], respectfully. The resulting *BCR-ABL* fusion gene encodes for a protein with tyrosine-kinase activity that has been shown to be necessary and sufficient to cause CML (Figure 22-1).

The clinical course of CML is divided into three phases: the chronic phase, the accelerated phase, and blast crisis. Most patients present during the chronic phase, which is characterized by myeloid hyperplasia with marked leukocytosis and circulating immature cells of the granulocytic lineage. Thrombocytosis is common, and there is invariably some degree of basophilia. Up to 50% of patients are asymptomatic at the time of diagnosis, and they are identified through routine blood tests. Common presenting symptoms include fatigue, night sweats, and splenomegaly with abdominal discomfort and early satiety. The survival of patients with CML is primarily determined by the length of time spent in the chronic phase, which lasts an average of 3 to 4 years. As the disease progresses, there is an increase in the white blood cell count (WBC) and in the percentage of basophils and blasts in the peripheral blood and bone marrow. The accelerated phase is the transition between the chronic phase and blast crisis; it typically lasts 6 to 18 months. Blast crisis is the usual terminal event in the natural course of CML. It is characterized by the presence of fever, sweats, weight loss, bone pain, and more than 30% blasts in the peripheral blood or bone marrow. It typically lasts 3 to 6 months.

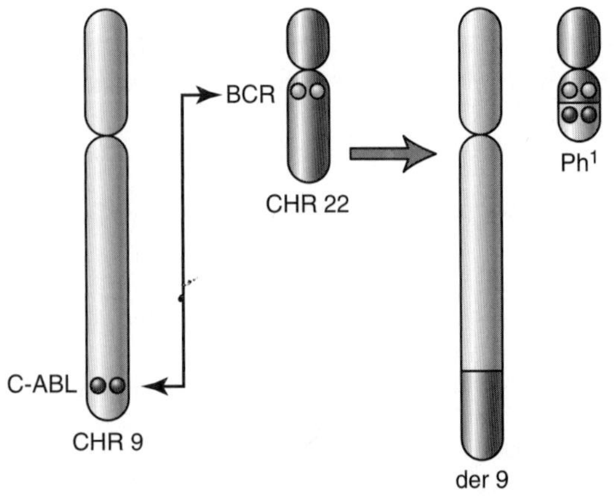

Figure 22–1. The Philadelphia chromosome (Ph1) is the result of a reciprocal translocation between chromosomes 9 and 22. This results in a fusion of the *C-ABL* proto-oncogene and the *BCR* gene. The resulting fusion protein (a tyrosine kinase) has been implicated in the etiology of chronic myelogenous leukemia and other malignancies.

The diagnosis of CML includes the evaluation of the peripheral blood and the bone marrow. The WBC will be increased, with a shift to immaturity (i.e., left shift) of the granulocyte lineage and with the presence of granulocytic precursors in the peripheral blood. Absolute basophilia is characteristic of CML. The leukocyte alkaline phosphatase score in the WBC is decreased in patients with CML. Diagnosis is confirmed by demonstration of the *BCR-ABL* fusion gene by cytogenetic evidence of the Ph chromosome and/or by fluorescence in situ hybridization and reverse transcriptase polymerase chain reaction analysis.

The treatment of CML is dependent on the phase of the disease. The most impact on survival and quality of life occurs with treatment that occurs during the chronic phase. Allogeneic hematopoietic stem-cell transplantation is the only known curative therapy for CML. Although its curative potential is unknown, imatinib mesylate (Gleevec, a bcr-abl tyrosine kinase inhibitor) has become the initial therapy for most patients with chronic-phase CML. Cytotoxic chemotherapy and interferon-α can also be used to obtain hematologic remission with the elimination of symptoms and signs of disease.

CML blast crisis is treated with induction chemotherapy regimens similar to those used for acute leukemias. However, complete remission rates are lower, and the relapse rate is much higher. Allogeneic hematopoietic stem-cell transplantation is effective for some, but it is associated with low response rates and high relapse rates.

Lymphomas

Lymphomas are neoplasms of cells derived from lymphocytes or lymphocyte precursors. The differentiation between lymphomas and lymphocytic leukemias rests primarily on the predominant location of the malignant cells (i.e., lymph nodes or related organs as compared with blood or bone marrow, respectively). There are two main categories of lymphomas: non-Hodgkin lymphoma (NHL) and Hodgkin disease; both have unique characteristics.

NHLs are classified on the basis of the malignant cells' apparent cell of origin and on the lymphoma cell's B or T cell phenotype. Flow cytometry and the immunohistochemical staining of biopsied tumor samples are very useful for determining the lymphoma cell of origin and the phenotype. The WHO classification system also takes into account cytogenetic abnormalities that are associated with specific lymphoma types (e.g., t(14;18) in follicular lymphomas, t(8;14) in Burkitt's lymphomas).

The biologic behavior of the different NHLs varies from indolent, incurable diseases to aggressive, curable neoplasms. NHLs are considered to spread in a noncontiguous manner (i.e., lymph nodes contiguous to involved nodes may not contain lymphoma). The classification and characterization of the lymphoma, the sites of involvement, and the characteristics of the patient direct the treatment and prognosis of the disease.

Hodgkin's disease has unique histologic characteristics that contrast it from NHL. The neoplastic cell in Hodgkin's disease is known as the Reed-Sternberg cell, which is a distinct type of B-lymphocyte. Hodgkin's disease is subclassified based on the morphologic appearance and distribution of cells present (Table 22-4). Hodgkin's disease typically spreads between lymph nodes contiguously.

The diagnosis of NHL or Hodgkin's disease is made after the pathologic evaluation of a biopsy of an abnormal lymph node or a neoplastic mass. Because much of the morphologic diagnosis of a lymphoma is based on the appearance of the neoplastic cells in the context of surrounding non-neoplastic cells, fine-needle aspirations are inadequate for diagnosis. A core-needle biopsy or, preferably, an excisional biopsy is usually necessary for diagnosis.

NHL and Hodgkin's disease usually present as an enlarged lymph node(s) that does not resolve with time or with treatment of benign conditions. Malignant lymph nodes tend to be large (>1 cm), firm, nontender, and occasionally matted, and they typically progressively enlarge. Patients may also experience fever, drenching night sweats, and/or weight loss (i.e., B symptoms). Other symptoms and signs are dependent on the sites with neoplastic involvement.

BOX 22-3 B SYMPTOMS

- Fever
- Drenching night sweats
- Unexplained weight loss (≥10% of body weight during the preceding 6 months)

The evaluation of a patient with lymphoma involves identifying the extent and sites of lymphoma involvement, a process known as *staging*. The Ann Arbor Staging System (see Table 22-4) guides the evaluation of patients with NHL and Hodgkin's disease. This evaluation will usually include a thorough history and physical examination, a complete blood count with differential, a comprehensive chemistry panel, a lactate dehydrogenase level, an erythrocyte sedimentation rate (especially for Hodgkin's disease), bilateral bone-marrow aspiration and biopsy, and computed tomographic scans of the chest, abdomen, and pelvis.

The treatment of NHL and Hodgkin's disease is dependent on the histologic subclassification, stage, and expected prognosis of the lymphoma. External-beam radiation therapy is useful for disease that is confined to a single radiation field (i.e., limited disease) or to decrease the risk of local recurrence of bulky lymphomatous masses. Chemotherapy, either with single agents or combinations, plays a major role in the treatment of all types of lymphomas. The role of surgery in the management of lymphomas is limited to obtaining

TABLE 22-4 • *Ann Arbor Staging Classification*

Stage*	Description
I	Involvement of a single lymph-node region (I) or a single extralymphatic organ or site (IE)
II	Involvement of two or more lymph-node regions on the same side of the diaphragm (II) or local involvement of an extralymphatic organ or site and one or more lymph-node regions on the same side of the diaphragm (IIE)
III	Involvement of lymph-node regions on both sides of the diaphragm (III), which may also be accompanied by involvement of the spleen (IIIs) or by local involvement of an extralymphatic organ or site (IIIE) or both (IIIsE)
IV	Diffuse or disseminated involvement of one or more extralymphatic organs or tissues, with or without lymph-node involvement

*Letters after the roman numerals are used to subclassify the stage. Fever, night sweats, or unexplained loss of 10% or more of body weight in the 6 months preceding diagnosis is denoted by the letter *B* (i.e., "B symptoms"); the letter *A* indicates the absence of these symptoms. The letter *E* indicates the involvement of an extralymphatic site; the letter *S* indicates splenic involvement.

BOX 22–4 STAGING WORKUP OF LYMPHOMA

- Thorough history and physical
- Complete blood cell count, with differential
- Comprehensive chemistry panel
- Lactate dehydrogenase level
- Erythrocyte sedimentation rate
- Bilateral bone-marrow aspiration and biopsy
- Computed tomographic scans of chest, abdomen, and pelvis

BOX 22–5 CLASSIFICATION OF HODGKIN'S DISEASE

- Lymphocyte depleted
- Lymphocyte-rich classical
- Mixed cellularity
- Nodular lymphocyte predominant
- Nodular sclerosis

diagnostic biopsies and, rarely, to managing localized sites of disease-associated complications that are not responsive or amenable to radiation therapy or chemotherapy.

Indolent NHLs are usually incurable and tend to grow slowly or to spontaneously regress for significant lengths of time. Because survival does not appear to be influenced by early intervention, many patients can be observed without treatment for a period of time. Chemotherapy and monoclonal antibody therapy are the mainstays of treatment for this disease. Mucosa-associated lymphoid tissue lymphomas of the stomach, which are a particular form of indolent lymphoma, may be curable with antibiotics directed against *Helicobacter pylori* (see Chapter 16: Neoplasms of the Stomach and the Small Intestine). NHL that occurs in a post-solid organ transplant setting may regress with the reduction of pharmacologic immunosuppression.

Aggressive NHL that responds to treatment results in longer survival and potential cure. Because these lymphomas tend to grow rapidly and to invade vital organs, the staging and treatment of these types of lymphomas should be initiated soon after diagnosis. Combination chemotherapy with or without monoclonal antibody therapy and with or without involved field radiation therapy to isolated or bulky disease sites is the mainstay of treatment. For those patients who do not achieve a complete remission or who relapse, salvage therapies with combination chemotherapy and/or hematopoietic stem-cell transplantation (usually autologous) can be used.

Highly aggressive NHL (e.g., Burkitt's and lymphoblastic lymphomas) very rapidly proliferate, and they need to be treated as soon as possible after diagnosis. These lymphomas are potentially curable with combination chemotherapy, and they require central nervous system prophylaxis with intrathecal chemotherapy with or without cranial radiation. Tumor lysis is a real concern in these patients, who must be monitored closely.

The treatment of Hodgkin's disease depends on the stage of disease, and it may include radiation therapy and/or chemotherapy. Radiation therapy alone is potentially curative for early-stage disease (i.e., stages IA, IB, and IIA). This approach resulted in the development of standard radiation fields (Figure 22-2). Later stages of Hodgkin's disease (i.e., stages IIB, IIIA, IIIB, IVA, and IVB) are treated primarily with combination chemotherapy. Salvage therapy for relapsed or refractory Hodgkin's disease consists of either combination chemotherapy or high-dose chemotherapy with autologous hematopoietic stem-cell transplantation.

The prognosis of the lymphomas is dependent on the histologic type of lymphoma, the stage of disease, and a variety of clinical factors. For indolent NHLs, the median survival is 7 to 10 years, despite the incurability of these diseases. Survival for aggressive NHL is predicted by the International Prognostic Index (Table 22-5). A similar prognosticating index has been identified for Hodgkin's disease. Despite their high rate of proliferation, the highly aggressive NHLs, such as Burkitt's lymphoma and lymphoblastic lymphoma, tend to be very responsive to chemotherapy and to typically have very good prognoses.

For early-stage Hodgkin's disease with no unfavorable factors, there is an 80% or higher 5-year freedom from relapse rate. For patients with advanced Hodgkin's disease, there is at least a 60% chance of cure.

Summary

The malignancy of hematopoietic cells can result in a wide variety of leukemias or lymphomas. These diseases have unique clinical and pathogenic characteristics that require pathologic evaluation for diagnosis. Knowledge of the natural behavior, the extent (stage) of

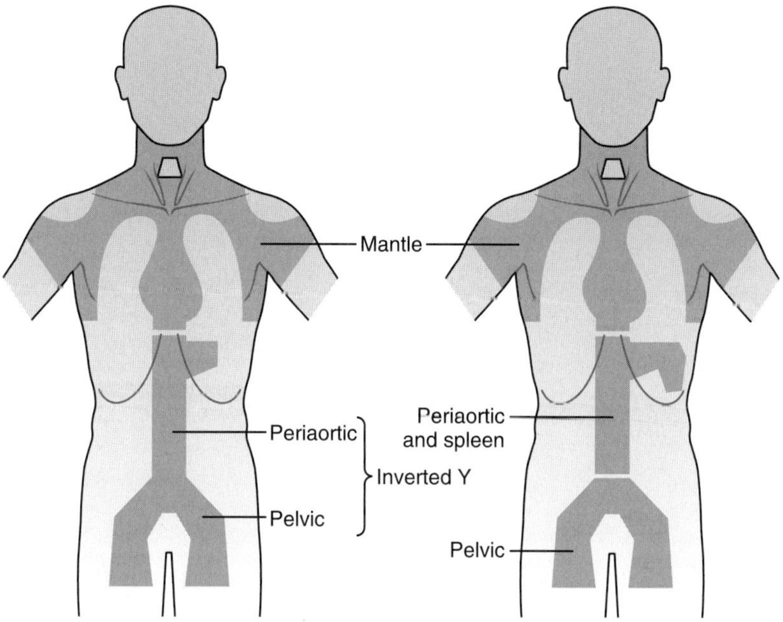

Figure 22-2. Radiation therapy fields commonly used for the treatment of Hodgkin's disease. Lymphoid irradiation fields include mantle, paraaortic (and spleen, if spleen still present), and pelvic. An inverted Y field consists of a combination of paraaortic and pelvic fields. A total lymphoid irradiation field consists of the combination of all of the above fields.

TABLE 22-5 • *International Prognostic Index for Aggressive Non-Hodgkin Lymphoma*

International Prognostic Index Score	Expected Complete Remission Rate	Predicted 2-Year Survival Rate	Predicted 5-Year Survival Rate
0-1	87%	84%	73%
2	67%	66%	51%
3	55%	54%	43%
4-5	44%	34%	26%

The International Prognostic Index is the sum of points based on the number of prognosis-influencing risk factors that are present. Each risk factor is assigned a value of 1 point. Risk factors include age of more than 60 years, stage III or IV disease, lactate dehydrogenase level elevation, two or more extralymphatic sites of disease, and performance status of 2 or more (on a 0-4 scale).

disease involvement, and the associated physiologic effects and an understanding of the prognostic factors of these diseases allow for the optimal selection of therapy. Awareness of the "curability" of these diseases is important for the optimal management of patients who have them.

Selected Readings

Chiorazzi N, Rai KR, Ferrarini M. Chronic lymphocytic leukemia. *N Engl J Med* 2005;352:804–815.

Connors JM. State-of-the-art therapeutics: Hodgkin's lymphoma. *J Clin Oncol* 2005;23:6400–6408.

Goldman JM, Melo JV. Chronic myeloid leukemia—advances in biology and new approaches to treatment. *N Engl J Med* 2003;349:1451–1464.

Löwenberg B, Downing JR, Burnett A. Acute myeloid leukemia. *N Engl J Med* 1999;341:1051–1062.

Pui C-H, Evans WE: Acute lymphoblastic leukemia, *N Engl J Med* 1998;339:605–615.

Oscier D, Fegan C, Hillmen P, *et al*. Guidelines on the diagnosis and management of chronic lymphocytic leukaemia. *Br J Haematol* 2004;125:294–317.

Sawyers CL: Chronic myeloid leukemia. *N Engl J Med* 1999;340:1330–1340.

Thomas RK, Re D, Wolf J, Diehl V. Part I: Hodgkin's lymphoma—molecular biology of Hodgkin and Reed-Sternberg cells. *Lancet Oncol* 2004;5:11–18.

Jaffe ES, Harris NL, Stein H, Vardiman JW, eds. *World Health Organization classification of tumours: pathology and genetics of tumours of haematopoietic and lymphoid tissues*. Lyon, France: IARC Press, 2001.

Pui C-H, Evans WE. Treatment of acute lymphoblastic leukemia. *N Engl J Med* 2006;354:166–178.

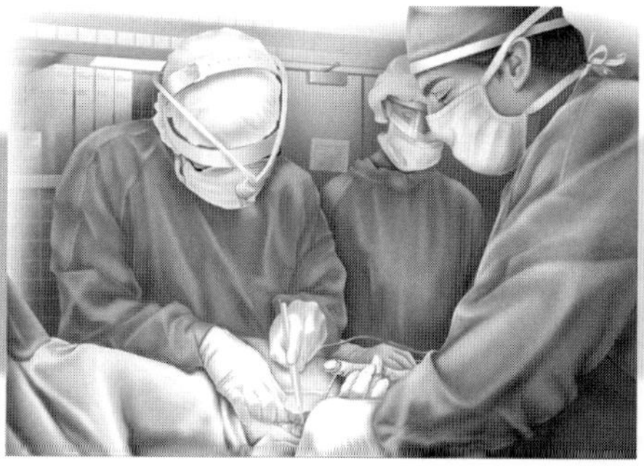

23

Gynecologic Cancers

Carolyn Johnston and William M. Burke

Gynecologic Cancers: Key Points

- Describe the assessment of a suspicious pelvic mass.
- Discuss the staging and management of ovarian cancer.
- Review the approaches to nonresectable and recurrent ovarian cancer.
- Outline the symptoms, clinical evaluation, staging, and surgical management of endometrial cancer.
- Detail the incidence and treatment of cervical cancer.
- Give an account of the clinical evaluation and treatment of vaginal cancer.
- Describe the sequelae that may develop after pelvic radiation and their appropriate management.

With the significant overlap of organ involvement and disease processes that each specialty manages and treats, it is imperative that there exist a good working relationship between the disciplines of gynecologic oncology and surgical oncology. Approximately 78,000 women will be diagnosed with a gynecologic cancer in 2006 (Table 23-1). It is important for surgical oncologists to be cognizant of the indications for and the surgical approaches to managing gynecologic malignancies, especially those involving the ovary, uterus, cervix, and vagina (Figure 23-1). The most common cell types of cancer in each organ are endometrioid endometrial adenocarcinoma, epithelial ovarian adenocarcinoma, and squamous cell

TABLE 23–1 • *The 2006 Estimated Annual Incidence and Deaths Attributed to the Five Most Common Gynecologic Malignancies*

Organ of Origin	Estimated Cases in 2006	Estimated Number of Deaths in 2006
Endometrium	41,200	7,350
Ovary	20,180	15,310
Cervix	9,710	3,700
Vulva	3,740	880
Vagina	2,420	820

From the American Cancer Society. *Cancer facts & figures 2005*. Available at: www.cancer.org/docroot/STT/content/STT_1x_Cancer_Facts__Figures_2005.asp. Accessed May 10, 2006.

cervical, vulvar, and vaginal carcinoma. Sarcomas of gynecologic origin are uncommon and most often occur in the uterus. Primary peritoneal cancer is diagnosed, occurs at a similar age, and is managed and treated identically to ovarian cancer. It is, by definition, at an advanced stage at diagnosis. Fallopian tube cancer is most often a diagnosis made in retrospect, but it is also managed and treated identically to ovarian cancer. Currently, ovarian, primary peritoneal, fallopian tube, endometrial, and vulvar carcinoma are surgically and pathologically staged, whereas cervical and vaginal carcinoma are clinically staged.

Ovarian Cancer

The risk in the female population of developing ovarian cancer is approximately 1 in 70. It is most commonly a disease of postmenopausal women, with the median age of diagnosis at 63 years. Prior tubal ligation and the use of oral contraceptives for more than 5 years reduce the risk of ovarian cancer by nearly 50%. Because ovarian cancer is not common and the presenting symptoms are sufficiently nonspecific, it is not unusual for a gastrointestinal source to be presumed, so the diagnosis may not be made

BOX 23–1 RISK FACTORS FOR THE DEVELOPMENT OF OVARIAN CANCER

- Older age
- Nulligravid
- Infertility
- Early age at menarche
- Late age at menopause
- Perineal talc exposure
- Higher socioeconomic level
- Caucasian race
- Family history of breast and ovarian cancer
- Family history of hereditary nonpolyposis colon cancer

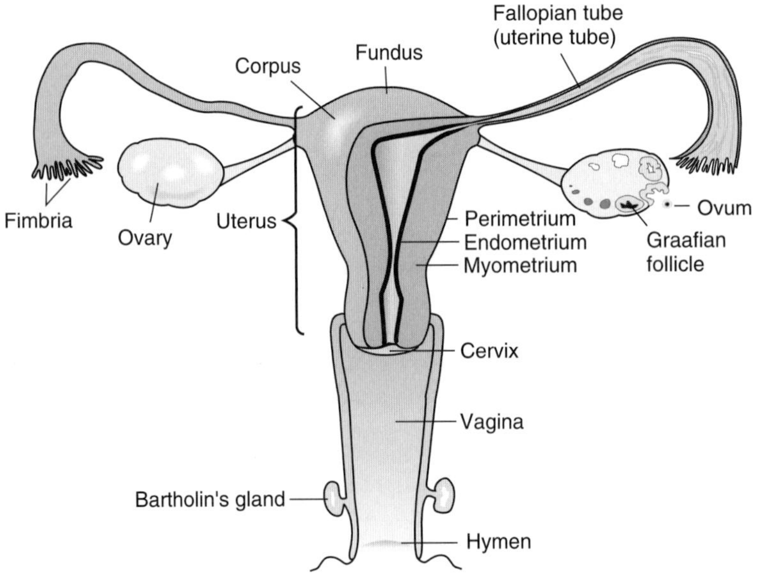

Figure 23–1. Organs of the female reproductive system. (From McSwain NE, Paturas JL. *The basic EMT,* ed 2. St. Louis: Mosby, 2001:374. Figure 21-2.)

until quite late in the disease's course; it is for this reason that 75% of women present with advanced-stage disease. Often patients will be referred to a general surgeon for nonspecific abdominal complaints. With a thorough history and physical examination, the presence of a pelvic mass should be detected before laparotomy, thereby allowing for an appropriate workup and consideration of the patient's age, her fertility desires, and coexisting diseases when selecting a course of treatment. However, this is not always the case, and general surgeons occasionally find themselves confronted in the operating room with an unexpected gynecologic malignancy.

BOX 23-2 COMMON SYMPTOMS OF OVARIAN AND PRIMARY PERITONEAL CARCINOMAS

- Abdominal discomfort or pain
- Abdominal distention
- Nonspecific bowel complaints, such as bloating, flatulence, and change in bowel function
- Early satiety
- Nausea/emesis
- Pelvic pressure
- Vaginal bleeding and urinary complaints are less common

BOX 23-3 SUGGESTIONS TO AVOID A SURPRISE PELVIC MASS AT LAPAROTOMY

1. Take a gynecologic history preoperatively.
2. Perform a pelvic examination.
3. Test for pregnancy preoperatively in premenopausal women.

Evaluation of the Suspected Pelvic Mass

When an adnexal mass is discovered on physical examination, the most useful radiologic tool for evaluating the ovary is transvaginal ultrasound. Characteristics noted on preoperative ultrasound that relate to the likelihood of malignancy include size, complexity, and the presence of septations and solid elements. CT scanning is useful for evaluating the remainder of the peritoneal cavity and the retroperitoneum. A chest radiograph provides an adequate evaluation of the chest, unless it is abnormal, and then a CT scan is also indicated.

BOX 23-4 COMMON SOURCES OF PELVIC MASSES

Nongynecologic

- GI
  - Cancer
  - Abscess
  - Diverticulum
- Urinary Tract
  - Cancer
  - Pelvic Kidney
- Retroperitoneal tumors
- Vascular
  - Aneursym
  - AVM
- Metastatic cancers

Gynecologic

- Ovary
  - Benign neoplasms
  - Malignant neoplasms
- Fallopian tube
  - Benign neoplasms
  - Malignant neoplasms
  - Tubo-ovarian abscess
  - Ectopic pregnancy
- Uterus
  - Leiomyomata
  - Adenomyosis
  - Pregnancy
  - Myometrial cysts
  - Malignant neoplasms

Ancillary studies such as barium enema, intravenous pyelogram, colonoscopy, and upper gastrointestinal studies are performed when indicated by clinical findings. Younger women, particularly those who are less than 40 years old, are less likely to have malignant ovarian neoplasms as the cause of an ovarian mass (Table 23-2). In large reviews, the reported incidence of ovarian malignancy in patients with a preoperative diagnosis of a pelvic mass is 13% to 21%. Figures 23-2 and 23-3 show the accepted management of pelvic masses and ovarian masses that are detected preoperatively.

Special mention should be made of ovarian masses that are discovered in pregnant patients. Most ovarian neoplasms during pregnancy are benign. Malignant neoplasms represent only 0.8% to 13% of masses. Because of the age group involved, most malignancies are low-malignant-potential (LMP) or germ-cell

TABLE 23-2 • *The Most Common Ovarian Neoplasms, Average Age of Occurrence, and Bilaterality*

Type of Neoplasm	Average Age of Occurrence (Years)	Percentage That Are Bilateral
Benign		
Functional	Premenopausal	
Dermoid	32	10–15%
Endometrioma	40	14–27%*
Serous	45	17%
Mucinous	44	2%
Malignant Epithelial		
Serous	56	73%
Mucinous	52	47%
Endometrioid	57	33%
Borderline		
Serous	48	34%
Mucinous	49	5–6%
Endometrioid	48	7%
Germ-cell tumors		
Dysgerminoma	10–30	10–15%
Yolk sac	17	<5%
Embryonal	First two decades of life	<5%
Mixed	First two decades of life	<10%
Immature teratoma	First two decades of life	<5%

From Parazzini F. Left:right side ratio of endometriotic implants in the pelvis. Italian Study Group for the Study of Endometriosis. *Eur J Obstet Gynecol Reprod Biol* 2003;111:65–67. The remainder of the table is adapted from Hoskins WJ, Perez CA, Young RC, eds. *Principles and practice of gynecologic oncology,* 2nd ed. Philadelphia: Lippincott-Raven Publishers, 1997.

cancers. The majority of the neoplasms are benign teratomas or serous cystadenomas. Tumor markers must be interpreted with caution in pregnancy as a result of normal elevations associated with the gravid state. Masses of less than 6 cm are usually managed expectantly throughout gestation with pelvic examinations and serial ultrasounds. Ultrasound characteristics can be helpful for predicting the likelihood that a pelvic mass is malignant. Indications for surgical intervention in pregnancy have been developed. Preferentially this surgery is performed at 16 to 18 weeks' gestation. Treatment and staging are similar to that of the nongravid state, which demonstrates that cystectomy or unilateral oophorectomy with staging is often adequate treatment of an LMP tumor.

BOX 23-5 INDICATIONS FOR SURGICAL INTERVENTION FOR A PELVIC MASS DURING PREGNANCY

- Size >6 cm
- Increasing size of mass
- Symptomatic mass
- Obvious metastatic spread

Conservative surgery and staging without hysterectomy is also most often appropriate for a germ-cell tumor. For early-stage epithelial disease that is either an LMP or invasive carcinoma, a hysterectomy is not mandatory. For stage III or IV ovarian carcinomas, the extent of surgery depends on the patient's desires and consent and the gestational age and relative viability of the fetus. Ideally, both an obstetrician and a gynecologic oncologist should be consulted for management.

Management of the Incidental Ovarian Mass at Laparotomy

It is not unusual for a surgeon to discover an ovarian mass at the time of laparotomy. Appropriate management is essential, because errors can worsen the prognosis when malignancy is discovered. If an unsuspected ovarian mass is encountered, the first step is to determine whether it is cystic or solid. Septations and solid areas can often be identified by transillumination of the cyst. If the mass is discovered to be a unilocular cyst, the likelihood of malignancy is extremely low (<1%). A cystectomy is rarely indicated in a postmenopausal woman. In premenopausal women, approximately 70% of masses that are less than or equal to 6 to 8 cm will resolve spontaneously. Thus, the presence of a simple cyst of this size is not an indication for resection, and it can be followed postoperatively through one to three menstrual cycles with serial pelvic examinations or ultrasounds. If the mass is larger than this, if there is no suspicion of extra-ovarian spread, and if the woman is premenopausal with unknown fertility desires, then cystectomy performed in a manner that does not rupture the cyst is recommended.

If the mass has a solid component, the likelihood of malignancy increases, especially in a postmenopausal woman, in whom a cyst with a solid component has a 70% chance of malignancy.

A random biopsy of an ovarian tumor is inappropriate because of the potential for spreading a confined process and thus worsening

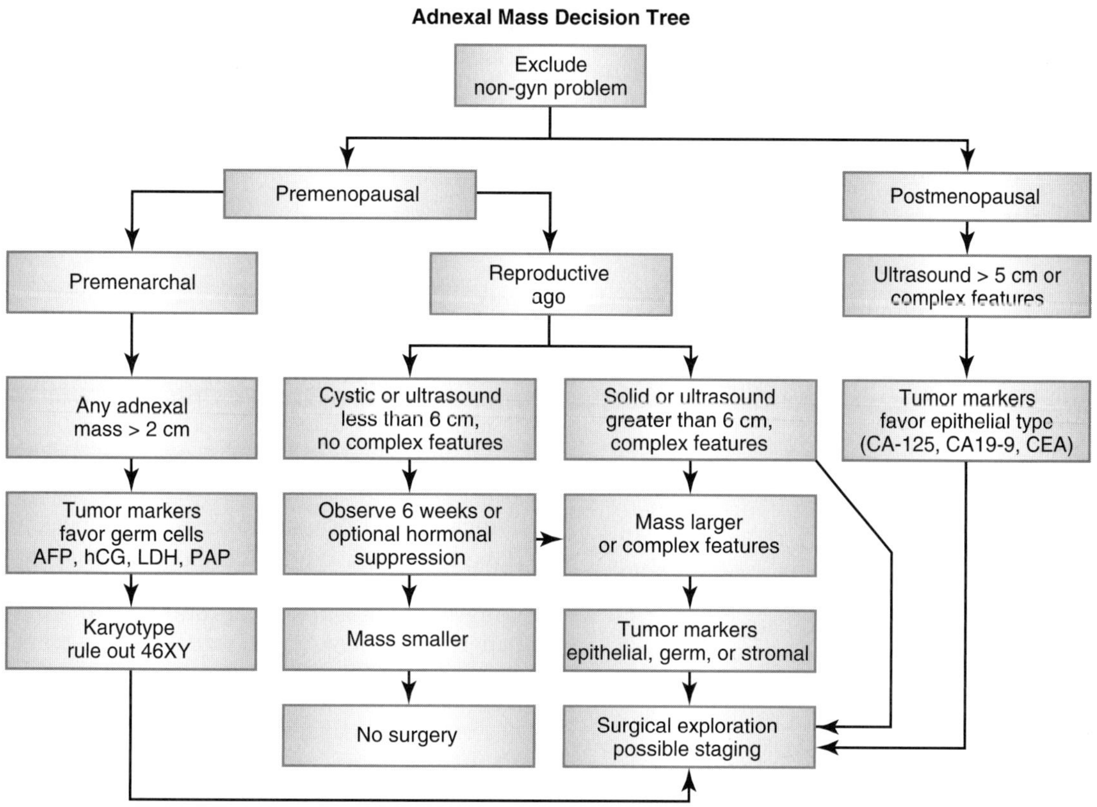

Figure 23–2. The accepted management of pelvic masses identified preoperatively.

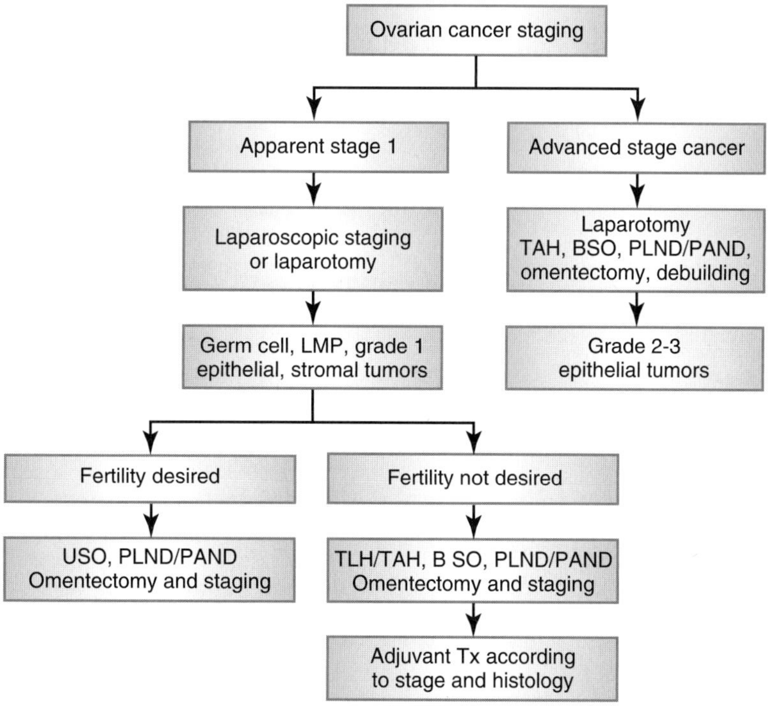

Figure 23–3. The accepted surgical management of an ovarian mass discovered preoperatively. *BSO,* Bilateral salpingo-oophorectomy; *PAND,* para-aortic node dissection; *PLND,* pelvic lymph node dissection; *TAH,* total abdominal hysterectomy; *TLH,* total laparoscopic hysterectomy; *USO,* unilateral salpingo-oophorectomy.

prognosis. The options for the management of an unsuspected ovarian mass in a premenopausal or postmenopausal woman include oophorectomy with frozen section and complete surgical staging if indicated or oophorectomy with further treatment to be performed at another procedure. In premenopausal patients who desire future fertility, preservation of the uterus and the remaining ovary would be appropriate, even if a complete staging procedure was required. Consultation with a gynecologic oncologist and with a family member at the time of surgery is ideal, particularly if this issue had not been discussed with the patient.

Ovarian Cancer Staging

If an unsuspected ovarian cancer is detected intraoperatively, a gynecologic oncologist should ideally be consulted. Comprehensive surgical evaluation, adequate debulking, and survival are most optimally achieved by gynecologic oncologists or obstetrician/gynecologists. Despite this observation, the surgical staging of ovarian cancer is within the surgical scope of a surgical oncologist, and a gynecologic oncologist may not always be available. The relative frequency of lymph node metastases in ovarian carcinomas is presented in Table 23-3. Thirty-one percent of apparent clinical stage I ovarian cancers are upstaged by retroperitoneal lymph node dissection and omentectomy, and 77% of those are stage III. Long-term prognosis for and treatment of patients with stage I and stage III disease are different, thereby making accurate surgical staging a critical component of caring for women with ovarian malignancies (Table 23-4).

TABLE 23-3 • *The Incidence of Lymph-Node Metastases in the Clinical Stages of Ovarian Cancer*

Germ cell tumors	Uncertain
Low malignant potential tumors	27%*/7%†
Epithelial tumors	
Clinical stage I	0–4%
Clinical stage II	20%
Clinical stages III and IV	71%

*Positive pelvic lymph nodes.
†Positive paraaortic lymph nodes.
From Buschbaum HJ, Brady, MF, Delgado G, *et al.* Surgical staging of ovarian carcinoma: stage I, II, and III (optimal): a GOG study. *Surg Gynecol Obstet* 1989;169:226.

BOX 23-6 SURGICAL STAGING OF EARLY OVARIAN EPITHELIAL CANCER

- Send ascites for cytology, or obtain washings of pelvis, both paracolic gutters, and upper abdomen
- Inspect the entire peritoneal cavity with biopsies, as indicated
- Unilateral oophorectomy or bilateral oophorectomy (with intact tumor removal)
- Bilateral pelvic and paraaortic lymph-node dissection
- Cytoreduction to microscopic disease
- Appendectomy for mucinous tumors
- Perform random biopsies of both para colic gutters, cul de sac, both lateral pelvic side walls, vesicouterine reflec tion, both diaphragms, and adhesions
- Infracolic omentectomy
- Total abdominal hysterectomy if the uterus is involved and/or if fertility is not a concern

Cytoreductive Surgery in Nonresectable Disease

In some cases, the surgeon will encounter advanced ovarian cancer when performing a laparotomy. In this case, in addition to diagnosis and staging, optimum cytoreduction is necessary. In 1995, a National Institutes of Health Consensus Panel opinion recognized the role of comprehensive staging and optimal cytoreduction (generally accepted as

BOX 23-7 SURGICAL STAGING OF ADVANCED OVARIAN CANCER

- Send ascites for cytology, or obtain washings of pelvis, both paracolic gutters, and upper abdomen
- Inspect the entire peritoneal cavity with biopsies, as indicated
- Total abdominal hysterectomy with bilateral salpingo-oophorectomy
- Omentectomy
- Optimal debulking to microscopic resid ual disease or to disease <1 cm in maximum diameter
- Bilateral pelvic and paraaortic lymph-node dissection if omental disease is <2 cm or if bulky lymph-node disease present

TABLE 23-4 • *International Federation of Gynecology and Obstetrics Staging Criteria for Ovarian Cancer*

Stage I	**Growth limited to the ovaries**
Ia	Growth limited to one ovary; no ascites; no tumor on the external surface; capsule intact
Ib	Growth limited to both ovaries; no ascites; no tumor on external surface; capsule intact
Ic	Tumor on the surface of one or both ovaries; capsule ruptured; malignant ascites present or positive peritoneal washings
Stage II	**Growth involving one or both ovaries, with pelvic extension**
IIa	Extension and/or metastases to the uterus and/or tubes
IIb	Extension to other pelvic tissues
IIc	Tumor stage II with tumor on surface of one or both ovaries; capsule(s) ruptured; malignant ascites or positive peritoneal washings present
Stage III	**Tumor involving one or both ovaries with peritoneal implants outside of the pelvis and/or positive retroperitoneal or inguinal lymph nodes; superficial liver metastases**
IIIa	Histologically confirmed microscopic seeding of abdominal and peritoneal surfaces
IIIb	Histologically confirmed implants of peritoneum less than or equal to 2 cm; negative lymph nodes
IIIc	Abdominal implants greater than 2 cm and/or positive retroperitoneal or inguinal lymph nodes
Stage IV	**Distant metastases; if pleural effusion is present, there must be positive cytologic test results to allot to a stage IV; parenchymal liver metastasis equals stage IV**

From Benedet JL, Hacker NF, Ngan HYS. *Staging classifications and clinical practice guidelines of gynaecologic cancers.* Available at: www.figo.org/content/PDF/staging-booklet.pdf. Accessed May 10, 2006.

BOX 23-8 SOME REPRESENTATIVE TECHNIQUES TO ACHIEVE OPTIMAL CYTOREDUCTION

- Lymph-node dissection of nodes >1 cm
- Peritoneal stripping
- Diaphragm stripping
- Use of the Cavitron Ultrasonic Surgical Aspirator®
- Use of the argon-beam coagulator
- Hepatic resection
- Splenectomy
- Bowel resection
- Anterior culdectomy

residual disease <1-1.5 cm) in ovarian cancer surgery, because the size of residual disease strongly affects survival. Methods used to achieve cytoreduction, in addition to total abdominal hysterectomy, bilateral salpingo-oophorectomy, and omentectomy, are listed.

If it is not possible to resect all of the disease, an oophorectomy or an intraoperative biopsy of an ovary or the omentum should be performed to confirm a diagnosis of ovarian or primary peritoneal cancer. Neoadjuvant chemotherapy with paclitaxel and carboplatin is then administered, and an interval cytoreduction is performed after three to four courses of chemotherapy, if the patient's cancer has responded. If optimal debulking is performed, then the survival outcome is at least similar to that of those patients for whom optimal cytoreduction to microscopic disease occurs primarily. As with primary cytoreduction, if optimum cytoreduction is not feasible, then the patient does not fare as well.

General Surgical Approaches

If the decision is made to proceed with resection, several surgical points should be mentioned. Caution should be taken when clamping the ovarian blood vessels contained in the infundibulopelvic ligament and when clamping the uterosacral and cardinal ligaments of the uterus so as to avoid either obstructing or kinking the ureter. Avoidance of ureteral damage is facilitated by opening the posterior sheath of the broad ligament and identifying the ureter as it runs along the medial aspect of the peritoneum, below the level of the ovarian vessels, and by always placing clamps on the cardinal ligament pedicles medial to the previously created pedicle. Similarly, dissection of the bladder off of the cervix and its retraction with a Deaver retractor will reduce ureteral and bladder damage at the level of the vaginal cuff. Grasping both uterine cornua with hysterectomy clamps and keeping the uterus elevated also increases the distance between the clamps placed on the cardinal ligaments and the ureters. Unlike endometriosis, which can cause retroperitoneal scarring, ovarian cancer rarely does; thus, entering the retroperitoneum can be an effective means of mobilizing masses that are adherent to the peritoneum and its contents.

The borders of the pelvic and paraaortic lymph-node dissections are similar for all of the gynecologic cancers (Figure 23-4). For a dissection, fatty and nodal tissue is removed completely with the use of clips and cautery for hemostasis. The borders of the pelvic lymphadenectomy are the bifurcation of the common iliac artery superiorly, the psoas muscle laterally, the anterior division of the internal iliac artery medially, and the deep circumflex iliac vein as well as the obturator nerve inferiorly. The paraaortic lymph-node dissection for both endometrial and ovarian cancers should be carried at least to the level of the origin of the inferior mesenteric artery on the aorta and higher for removal of any bulky lymph nodes. Many of the lymph nodes are located in the space between the aorta and the vena cava. Care is taken to avoid the ureters on either side of the great vessels. The role of debulking lymph nodes is clearly related to survival for ovarian carcinoma, but it is less well established for endometrial and cervical carcinomas. The

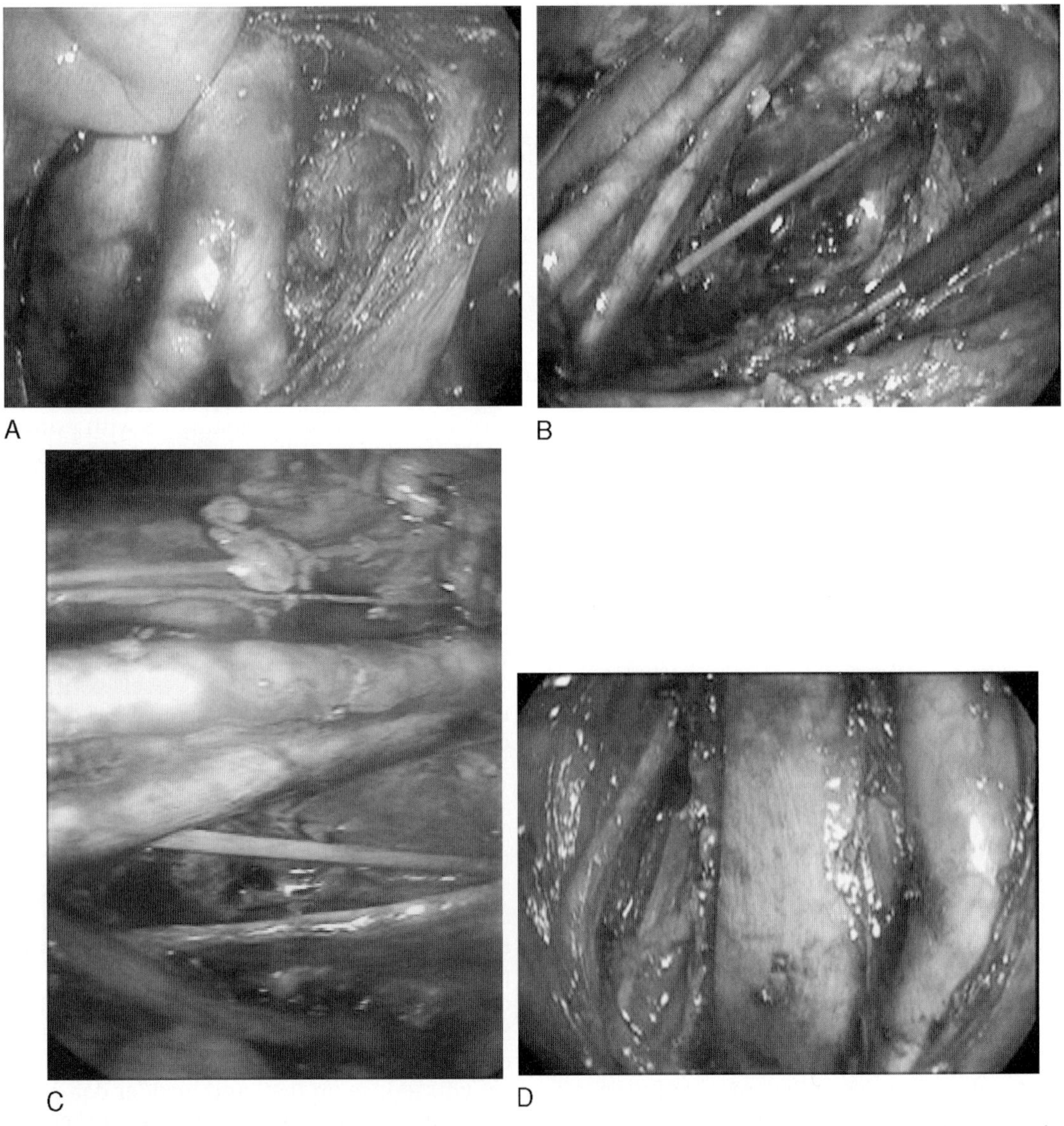

Figure 23–4. Borders of pelvic and paraaortic lymph-node dissection. **A,** Left paraaortic boundary. **B** and **C,** Pelvic lymph-node boundary. **D,** Right paraaortic boundary.

level of lymph node involvement does, however, define the radiation ports for endometrial and cervical cancers.

Recurrent Ovarian Carcinoma

Recurrent ovarian cancer is usually treated with chemotherapy, although surgery is sometimes indicated. Isolated hepatic recurrences are amenable to surgical resection and should be followed by a course of chemotherapy. The criteria for resection are nearly identical to those applied to colorectal patients with hepatic metastases. Another indication for surgery is the patient with a history of early-stage disease with a long disease-free interval between the original diagnosis and the recurrence.

BOX 23–9 CRITERIA FOR THE RESECTION OF OVARIAN HEPATIC METASTASES

- Patient is medically able to undergo surgery
- Number of metastases is <4
- No preoperative evidence of extrahe patic tumor
- Able to remove all tumor, with negative margins

The survival impact of secondary debulking, especially for advanced disease, has not been evaluated prospectively. The impact of secondary debulking to the level of microscopic disease is also uncertain, but more current studies have suggested a role in chemosensitive disease. The key point here is to obtain microscopic residual disease at this secondary laparotomy; otherwise, the patient should just receive chemotherapy. Partial debulking is not useful and should not be performed unless it is done concurrently with bowel surgery to relieve an obstruction and to improve quality of life. Patients whose disease progresses on first-line chemotherapy or in whom it recurs fewer than 6 months after completing initial chemotherapy are not likely to achieve a complete clinical response to further chemotherapy and should not generally be considered for surgical debulking. However, they can be treated with second-line chemotherapy or enrolled in a clinical trial.

Most women with recurrent ovarian cancer will eventually have spread of the disease within the peritoneal cavity and develop obstructive bowel symptoms. The small intestine is most often affected. The decision of whether or not to intervene surgically is based on several factors, including performance status, remaining treatment options, site of obstruction, and prior treatment. Experience suggests that poor nutritional status, multiple levels of partial small bowel obstruction, diffuse carcinomatosis, and extraabdominal disease are all predictive of failure of surgical outcome. Successful palliative bowel surgery has been achieved in 51% to 71% of patients, with a median survival of 8 months. Gastrojejunostomy may be indicated for select patients with a proximal intestinal obstruction, especially for chemosensitive or chemotherapy-naïve patients and for those who have an expected longevity that exceeds 6 months.

Chemotherapy, outside of a clinical trial, is ineffective for women who are heavily pretreated, and it will do little to alleviate a bowel obstruction. In this situation, chemotherapy should be reserved for women who are chemotherapy naïve. Total parenteral nutrition is also best reserved for chemotherapy-naïve women with a bowel obstruction or for short-term use for perioperative support in women undergoing debulking and bowel surgery; it is not a long-term solution. If surgery is not an option, then consideration should be given to palliation with a percutaneous endoscopically or radiologically placed gastrostomy tube. This is much less morbid for the patient and can be successfully placed in the presence of ascites and carcinomatosis. Alternatively, if this type of gastrostomy tube is not an option and emesis predominates, octreotide has been reported to effectively halt emesis within 2 to 3 days of initiating treatment at a dose of 0.3 to 0.6 mg per day, thereby avoiding prolonged nasogastric tube decompression.

Management of Ascites

Ascites is common at the time of diagnosis and recurrence of ovarian cancer. It often responds to primary chemotherapy, but, as the disease becomes refractory, it may need to be drained when the patient becomes symptomatic. The

BOX 23–10 TREATMENT OF ASCITES IN OVARIAN CANCER

- Intravenous chemotherapy
- Intraperitoneal chemotherapy
- Intermittent paracentesis
- Placement of indwelling catheter (e.g., Tenckhoff, pigtail)
- Peritoneovenous shunt

most common associated symptoms are early satiety, nausea, solid food intolerance, abdominal pain, and shortness of breath. Paracentesis can safely be performed intermittently and rapidly without concern for hemodynamic instability. Patients should be counseled that tumor nodules may develop in the skin at the paracentesis site. For this reason, if paracentesis is performed before a primary surgical debulking, then the ideal approach is in the midline so that the site can be easily excised with the incision.

Paracentesis or placement of a Tenckhoff catheter (Tyco Healthcare, Mansfield, MA), an intraperitoneal port, or a pigtail catheter for individualized drainage by the patient is more useful than intraperitoneal instillation of sclerosing agents or peritoneovenous shunts. These catheters can be placed surgically, but placement by the members of the dialysis unit or interventional radiologists may be easier for the patient. These indwelling catheters are usually placed after the patient has required two or three paracenteses in rapid succession. For the women who obtain several weeks of relief after a single paracentesis, these catheters are not indicated.

Ovarian Germ Cell Tumors

Germ cell tumors deserve special comment, because, with the exception of dysgerminoma, they are unilateral 95% of the time or greater. These tumors generally occur during the first and second decades of life, so conservative surgery with unilateral oophorectomy or salpingo-oophorectomy and staging is the preferred surgical approach. Postoperative chemotherapy with bleomycin, etoposide, and cisplatin is associated with high subsequent survival and fertility rates. Optimal cytoreduction should be attempted, because it positively affects ultimate outcome. Second-look laparotomy is indicated for those tumors without a tumor marker, those with gross residual disease after the original surgery, and those that contain elements of immature teratoma.

BOX 23–11 SURGICAL STAGING OF GERM-CELL TUMORS OF THE OVARY

- Vertical incision
- Send ascites for cytology, or obtain wash ings of pelvis, both paracolic gutters, and upper abdomen
- Inspect the entire peritoneal cavity with biopsies, as indicated
- Unilateral oophorectomy (with intact tumor removal)
- Bilateral salpingo-oophorectomy for bilateral involvement, dysgerminoma, or patient desire
- Bilateral pelvic and paraaortic lymph-node dissection
- Cytoreduction to microscopic disease
- For localized disease, perform random biopsies of both paracolic gutters, cul de sac, both lateral pelvic side walls, vesicouterine reflection, both diaphragms, and any adhesions
- Omentectomy

Prophylactic Bilateral Salpingo-oophorectomy

Prophylactic bilateral salpingo-oophorectomy is considered for women with a strong family history of ovary and/or breast cancer, particularly women with a known BRCA1 or BRCA2 mutation, in whom the lifetime risk of ovarian cancer is estimated to be 16% to 30%. It is important to point out that, even after a bilateral oophorectomy, an estimated 3.5% of these women can still develop a primary peritoneal carcinoma. In women with hereditary non-polyposis colon cancer, because of their increased risk of endometrial and ovarian cancer, total abdominal hysterectomy and bilateral salpingo-oophorectomy may also be indicated at the time of colectomy if fertility is not a concern. Women with a mismatch repair gene mutation have a lifetime risk of 25% to 50% of developing endometrial cancer and an 8% to 12% risk of developing ovarian cancer.

Bilateral prophylactic oophorectomy may also be considered at the time of surgery for gastrointestinal cancer, because only 50% of the metastases are detected prospectively. The risk of metastases to the ovaries in colon and gastric cancer is estimated to be between 3% and 8%. As many as 50% of the metastases occur in premenopausal women. It is possible that premenopausal women develop ovarian metastases at a higher rate than do postmenopausal women and that metastectomy may improve survival. Ideally, the possibility of bilateral salpingo-oophorectomy should be discussed preoperatively, especially in premenopausal women; this is because, despite a higher potential risk of colorectal metastases, their fertility will be affected, and this may be an unacceptable tradeoff.

Endometrial Cancer

Endometrial cancer has easily identifiable risk factors and typically presents with symptoms

BOX 23-12 POSSIBLE SITUATIONS FOR PROPHYLACTIC BILATERAL SALPINGO-OOPHORECTOMY

- Known BRCA1 or BRCA2 mutation in women past childbearing or >35 years old
- Hereditary nonpolyposis colon cancer (Lynch 2 syndrome) in women past childbearing age (a total abdominal hysterectomy and bilateral salpingo-oophorectomy should be considered)
- At the time of surgery for gastric or colon cancer in postmenopausal women and possibly in premenopausal women

that lead to an early diagnosis. The average age at diagnosis is 60 years, with only 25% of patients diagnosed when they are less than 40 years old. A significant risk factor for developing endometrial cancer is an excess exposure to both endogenous and exogenous estrogens. Other risk factors include obesity, hypertension, a family history of endometrial cancer, and a personal history of hereditary nonpolyposis colon cancer. In the United States, the disease is more prominent among white women; however, the overall 5-year survival is significantly worse in black women. This survival disparity is true for all stages of the disease. Although, stage for stage, endometrial cancer is as deadly as ovarian cancer, 73% of women diagnosed with endometrial cancer will be found to have local disease, and 96% of these patients will achieve long-term survival.

BOX 23-13 CLINICAL RISK FACTORS FOR ENDOMETRIAL CANCER

- Early menarche
- Late menopause
- Nulliparity
- Anovulation
- Tamoxifen
- Hormone-replacement therapy

Symptoms

The most common clinical finding in women with endometrial cancer is abnormal uterine bleeding. The incidence of endometrial cancer in women presenting with postmenopausal bleeding ranges from 4% to 25%. However, of the women who are ultimately diagnosed with endometrial cancer, 90% report a history of abnormal bleeding.

BOX 23-14 PRESENTING SIGNS AND SYMPTOMS OF ENDOMETRIAL CANCER

- Vaginal bleeding (especially postmenopausal)
- Purulent vaginal discharge
- Pyometra
- Enlarged uterus
- Adnexal mass
- Pelvic pain
- Abnormal PAP smear

Women presenting with postmenopausal or abnormal bleeding should undergo a careful visual and speculum examination to rule out a vaginal, cervical, or urethral source. If negative, this examination is followed by evaluation with either an office endometrial sampling or a fractional dilatation and curettage. Endometrial sampling is a sensitive technique for the diagnosis of endometrial carcinoma, with a detection rate as high as 99% in postmenopausal women and 91% in premenopausal women. In addition to the accuracy of an endometrial biopsy, its lack of invasiveness, ease of performance, low morbidity, and low cost make this technique the preferred method for obtaining a clinical diagnosis. However, in a woman who has persistent symptoms that are suggestive of an underlying endometrial malignancy (despite having a negative biopsy), it is recommended to proceed with a fractional dilatation and curettage. Premenopausal women must have a negative pregnancy test before undergoing endometrial biopsy.

Clinical Evaluation and Staging

If a careful clinical gynecologic examination suggests that the carcinoma is likely of an early stage, minimal pretreatment evaluation is necessary. A preoperative CA-125 level is useful for predicting patients who are likely to have extrauterine spread, and obtaining this is recommended. If the CA-125 level is elevated, there is approximately an 80% chance that a woman will harbor disseminated disease, and further evaluation by CT or positron emission tomography scanning is indicated. When there is a low suspicion for advanced disease, then CT scanning, magnetic resonance imaging, positron emission tomography scanning,

BOX 23–15 PREOPERATIVE EVALUATION OF WOMEN WITH PRESUMED EARLY ENDOMETRIAL CANCER

- History and physical
- Pelvic examination
- Chest radiograph
- Complete blood cell count
- Serum chemistries
- CA-125 level
- Electrocardiogram, if clinically indicated
- Consider pelvic ultrasound

and other invasive and costly tests are not indicated. Since 1988, endometrial cancer has been surgically staged according to the guidelines issued by the International Federation of Gynecologists and Obstetricians (Table 23-5)

BOX 23–16 PROGNOSTIC VARIABLES FOR ENDOMETRIAL CANCER

- Patient age
- Tumor grade
- Depth of myometrial invasion
- Presence of lymphovascular space invasion
- Positive peritoneal cytology
- Cervical involvement
- Extrauterine extension

Surgical Management

The initial management of early-stage disease is surgical exploration and staging. When surgically treated in the appropriate manner, 5-year survival rate for women found to have stage I disease is more than 90%. The recommended surgical approach is to enter the abdomen through either a midline vertical or a Maylard incision. A Maylard incision is a transverse abdominal incision that involves the isolation and transaction of the inferior epigastric vessels and the transaction of the rectus abdominus muscles. Upon entering the peritoneal cavity, peritoneal washings for cytology should be obtained from both paracolic gutters and the pelvis. A thorough exploration of all intraabdominal surfaces and organs for evidence of metastatic disease is completed; following this with a careful examination of the aortic and pelvic lymphatic regions for any enlarged or suspicious lymph nodes is recommended. Critical components of the surgical approach are the extrafascial total abdominal hysterectomy, the bilateral salpingo-oophorectomy, and the pelvic and paraaortic lymphadenectomy. An omentectomy is indicated in patients with obvious metastatic disease or a high-grade lesion on initial biopsy. Because the majority of patients found to have metastatic spread to the lymphatic system have microscopic disease, the palpation of nodal regions alone is not an acceptable alternative to completing a lymphadenectomy. Therefore, when technically feasible, all patients should undergo pelvic and paraaortic lymphadenectomy.

TABLE 23–5 • *International Federation of Gynecology and Obstetrics Staging Criteria for Endometrial Cancer*

Stage I	**Tumor confined to the uterine corpus**
Ia	Tumor limited to the endometrium
Ib	Tumor invades up to less than half the myometrium
Ic	Tumor invades to more than half the myometrium
Stage II	**Tumor invades the cervix but does not extend beyond the uterus**
IIa	Endocervical glandular involvement only
IIb	Cervical stromal invasion
Stage III	**Local and/or regional spread**
IIIa	Tumor involves serosa and/or adnexa (direct extension or metastasis) and/or cancer cells in ascites or peritoneal washings
IIIb	Vaginal involvement
IIIc	Metastasis to retroperitoneal lymph nodes
Stage IVa	**Tumor involves bladder mucosa and/or bowel mucosa**
Stage IVb	**Distant metastasis**

From Benedet JL, Hacker NF, Ngan HYS. *Staging classifications and clinical practice guidelines of gynaecologic cancers.* Available at: www.figo.org/content/PDF/staging-booklet.pdf. Accessed May 10, 2006.

An exception to this recommendation would be the patient who is found to have clear evidence of metastatic disease to one or more lymph nodes or pelvic structures and who will require postoperative pelvic radiation. In this case, the recommendation is to remove the enlarged lymph nodes and/or all evidence of macroscopic pelvic disease and to proceed with only the paraaortic lymphadenectomy. This refinement of technique spares the patient the morbidity associated with radiation therapy after lymphadenectomy, and it permits determination of the appropriate radiation ports.

Alternative surgical approaches to early endometrial cancer include a total vaginal hysterectomy with a bilateral salpingo-oophorectomy in women who are medically unstable or who have contraindications to major abdominal surgery. Ideally, this approach would only be used in patients with well-differentiated endometrioid adenocarcinomas, and it would be avoided in patients with high-grade lesions or aggressive cell types, such as clear-cell or papillary serous carcinomas. In women who desire a less-invasive procedure, a total laparoscopic hysterectomy, a bilateral salpingo-oophorectomy, and a pelvic and paraaortic lymphadenectomy is an option. Early studies suggest that the laparoscopic approach has similar outcomes with respect to disease recurrence and overall survival. However, to date, there are no randomized, prospective studies that have compared laparotomy with laparoscopy for treating endometrial cancer. The Gynecologic Oncology Group is currently conducting a phase III randomized trial to address this question. Until this study is completed, the laparoscopic management of endometrial cancer must be considered experimental.

Cervical Cancer

Screening for cervical cancer in the United States with Pap smears has reduced the incidence by nearly 80%, and it has improved overall survival rates. The overall survival rate for cervical cancer is approximately 71% to 92% for stage I disease. The most common age at the diagnosis of carcinoma in situ, which is the precursor lesion to invasive carcinoma, is 30 to 35 years, whereas invasive disease most commonly occurs after the age of 40 years. The most common symptom of cervical cancer is posttraumatic or intermenstrual bleeding. The diagnosis is made by biopsy, and the staging is clinical. Squamous cell carcinoma is the most frequent histology, but adenocarcinoma now represents approximately 25% of cases, and it seems to be rising in incidence.

BOX 23-17 RISK FACTORS FOR THE DEVELOPMENT OF CERVICAL CANCER

- Early coitarche
- Multiple sexual partners
- High-risk sexual partners
- Smoking
- History of human papilloma virus infection
- History of an abnormal PAP smear
- Low socioeconomic status
- Immunosuppression
- Intravenous drug abuse
- Multiple pregnancies
- In utero diethylstilbestrol exposure

Treatment

Treatment for women diagnosed with cervical cancer depends on the clinical stage of the lesion. Table 23-6 presents the International Federation of Gynecology and Obstetrics staging system. For microinvasive lesions, surgical options include cold-knife conization of the cervix, trachelectomy (surgical removal of the cervix), and simple hysterectomy. For International Federation of Gynecology and Obstetrics stages IA2 to IIA, treatment is either a radical hysterectomy and bilateral pelvic lymphadenectomy or external-beam pelvic radiation and intracavitary implants with concurrent chemosensitization. The efficacy of both treatments for localized disease is similar. Radical trachelectomy with pelvic lymphadenectomy may be used in select patients with cancer in stages IA2 to IB1. For more advanced stages of disease, treatment should consist of a combination of chemotherapy and radiation.

Recurrent Cervical Cancer

When cervical cancer recurs, there are several therapeutic options, with individual treatment depending on the site of the recurrence, the type of prior therapy, and the patient's overall medical health. For distant recurrences, patients are treated with chemotherapy. Response rates to chemotherapy are typically 10% to 50% and of short duration. Disease outside of the previously radiated field is much more likely to respond to chemotherapy.

TABLE 23–6 • *International Federation of Gynecology and Obstetrics Staging Criteria for Cervical Cancer*

Stage 0	**Carcinoma in situ**
Stage I	**Carcinoma confined to the cervix**
Ia1	Invasion ≤3 mm in depth and ≤7 mm in diameter
Ia2	Invasion >3 mm in depth and ≤5 mm in depth and ≤7 mm in diameter
Ib1	Lesion >5 mm in depth and/or >7 mm in diameter but ≤4 cm in diameter
Ib2	Lesion >4 cm
Stage II	**Tumor extends beyond cervix but not to pelvic wall; may involve the vagina, but not the lower third**
IIa	No parametrial involvement
Iib	Parametrial involvement
Stage III	**Tumor extends to the pelvic side wall; may involve the lower third of the vagina**
IIIa	No extension to side wall
IIIb	Extension to pelvic wall; includes all cases with hydronephrosis or a nonfunctioning kidney
Stage IV	**Spread beyond the true pelvis or involvement of the bladder and rectal mucosa**
IVa	Spread to the adjacent organs
IVb	Spread to distant organs

From Benedet JL, Hacker NF, Ngan HYS. *Staging classifications and clinical practice guidelines of gynaecologic cancers.* Available at: www.figo.org/content/PDF/staging-booklet.pdf. Accessed May 10, 2006.

An exception would be patients who are found to have metastatic bone lesions; these patients are treated with focal radiation. For local pelvic recurrences in patients who were initially treated with surgery, radiation with chemosensitization is the treatment of choice. For patients with a central pelvic recurrence who have received radiation therapy and who have no evidence of metastatic disease, a potentially curative surgical option is a total pelvic exenteration. Pelvic exenteration, when performed on properly selected patients, is associated with a 5-year survival rate of 61%, which is a much better outcome that that seen with chemotherapy. Pelvic reconstruction after the initial surgical resection typically includes the formation of either an ileal conduit or a continent urinary pouch, the completion of an end colostomy, or, if a supralevator total pelvic exenteration is performed, a primary colorectal reanastomosis using a circular stapling device. A vaginal reconstruction may also be completed.

Vaginal reconstruction after a pelvic exenteration should be performed in women who want to retain sexual function. Many types of vaginal reconstruction have been described in the literature, including myocutaneous flaps, split-thickness skin grafts, and bowel interposition. Split-thickness skin graft vaginoplasty is a straightforward surgical option. The skin graft is harvested from the anterior or medial thigh. The recommended thickness of the graft is .015 to .017 of an inch. The length of the graft needs to be sufficient to cover the entire vaginal vault, without tension. To avoid complications resulting from contracture of the graft and the formation of hematomas and seromas, it is generally recommended to complete a meshed graft with a 1.5 to 3:1 ratio. An omental J-flap is created and serves as a vascular bed for the graft. Alternatively, a peritoneal patch may serve to cover the upper vagina. The graft is then stabilized using gauze packing to ensure close apposition of the graft to the bed. The distal edges of the graft are sutured to the introitus. The surgeon's preference determines whether the graft should be performed at the time of the pelvic exenteration or after a delay of 1 week. There is no significant difference in the surgical outcome or percentage of graft take in patients who underwent immediate reconstruction as compared with those who underwent a delayed reconstructive procedure.

Regardless of the procedure used to complete the reconstruction of the vagina, patients should be selected carefully preoperatively, and they should be counseled appropriately with regard to the psychosexual changes after a pelvic exenteration. Patients should be made aware of the necessity for the diligent postoperative use of a vaginal obturator and/or the need for the resumption of sexual intercourse to ensure the formation of an adequate vaginal vault. There should be a clear understanding of the potential long-term complications, including abnormal vaginal discharge, vaginal stenosis, dyspareunia, and pelvic pain.

Vaginal Cancer

Primary vaginal cancer is the least common gynecologic malignancy. The risk factors, natural history, and underlying etiology of vaginal cancer are not well defined, largely as a result of the relative infrequency of the disease. However, it is recognized that women who have undergone a hysterectomy for cervical dysplasia or carcinoma have an increased risk of developing a vaginal malignancy. Therefore, it is recommended that these patients continue to undergo Pap smears, despite having undergone a hysterectomy.

Patients with vaginal cancer typically present with complaints of abnormal vaginal bleeding. Other common symptoms include urinary complaints, pelvic pain, and abnormal vaginal discharge. Most women who develop vaginal cancer are between the ages of 50 and 70 years. The most common histologic type is squamous. An initial careful gynecologic examination with the evaluation of all vaginal surfaces, followed by tissue biopsy of an obvious lesion, is essential for making the diagnosis. The most common site for a vaginal cancer is the posterior aspect of the upper third of the vagina.

Clinical Evaluation

Further workup typically includes a careful history and physical examination, a chest radiograph, a complete blood cell count, a comprehensive serum chemistry panel, and an abdominopelvic CT scan or magnetic resonance image that includes imaging of the entire vaginal vault. As with cervical cancer, when there is suspicion of locally advanced disease, cystoscopy and sigmoidoscopy should be used to evaluate for bladder and bowel involvement. Staging of each lesion should be performed clinically according to the International Federation of Gynecology and Obstetrics or American Joint Committee on Cancer staging systems (Table 23-7). The majority of patients are diagnosed with stage I or II disease. Five-year survival rates for patients with stage I and stage II lesions are approximately 73% and 58%, respectively. Women with more advanced lesions generally have a poor outcome.

Treatment Considerations

The standard of care for the majority of vaginal cancers is whole pelvic radiation and vaginal brachytherapy. Exceptions to this approach include vaginal cancers that arise in the upper third of the vagina, localized stage IV lesions, and pelvic recurrences. Lesions in the upper third of the vagina can be treated with a radical abdominal hysterectomy and bilateral pelvic lymphadenectomy. Stage IV lesions and central pelvic recurrences can be extirpated with a total pelvic exenteration.

Posttreatment Sequelae for Lower Genital Tract Malignancies Treated with Radiation Therapy

Many of the treatment regimens for ovarian, cervical, endometrial, and vaginal cancer incorporate radiation therapy. The surgical

TABLE 23-7 • *International Federation of Gynecology and Obstetrics Staging Criteria for Vaginal Cancer*

Stage 0	**Carcinoma in situ**
Stage I	**Tumor confined to the vaginal mucosa**
Stage II	**Tumor invades the paravaginal tissues but does not extend to the pelvic sidewall**
IIa	Subvaginal infiltration, but not to parametrium
IIb	Parametrial infiltration, but not extending to the pelvic sidewall
Stage III	**Tumor extends to the pelvic sidewall**
Stage IV	**Tumor involves the adjacent organs or distant metastases**
IVa	Tumor invades the mucosa of the bladder or rectum and/or extends beyond the true pelvis (bullous edema is not included)
IVb	Distant metastases

From Benedet JL, Hacker NF, Ngan HYS. *Staging classifications and clinical practice guidelines of gynaecologic cancers.* Available at: www.figo.org/content/PDF/staging-booklet.pdf. Accessed May 10, 2006.

oncologist might encounter several side effects of radiation, including proctitis, sigmoiditis, bowel obstruction or stricture, and fistulas. Side effects are more likely if the patient has undergone both radiation and radical surgery.

Gastrointestinal side effects occur usually within the first 2 years after radiation therapy, whereas genitourinary side effects occur most commonly after 3 to 4 years. Rectal and vaginal complications are associated with brachytherapy, whereas small bowel and sigmoid disease are more likely related to the teletherapy. Radiation proctitis that is unresponsive to conservative therapy may require resection and reanastomosis. A diverting colostomy or ileostomy is recommended after the resection and reanastomosis of irradiated colon. The terminal ileum is most vulnerable to radiation-induced damage because of its position in the peritoneal cavity. Resection of the terminal ileum and the ascending colon with ileocolonic reanastomosis is the preferred approach to minimize the use of heavily irradiated bowel in the anastomosis.

It is not uncommon to encounter an agglutinated mass of small bowel adherent in the pelvis as the cause of a small bowel obstruction. In this case, wide resection of the involved small bowel is a surgical option. If the loops of small bowel are involved in an enterovaginal fistula and cannot be resected, then total exclusion from the fecal stream is recommended, with the creation of an ileal mucous fistula proximal to the enterovaginal fistula to reduce vaginal drainage and irritation. The exposure of the vagina and the vulva to enteric fluid causes significant pain and a reduction in the quality of life.

Primary rectovaginal fistula repair of previously radiated tissue without diverting colostomy or the introduction of a new blood supply often fails as a result of extensive scarring, inflammation, and poor blood supply. Repair can be attempted after diverting colostomy has allowed for the resolution of the inflammation and after a biopsy has excluded recurrent cancer. Sources of a fresh blood supply to supplement the repair include the bulbocavernosus fat pad, gracilis and rectus myocutaneous grafts, and the colonic patch. This colonic patch uses an adjacent portion of normal colon to cover the fistula.

Brachytherapy can also lead to vaginal and cervical stenosis. The vaginal effects can be reduced by encouraging diligent use of a vaginal dilator with or without vaginal estrogen cream. An agglutinated vagina should be treated with dilatation with dilators of progressively increasing size, with surgical cannulation reserved for unresponsive cases. Operative reestablishment of the vaginal canal is associated with the potential for bleeding and fistula formation, and it can be difficult to perform in the presence of dense adhesions. Performing it under ultrasound guidance with saline distension of the bladder and frequent assessment of the rectal lumen can reduce these complications.

Cervical stenosis can lead to a fluid collection in the endometrial cavity, with concomitant symptoms of pelvic pain and a palpable mass. Although a CT scan is often ordered, the diagnosis is easily made by recognition of symptoms, pelvic examination, and ultrasound. The first line of treatment is cervical dilatation, curettage, and drainage under ultrasound guidance. As a result of the low but real risk of endometrial cancer and the possibility of cervical cancer recurrence, the specimens should be sent for pathologic analysis.

Key Selected Reading

Hoskins WJ, Young RC, Markman M, *et al. Principles and practice of gynecologic oncology,* 4th ed. Philadelphia: Lippincott Williams & Wilkins, 2004.

Selected Readings

Acs G, Gombos Z. Prognostic factors and new methods in cervical carcinoma. *Pathology Case Reviews* 2006;11:130–139.

Amant F, Moerman P, Neven P, *et al.* Endometrial cancer. *Lancet* 2005;366:491–505.

Armstrong DK, Bundy B, Wenzel L, *et al.* Intraperitoneal cisplatin and paclitaxel in ovarian cancer. *N Engl J Med* 2006;354:34–43.

Brooks SE, Zweizig SL, Wakely K. Ovarian cancer: a clinician's perspective. *Pathology Case Reviews* 2006;11:3–8.

Cannistra SA. Medical progress: cancer of the ovary. *N Engl J Med* 2004;351:2519–2529.

Curtin JP. Management of the adnexal mass. *Gynecol Oncol* 1994;55:S42–S46.

Hopkins MP, Morely GW. Radical hysterectomy versus radiation therapy for stage IB squamous cell cancer of the cervix. *Cancer* 1991;1:173–177.

Morice P, Dubernard G, Rey A, *et al.* Results of interval debulking surgery compared with primary debulking surgery in advanced stage ovarian cancer. *J Am Coll Surg* 2003;197:955–963.

Morrow PC, Curtin JP. *Gynecologic cancer surgery.* New York: Churchill Livingstone, 1996.

Munkarah AR, Coleman R. Critical evaluation of secondary cytoreduction in recurrent ovarian cancer. *Gynecol Oncol* 2004;95:273–280.

Pothuri B, Vaidya A, Aghajanian C, *et al.* Palliative surgery for bowel obstruction in recurrent ovarian cancer: an updated series. *Gynecol Oncol* 2003;89:306–313.

Sherard GB, Hodson CA, Williams J, *et al.* Adnexal masses and pregnancy: a 12-year experience. *Am J Obstet Gynecol* 2003;189:358–363.

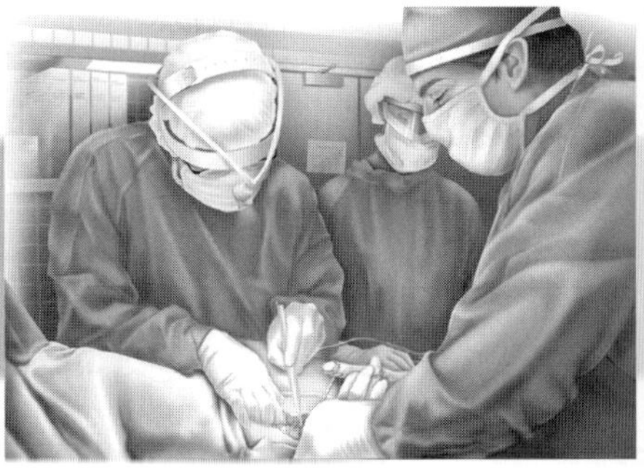

24

Urologic Oncology

Alejandro Rodriguez and Julio M. Pow-Sang

PROSTATE CANCER	KIDNEY CANCER
BLADDER CANCER	

Urologic Oncology: Key Points

- Describe the presentation, diagnosis, staging, and treatment of prostate cancer.
- Discuss the presentation, diagnosis, treatment, and outcomes of bladder cancer.
- Detail the risk factors, presentation, diagnosis, staging, and treatment of kidney cancer

Prostate Cancer

Prostate cancer is the most common cancer in the United States. It is estimated that 234,000 men will be diagnosed in 2006 and that 27,000 will die from this cancer, making it the third most prevalent cause of cancer mortality among American men. Despite these dire statistics, the presentation of the disease has changed dramatically over the last 15 years. Before the 1990s, two thirds of the cancers were diagnosed as advanced and not amenable to long-term cure. Today, more than two thirds present at an early stage and are curable with local treatment modalities. Improvements in techniques and technology within the last two decades are improving the quality of life of those treated, with shorter convalescence and decreased complication rates.

Presentation

The majority of patients present today with elevation of the prostate-specific antigen (PSA) test. The most common scenario is a man who is evaluated by his primary care physician. The practitioner obtains a PSA level as part of the general medical evaluation. The second most common presentation is the presence of an abnormal digital rectal examination discovered as part of the patient's evaluation by the primary care physician. In either of these two

BOX 24–1 RECOMMENDATIONS FOR PROSTATE CANCER SCREENING BY THE AMERICAN CANCER SOCIETY, THE NATIONAL CANCER COMPREHENSIVE NETWORK, AND THE AMERICAN UROLOGIC ASSOCIATION

Both the prostate-specific antigen blood test and the digital rectal examination should be offered annually, beginning at age 50, to men who have at least a 10-year life expectancy. Men at high risk (African-American men and men with a strong family history of one or more first-degree relatives [father, brothers] diagnosed at an early age) should begin testing at age 45. Men at even higher risk as a result of having multiple first-degree relatives affected at an early age could begin testing at age 40. Depending on the results of this initial test, no further testing might be needed until age 45.

cases, the patient is referred to a urologist, who proceeds with a transrectal ultrasound of the prostate with biopsies. Although it is rarely seen today, the patient may present with lower urinary tract symptoms such as decreased force or urinary stream, frequency, urgency, nocturia, or sensation of incomplete bladder emptying.

Diagnosis

The diagnosis is established by performing a transrectal ultrasound of the prostate with biopsies of the organ (Figures 24-1 and 24-2). It is important that at least 10 biopsies are obtained, because the yield of the outdated "sextant" biopsies is low and likely to miss

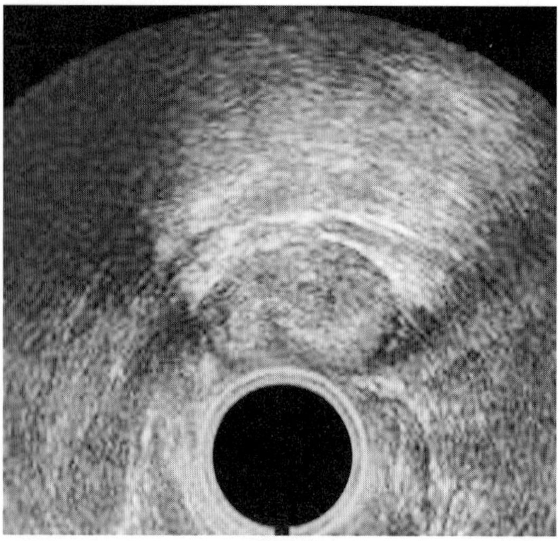

Figure 24–1. Transrectal ultrasound of the prostate.

BOX 24–2 SIGNS AND SYMPTOMS OF LOCALIZED PROSTATE CANCER

- Abnormal digital rectal examination
- Lower urinary tract obstruction
  - Decreased force of urinary stream
  - Frequency
  - Urgency
  - Nocturia
  - Sensation of incomplete bladder emptying
- Hematuria
- Rectal obstruction (rare)
- Priapism (rare)

significant cancers. It is also important to map the location of the specimen as it relates to the prostate area in which each biopsy was obtained so that the exact location and extent of the cancer is established, because this will better tailor the delivery of nonsurgical treatments of the cancer. The described areas are the right base, mid prostate, and apex and the left base, mid prostate, and apex.

Staging

Today, because the majority of cancers present at a very early stage, there is rarely a need to

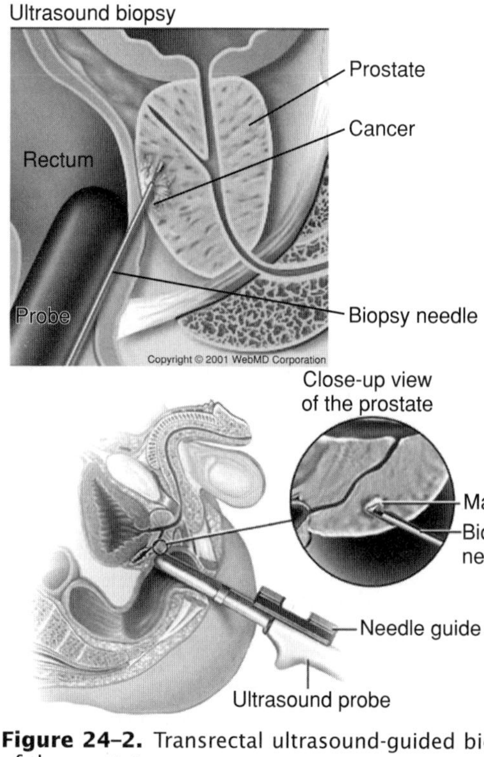

Figure 24–2. Transrectal ultrasound-guided biopsy of the prostate.

perform additional staging studies, such as a bone scan or a computed tomography (CT) scan of the pelvis (Table 24-1). For cases in which the PSA level is greater than 20 or there is significant Gleason 7 cancer or the presence of a Gleason 8, 9, or 10 cancers (Figure 24-3), these studies then should be obtained. Using predictive algorithms, the practitioner may establish the probability of extracapsular extension, the presence of cancer in regional lymph nodes, and the probability of recurrence 5 years after definitive treatment (Figure 24-4).

Treatment

Localized Disease

There are four major management options for localized prostate cancer.

BOX 24-3 TREATMENT OPTIONS FOR PROSTATE CANCER

- Surgery
  - Open radical prostatectomy
  - Laparoscopic prostatectomy
- Radiation therapy
  - External beam radiation
  - Brachytherapy
  - Combined external beam radiation and brachytherapy
- Cryosurgery
- Active surveillance

Surgery

The surgical management of prostate cancer is rapidly evolving. Up to the year 2000, the major surgical approach was with the open retropubic prostatectomy, popularized by Dr. Patrick Walsh in 1980. He described the anatomical radical prostatectomy as consisting of early control of the dorsal vein complex (Santorini's plexus), with preservation of the neurovascular bundles. These improvements in technique decreased the incidence of intraoperative bleeding and improved continence and potency rates.

BOX 24-4 POSSIBLE COMPLICATIONS OF PROSTATECTOMY

- Anastomotic stricture
- Incontinence
- Erectile dysfunction

In 1997, two French surgeons named Guillonneau and Vallencien reported on their experience with laparoscopic radical prostatectomy. Since their initial report, the majority of centers in Europe and now major centers in the United States perform the procedure by laparoscopy. A recent development to assist in the laparoscopic procedure is the introduction of the DaVinci robot as an interface to augment the surgeon's skills.

Table 24-1 • American Joint Committee on Cancer Prostate Primary Tumor Staging System

Primary tumor (T)	
TX	Primary tumor cannot be assessed
T0	No evidence of primary tumor
T1	Clinically inapparent tumor not palpable nor visible by imaging
T1a	Tumor incidental histologic finding in ≤5% of tissue resected
T1b	Tumor incidental histologic finding in >5% of tissue resected
T1c	Tumor identified by needle biopsy (e.g., because of elevated prostate-specific antigen level)
T2	Tumor confined within prostate*
T2a	Tumor involves 50% of one lobe or less
T2b	Tumor involves >50% of one lobe but not both lobes
T2c	Tumor involves both lobes
T3	Tumor extends through the prostate capsule†
T3a	Extracapsular extension (unilateral or bilateral)
T3b	Tumor invades seminal vesicle(s)
T4	Tumor is fixed or invades adjacent structures other than seminal vesicles: bladder neck, external sphincter, rectum, levator muscles, and/or pelvic wall

*Tumor found in one or both lobes by needle biopsy but not palpable or reliably visible by imaging is classified as T1c.
†Invasion into the prostatic apex or into (but not beyond) the prostatic capsule is not classified as T3 but rather as T2.

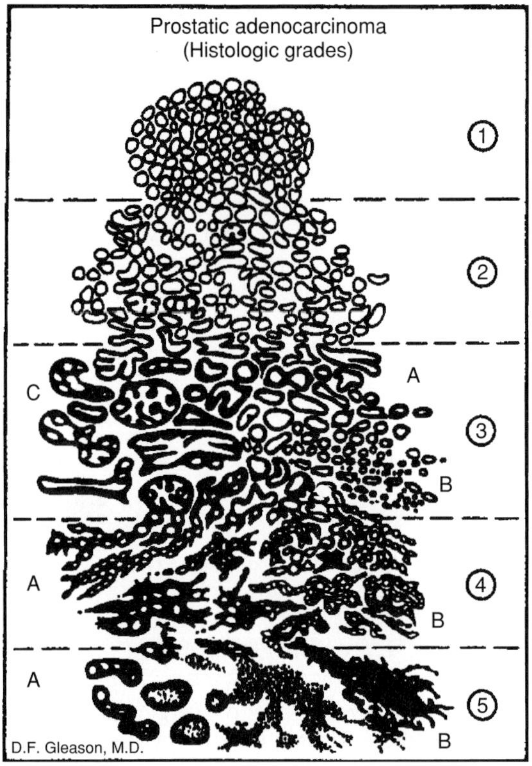

Figure 24–3. The Gleason grading system includes five histologic patterns distinguished by the glandular architecture of the cancer under low to medium magnification. The final Gleason score is the sum of the grades of the primary and secondary growth patterns. Thus, the Gleason score can range from 2^{1+1} to 10^{5+5}.

If the likelihood of finding nodal disease is high (increasing PSA, Gleason score, clinical stage), a pelvic lymph node dissection is warranted. This can be performed in an open manner or laparoscopically.

Radiation Therapy

External Beam Radiation Therapy

Radiation therapy is an effective treatment for localized prostate cancer. Newer technologies consisting of better collimators and computers allow for more precise delivery of the radiation beam to the prostate while minimizing exposure to structures around it (e.g., bladder, rectum), so toxicity is controlled. The most recent development has been the introduction of intensity modulated radiation therapy (IMRT).

Brachytherapy

An alternative means of radiation therapy delivery is the direct placement of radiation sources into the organ. This is today the most common treatment for localized prostate cancer. Two radioactive sources are used: iodine-125 and palladium-103.

Combination External Beam Radiation Therapy with Brachytherapy

To minimize toxicity and increase delivery outside and around the prostate, some practi-

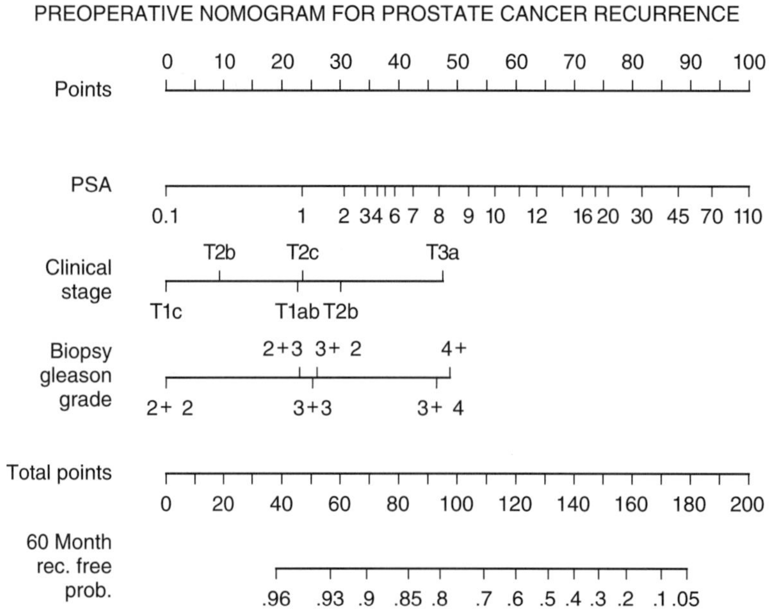

Figure 24–4. Using a nomogram based on the prostate-specific antigen level, the Gleason score, and the clinical stage, one can predict the probability of recurrence after prostatectomy. (From Kattan MW, Eastham JA, Stapleton AMF, *et al.* A preoperative nomogram for disease recurrence following radical prostatectomy for prostate cancer. *J Natl Cancer Inst* 1998;90;766–771.)

BOX 24-5 POSSIBLE COMPLICATIONS OF PROSTATE IRRADIATION

- Rectal complications
  - Diarrhea
  - Rectal bleeding
  - Obstruction
  - Fistula
- Urinary complications
  - Frequency of urination or nocturia
  - Bladder spasm
  - Dysuria
  - Urgency
  - Hematuria
  - Severe hemorrhagic cystitis
  - Erectile dysfunction

tioners combine the two radiation modalities, especially for cancers that are considered to be at intermediate or high risk of failure after treatment with either of the single modalities.

Cryosurgery

Subfreezing temperatures to destroy tumors have been used since the turn of the century. For prostate cancer, the procedure was first used more than 30 years ago, with the delivery of liquid nitrogen directly into the prostate through an open transperineal approach. With the advent of transrectal ultrasound and percutaneous techniques, the procedure is now performed in a way that is similar to brachytherapy.

Observation

Prostate cancer is a slow-growing cancer, especially during the early stages. In addition, many of these cancers will be diagnosed in elderly men in whom the cancer will never manifest clinical symptoms (clinically insignificant cancers). In these men, expectant management with PSA and biopsy follow up is recommended, with treatment offered when the cancer becomes more biologically active. It is estimated that 10% of men are amenable to this management alternative and that one third will require treatment within the first 3 to 5 years of follow up.

Advanced Disease

The primary treatment for advanced prostate cancer is hormonal therapy. Prostate cancer is a hormone-sensitive cancer, and it depends on testosterone for growth. Thus, testosterone withdrawal is the goal of treatment. This may be achieved by surgical or medical castration. The latter is currently the most common treatment, because it is reversible and does not subject the patient to the psychological impact of orchiectomy. Luteinizing-hormone-releasing hormone agonists are used with or without an antiandrogen. For patients with hormore-refractory cancer, chemotherapy with docetaxel or docetaxel and estramustine should be considered.

Bladder Cancer

Bladder cancer is the second most common urologic malignancy, after prostate cancer. The majority of these cancers (93%) are transitional cell carcinomas, with only 5% presenting as squamous cell carcinomas and 2% as adenocarcinomas. Eighty percent of bladder cancers present as superficial, 15% present as invasive, and 5% present as metastatic disease.

Superficial bladder cancers are a heterogeneous group of cancers with variable biologic potentials. Three substages of superficial bladder cancer are defined: *Ta,* papillary and limited to the urothelium; *T1,* papillary tumor invading the underlying lamina propria; and *Tcis* (carcinoma in situ), flat, reddened lesions on cystoscopy, with high-grade histologic features (i.e., changes throughout the whole thickness of the urothelium, marked loss of polarity, and easily found mitotic figures) (Table 24-2).

Presentation

The most common clinical presentation is asymptomatic gross or microscopic hematuria. Occasionally, patients present with irritative voiding symptoms such as dysuria, frequency, and urgency.

Diagnosis

When the presence of transitional cell carcinoma is suspected, a full urologic evaluation consisting of cystoscopy, urinary cytology, and intravenous pyelogram is mandatory. This evaluation allows for the assessment of the whole urinary tract, because tumor lesions may be located anywhere along the upper urinary tract (calyces, renal pelvis, ureters), the lower urinary tract (bladder, proximal urethra), or both. When a lesion is noted on cystoscopy, the configuration (flat, sessile, papillary),

TABLE 24-2 • American Joint Committee on Cancer Bladder TNM Staging System

Primary Tumor (T)	
Superficial bladder cancer	
TX	A primary tumor cannot be assessed
T0	No primary tumor seen
Ta	Superficial cancer is found only in polyps (papillary) on the surface of the inner lining of the bladder; lymph nodes are not involved, and cancer has not spread (metastasized)
Tis	Carcinoma in situ; tumor is found only in flat lesions on the surface of the inner lining of the bladder; lymph nodes are not involved, and cancer has not spread (metastasized)
T1	Tumor is found in the connective tissue below the lining of the bladder but has not spread to the bladder muscle; lymph nodes are not involved, and cancer has not spread (metastasized)
Invasive bladder cancer	
T2a	Tumor has spread to the inner half of the smooth muscle layer (superficial layer), below the lining of the bladder
T2b	Tumor has spread to the outer half of the smooth muscle layer (deep layer) of the bladder
T3a	Tumor has spread through the muscular wall of the bladder into the fatty tissue layer, as identified by microscopic examination
T3b	Tumor has spread through the muscular wall of the bladder, into the fatty tissue layer, and a mass is visible to the eye
T4a	Tumor has spread to the prostate in men and to the uterus or vagina in women
T4b	Tumor has spread to the pelvic or abdominal wall
Regional Lymph Nodes (N)	
NX	Lymph nodes in the pelvis cannot be assessed
N0	No bladder cancer is found in lymph nodes
N1	Bladder cancer is found in one lymph node, 2 cm or less in size
N2	Bladder cancer is found in one lymph node and is more than 2 cm but less than 5 cm in size, or cancer is found in multiple lymph nodes, but none are more than 5 cm in size
N3	Bladder cancer is found in one or more lymph nodes and is more than 5 cm in size
Distant Metastases (M)	
MX	Metastasis cannot be evaluated
M0	No evidence of metastasis
M1	Distant metastases

location (trigone, base, right lateral wall, left lateral wall, dome), size (in centimeters), and number should be noted. The lesion is then removed by a transurethral resection. It is important to completely remove the lesion and to obtain adequate depth of resection into the bladder wall for the pathologist to give an adequate tumor staging of the cancer.

Treatment

Superficial Bladder Cancer

The initial management consists of the complete transurethral resection of any visible tumors and selected biopsies of the bladder mucosa, including the prostatic urethra. An examination under anesthesia is performed both before and after resection. The presence of a palpable mass suggests muscle invasion by tumor. With the cystoscopic and pathology findings, the clinician can determine if further treatment with intravesical therapy is required (if the cancer is superficial and high risk) or if cystectomy or bladder-sparing treatment with chemotherapy and radiation therapy is warranted (if the cancer is invasive with no evidence of metastasis).

If the patient has only superficial bladder cancer, the disease may be stratified as either low risk or high risk for recurrence and progression (Table 24-3).

TABLE 24–3 • *Low-Risk Versus High-Risk Bladder Cancer*

Low-Risk Features	High-Risk Features
First occurrence or long interval since initial therapy	Multiple recurrences overa short period of time
Up to three lesions	Four or more lesions
No lesion >3 cm in size	Any lesion >3 cm
Papillary configuration	Sessile configuration
No invasion of lamina propria	Invasion of lamina propria
Well or moderately differentiated (grade I or II)	Poorly differentiated (grade III)
	Diffuse bladder involvement
	Incomplete resection
	Presence of carcinoma in situ

Low-Risk Group

In most cases, patients present either with a bladder tumor for the first time or with a long interval of time without recurrence. On cystoscopy, there may be up to three lesions up to 3 cm in size and with a papillary configuration. On histopathology, the lesions do not invade the lamina propria (stage Ta), and they are well or moderately differentiated (grade I or II).

Patients with low-risk tumors are managed by transurethral resection (TUR) alone. Patients are followed with periodic cystoscopies and urine cytologies. These examinations are performed every 6 months for the first 2 years and then yearly for at least 5 years.

High-Risk Group

Patients in this group may present with a bladder tumor for the first time, or they may have had multiple recurrences in a short period of time. On cystoscopy, there may be more than three lesions, any of which may be larger than 3 cm, and they will have a less papillary (sessile) appearance. Additional unfavorable findings include incomplete resection as a result of technical problems (e.g., tumor located in an area that is difficult to resect) or diffuse bladder involvement. Pathologically, tumors are high grade and/or invade the lamina propria (T1 lesions). The presence of carcinoma in situ alone or tumor associated with papillary tumors is also an adverse prognostic sign.

Newer assays for the presence of bladder tumor antigen and nuclear matrix protein 22 in voided urine have recently been introduced into clinical practice to supplement the cystoscopic and cytologic evaluation. However, the true role of these newer tumor assays in the routine management of bladder cancer has yet to be defined as a result of their poor specificity. Tumors at high risk of recurrence and progression are treated with intravesical therapy after complete resection of all visible tumors.

Intravesical Therapy Agents

Agents commonly used in the United States are mitomycin C, bacillus Calmette-Guérin (BCG), and interferon. The first-line intravesical agents for superficial bladder cancer are either BCG or mitomycin C. For carcinoma in situ, BCG is the first agent of choice. The optimal dose and treatment schedules for any of the intravesical agents are unknown, but a 6- to 8-week course is usually recommended. Patients for whom primary treatment fails may be treated with a different agent. In the case of BCG, a second course with the same agent may be considered.

Mitomycin C The alkylating agent mitomycin C is used in doses ranging from 20 mg to 60 mg diluted in water at concentrations ranging from 0.5 mg/mL to 2.0 mg/mL. Mitomycin C is administered weekly for 6 to 8 weeks as induction therapy with or without maintenance for 1 year. In one study, the overall response rate was 43% for papillary lesions and 58% for carcinoma in situ. Tolley and colleagues reported on 502 patients after complete resection. Patients were randomized to one of three treatment arms: no further treatment, a single instillation at resection, and immediate instillation of mitomycin C within 24 hours of resection followed by 1 year of maintenance therapy. A benefit was observed for the immediate-instillation group with or without maintenance with regard to recurrence-free survival during the first 2 years of a median follow up of 7 years. A study by Solsona confirmed the beneficial effect of a single instillation of mitomycin C after TUR.

The most common side effects from the intravesical use of mitomycin C are chemical cystitis and allergic skin reactions (Table 24-4).

Bacillus Calmette-Guérin BCG is a live, attenuated form of *Mycobacterium bovis*. The exact mechanism by which BCG produces its antitumor effect is unknown. BCG is considered the most active agent in the treatment of superficial bladder cancer, especially for carcinoma in situ. Morales and associates first reported on the use of BCG for the treatment of superficial bladder cancer in 1976. Since then, multiple studies have confirmed the efficacy of BCG for decreasing tumor recurrences from 83% to 44% and tumor progression from 35% to 7% as compared with TUR alone. A recent study by Herr also demonstrated an improved long-term progression-free survival at a minimum follow up of 15 years with the use of BCG in high-risk patients. Of concern was the finding that 35% of treated patients eventually died of bladder cancer when evaluated for many years. A recent Southwest Oncology Group study addressed the use of maintenance BCG. Standard induction therapy alone (6 weekly treatments) was compared with induction plus maintenance over a period of 3 years. Median recurrence-free survival time was twice as long and progression-free survival was significantly longer in the maintenance arm. Local toxicity as a result of BCG therapy is common but self-limited. Cystitis occurs in 90% of patients, and hematuria occurs in one third of patients. Severe complications such as fever, allergic reactions, and sepsis are rare, and they are usually associated with traumatic catheterization at the time of the BCG instillation. Prompt antituberculosis therapy can be lifesaving if a patient develops a severe reaction to BCG.

TABLE 24-4 • *Potential Side Effects of Intravesical Therapeutic Agents for Bladder Cancer*

Drug	Side Effects
Mitomycin C	Cystitis
	Allergic skin reactions
Bacillus Calmette-Guérin	Cystitis
	Hematuria
	Fever
	Joint pain
	Allergic reactions
	Granulomatous prostatitis
	Tuberculosis
Interferon-α	Cystitis
	Flu-like symptoms
Thiotepa	Cystitis
	Myelosuppression
Doxorubicin	Cystitis
	Gastrointestinal upset
	Allergic reactions

Interferon IFN-α is the most commonly studied interferon for the treatment of superficial bladder cancer. An initial study with IFN-α reported a 38% complete response in eight patients at a dose of 50 million units. A randomized controlled study compared 10 million and 100 million units of IFN-α2b given weekly for 12 weeks and then monthly for 1 year for the treatment of carcinoma in situ. High-dose and low-dose groups achieved complete response rates of 43% and 5%, respectively.

Six of nine patients (67%) who failed prior BCG therapy had a complete response to interferon. Toxicity was low, and only 17% of patients had flu-like symptoms at the higher interferon dose. A recent study evaluated the combined use of low-dose BCG and IFN-α2b. Twelve patients were treated with 60 mg of BCG weekly in combination with IFN-α2b. Four groups of three patients each received interferon in doses of 10 million, 30 million, 60 million, or 100 million units. There were no tumor progressions 12 months after treatment. Two patients had solitary recurrences. The treatment was safe and well tolerated.

Outcomes and Follow-Up

Among patients with superficial bladder cancer, 70% will respond to intravesical therapy, whereas 30% will not and will instead develop a recurrence or progress to invasive disease. Surveillance of all patients with a diagnosis of bladder cancer is mandatory. Evaluation consists of cystoscopy and urine cytology. The frequency of examinations is dependent on risk. For low-risk patients, cystoscopy at 6-month intervals for the ensuing 3 to 5 years is adequate. For high-risk patients, cystoscopy is recommended every 3 months for the first year, every 6 months for 5 years, and yearly for 10 years. Patients with low-grade and low-stage tumors who fail BCG are candidates for a subsequent treatment with other intravesical agents. These patients have a low risk of progression, with multiple recurrences being the major clinical challenge. Of the patients with high-grade tumors and carcinoma in situ for whom a first course of BCG is not effective, 50% will respond to a second course of BCG. Patients who do not respond to this second course of treatment should undergo cystectomy, because they are at a high likelihood (30%-60%) of developing invasive or metastatic disease.

Invasive Bladder Cancer

The standard treatment consists of cystectomy and urinary diversion. Urinary diversion may be achieved by continent or noncontinent techniques. For many years, the ileal conduit urinary diversion was the standard type of urinary diversion. In 1985, Rowland described the cecoileal continent urinary reservoir "Indiana pouch," in which approximately 8 cm to 10 cm of terminal ileum and 25 cm to 30 cm of cecum and ascending colon are isolated (Figure 24-5). The colonic segment is detubularized either by incising along its antimesenteric surface with scissors or cautery or by placing a 60-mm to 75-mm gastrointestinal anastomosis stapler between the two more lateral tenia. The continence mechanism is then created by tapering the efferent limb (terminal ileum) over a 12F red rubber catheter resting against the antimesenteric surface of the ileum. A 60-mm gastrointestinal anastomosis metal staple is applied to excise the redundant antimesenteric portion of the ileum and to create a smooth tube for catheterization using 16F to 18F catheters. The ureters are tunneled into the tenia of the colonic segment through an inverted "T" incision. A mucosal incision is then made for the orifice, the ureter is cut either obliquely or spatulated, and a ureter-to-mucosa anastomosis is performed over a 5F to 8F stent using interrupted 5-0 absorbable, synthetic, monofilament sutures. The cephalad end of the pouch is folded to the caudal end, and the reservoir is closed with a single layer of running 3-0 braided synthetic absorbable suture. Hautman introduced the concept of the neobladder, which involves the creation of a reservoir based on terminal ileum and anastomosed to the urethra and with the ureters reimplanted into the reservoir. The choice of urinary diversion is based on patient preference.

BOX 24-6 POSSIBLE COMPLICATIONS OF CYSTECTOMY AND URINARY DIVERSION

- Electrolyte abnormalities, acidosis
- Urinary complications
  - Urine leak
  - Ureteral obstruction
  - Pyelonephritis
  - Renal failure
  - Failure of continence mechanism/ stoma problems
- Bowel complications
  - Bowel obstruction
  - Bowel perforation/fistula/sepsis

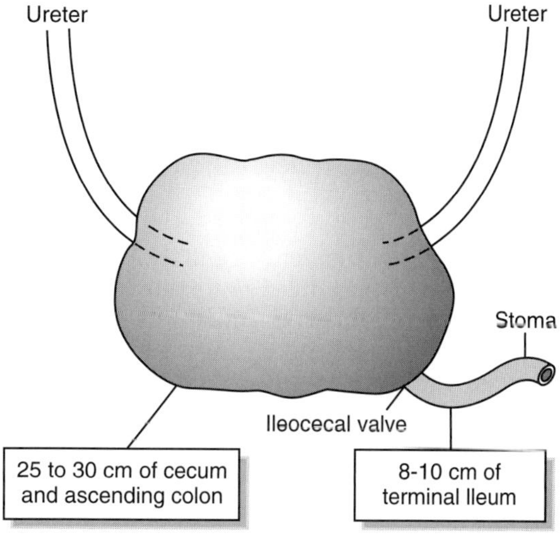

Figure 24-5. Indiana pouch made from the cecum and the terminal ileum. Approximately 8 cm to 10 cm of terminal ileum and 25 cm to 30 cm of cecum and ascending colon are isolated, and the colonic segment is detubularized. The continence mechanism is then created by tapering the terminal ileum. The natural ileocecal valve helps maintain continence. The ureters are tunneled into the tenia of the colonic segment.

Bladder Preservation

Several investigators have proposed using a combination of external-beam radiation therapy with concomitant systemic chemotherapy (using radiosensitizing drugs such as cisplatin, carboplatin, paclitaxel, or 5-fluorouracil). The outcomes for small solitary tumors that are completely resected are comparable to those of cystectomy.

Kidney Cancer

Renal-cell carcinoma (RCC) accounts for about 2% of all cancers, with a worldwide annual increase of 1.5% to 5.9%. The mean age at the time of diagnosis is about 70 years, and there is a predominance of men over women in the range of 1.5 to 3.1. The mortality from RCC is increasing at a rate that parallels trends in incidence. Worldwide mortality is expected to increase from 54,000 deaths in 1985 to 102,000 deaths in 2000, and it may reach or even exceed that of bladder cancer in certain areas. An estimated 38,890 new cases of kidney cancer will be diagnosed in 2006, and 12,840 will die of the disease that year in the United States.

The increased incidence of RCC is primarily a result of the enhanced detection of tumors by the expanded use of imaging techniques, such as ultrasound and CT. At present, 25% to 40% of clinically diagnosed RCC are found incidentally. A total of 25% to 30% of patients with RCC have overt metastases at initial presentation and, in addition, a substantial fraction of patients have subclinical metastases at that time, which explains the unsatisfactory outcome of treatment.

A slight to moderate improvement in survival has been observed in most countries. Survival is closely related to initial stage: 5-year survival is 50% to 90% for localized disease, and this decreases to 0% to 13% for metastatic disease.

RCC occurs in both sporadic and hereditary forms. Approximately 90% of renal tumors are RCCs, and 85% of these are clear cell tumors. Other, less common cell types include papillary, chromophobe, and Bellini duct (collecting duct) tumors. Medullary renal carcinoma is a variant of collecting duct renal carcinoma, and it was initially described as occurring in patients who are sickle cell trait positive. Collecting duct carcinoma comprises less than 1% of kidney cancer cases.

There are a number of hereditary types of RCC that are associated with different histologic types of renal carcinoma, including von Hippel-Lindau syndrome (Table 24-5). This syndrome is an hereditary form of clear-cell histology with autosomal dominant genetic changes on chromosome 3p. Affected individuals are predisposed to cancer development in different organs, including the kidney.

Smoking and obesity are among the risk factors for the development of RCC. Tumor grade and stage are important for predicting the patient's outcome after nephrectomy. RCC primarily metastasizes to the lungs, brain, liver, and adrenal glands.

Presentation and Diagnosis

Clinical symptoms of RCC, such as hematuria, palpable tumor, and flank pain, are becoming less frequent; asymptomatic tumors are more commonly diagnosed. Clinical examination has a limited role in diagnosis, but it may be valuable for assessing comorbidity. In cases involving hematuria, additional tumors of the genitourinary tract should be excluded. The most commonly assessed laboratory parameters are as follows:

BOX 24–7 POSSIBLE PRESENTING SYMPTOMS OF RENAL-CELL CARCINOMA

- Hematuria }
- Pain } "Classic triad"
- Flank mass }
- Abdominal mass
- Fever
- Weight loss
- Symptoms of metastases

TABLE 24–5 • *Inherited Forms of Renal Carcinoma*

Syndrome	Involved Gene	Renal Cancer Histology	Features
von Hippel-Landau	*VHL*	Clear cell	Also pheochromocytoma, islet cell tumors, retinal angiomas, hemangioblastomas, and inner ear tumors
Hereditary papillary renal carcinoma	*Met*	Papillary type 1	Often bilateral, multifocal cancers
Hereditary leiomyomatosis renal cell carcinoma	Fumarate hydratase	Papillary type 2	Also at risk of cutaneous and uterine leiomyomas
Birt-Hogg-Dube	*BHD*	Chromophobe renal-cell carcinoma/ oncocytoma	Also at risk of benign hair follicle tumors and pulmonary cysts; renal cancer is often bilateral and multifocal

- hemoglobin and erythrocyte sedimentation rate, for prognosis;
- creatinine, for overall kidney function;
- alkaline phosphatase, for liver or bone metastasis; and
- serum calcium, for its association with paraneoplastic manifestation, which may have clinical implications.

The majority of tumors are diagnosed by abdominal ultrasound performed for various reasons. Standard radiologic procedure is an abdominal CT scan with and without contrast medium. It serves to document the diagnosis of RCC, and it provides information about the function and morphology of the contralateral kidney.

Additional diagnostic procedures, such as magnetic resonance imaging, angiography, or fine-needle biopsy, have a very limited role, but they may be considered in selected cases.

Abdominal CT scanning assesses primary tumor extension and provides information about venous involvement and metastatic spread to locoregional lymph nodes, adrenal glands, the contralateral kidney, and the liver. Chest x-ray is performed to assess pulmonary spread. If indicated by signs and symptoms, other diagnostic procedures may be applied, such as bone scanning, brain CT scanning, and chest CT scanning.

Staging

Patients who are in satisfactory medical condition and who are thought to have a localized tumor based on the clinical evaluation already outlined should undergo a nephrectomy. Patients with locally advanced, unresectable tumors, as well as most patients with evidence of distant metastases, should have a CT-guided needle biopsy of the kidney or other accessible sites for diagnosis, or they should undergo cytoreductive nephrectomy for diagnosis. Diagnosis may be rendered in selected patients with metastases at the time of cytoreductive nephrectomy. Infrequently, patients present with a resectable primary tumor and solitary metastasis, in which case resection of both may be undertaken.

Before surgery, a clinical stage (T stage) is assigned. The final pathological stage (P stage) may vary from the clinical stage that was determined on the basis of the findings at nephrectomy. The American Joint Committee on Cancer TNM staging classification is shown in Table 24-6. The important prognostic determinants of 5-year survival are the local extent of the tumor, the presence of regional nodal metastases, and the evidence of metastatic disease at presentation.

Treatment

Surgical resection remains the only effective therapy for clinically localized RCC. Surgery is advised for patients with clinical stage I or II tumors. Surgery is also indicated for patients with clinical stage III disease (i.e., patients who have a tumor involving the renal vein or the vena cava). Patients with minimal regional adenopathy may also be considered for surgery, because lymph nodes that are suspicious for disease on CT may be hyperplastic and may not be involved by tumor. The management of stage IV disease is discussed later. Patients with lower-stage kidney cancer have a better prognosis. The estimated 5-year survival rate for stage I is 95%; for stage II, it is 88%. It is 59% for patients with stage III disease and 20% for patients who present with stage IV disease.

Radical Nephrectomy

A radical nephrectomy is defined as a perifascial resection of the kidney, the perirenal fat, the regional lymph nodes, and the ipsilateral adrenal gland. The lymph-node dissection may not be therapeutic, but it provides prognostic information, because virtually all patients with nodal involvement subsequently relapse with distant metastases, despite lymphadenectomy. Resection of the ipsilateral adrenal gland may be restricted to patients with large upper-pole lesions and/or abnormal-appearing adrenal glands on CT scan.

BOX 24-8 SURGICAL APPROACHES TO NEPHRECTOMY

- Flank approach: good for small tumors without venous involvement
- Anterior transperitoneal approach: good for large tumors or venous involvement
- Thoracoabdominal approach: good for larger tumors with venous involvement
- Laparoscopic nephrectomy

Radical nephrectomy with excision of tumor thrombus is indicated if the tumor has extended into the inferior vena cava. Long-term

TABLE 24–6 • *American Joint Committee on Cancer Renal-Cell Carcinoma TNM Staging System*

Primary Tumor (T)	
TX	Primary tumor cannot be assessed
T0	No evidence of primary rumor
T1	Tumor 7 cm or less in greatest dimension, limited to the kidney
T1a	Tumor 4 cm or less in greatest dimension, limited to the kidney
T1b	Tumor more than 4 cm but not more than 7 cm in greatest dimension, limited to the kidney
T2	Tumor more than 7 cm in greatest dimension, limited to the kidney
T3	Tumor extends into major veins or invades adrenal glands or perinephric tissues, but not beyond Gerota's fascia
T3a	Tumor directly invades the adrenal gland or perirenal and/or renal sinus fat, but not beyond Gerota's fascia
T3b	Tumor grossly extends into the renal vein, its segmental (muscle-containing) branches, or the vena cava below the diaphragm
T3c	Tumor grossly extends into the vena cava above the diaphragm, or it invades the wall of the vena cava
T4	Tumor invades beyond Gerota's fascia
Regional Lymph Nodes (N)*	
NX	Regional lymph nodes cannot be assessed
N0	No regional lymph-node metastases
N1	Metastases in a single regional lymph node
N2	Metastases in more than one regional lymph node
Distant Metastasis (M)	
MX	Distant metastasis cannot be assessed
M0	No distant metastasis
M1	Distant metastasis

Stage Grouping

Stage	T	N	M
I	T1	N0	M0
II	T2	N0	M0
III	T1	N1	M0
	T2	N1	M0
	T3	N0	M0
	T3	N1	M0
	T3a	N0	M0
	T3a	N1	M0
	T3b	N0	M0
	T3b	N1	M0
	T3c	N0	M0
	T3c	N1	M0
IV	T4	N0	M0
	T4	N1	M0
	Any T	N2	M0
	Any T	Any N	M1

*Note: Laterality does not affect the N classification. If a lymph node dissection is performed, then pathologic evaluation would ordinarily include at least eight nodes.

Used with the permission of the American Joint Committee on Cancer (AJCC), Chicago. The original and primary source for this information is AJCC, ed. *AJCC cancer staging manual,* 6th ed. New York: Springer-Verlag, 2002. (For more information, visit www.cancerstaging.net.)

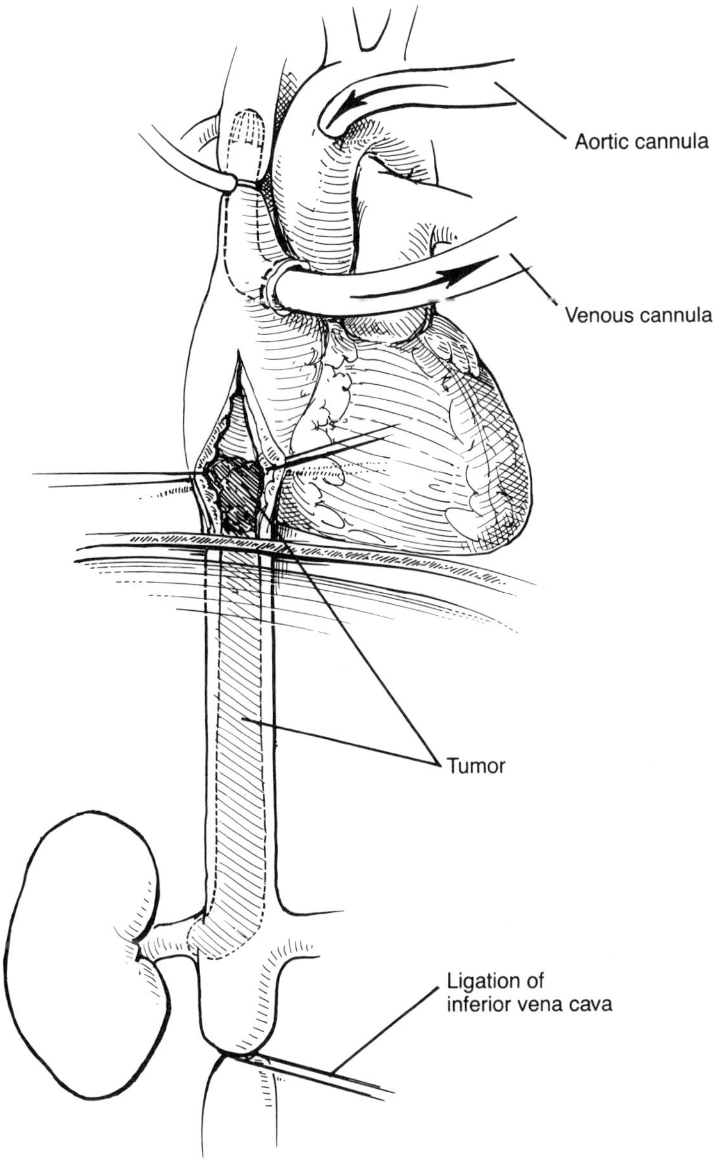

Figure 24–6. The aortic and superior vena caval cannulation technique for cardiopulmonary bypass. The right atrium is opened, revealing the renal-cell tumor. (From Bland KI, Karakousis CP, Copeland EM, eds. *Atlas of surgical oncology*. Philadelphia: WB Saunders, 1995.)

survival can be achieved in about half of patients with such tumors. Resection of a caval/atrial thrombus often requires the assistance of cardiovascular surgeons, and it may entail the techniques of venovenous or cardiopulmonary bypass, with or without circulatory arrest (Figure 24-6). Patients considered for the resection of a caval/atrial tumor thrombus should have surgery performed by experienced teams, because treatment-related mortality approaches 10%.

Nephron-Sparing Surgery

Nephron-sparing surgery is indicated in clinical settings in which a radical nephrectomy would render the patient functionally anephric, thereby necessitating dialysis. These settings include RCC in a solitary kidney, RCC in one kidney with inadequate contralateral renal function, and bilateral synchronous RCC. Nephron-sparing surgery is most appropriate under these circumstances for patients with tumors less than 4 cm in size that are situated at the upper or lower pole or in a peripheral location (Figures 24-7 and 24-8). Nephron-sparing surgery is also increasingly being used for small accessible tumors with a normal contralateral kidney. Patients with hereditary forms of RCC, such as von Hippel-Lindau syndrome, also should be considered for nephron-sparing therapy. After nephron-sparing surgery,

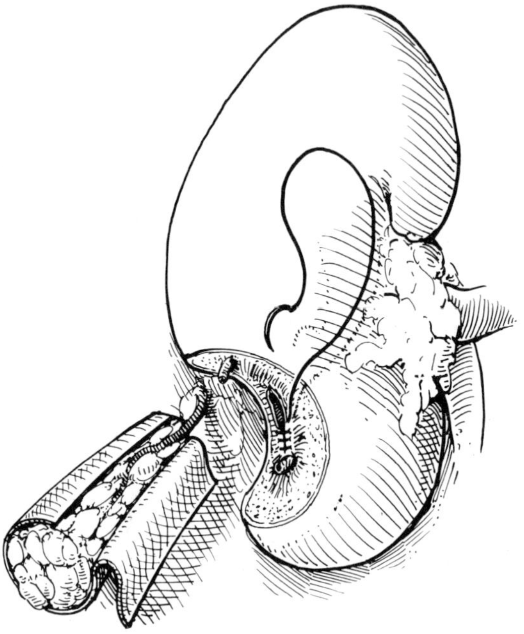

Figure 24-7. The tumor is resected with a 1-cm margin. The collecting system is being closed. A piece of retroperitoneal fat is placed within Surgicel (Johnson & Johnson, New Brunswick, NJ). (From Bland KI, Karakousis CP, Copeland EM, eds. *Atlas of surgical oncology*. Philadelphia: WB Saunders, 1995.)

local recurrences within the operated kidney occur in less than 5% of patients. The cancer-specific survival rate after partial nephrectomy is 90% to 100% in patients with a unifocal tumor of 4 cm or less.

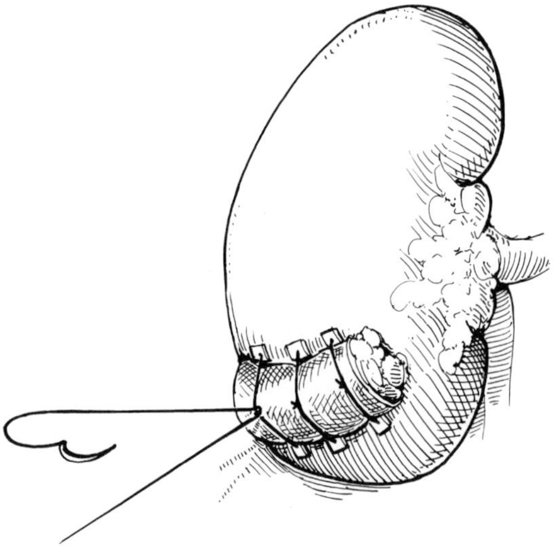

Figure 24–8. The kidney defect is closed over the piece of fat and Surgicel (Johnson & Johnson, New Brunswick, NJ) and tied with pledgets, thereby preventing it from cutting through the kidney tissue. (From Bland KI, Karakousis CP, Copeland EM, eds. *Atlas of surgical oncology*. Philadelphia: WB Saunders, 1995.)

Management After Nephrectomy

After nephrectomy, 20% to 30% of patients with localized tumors relapse. Lung metastasis is the most common site of distant recurrence, occurring in 50% to 60% of patients. The median time to relapse after nephrectomy is 1 to 2 years; most relapses occur within 3 years. The longer the disease-free interval between the diagnosis and the recognition of metastatic disease, the longer the projected long-term survival.

There is no established role for adjuvant treatment after nephrectomy in patients who have undergone complete resections of their tumors. Radiation therapy after nephrectomy is not beneficial, even for patients with nodal involvement or incomplete tumor resection.

Role of Surgery in Stage IV Disease

Depending on the number and location of metastatic lesions, patients may be considered for resection of the metastasis if they can be rendered free of tumor by surgery. Patients with hematuria or other symptoms related to the primary tumor may be considered for palliative nephrectomy or embolization. Immunotherapy is appropriate for patients with good performance status.

Selected patients with stage IV disease may be considered for resection of the metastatic site. Candidates include patients who initially present with primary RCC and a solitary site of metastasis or who develop a solitary recurrence after nephrectomy. Sites amenable to this approach include the lung, the bone, and the brain. Long-term survival has been observed in some patients. In some instances, after bone metastases, radiation therapy may be administered.

Some patients may undergo palliative nephrectomy to improve their quality of life. Treatment for the palliation of symptoms, especially for patients with marginal performance status and evidence of metastatic disease, includes optimal pain management.

Patient selection is important to identify patients who might benefit from cytoreductive therapy. Patients who are most likely to benefit from nephrectomy before systemic therapy are those with lung-only metastases, good prognostic features, and good performance status.

Key Selected Reading

Walsh PC, Retik AB, Vaughan ED, Wein AJ, eds. *Campbell's urology*. Philadelphia: WB Saunders, 1998:2283–2326.

Selected Readings

Bechtold RE, Zagoria RJ. Imaging approach to staging of renal cell carcinoma. *Urol Clin North Am* 1997; 24:507–522.

Bill-Axelson A, Holmberg L, Ruutu M, *et al*. Radical prostatectomy versus watchful waiting in early prostate cancer. *N Engl J Med* 2005;352:1977–1984.

Chawla SN, Crispen PL, Hanlon AL, *et al*. The natural history of observed enhancing renal masses: meta-analysis and review of the world literature. *J Urol* 2006;175:425–431.

Cohen HT, McGovern FJ. Renal-cell carcinoma. *N Engl J Med* 2005;353:2477–2490.

Diblasio CJ, Kattan MW. Use of nomograms to predict the risk of disease recurrence after definitive local therapy for prostate cancer. *Urology* 2003;Suppl 1:9–18.

Herr H. Tumour progression and survival in patients with T1G3 bladder tumours: 15 year outcome. *Br J Urol* 1997;80:762–765.

Lamm DL, Blumenstein BA, Crissman JD, Montie JE, Gottesman JE, Lowe A, *et al*. Maintenance bacillus Calmette-Guérin immunotherapy for recurrent Ta, T1 and carcinoma in situ transitional cell carcinoma of the bladder: a randomized Southwest Oncology Group Study. *J Urol* 2000;163:1124–1129.

Nelson WG, De Marzo AM, Isaacs WB. Prostate cancer. *N Engl J Med* 2003;349:366–381.

Linehan WM, Walther MM, Zbar B. The genetic basis of cancer of the kidney. *J Urol* 2003;170:2163–2172.

Pow-Sang JM, Seigne JD. Contemporary management of superficial bladder cancer. *Cancer Control* 2002;7:335–339.

Routh JC, Leibovich BC. Adenocarcinoma of the prostate: epidemiological trends, screening, diagnosis and surgical management of localized disease. *Mayo Clin Proc* 2005;80:899–907.

Stein JP, Lieskovsky G, Cote R, *et al*. Radical cystectomy in the treatment of invasive bladder cancer: long-term results in 1,054 patients. *J Clin Oncol* 2001;19:666–675.

Tooher R, Swindle P, Woo H, *et al*. Laparoscopic radical prostatectomy for localized prostate cancer: a systematic review of comparative studies. *J Urol* 2006;175:2011–2017.

Uzzo RG, Novick AC. Nephron sparing surgery for renal tumors: indications, techniques and outcomes. *J Urol* 2001;166:6–18.

25

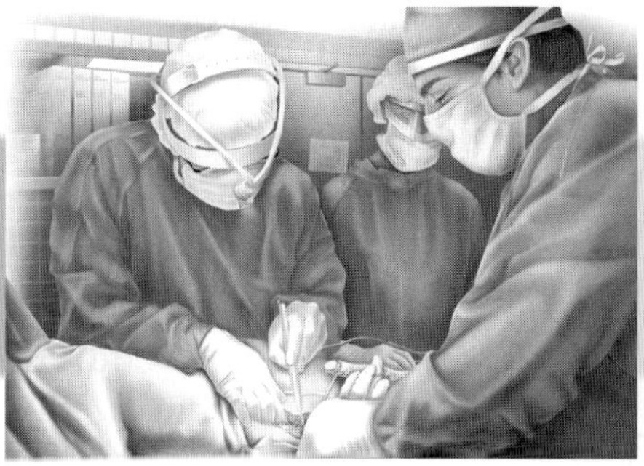

Childhood Cancers

Kathleen Graziano and James D. Geiger

Childhood Cancer: Key points

- Be aware that a high index of suspicion is required for the early diagnosis of childhood cancer because of vague or unusual presenting symptoms.
- Detail the incidence, clinical manifestations, and treatment of central nervous system tumors.
- Detail the incidence, clinical manifestations, and treatment of neuroblastoma.
- Outline the incidence, clinical manifestations, staging, and treatment of Wilms' tumor.
- Describe the incidence, clinical manifestations, staging, and prognosis of rhabdomyosarcoma.
- List the pertinent facts about childhood leukemia and lymphoma.

Childhood cancer, although a relatively uncommon cause of death among children between the ages of 0 and 15, is the leading cause of disease-related mortality; the highest non-disease cause is accidental death. The likelihood of being diagnosed with cancer during childhood is 1 in 300 for males and 1 in 333 for females. Mortality rates for all childhood cancers have decreased significantly since the 1950s, when there were 80 deaths per million children diagnosed with a neoplasm. During the late 1990s, the number of deaths had declined to 30 per million. Still, more than 2,000 children die each year of some type of cancer, and there is significant morbidity associated with cancer treatments. Because many types of pediatric cancers are so rare, enrollment in multicenter trials is critical for further advances in treatment to occur.

The leukemias—acute lymphoblastic and acute myeloid—continue to be the most frequently diagnosed malignancy among children under the age of 15 years, comprising 28% of the total number of neoplasms diagnosed each year. Tumors of the central nervous system are the second most common (22%), followed by lymphoma (8%), neuroblastoma (8%), and Wilms' tumor (6%). Other tumors comprise from 2% to 4% of the total and consist of rhabdomyosarcoma, other soft-tissue sarcomas, germ-cell tumors, retinoblastoma, osteosarcoma, and hepatoblastoma.

Unfortunately, there is often a delay in the diagnosis of pediatric cancers (Table 25-1). The reason for the apparent delay is the vague nature of the symptoms associated with many cancers. Neuroblastoma can present with unusual signs or symptoms that may not raise a specific concern for the disease, including failure to thrive, chronic diarrhea, or Horner's syndrome from tumor compression in the chest.

There is a broad range of hereditary abnormalities that play a role in childhood cancer. It is important to recognize certain syndromes, such as Beckwith-Wiedemann syndrome, so that appropriate monitoring for associated neoplasms can be performed. The types of genetic abnormalities that may predispose a child to the development of cancer include constitutional chromosomal anomalies (trisomy 21), sex-chromosome abnormalities, structural chromosomal abnormalities, and mendelian inheritance of a predisposition to cancer.

BOX 25-1 HEREDITARY ABNORMALITIES CONTRIBUTING TO CANCER RISK

Trisomy 21

- Leukemia

Sex-chromosome abnormalities

- Gonadoblastoma in streak gonads

Structural-chromosomal abnormalities

- WAGR syndrome: Wilms' tumor, aniridia, genital abnormalities, retardation
- Beckwith-Wiedemann syndrome: Wilms' tumor, hepatoblastoma

Mendelian inheritance of a predisposition

- Li-Fraumeni syndrome
- Neurofibromatosis-1
- von Hippel-Lindau syndrome
- Multiple endocrine neoplasia syndromes

Tumors of the Central Nervous System

Incidence

Neoplasms of the central nervous system (CNS) are the second most common pediatric cancer. There are 1,700 new cases diagnosed each year in children less than 14 years old. There is a slightly increased ratio of males to females among those affected with medulloblastoma and ependymoma. Less than 10% are associated with other syndromes. The nomenclature of CNS tumors is problematic, depending on whether tumors are categorized by morphology, histology, or phenotype. Medulloblastoma is the most common and accounts for 20% of CNS tumors. This entity can metastasize, most commonly to bone. A near-total resection is possible in 80% of cases. The gliomas are a diverse group of tumors that includes astrocytomas, both high grade and low grade. Less common tumors include ependymomas (which have only a 50% resectability rate), primitive neuroectodermal tumors, optic pathway tumors, pineal region tumors, and craniopharyngiomas.

TABLE 25-1 • ***Median Time to the Diagnosis of Childhood Cancers***

Wilms' tumor	31 days
Leukemia	52 days
Neuroblastoma	58 days
Osteosarcoma	127 days
Rhabdomyosarcoma	127 days
Hodgkin's lymphoma	223 days

BOX 25-2 TYPES OF PEDIATRIC CENTRAL NERVOUS SYSTEM TUMORS

Supratentorial
- Gliomas
- Primitive neuroectodermal tumor
- Ependymoma
- Choroid plexus tumors
- Craniopharyngioma
- Germinoma
- Malignant germ-cell tumor
- Pineal tumor

Infratentorial
- Medulloblastoma (primitive neuroectodermal tumor)
- Cerebellar astrocytoma
- Ependymoma
- Brainstem glioma

Signs and Symptoms

Because neoplasms of the CNS are common, one should have a high index of suspicion when children present with neurological complaints. Headaches are not uncommon in children, but there are some associated symptoms that should prompt a computed tomographic (CT) scan, including the presence of an abnormal neurological finding, visual changes, persistent vomiting, morning headaches, or headaches that awaken a child from sleep. Infants commonly present with more subtle signs than older children may have. An infant may have increased irritability, failure to thrive, anorexia, or a bulging fontanel. They may present with Parinaud's syndrome (see Box 25-4), which is a constellation of findings that is suggestive of a dorsal midbrain lesion. Certain symptoms may help to localize a lesion to the supratentorial or infratentorial location (see Box 25-5).

Treatment

The general principles of surgical intervention for pediatric brain tumors are to achieve gross total resection whenever possible while preserving as much functional brain tissue as possible. Stereotactic biopsy techniques may be used for certain tumors that have not been shown to be amenable to surgery, such

BOX 25-3 SIGNS AND SYMPTOMS THAT SHOULD RAISE SUSPICION FOR BRAIN TUMOR IN CHILDREN WITH HEADACHES

- Presence of neurologic abnormality
- Visual changes
- Persistent vomiting
- Morning headaches
- Diabetes insipidus
- Age of less than 3 years
- Presence of neurofibromatosis
- History of central nervous system irradiation

BOX 25-4 PARINAUD'S SYNDROME: A CONSTELLATION OF SYMPTOMS FOUND WITH DORSAL MIDBRAIN LESIONS

- Impaired upward gaze in infants
- Large pupils
- Nystagmus with gaze convergence
- Head tilt to accommodate trochlear nerve palsy

BOX 25-5 LOCALIZING SYMPTOMS IN PEDIATRIC CENTRAL NERVOUS SYSTEM TUMORS

Supratentorial
- Hemiparesis
- Hemisensory loss
- Hyperreflexia
- Seizures
- Visual complaints

Infratentorial (cerebellum and brainstem)
- Ataxia
- Difficulty hopping or running
- Clumsiness
- Worsening handwriting
- Slow speech

as diffuse brainstem gliomas. Certain tumors tend to be well circumscribed (e.g., craniopharyngiomas), and total or near-total resection may be achieved. Preoperative steroids are often given to reduce edema and to improve symptoms. The drainage of obstructive hydrocephalus preoperatively can be helpful, and a temporary or permanent shunt is often placed.

Neuroblastoma

Incidence

Neuroblastoma is the most common extracranial solid tumor, accounting for 8% to 10% of all childhood tumors. There are about 600 new cases diagnosed each year, or approximately 1 in 7,000 children. About 2% of patients have a family history, and most of these patients have no associated syndromes. Neuroblastoma arises from primordial neural crest cells, and it is found in locations typical for these cells: 65% of these tumors are located in the abdomen, and the remainder are found in the mediastinum, the paraspinal region, the neck, and the pelvis (Figure 25-1; Table 25-2). Half of patients are diagnosed when they are less than 2 years old, and 90% are diagnosed when they are less than 8 years old. The adrenal gland is frequently involved, more so in older children (40%) than in infants (25%).

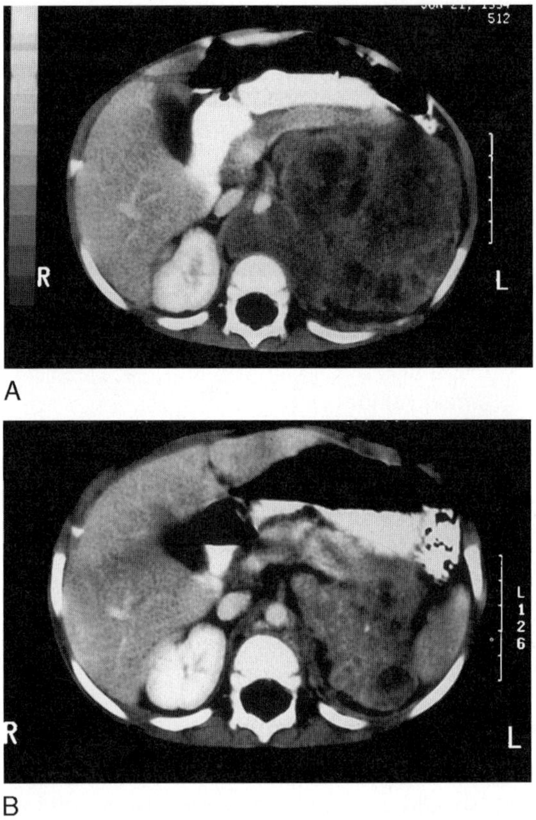

Figure 25-1. A, Abdominal CT scan demonstrating large retroperitoneal neuroblastoma, with tumor encasing the aorta and the superior mesenteric artery. **B,** After chemotherapy, the tumor is significantly smaller. An excellent response of the disease around the vessels allowed for total resection.

Clinical Manifestations

Half of patients will have a fixed, hard abdominal mass on examination, but there are many presenting symptoms that are related to the location of the primary tumor and to metastatic disease. Mediastinal tumors may present with Horner's syndrome or, less commonly, with respiratory distress. About 35% of abdominal tumors present with hypertension from catecholamine release or renal compression. Spinal cord compression may be present if there is tumor extension into the extradural space. Children with metastatic disease may present with proptosis or bilateral orbital ecchymoses not related to trauma. Bone metastasis may cause a child to refuse to walk. Children with advanced cases have weight loss, anemia, and failure to thrive. The dancing eye syndrome refers to cerebellar ataxia and opsomyoclonus, and it may fail to resolve after resection of the primary tumor. Secretion of vasoactive intestinal peptide may produce a syndrome of dehydration and hypokalemia from secretory diarrhea. Most patients will have an elevation of serum catecholamines.

TABLE 25-2 • *Neuroblastoma Primary Tumor Sites*

Adrenal gland	50%
Paraspinal	24%
Mediastinum	20%
Cervical	4%
Pelvic	2%

Staging and Treatment

The international neuroblastoma staging system is used in clinical trials and defines stage I as a localized tumor that is completely excised, stage II as unilateral disease that is incompletely

BOX 25-6 PRESENTING SYMPTOMS IN PATIENTS WITH NEUROBLASTOMA

Abdominal primary site
- Abdominal mass
- Hypertension

Thoracic primary site
- Respiratory distress
- Horner's syndrome: ptosis, myosis, anhidrosis
- Superior vena cava syndrome

Signs and symptoms not related to tumor site
- Chronic diarrhea
- Polymyoclonus-opsoclonus ("dancing eyes")
- Failure to thrive
- Proptosis or bilateral orbital ecchymoses ("panda eyes")
- Paraplegia

excised, stage III as tumor that infiltrates across the midline, and stage IV as the presence of distant metastasis. Surgical staging includes the resection of the tumor (if possible), the biopsy of any suspicious liver lesions, and the extensive sampling of lymph nodes (Table 25-3). A unique stage, IV-S, applies to infants less than 1 year old who have localized tumor that would be classified as stage I or II along with liver, skin, or bone marrow involvement (Figure 25-2). These patients have an excellent prognosis despite the presence of disseminated disease.

N-myc is a protooncogene that is found to be amplified in 25% of tumors and that is

TABLE 25-3 • *International Neuroblastoma Staging System*

Stage	Definition
I	Localized tumor, completely excised; lymph nodes negative
IIA	Unilateral tumor; gross tumor left after resection
IIB	Same as IIA, with positive regional lymph nodes
III	Tumor infiltrating across midline
IV	Dissemination of tumor to distant sites
IV-S	Localized tumor as in stages I or II, with dissemination to liver, skin, or bone marrow in infants less than 1 year old

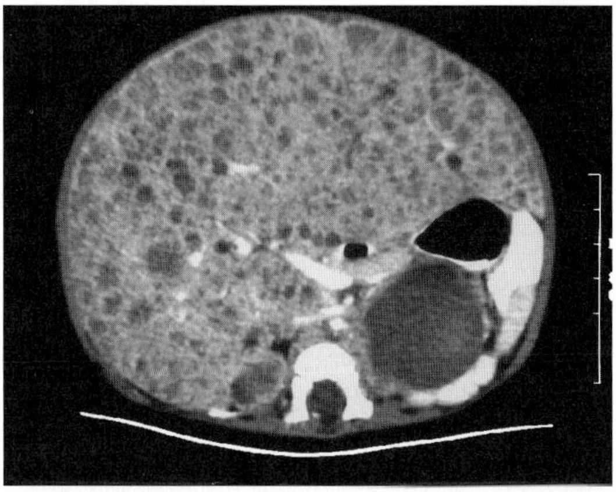

Figure 25-2. CT scan of the abdomen demonstrates "salt and pepper" metastases of the liver as well as a left adrenal mass in a newborn with stage IV-S neuroblastoma.

prognostically important. Approximately 30% to 40% of patients with advanced-stage disease have amplification of *N-myc* as opposed to 5% to 10% of low-stage or IV-S patients. The DNA index is a measure of the ploidy of the tumor. Hyperdiploidy carries a favorable prognosis among children less than 1 year old.

Surgical specimens are evaluated histologically using the Shimada classification system that describes two basic histologic groups: stroma rich and stroma poor. Most tumors that are classified under this system as having unfavorable histology are stroma poor. Other prognostic factors include the age of the patient, neuroblast differentiation, and the mitosis-karyorrhexis index. This classification—along with the International Neuroblastoma Staging System (INSS) stage, the N-myc status, and DNA ploidy—allow for the placement of patients into low-, intermediate-, and high-risk groups. Low-risk patients may benefit from surgery alone, whereas intermediate-risk patients will undergo surgery, chemotherapy, and radiotherapy. High-risk patients undergo more intense regimens of chemotherapy, and they often undergo delayed resections of the primary tumor. The role of surgery for the survival in high-risk patients is not clear, but, in general, patients should be able to undergo an attempt at complete resection without taking on significant morbidity.

Prognosis

The most important prognostic factors for patients with neuroblastoma are the age at diagnosis and the stage of the disease at diagnosis. In one series, overall survival in children less than 1 year old was 76%, and survival in children more than 1 year old was 32%. Patients with disease in stages I and II clearly fare much better than those with disease in stages III and IV.

Wilms' Tumor

Incidence

Renal tumors are relatively frequent, and they make up 6% of all childhood cancers. There are 500 new cases diagnosed each year, which corresponds with 7 to 8 per 1 million children under the age of 15 years. The incidence of bilateral tumors is slightly higher among girls. The tumor tends to present earlier in boys, with an average age at diagnosis of 41 months in boys and 47 months in girls. Bilateral disease presents even earlier, with an average age at diagnosis of 29 months in boys and 32 months in girls. Several genetic syndromes are associated with the development of Wilms' tumor, including Beckwith-Wiedemann syndrome, Denys-Drash syndrome, and WAGR syndrome (Wilms' Tumor, aniridia, genitourinary malformations, and mental retardation).

BOX 25–7 GENETIC SYNDROMES WITH INCREASED RISK FOR WILMS' TUMOR

- Beckwith-Wiedemann syndrome: visceromegaly, macroglossia, hypoglycemia
- WAGR syndrome: aniridia, genitourinary malformations, mental retardation
- Denys-Drash syndrome: intersex anomalies, renal failure

Clinical Presentation

Most patients present with an asymptomatic abdominal mass noted by a parent, a caregiver, or a healthcare worker. Some patients will complain of abdominal pain or have fevers and/or hematuria. Hypertension will be present in up to 25% of patients at presentation. Males may present with a varicocele, which is associated with abdominal venous obstruction. A CT scan of the abdomen should be obtained, and a plain radiograph or CT scan of the chest should be used for staging purposes (Figure 25-3).

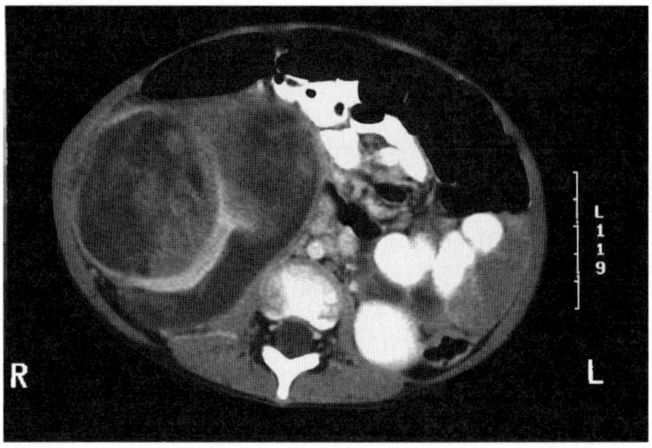

Figure 25–3. Abdominal CT scan demonstrating a large, lobulated Wilms' tumor, which is inhomogeneous as a result of a recent hemorrhage into the mass.

Staging and Treatment

Stage I tumors are those that are completely resected, with the tumor confined to the kidney. Stage II involves one or more of the following situations: tumor extension beyond the capsule of the kidney, invasion of the renal veins, biopsy of the tumor before removal, or spillage of the tumor during removal. Stage III includes the presence of gross or microscopic tumor postoperatively. Stage IV lesions have metastasized, most commonly to the lungs, and stage V consists of bilateral disease (Table 25-4). Treatment

TABLE 25–4 • *Staging for Wilms' Tumor*

Stage	Definition
I	The tumor is limited to the kidney and is excised completely.
II	The tumor extends beyond the kidney but is excised completely. Capsular penetration, renal vein involvement, and renal sinus involvement may also be found. A biopsy of the tumor is performed, and local spillage ocurs.
III	Residual intra-abdominal tumor (nonhematogenous) exists after the completion of surgery. Lymph node findings are positive or peritoneal implants are found. The resected specimen has histologically positive margins or the tumor has been spilled into the abdominal cavity.
IV	Hematogenous or lymph node metastasis has occurred outside the abdomen or pelvis.
V	Synchronous bilateral involvement has occurred. Each side is assigned a stage from I to III, and histology is based on biopsy findings.

is resection and must include regional lymph nodes for staging. En bloc resection of surrounding organs is rarely necessary.

There is a diverse pattern of histologic findings in these tumors, which are classically made up of three cell types: blastemal, stromal, and epithelial. Some tumors may be made up of one or two predominant cell types. The histologic pattern is then divided into favorable and unfavorable histologies. About 5% of tumors are found to be anaplastic, which has the same prognosis for stage I disease but is a worse prognostic factor for higher stages. Roughly 35% of patients with unilateral disease and 100% of patients with bilateral disease are found to have nephrogenic rests in the specimen. These are thought to be embryonal nephroblastic tissue, and they are found at autopsy in 1% of children who do not have a history of renal tumors.

Renal tumors other than Wilms' tumor exist in the pediatric population. These include clear-cell sarcoma, which carries a worse prognosis as compared with Wilms' tumor, with frequent metastasis to bone. Rhabdoid tumors of the kidney also tend to present with metastasis at diagnosis. Renal-cell carcinoma is seen less commonly; the incidence increases during adolescence. Congenital mesoblastic nephroma is an entity that is found in very young infants, with a median age at diagnosis of 2 months. Recurrence or metastasis has been noted in 20% of cases.

Bilateral Disease

The involvement of both kidneys is not uncommon, and it is seen in 4.5% to 7% of cases. Exploration of the opposite kidney is currently mandatory in an operation for resection of what is thought to be a unilateral tumor, because preoperative imaging has historically missed 7% of tumors that were present in the contralateral kidney. Improved imaging may eliminate the need for contralateral exploration in the future. The treatment if tumors are found in both kidneys is the biopsy of both sides and of any enlarged lymph nodes. The patient then undergoes 4 to 6 weeks of preoperative chemotherapy in an attempt to cytoreduce the tumors. A bilateral resection of the tumors is then performed, with the preservation of as much normal renal tissue as possible on both sides.

Prognosis

The National Wilms' Tumor Study Group, now a part of the Children's Oncology Group, has conducted multiple clinical trials with protocols based on tumor stage and histology. Dramatic improvements in survival for this disease have occurred over the last 40 years. In patients who have favorable histology, the 2-year disease-free survival rate is 95% for stage I, 85% to 90% for stages II and III, and 80% for stage IV.

Rhabdomyosarcoma

Incidence

A sarcoma is a malignant tumor of mesenchymal cell origin. Rhabdomyosarcoma is the third most common extracranial solid tumor in children, after neuroblastoma and renal tumors. There are 350 new cases each year, which means that 4.3 children out of every 1 million individuals under the age of 20 years will be affected. Two thirds of the patients are less than 6 years old. The site of the tumor can vary in different age groups, with head and neck tumors being more common in children less than 8 years old and extremity tumors being more common in adolescents (Table 25-5). A type of tumor that occurs most often in infants and in the genitourinary tract is called *botryoid,* and it has an appearance similar to that of a cluster of grapes. Some patients have associated syndromes, such as neurofibromatosis or Li-Fraumeni syndrome.

Presentation

About 25% of patients will have evidence of metastasis at the time of diagnosis. Sites of metastasis include the lung in 40% to 50% of cases and the bone or bone marrow less

TABLE 25-5 • *Site of Primary Tumor in Children With Rhabdomyosarcoma*

Site	Percentage
Genitourinary	22%
Extremity	18%
Parameningeal	16%
Head and neck	10%
Orbit	9%
Other	25%

commonly. Most patients will present with complaints of a mass and no history of trauma. The mass is frequently nontender, and there is usually no discoloration or ecchymosis. The diagnosis is made by biopsy, and imaging studies are important for staging.

Staging and Prognosis

The staging for rhabdomyosarcoma is divided into favorable and unfavorable sites, with extremity sites faring better than truncal or retroperitoneal sites. Patients with completely resected disease are stage I. Stage II patients have microscopic residual disease, stage III patients have gross residual disease, and stage IV patients have metastatic disease.

TABLE 25-6 • *Features of Hepatic Tumors in Children*

Hepatoblastoma
Most common
Seen in children less than 4 years old
90% have elevated α-fetoprotein levels
May be associated with prematurity
Overall survival, 70%
Hepatocellular carcinoma
Less common
Seen in older children and adolescents
50% have elevated α-fetoprotein levels
Associated with chronic hepatitis and cirrhosis
Overall survival, 15%

Hepatic Tumors

Incidence

There are between 100 and 150 new cases of hepatic neoplasms diagnosed in children each year, which account for only 1.1% of all childhood tumors. Of all of the liver masses that are detected in children, two thirds are found to be malignant. Children less than 3 years old are more likely to have hepatoblastoma, rhabdomyosarcoma, or a benign process such as a mesenchymal hamartoma or a teratoma. The mean age at diagnosis for hepatoblastoma is 19 months, and only 5% of cases involving this type of tumor are seen in children more than 4 years old. There is a slight male predominance. Older children are more likely to have hepatocellular carcinoma or sarcoma (Table 25-6).

Diagnosis

Hepatoblastoma is associated with certain genetic syndromes such as Beckwith-Wiedemann and familial adenomatous polyposis, and children with these syndromes are monitored for the development of a hepatic mass by serial ultrasounds. Hepatocellular carcinoma is associated with syndromes that produce cirrhosis, such as hepatitis B infection or enzyme deficiencies.

Patients present with an asymptomatic abdominal mass. Patients with advanced disease may report abdominal pain, weight loss, anorexia, nausea, or vomiting, and they will rarely have jaundice. A CT scan should be obtained, and laboratory values including a complete blood count (one fifth will have thrombocytosis) and an α-fetoprotein level, which will be markedly elevated in most patients with hepatoblastoma.

Staging

Staging of hepatoblastoma depends partly on histology, so a tissue biopsy should be obtained. Stage I tumors are those of favorable histology that can be completely resected. These are typically of a purely fetal histologic pattern, with a low mitotic index. Tumors that fall into the other stages are of other than purely fetal type, and they have a wide range of histologic differentiation, ranging from undifferentiated small-cell types to embryonal to well-differentiated types. Stage II tumors are grossly resected with microscopic margins, or they experience preoperative rupture. Stage III tumors are of one of three types: (1) unresectable tumors; (2) partly resected tumors with measurable tumor left behind; and/or (3) tumors with lymph node involvement. Stage IV tumors present with metastatic disease.

Treatment/Prognosis

Recommended treatment includes aggressive resection whenever possible. Factors that prevent initial surgical resection include the involvement of both lobes or the involvement of the porta hepatis. Lymph nodes around the porta should be sampled regardless of size; celiac and paraaortic lymph nodes should be sampled if they are clinically enlarged.

Survival is improved if pulmonary lesions are resected. Chemotherapy can convert unresectable to resectable tumors in some cases. A cisplatin-based chemotherapy regimen is recommended, and it has improved survival. Patients with tumors that are multifocal and that are not resectable by standard liver resections should undergo liver transplant if distant metastatic disease has been controlled. Only 10% to 20% of hepatocellular carcinomas are found to be resectable at presentation. Overall, the 5-year survival rate for hepatoblastoma is 65% to 75%.

Leukemia

Incidence

Acute lymphoblastic leukemia is the most common malignancy of childhood, with 2,500 to 3,500 new cases diagnosed each year. The peak age group is from 3 to 5 years old. There is an association of leukemia with certain genetic syndromes, especially trisomy 21, which carries 15 times the risk as compared with genetically normal children. Acute myeloblastic leukemia accounts for 15% to 25% of all leukemias (500 new cases per year). Acute myeloblastic leukemia is more lethal, and it is responsible for 30% of all deaths from leukemia.

Diagnosis

Clinical symptoms are often vague, and they include fever in more than half of patients and bleeding or petechiae in more than 40% of patients. Lymphadenopathy and hepatosplenomegaly are often present. Laboratory abnormalities include anemia, thrombocytopenia, and, frequently, leukocytosis. A high white blood cell count at diagnosis carries a worse prognosis. The surgeon's involvement in the care of patients with acute lymphoblastic leukemia or acute myeloblastic leukemia is often limited to establishing vascular access for induction and maintenance chemotherapy. Some patients will undergo stem-cell transplantation for disease that is unresponsive to chemotherapy. These patients will sometimes develop complications from this aggressive therapy that require surgical intervention, specifically graft-versus-host disease, which requires biopsy for diagnosis, or typhlitis, which is an inflammatory condition of the ileum and the colon that may progress to perforation.

Lymphoma

Incidence

Hodgkin's disease and non-Hodgkin lymphoma have a bimodal age distribution, with an early peak in the middle to late 20s. These disorders make up 10% of all childhood cancers. The childhood form usually occurs in patients who are less than 14 years old and who usually present with lymphadenopathy (frequently involving the mediastinal nodes), fatigue, anorexia, fevers, night sweats, and slight weight loss. A diagnostic workup is important for staging, and the surgeon is involved in obtaining tissue. A staging laparotomy is largely historical given modern imaging techniques.

Mediastinal Lymphadenopathy

Patients who present with anterior mediastinal mass effect from enlarged lymph nodes require careful perioperative management. If the history reveals orthopnea or if stridor or wheezing are present on examination, one should look for the presence of extrathoracic tumor compromising the airway. Evaluation of the amount of airway compromise should include a CT scan to define the diameter of the trachea and an evaluation of the peak expiratory flow rate. If either of these measurements is less than 50% of predicted values, attempts should be made at biopsy without general anesthesia. Pleural effusions should be tapped under local anesthesia, and CT-guided needle biopsies can be obtained. If a transthoracic approach is still necessary, a Chamberlain procedure can be performed with minimal anesthesia.

Abdominal Lymphoma

Certain B cell lymphomas can present in the small bowel, especially the ileum, and they are thought to arise in Peyer's patches. Up to 25% of patients with Burkitt's lymphoma can present with a mass in the right lower quadrant; the symptoms can also mimic acute appendicitis. Patients with an acute abdominal examination or intussusception will require laparotomy, and the lesions should be resected when possible. Extensive resection of very large lesions should be avoided, and chemotherapy should be instituted to relieve the obstruction.

Staging

The Ann Arbor staging classification for Hodgkin's disease defines stage I as involvement of a single nodal region or organ, stage II as involvement of two or more regions on the same side of the diaphragm, stage III as involvement of nodal regions on both sides of the diaphragm, and stage IV as diffuse extralymphatic involvement. The presence of high fevers, night sweats, or significant weight loss designates any given stage as "B" (e.g., IIB) for the purposes of treatment and prognosis. Overall survival in the various clinical trials is 85% to 95%.

Germ Cell Tumors

Incidence

This diverse group of tumors accounts for 1% of childhood tumors or 2.4 cases per 1 million children. Pathology can range from benign mature teratomas to malignant yolk sac tumors or germinomas. Clinical serum markers include the oncofetoproteins: α-fetoprotein and the β subunit of human chorionic gonadotropin. Treatment depends on the site of the tumor.

Ovarian Tumors

Two thirds of ovarian tumors will be of germ cell origin, and they occur most commonly in girls between the ages of 10 and 14 years. Most will present with abdominal pain (80%), and torsion of the ovary is a frequent occurrence. Ultrasound or CT scanning is followed by resection (Figure 25-4). Ovarian teratomas are managed in accordance with the most malignant element present.

Testicular Tumors

One in 100,000 males under the age of 15 years will present with a testicular mass, and that mass will usually be irregular and nontender. About 75% of these tumors will be of germ cell origin, and serum markers should be evaluated. A cryptorchid or undescended testis has a prevalence of 0.25% of the population, and the risk of developing a testicular tumor in this group of patients is 10 to 50 times higher than that of the unaffected population. Up to 45% of testicular malignancies occur in cryptorchid testes. For this reason, orchidopexy is advised after 6 months of age and before 18 months of age if the testis has not descended. The need for close follow up, even after orchidopexy, is emphasized.

Extragonadal Tumors

This group of germ cell tumors usually occurs in the midline in the intracranial, mediastinal, or sacrococcygeal regions. Sacrococcygeal tumors account for 40% of all germ cell tumors and for 80% of all extragonadal germ cell tumors. Seventy-five percent of sacrococcygeal tumors are seen in females, and 18% are associated with other anomalies. Mediastinal germ

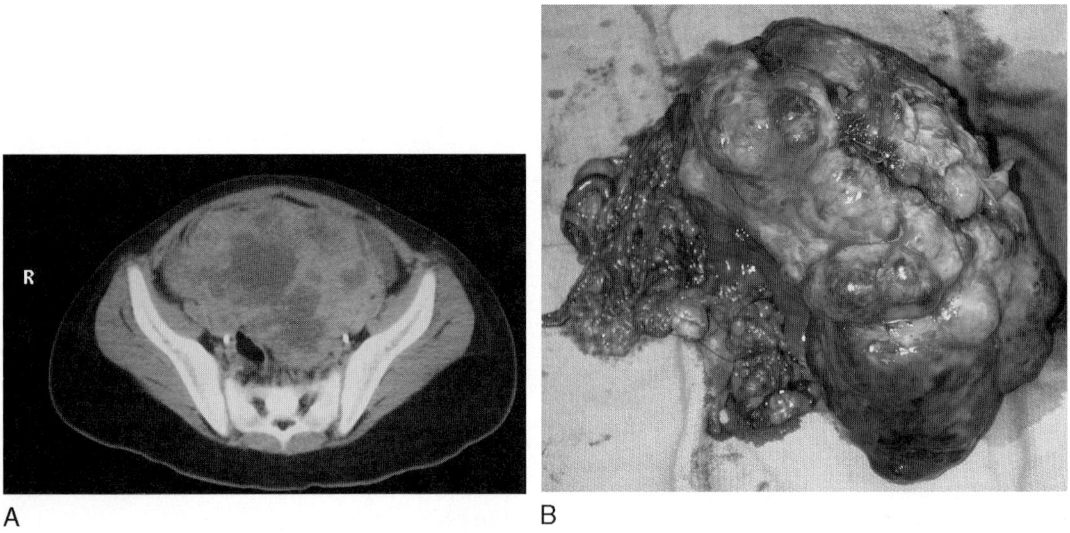

Figure 25-4. A, A large, ovarian, mixed germ-cell tumor is seen in the pelvis on a preoperative CT scan. **B,** The gross specimen in the operating room, after resection.

cell tumors are usually in the anterior mediastinum, and they occur more frequently in males; they have an association with Klinefelter's syndrome.

Other Tumors

Retinoblastoma

The incidence of retinoblastoma is 11 of every 1 million children less than 5 years old. Approximately 200 new cases are diagnosed each year, with about 50 of those consisting of bilateral involvement. Diagnostic signs include strabismus and/or leukocoria, which is defined as a pupil that appears white when light is shone into it (normally the retinal vessels cause a red papillary reflex). Useful imaging studies include ultrasound or CT scanning, and examination under anesthesia is important to establish the diagnosis. There is a 90% 5-year survival rate with aggressive treatment, which consists of enucleation of the eye and/or radiation therapy, and chemotherapy for metastatic disease.

Endocrine Tumors

This group of tumors arises from endocrine organs and it includes tumors of the hypothalamic-pituitary unit, thyroid and parathyroid tumors, adrenal tumors, and pancreatic tumors. Together, they constitute 4% to 5% of all childhood cancers. The multiple endocrine neoplasia syndromes type I and II are hereditary syndromes that are associated with more than one endocrine tumor in predictable locations.

The treatment of thyroid tumors in children is similar to treatment in adults except that thyroid nodules in children carry a higher likelihood of being cancerous, with 20% to 40% of nodules that come to surgical exploration having malignant elements. Despite this, the prognosis for treated disease is excellent.

Adrenal tumors include adrenocortical adenomas, adrenal carcinomas, pheochromocytomas, and paragangliomas. Pheochromocytomas require careful perioperative management, because most of these patients will have hypertension that is sustained and that is often refractory to medical therapy. Patients are placed on α-blockers for 1 to 2 weeks preoperatively, and careful intraoperative management is required during manipulation of the tumor.

Pancreatic tumors include insulinomas, gastrinomas, VIPomas (vasoactive intestinal peptide), and glucagonomas.

Osteosarcoma

A primary malignant tumor of the bone, osteosarcoma is diagnosed in approximately 400 children each year, with the peak time of diagnosis being adolescence. Patients present with a history of pain (3 months on average), and 15% to 20% of these patients have metastasis upon diagnosis. A longitudinal biopsy is obtained after plain films and CT scanning or magnetic resonance imaging. Staging is based on histologic grade, and treatment involves limb salvage, whenever possible. These tumors are highly radioresistant, but, with current chemotherapy, at least 60% to 70% of patients with nonmetastatic disease will survive without recurrence.

Ewing's Sarcoma Family of Tumors

These tumors are considered to be a spectrum of a single neoplastic entity arising from primitive neural crest tissue. They classically originate in the bone, but they can arise in soft tissue, and they affect 2 out of every 1 million children each year, most of whom are between the ages of 10 and 20 years. The site of disease is most often the extremity, with pelvic and chest-wall sites commonly seen. A surgical biopsy is obtained first, and this is followed by delayed resection in a significant percentage of cases. Prognosis depends on the site of origin, with extremity tumors faring better than pelvic tumors. Overall 5-year survival is in the range of 60% to 70%.

Key Selected Reading

O'Neill JA, Grosfeld JL, Fonkalsrud EW, *et al. Principles of pediatric surgery,* 2nd ed. St. Louis: Mosby, 2003.

Pizzo PA, Poplack DG. *Principles and practice of pediatric oncology,* 4th ed. Philadelphia: Lippincott, Williams and Wilkins, 2002.

Selected Readings

Altman RP, Randolph JG, Lilly JR. Sacrococcygeal teratoma: American Academy of Pediatrics surgical section survey?1973. *J Pediatr Surg* 1974;9:389–398.

Kim S, Chung DH. Pediatric solid malignancies: neuroblastoma and Wilms' tumor. *Surg Clin North Am* 2006;86:469–487.

Shimada H, Chatten J, Newton WA Jr, *et al.* Histopathologic prognostic factors in neuroblastic tumors: definition of subtypes of ganglioneuroblastoma and an age-linked classification of neuroblastoma. *J Natl Cancer Inst* 1984;73:405–416.

26

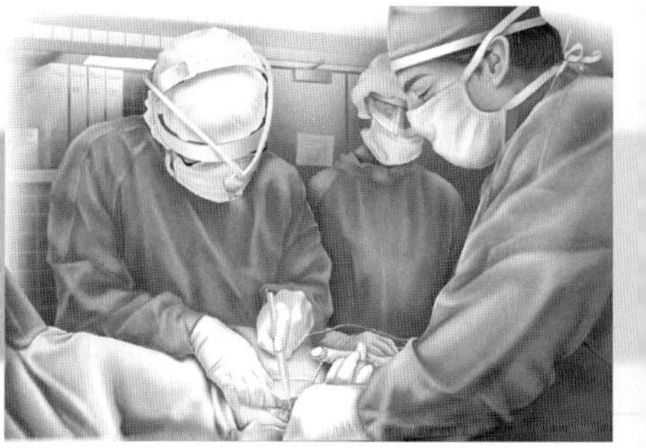

Surgery for Advanced Cancer

Jeffrey J. Sussman

Surgery for Advanced Cancer: Key Points

- Identify several commonly seen patterns in tumor behavior that affect outcomes.
- List factors to consider when choosing which studies to undertake when assessing metastatic disease.
- Describe situations in which surgical debulking or the cytoreduction of tumors is warranted.
- Discuss possible uses for surgically administered regional therapy.
- List palliative and adjunctive surgical procedures used on an emergency basis.

Surgery is often reflexively disregarded after a patient has been diagnosed with distant metastatic disease. Although traditionally surgery has been used primarily in the setting of localized or local-regional disease, there is a clear and increasing role for surgeons to play for the cure and palliation of patients with advanced cancer.

This chapter addresses three applications for surgery for patients with advanced disease: (1) surgical treatments that attempt to remove all distant metastatic disease; (2) surgical treatments to cytoreduce distant disease (often used a multimodality setting); and (3) surgical treatments used to palliate or to assist with other treatments. It is important for the surgical oncologist to recognize the utility of these approaches, but it is equally important to recognize their limitations and thus be able to appropriately counsel patients who are both seeking hope and desiring to maximize the quality of their remaining life, which may be quite limited.

Surgical Cure of Distant Disease

Cancers often will metastasize widely, thereby limiting any usefulness of surgery. The natural history of cancer progression, however, differs according to tumor type, and it also differs for individuals with the same specific type of cancer. The behavior of the tumor with regard to growth rate, site of metastases, response to treatment, and so on can vary widely. Despite these variations, there are certain routinely seen patterns that have been appreciated. Although there are often exceptions, these patterns—when recognized—can be taken advantage of by surgeons to affect the eventual outcome of the cancer patient.

For example, colorectal cancer has a propensity to develop liver metastases. Whether this is a result of portal vein drainage of the colon, of genetic influences, or of a combination of factors is not completely understood. Not uncommonly, the metastases will be limited to the liver, and the disease within the liver can be resected. When initial reports about liver resection extending the lives of colon cancer patients became available, they were criticized as flawed as a result of selection bias. The patients who underwent resection were likely healthier and had less disease than the historical controls they were compared with and who did not undergo operations. Although there still has not been a randomized study demonstrating improved survival with liver resection, there is now substantial evidence that liver resection in selected patients will indeed cure some patients and that it will prolong the survival of many others. This is shown by more careful analysis of the historical studies, in which there are many reports of documented cures and very prolonged survivals of patients who undergo resection as compared with the uniformly limited survival in closely matched controls. This is true not just for colorectal liver metastases but for other cancers as well (Table 26-1). In a similar fashion, the resection of pulmonary metastases from a variety of cancers has been described, with a potential benefit reported as compared with the historical controls of untreated patients (Table 26-2).

The means by which to select patients who can benefit from surgical resection is still an ongoing debate. Some have proposed specific cutoffs (e.g., less than four hepatic metastases), but such thresholds are somewhat arbitrary. There are, however, several factors that can be broadly understood to help with the making of these decisions.

TABLE 26-1 • *Survival After Resection of Liver Metastases*

Author	Year	Cancer	N	5-Year Survival
Harrison	1997	Multiple	41	26%
Raab	1998	Breast	34	18%
Bakalakos	1998	Colorectal	238	29%
Fong	1999	Colorectal	1,001	37%
Ambiru	1999	Colorectal	168	26%
DeMatteo	2001	Sarcoma	56	30%
Pocard	2001	Breast	65	46%

BOX 26-1 FACTORS IN DETERMINING THE ADVISABILITY OF RESECTING METASTATIC DISEASE

- Tumor biology
- Ability to address all disease
- Number of metastatic sites
- Disease-free interval
- Medical condition of the patient

Tumor Biology

There are some cancers that are inherently much more aggressive, and the resection of metastatic disease historically has had no effect as a result of the rapid appearance of widespread disease. Other cancers, although they may be slow growing, are almost never isolated to single or few sites that are amenable to resection. Examples of these cancer types include pancreatic, bile duct, lung, esophageal, and prostate cancers. This is contrasted with melanomas, sarcomas, colorectal, and renal cell cancers, which often can present with isolated metastatic lesions that are amenable to resection, with good long-term survivals (Tables 26-3 and 26-4). Moreover, as systemic chemotherapy improves, some traditionally aggressive tumors may be turned into a more indolent processes, for which the aggressive surgical resection of metastatic sites may become more fruitful.

TABLE 26–2 • *Survival After Resection of Lung Metastases*

Author	Year	Cancer	N	5-Year Survival
Ris	1991	Multiple	83	38%
Skinner	1992	Osteogenic sarcoma	114	37%
McCormack	1992	Colorectal	144	40%
McAfee	1992	Colorectal	139	31%
Choong	1995	Soft-tissue sarcoma	214	40%
Okumura	1996	Colorectal	159	41%
Van Geel	1996	Soft-tissue sarcoma	255	35%
Liu	1999	Head and neck	83	50%
Billingsley	1999	Soft tissue sarcoma	213	37%
Zink	2001	Colorectal	110	33%
Murabito	2000	Breast	86	80%
Friedel	2002	Breast	467	38%
Pfann-schmidt	2002	Renal cell	185	37%
Piltz	2002	Renal cell	105	40%

All Disease Can Be Addressed

Debulking surgery has a very restricted role (see below). Subjecting a patient to a major surgery and a prolonged recuperation period knowing that gross disease will be left behind is not usually beneficial. Often the residual disease expands very quickly, and the natural history of tumors that are extensive enough to preclude complete resection also predicts more rapid and widespread recurrences. Detailed imaging studies to detect common areas of metastatic spread are reasonable to prevent operative procedures that are not helpful. There is some debate regarding the cost of these studies and how often they change therapy, so some thought is necessary about which tests are ordered. Take the example of colon cancer: CT scanning of the chest, abdomen, and pelvis and colonoscopy are reasonable to select to screen for lung metastases, the extent of abdominopelvic disease, and metachronous tumor formation or suture-line recurrence. Additional studies directed by patient symptoms are also indicated. Isolated brain metastases are rare enough that obtaining a screening scan of the brain is not particularly helpful. Some advocate a positron emission tomography scan as well, but evidence is still accumulating and may depend in part on the quality of the CT imaging. Some may request a chest x-ray rather than a CT scan of the chest, but, given the low cost of noncontrast CT scanning and its much higher sensitivity, others find obtaining the CT scan reasonable. If lesions in separate organs are identified (e.g., a liver lesion

TABLE 26–3 • *Common Sites of Resectable Metastases*

Primary Cancer	Common Site of Resectable Metastasis
Colorectal	Liver, lung
Sarcoma	Lung
Melanoma	Lung, small bowel, distant lymph node, soft tissue
Renal cell carcinoma	Lung, pancreas

TABLE 26–4 • *Survival After Resection of Melanoma Metastases*

Author	Year	Site	N	5-Year Survival
Markowitz	1991	Distant lymph nodes	72	45%
Markowitz	1991	Soft tissue	60	61%
Gorenstein	1991	Lung	56	25%
Gadd	1992	Skin, soft tissue	190	14%
Harpole	1992	Lung	84	20%
Karakousis	1994	Distant lymph nodes	23	22%
Karakousis	1994	Skin, soft tissue	27	33%
Tafra	1995	Lung	106	27%
Ricaniadis	1995	Gastroin-testinal tract	47	28.3%
La Hei	1996	Lung	83	22%
Ollila	1996	Gastroin-testinal tract	46	41%
Haigh	1999	Adrenal glands	18	27%
Meyer	2000	Distant lymph nodes	45	20%
Meyer	2000	Skin, soft tissue	30	17.8%
Leo	2000	Lung	282	22%
Rose	2001	Liver	24	29%

and a lung lesion) and both are resectable, surgery may still be considered (Table 26-5).

Newer technology has also expanded the number of patients who are able to undergo potentially curative resections. Laparoscopy offers a low-morbidity method to visually inspect the abdomen. Radiofrequency ablation can treat lesions that are not readily resectable to preserve surrounding liver tissue or to minimize morbidity. Portal vein embolization of the affected liver lobe can expand the amount of anticipated residual liver so that a large resection would be possible. Rarely, whole liver resection and transplantation can also be of value, particularly when underlying cirrhosis is present.

Prolonged Disease-Free Interval

The longer the period from primary treatment until disease recurrence, the more likely that any metastatic lesions identified will be the only ones that exist or at least that a significant additional disease-free interval will be obtained. In some settings, preoperative systemic chemotherapy can be used to both determine if the metastatic diseases is responsive and also to determine if widespread metastases appear during the systemic therapy treatment period. If the latter is true, then surgery would not have been helpful.

Limited Metastatic Sites

Although there is no absolute limit on the number of metastases that should be resected, the more tumor deposits that are known to exist the greater the likelihood that there is additional disease that is subclinical and that will appear in the near future, thereby making surgery less helpful. The best results are seen with a single metastatic site.

TABLE 26–5 • *Survival After Resection of Lung and Liver Metastases in Colorectal Cancer*

Author	Year	N	5-Year Survival
Regnard	1998	43	11%
Kobayashi	1999	47	31%
Robinson	1999	25	43%
Headrick	2001	58	30%
Nagakura	2001	27	27%
Mineo	2003	29	51%

Patient Factors

Many patients have significant comorbidities that are competing causes for their demise. These comorbidities also complicate and increase the risks for attempts at surgical resection. One must balance the risks of surgery and the risks of major complications and prolonged recovery with the potential for improved survival and the potential that the procedure will have no significant survival benefit, even without any complications. In most circumstances, the chance of "curing" the patient of metastatic disease with surgery is much less than that with surgery performed to treat the primary. On the other hand, young patients facing almost certain death from metastatic disease may undergo surgically aggressive procedures that have small odds of success; in these cases, if the procedures are successful, the long-term benefit is great enough to warrant the attempt. In all cases, any specific individual's tumor biology is difficult to predict exactly.

Indications for Surgery in the Presence of Metastatic Disease

As already discussed, it is only under unusual circumstances that a tumor is debulked or cytoreduced to achieve a survival benefit or a hope of cure. However, as chemotherapy improves, this may become a more active area of surgical practice.

Aside from resections under emergency conditions (e.g., for bowel perforations, obstructions, or actively bleeding lesions), there is still a role for the surgical removal of metastatic lesions or primary cancers in the setting of distant disease when patients are symptomatic. For example, metastatic melanoma to the intestine can cause slow but ongoing bleeding, and it can often be resected to good effect in patients of adequate performance who do not have overwhelming additional disease. Carcinoid and neuroendocrine metastases can cause symptoms from their hormone secretion, and they can be so slow growing that debulking these tumors and removing significant gross disease will also remove a significant source of the hormonal secretions for prolonged periods of time.

There are also circumstances in which the primary tumor should be addressed, even in the presence of metastatic disease. Gastric cancer causing an immotile stomach and/or slow

BOX 26-2 CYTOREDUCTION

- Improves effects of systemic therapy on residual metastatic disease
- Extent of cytoreduction correlates with survival
- Possible added benefit with the addition of regional systemic therapy, which may include:
  - Heated intraperitoneal chemotherapy
  - Surgically administered regional therapy
  - Isolated limb perfusion or infusion
  - Hepatic infusion or isolated hepatic perfusion

bleeding may benefit from resection—even with distant disease—to relieve these symptoms. Locally advanced breast cancers or sarcomas may need surgery for wound care concerns in a stage IV setting, particularly if the local disease is causing distressing symptoms and/or the distant disease is progressing slowly. Traditionally, colon and rectal cancers were recommended to be resected—even when they were widely metastatic—to prevent obstruction. In many instances, chemotherapy or endoscopic stenting/ablation can delay or alleviate the need for primary surgical resection. However, these patients need to be carefully evaluated. With good systemic response to chemotherapy which is increasingly common, primary resection can be reconsidered.

Another area of active interest is in tumor cytoreduction to improve the effects of systemic therapy on any residual metastatic disease. This has been demonstrated in ovarian cancer, in which the cytoreduction of the tumor (while leaving small amounts of gross and microscopic tumor behind) improves survival after systemic chemotherapy administration. Similarly, removing the primary tumor in renal cancer improves survival in selected patients with known metastatic disease. Presumably, systemic therapy can work better on smaller volumes of disease. Whether this is the result of the immunological effects of decreased tumor burden or of reducing the pool of resistant tumor cell subpopulations is unknown.

The cytoreduction of intraperitoneal-restricted metastatic cancers (e.g., appendiceal and selected colorectal cancers) performed in conjunction with heated intraperitoneal chemotherapy administration has also been shown to be beneficial (Figure 26-1). The gross tumor is surgically removed by multiorgan resections and by stripping involved peritoneal surfaces. After the reduction of tumor to microscopic levels or nodules less than 2 mm, heated chemotherapy at high concentrations is infused into the abdomen for approximately an hour during the surgical procedure (Figures 26-2 and 26-3). The chemotherapy may then destroy the residual disease without being absorbed to a great extent. This has been shown to be effective for appendiceal cancer in retrospective studies, and it prolonged survival in a randomized trial of colorectal cancer patients. Morbidity is considerable, and patient selection is important to maximize benefits. Heated intraperitoneal perfusion experience also exists for ovarian cancer, sarcomas, mesotheliomas, and primary peritoneal cancers. Intraperitoneal chemotherapy administered prophylactically during surgery for high-risk gastric cancers has also been explored in Japan, with promising results. The extent to which the chemotherapy, the heat, and the surgical cytoreduction each contribute to the observed survival benefit is not clear; upcoming studies may clarify this.

Surgically administered regional therapy can also be thought of as a cytoreductive technique. Examples of this are isolated hyperthermic limb perfusion for local-regional advanced melanoma and sarcoma patients and hepatic artery infusion or isolated hepatic perfusions for unresectable liver metastases.

Isolated limb perfusion involves the surgical isolation and control of the inflow and outflow of the affected limb using an oxygenated bypass pump bypass circuit. Hyperthermic chemother-

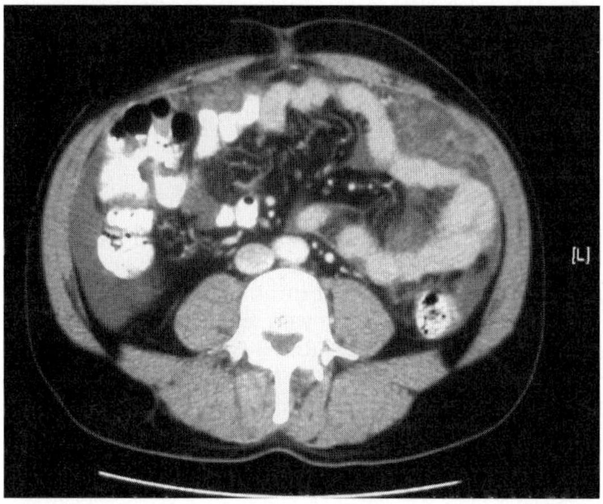

Figure 26-1. CT slice of advanced carcinomatosis.

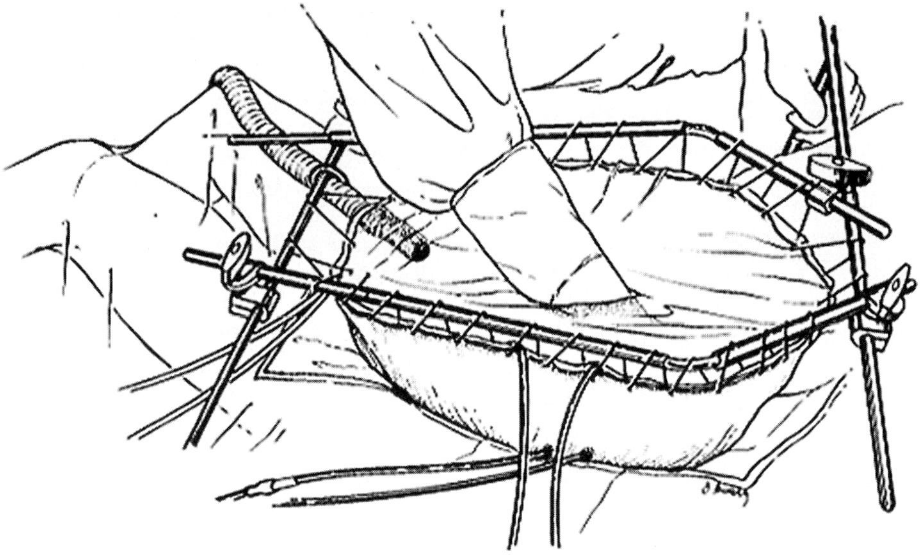

Figure 26-2. Schematic of intraperitoneal hyperthermic perfusion. Through a long midline incision, a complete cytoreduction of all macroscopic tumor is performed. This may include multiple organ resections and/or peritoneum stripping of the involved areas. A silastic sheet is sewn to the skin edges and suspended from a fixed retractor system to create a bowl into which high dose chemotherapy is continuously circulated through a heat exchanger to maintain a perfusate temperature of 42°C to 44°C. The contents of the abdomen are agitated by hand to evenly distribute the perfusate. After 90 minutes, the perfusate is washed out and the operation is completed.

apy (usually melphalan) is administered for 60 minutes at relatively high doses that could not be well tolerated if given systemically. After treatment, the limb is washed out, the vessels

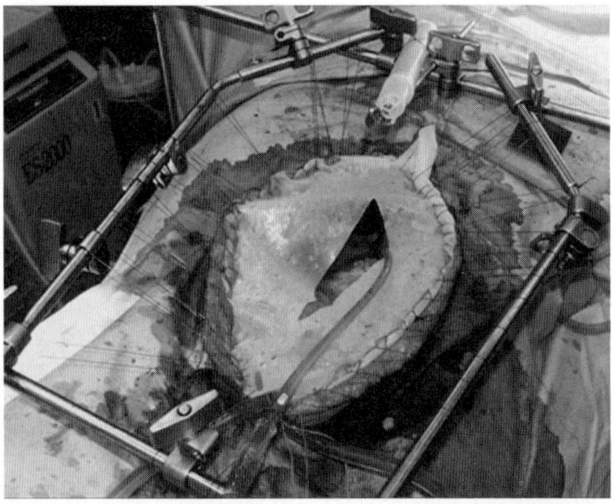

Figure 26-3. Schematic of an isolated limb infusion. Arterial and venous catheters are placed through the contralateral groin and into the superficial femoral artery and vein of the affected limb. A tourniquet is inflated above the catheter tip locations and heated high dose chemotherapy is pumped using a hand syringe and 3-way stopcock through the heat exchanger and into the leg. The leg is also heated externally with hot air and hot water blankets. An esmarch bandage can be used on the foot to limit chemotherapy perfusion and the associated toxicity if the foot is not affected by the disease.

are repaired, and normal blood flow is reestablished to the limb. Similar to this (but less complex) are limb infusion techniques that involve percutaneous vascular access, with tourniquet control of the limb and nonoxygenated chemotherapy administration for a shorter period of time (Figure 26-4). The potential leak of agent into the systemic circulation is higher, but the overall results appear to be similar.

Hepatic artery infusion therapy via an implanted port or, more commonly, an implanted pump has been used to treat unresectable hepatic metastases. This method offers a greater response rate as compared with systemic therapy. Survival benefits have been more difficult to demonstrate, and complication rates are significant. Ongoing trials may clarify the role of hepatic arterial infusion, and they may determine whether it can be a supplement to resection for treating the residual liver or whether newer systemic chemotherapy agents are more simply administered and more effective in these situations.

Isolated hepatic perfusion techniques are currently experimental and involve either surgical vascular control or percutaneous angiographically guided control via balloon catheters, with the administration of chemotherapy into the liver directly through the hepatic artery. Systemic exposure is greater than it is in limb

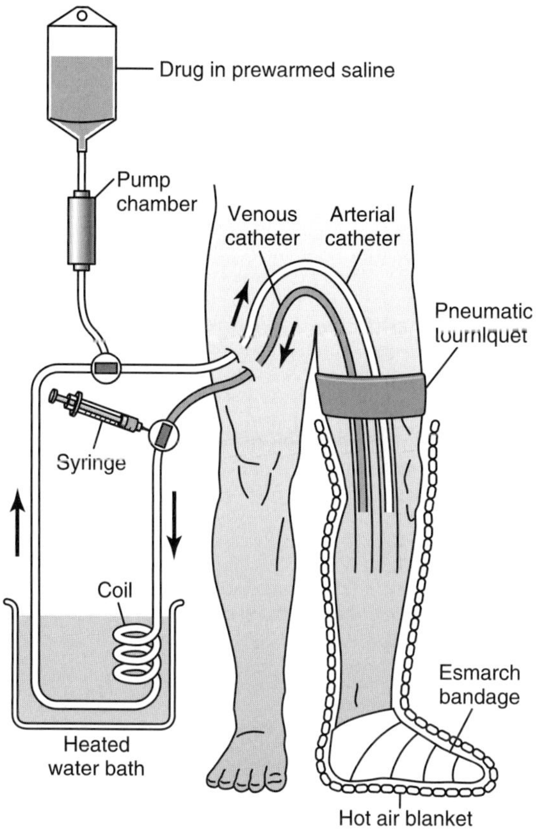

Figure 26–4. Diagram of isolated extremity infusion.

perfusion protocols, and the tumors may not be as responsive; however, trials are ongoing.

Palliative and Adjunctive Surgical Procedures

Palliative and adjunctive procedures include surgeries for symptom relief and those that are performed under emergency conditions.

BOX 26–3 POSSIBLE PALLIATIVE AND ADJUNCTIVE PROCEDURES

- Placement of feeding tube or decompression tube
- Pain-control procedures
- Drainage procedures, including the following:
  1. Paracentesis
  2. Catheter drainage
  3. Peritoneovenous shunting
  4. Hyperthermic intraperitoneal heated chemotherapy without cytoreduction

Selected patients may achieve a significant period of quality survival out of the hospital. A common example is the placement of a feeding or decompressive tube either by percutaneous, laparoscopic, or open methods. Palliative procedures may be considered during an operation when the planned resection is terminated as a result of advanced disease. Surgical treatments may not have otherwise been indicated, but, because the patient had undergone the laparotomy already, surgical decompression of the bowel or biliary system, regional neurolytic injections, or tube decompressive procedures may be more durable, and they may preclude multiple radiologic or endoscopic procedures.

Pain control can sometimes be helped with surgery. Examples include splanchnicectomy, neurolysis, decompressive tumor debulking, and pain-pump implantation. Tumor can be harvested for clinical trial protocols or chemotherapy sensitivity testing.

Drainage procedures can be palliative, and they may include treatments of pleural and pericardial effusions and ascites. Thoracentesis and pleurodesis are effective in the majority of patients with malignant effusions. Repeated paracentesis, catheter drainage, and peritoneovenous shunting can all be used to control ascites. The chosen procedure often depends on the difficulty of controlling the symptoms versus the increasing morbidity of these procedures with the level of invasiveness. Often the procedures are used in sequence, escalating with the persistence of the ascites and associated symptoms. For extreme cases of malignant ascites (particularly with more indolent tumors), hyperthermic intraperitoneal heated chemotherapy without cytoreduction is very effective for controlling persistent ascites in 80% of patients.

In summary, surgeons can play an active and helpful role in the treatment of cancer patients, despite the existence of distant disease. Surgical therapy can cure some patients, prolong survival in others, and alleviate suffering and assist with other therapies in the vast majority.

Key Selected Reading

Wagman LD. Palliative surgical oncology. *Surg Oncol Clin N Am* 2004;13:401–548.

Selected Readings

Ahmad SA, Kim J, Sussman JJ, *et al.* Reduced morbidity following cytoreductive surgery and intraperitoneal hyperthermic chemoperfusion. *Ann Surg Oncol* 2004;11:387–392.

Alexander HR, Jr., Fraker DL, Bartlett DL. Isolated limb perfusion for malignant melanoma. *Semin Surg Oncol* 1996;12:416–428.

Dunn GP. The surgeon and palliative care. *Surg Oncol Clin N Am* 2001;10:1–232.

Eggermont AMM, Koops HS, Klausner JM, *et al.* Isolation limb perfusion with tumor necrosis factor alpha and chemotherapy for advanced extremity soft tissue sarcomas. *Semin Oncol* 1997;24:547–555.

Glehen O, Kwiatkowski F, Sugarbaker PH, *et al.* Cytoreductive surgery combined with perioperative intraperitoneal chemotherapy for the management of peritoneal carcinomatosis from colorectal cancer: a multi-institutional study. *J Clin Oncol* 2004;22: 3284–3292.

Hofmann B, Haheim LL, Soreide JA. Ethics of palliative surgery in patients with cancer. *Br J Surg* 2005;92:802–809.

Krouse RS. Advances in palliative surgery for cancer patients. *J Support Oncol* 2004;2:80–87.

Maltoni M, Caraceni A, Brunelli C, *et al.* Prognostic factors in advanced cancer patients: evidence-based clinical recommendations—a study by the Steering Committee of the European Association for Palliative Care. *J Clin Oncol* 2005;23:6240–6248.

Miner TJ. Palliative surgery for advanced cancer. Lessons learned in patient selection and outcome assessment. *Am J Clin Oncol* 2005;28:411–414.

Ollila DW, Caudle AS. Surgical management of distant metastases. *Surg Oncol Clin N Am* 2006;15: 385–398.

Sugarbaker PH. Strategies for the prevention and treatment of peritoneal carcinomatosis from gastrointestinal cancer. *Cancer Invest* 2005;23:155–172.

Thompson JF, Hunt JA, Shannon KF, *et al.* Frequency and duration of remission after isolated limb perfusion for melanoma. *Arch Surg* 1997;132:903–907.

Thompson JF, Kam PC. Isolated limb infusion for melanoma: a simple but effective alternative to isolated limb perfusion. *J Surg Oncol* 2004;88:1–3.

Vauthey JN, ed. Primary and metastatic liver cancer: *Surg Oncol Clin N Am* 2003;12:1–11, vii.

Verwaal VJ, van Ruth S, de Bree E, *et al.* Randomized trial of cytoreduction and hyperthermic intraperitoneal chemotherapy versus systemic chemotherapy and palliative surgery in patients with peritoneal carcinomatosis of colorectal cancer. *J Clin Oncol* 2003;21:3737–3743.

Vogelbaum MA, Suh JH. Resectable brain metastases. *J Clin Oncol* 2006;24:1289–1294.

Young SE, Martinez SR, Essner R. The role of surgery in treatment of stage IV melanoma. *J Surg Oncol* 2006;94:344–351.

27

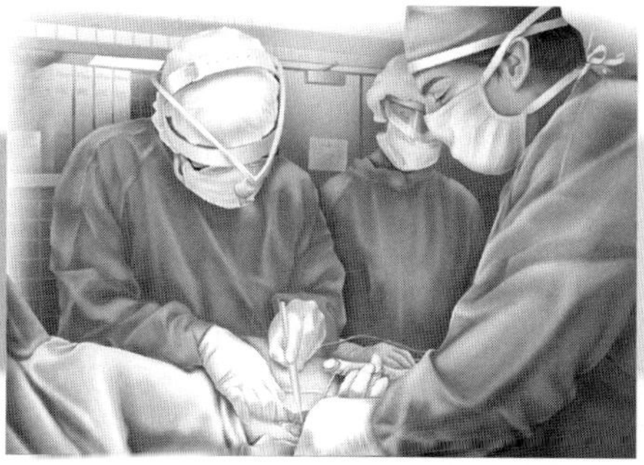

Surgical Emergencies in the Cancer Patient

Jeffrey J. Sussman

Surgical Emergencies in the Cancer Patient: Key Points

- Discuss how the basic tenets of general surgery differ for surgical emergencies in cancer patients.
- List the emergency surgical approaches for esophageal, gastric, small-bowel, colorectal, and biliary obstructions.
- Detail the causes of perforation.
- Outline the common approaches and cautions to be considered when treating perforations.
- Describe the causes and treatments of fistulas.
- Identify the causes and management of bleeding problems in cancer patients.
- Outline effective pain-control techniques and practice considerations.
- Describe neutropenic enterocolitis and appropriate approaches to its treatment.

Emergency care is needed for cancer patients under various circumstances. These interventions can be divided into medical and surgical emergencies, and they can be further subdivided into those related to cancer diagnosis or cancer therapy and those unrelated to cancer specifically and only occurring incidentally in the cancer patient. Although it is tempting to always connect a new surgical problem to a cancer recurrence, in many instances, the new problem is unrelated and the cancer diagnosis is of no consequence.

BOX 27–1 GENERAL SURGICAL EMERGENCIES

- Obstruction
- Perforation
- Bleeding
- Neutropenic enterocolitis
- Fistulas
- Pain
- Airway compromise

BOX 27–2 OTHER SURGICAL EMERGENCIES IN THE CANCER PATIENT

- Metabolic/paraneoplastic syndromes
  - Syndrome of inappropriate antidiuretic hormone secretion
  - Hypoglycemia
  - Hypercalcemia
  - Hyperuricemia
  - Adrenal insufficiency
  - Lambert-Eaton syndrome
  - Polymyositis/dermatomyositis
- Brain edema/cord compression
  - Intracranial hemorrhage
  - Status epilepticus
- Deep venous thrombosis/pulmonary embolus
- Superior vena cava syndrome
- Cardiac complications
  - Pericardial tamponade
- Nonbacterial thrombotic endocarditis
- Urologic complications
  - Bleeding
  - Ureteral obstruction
  - Infections
  - Priapism
- Orthopedic (fractures)

The basic principles of general surgery are still used to deal with surgical emergencies in the cancer patient. The main difference is that these techniques and strategies are used with an eye toward the overall status of the patient, their cancer-related prognosis, and their need for ongoing cancer treatment, including chemotherapy, radiation, and/or additional surgery. Because of this, as much information relating to the patient's cancer diagnosis and current cancer stage as possible should be sought. Of particular importance is an assessment of the patient's tumor's biological aggressiveness. The pre-emergency performance status of the patient is critically important, and, ideally, frank conversations with the patient and his or her family in a nonemergency setting to clarify the patient's wishes regarding aggressive medical and surgical interventions in case of deterioration or an unexpected emergency should have already occurred. How aggressive an intervention should be undertaken in a particular patient varies from patient to patient and from tumor to tumor, even given the exact same complication. Living wills, power-of-attorney documents, and prior discussions with the patient all are useful for helping to determine the most appropriate intervention. It is necessary to balance the risks of surgical intervention with the

BOX 27–3 CONSIDERATIONS WHEN APPROACHING A SURGICAL EMERGENCY IN A CANCER PATIENT

- Medical condition of the patient
  - Age and comorbid conditions
  - Performance status
  - Nutritional status
- Prognosis of cancer
  - Type and stage of cancer
  - Quality and duration of life without treatment
  - Plans for additional radiation, chemo therapy, and/or surgery
- Risks and benefits of intervention
  - Treatment of emergency versus prognosis of patient
  - Cure versus palliation
  - Risks of therapy
  - Quality and duration of life with treatment
- Efficacy of nonsurgical interventions
  - Patient's and family's expressed wishes

risks—both short and long term—of more minimally invasive interventions and the potential benefits of these interventions with regard to the patient's cancer prognosis. Sound judgment and good communication skills are critical.

Obstruction

Obstructive problems in the cancer patient require emergent attention, but they often do not require emergent surgery. One third of obstructions are benign and unrelated to the cancer diagnosis. Many gastrointestinal (GI) obstructions can be decompressed with nasogastric suction. The patient can be rehydrated and staging studies performed to evaluate the location and nature of the obstruction and the extent of cancer involvement. Therefore, the best approach to the treatment and/or palliation of the patient as a whole can be considered.

Esophageal Obstruction

Locally advanced esophageal cancer can present initially with obstruction, or obstruction can occur as a result of recurrent disease. One needs to assess the degree of obstruction and whether the patient can handle his or her own salivary secretions. A nasogastric tube can be placed above the level of the obstruction to clear secretions and to prevent aspiration in the completely obstructed patient as a short-term solution. Most commonly, however, patients can manage their own secretions, but they are unable to adequately receive oral nutrition. Liquid dietary supplements can be used while obtaining staging imaging studies to determine the extent of disease both locally and distantly and while assessing the patient's performance status and comorbidities. If the patient is judged to be a potential surgical candidate, then he or she can be properly prepared for surgery. If nutritionally depleted, the patient may benefit from either a feeding tube placed past the obstruction, if possible, or a laparoscopically or radiologically placed percutaneous jejunostomy tube. A gastrostomy tube can be placed; however, if surgery is anticipated, a jejunostomy tube may be preferred to avoid repairing the usual conduit. Alternatively, intravenous nutrition can be instituted.

If primary or neoadjuvant chemotherapy/radiation therapy is planned, one should be prepared for treatment-related edema and initial worsening of the obstructive symptoms before esophageal patency improves. This may also require feeding-tube placement to help with nutritional support resulting from both tumor obstruction and treatment-related mucosal erosions.

For patients with a complete obstruction, advanced disease, or recurrent cancer after failed initial treatment, endoscopically placed self-expanding metal wire stents have been used successfully. Wire stents appear to be an improvement over previously placed plastic prostheses, which had significant problems with erosion and migration. Stents may be combined with endoscopic ablative techniques such as laser, photodynamic therapy, bipolar cautery, or the injection of sclerosing agents. These ablative techniques, however, risk perforation, and, even if they are successful, the patient's esophageal motility may still be decreased in the area of tumor treatment, thus requiring careful patient instructions for thorough mastication with plenty of liquids to prevent clogging of the newly formed passage. Subtotal palliative resection or substernal surgical bypass may rarely be necessary because of the typical aggressive biology of locally advanced esophageal cancers.

Gastric Obstruction

Because of the size of the body of the stomach, mechanical obstruction is uncommon in this location. Functional obstruction, however, can occur with tumor infiltration of the wall of the stomach or the neural structures, making it noncompliant and dysmotile. Physical obstruction can occur more commonly at the gastroesophageal junction (which can be treated similar to esophageal cancer; see above) or in the antrum, where the stomach is narrower.

Analogous to esophageal cancer, nasogastric decompression can be used for complete or near-complete obstructions to relieve the acute distention and patient emesis. The patient should be rehydrated, the electrolytes should be corrected as necessary, and proton-pump inhibitors should be used to decrease gastric fluid output. This provides time to properly stage the cancer patient and to discuss an overall treatment plan. Operative candidates can more electively undergo resection with consideration of neoadjuvant treatment. Some patients with good performance status may be candidates for a palliative resection, even in the setting of early metastatic disease, to relieve gastric obstruction. Consideration of the response to systemic chemotherapy may help define the tumor's biological aggressiveness before putting a patient through surgery and prolonged recovery if life expectancy is short.

Patients who are unresectable for cure may be palliated with endoscopic stent placement.

Migration and long-term durability of the stents are still problematic, however, and a surgical gastrojejunostomy bypass for distal obstructing lesions or a proximal resection and either gastroesophagostomy or jejunoesophagostomy for proximal lesions should be considered for patients with a life expectancy greater than several months. Often this is combined with a jejunostomy tube and/or a gastrostomy tube placement to help speed nutritional recovery, particularly if the stomach fails to empty promptly through the new anastomosis or becomes reobstructed.

Small Bowel Obstruction

If the small bowel obstruction is caused by the primary tumor, resection is recommended as the primary treatment option. Nasogastric decompression may also allow time for optimizing the patient's hydration, for electrolyte correction, and for staging the cancer for appropriate treatment planning. More commonly, small-bowel obstruction—if it is tumor related—is caused by carcinomatosis. Again, performance status, extent of metastatic tumor burden, and aggressiveness of the tumor biology must be considered in this situation. Bowel resection in the face of carcinomatosis can lead to perforation and fistula formation, so sound surgical judgment is required. Some patients are best served by hospice, without operative intervention. A percutaneous endoscopic gastrostomy tube can be placed for palliation in such situations to eliminate the need for nasogastric intubation. Intravenous nutrition decisions are left for the patient-physician discussion, with the recognition that, after they have been started, such feedings can be emotionally difficult for the patient and/or the patient's family to stop.

Carcinomatosis rarely leads to bowel ischemia, except with closed-loop obstruction. Therefore, time is often available for nasogastric decompression, prolonged observation, full cancer staging, and detailed patient-family discussions. CT scanning can often delineate the extent of tumor involvement and the level of obstruction. Many times, nasogastric decompression alone allows a partial small-bowel obstruction to resolve after a few days of supportive care. After it has resolved, however, an outpatient elective contrast study may be helpful to define the level and degree of a partial obstruction for either elective repair or if recurrence develops.

Nonresolving small-bowel obstructions in a patient with an otherwise good performance status should be operatively explored. Even with carcinomatosis, patients can often best be palliated for the longest period of time by surgical intervention. If a localized implant of tumor is causing the obstruction, resection of the bowel segment is preferred. In many instances, an adhesive band is the source of the obstruction, rather than tumor. If resection cannot be performed safely, bypass to a distal small-bowel loop or to the colon may be preferred. If extensive bowel involvement by cancer is noted, proximal decompression with an intestinal stoma or a gastrostomy tube may be in order. Care is needed to prevent inadvertent enterotomies and fistulas that may be difficult to heal and treat. Attention should be paid to additional more distal obstructing lesions or impending obstructions. Additional bypasses or resections may be necessary. The creation of mucous fistulas to decompress closed loops that are no longer in intestinal continuity may also be required. One should define in the operative report the extent of disease, and, if a reobstruction were to occur, whether the patient would likely benefit from an additional operation.

In highly selected patients, aggressive cytoreduction may be indicated. Ongoing trials appear to support this for appendiceal and colorectal cancer, sarcoma, mesothelioma, and ovarian cancers in which the spread is primarily based in the peritoneum. This is often combined with hyperthermic chemotherapy perfusion. Ideally, the patient should not be acutely obstructed when undergoing this procedure, and he or she may require an initial decompressive procedure before undergoing definitive cytoreduction. Complete or near-complete gross cytoreduction should be anticipated for this procedure to have any hope of effectiveness.

Colorectal Obstruction

Obstructing colorectal lesions are an emergency, because an intact ileocecal valve leads to a closed-loop situation with the risk of colonic perforation. In addition, pseudo-obstruction or an "Ogilvie's syndrome" may simulate a mechanical obstruction. CT or water-soluble contrast enema studies may differentiate the two conditions (Figure 27-1). Nonmechanical obstruction should be initially treated nonoperatively, if possible, by addressing the underlying cause of the colonic ileus with electrolyte correction, sepsis control, ambulation, and narcotic medication mini-

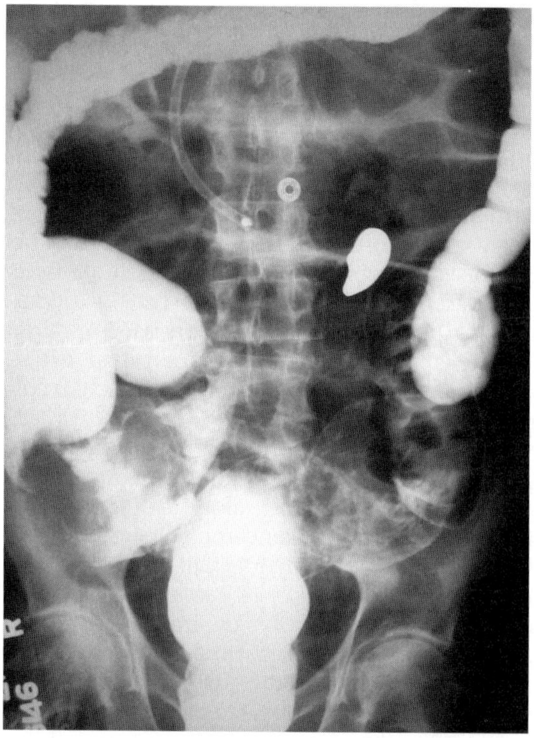

Figure 27-1. Contrast x-ray obstructing colon cancer. A barium contrast study image is shown that demonstrates a narrowing of the ascending colon from the obstructing colon cancer in this location. Proximal small bowel is dilated as a result of the obstruction.

mization. Neostigmine and/or endoscopic decompression may be necessary.

Mechanical obstruction may be amenable to decompression with endoscopy with or without stent placement or ablative techniques to allow for bowel preparation and elective resection in non–end-stage patients. If relief is not achieved expeditiously, then operative intervention for resection and/or diversion is mandated.

Biliary Obstruction

Endoscopic or transhepatic percutaneous drainage is often well tolerated when biliary obstruction is associated with sepsis. Initial decompression and stenting can be converted to a covered wire stent without the need for frequent plastic stent exchanges if definitive resectional therapy is not possible. If a long survival is anticipated or if surgical intervention is contemplated for other reasons, then a surgical biliary-enteric anastomosis provides good long-term durability, although with higher initial morbidity than endoscopic techniques. For patients with poor performance status, decompression and external drainage of bile flow via percutaneous transhepatic cholangiography provides better palliation. Biliary obstruction without cholangitis does not mandate immediate decompression, and patients can be fully staged and evaluated for definitive resection and treatment.

Perforation

Perforation of the GI tract and concomitant infectious complications are life-threatening events that can occur in cancer patients. Perforation may present after prolonged obstruction, which has led to distention and ischemia; it may also result from localized tumor replacement of the bowel wall with subsequent tumor necrosis or perforation from a lack of normal mucosal integrity. Occasionally, perforation may result from treatments (e.g., steroids) or from complications of chemotherapy (e.g., severe dehydration, decreased bowel perfusion).

If an abscess develops from a walled off, contained perforation, then image-guided percutaneous drainage may be preferred to control the infection and to convert the situation into a controlled enterocutaneous fistula, particularly in a palliative setting; the drain tract in this circumstance may now be seeded with tumor. In situations involving a primary tumor perforation and in which a formal resection can remove both the primary and the entire perforated space, then this would be preferred (Figure 27-2).

If an uncontrolled perforation exists into the chest or abdomen, surgery is usually necessary for the patient's survival. Surgical considerations are detailed below. Occasionally, in a patient with poor performance status and end-stage disease, palliative pain control is all that may be appropriate.

If perforation occurs during chemotherapy treatment and the patient is neutropenic, mortality is high. Treatment should include broad-spectrum antibiotics/antifungals and colony-stimulating factors to reverse the immunosuppression. Treatment responses in full-thickness bowel-wall tumor deposits do not typically lead to perforation; however, this may occur with very chemoradiation-sensitive tumors (e.g., lymphoma). The rapid necrosis of the malignant lymphocytes that have

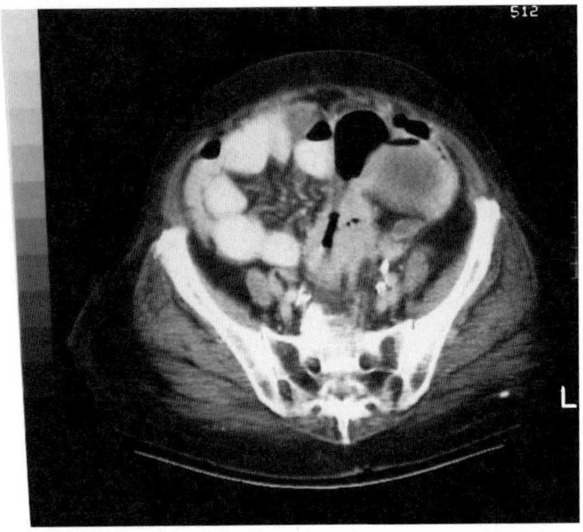

Figure 27–2. Computed tomography image of colon carcinoma and associated perforation with abscess formation. The image demonstrates a thickening in the sigmoid colon representing the patient's colon cancer and the associated fluid collection in the mesentery beside the cancer. The air-fluid level is outside of the bowel loops, and it represents an abscess formed by the perforation of the colon cancer.

replaced the bowel wall in certain areas can lead to a perforation. However, this scenario is not sufficiently common that prophylactic surgery is required in high-risk patients or that the chemotherapy regimens should be changed to be less efficacious.

Principles of treatment include drainage and control of the perforation. If resection of the tumor-involved area is possible, this is preferable, but the risk of a prolonged surgery, the patient's hemodynamic status, and the degree of intestinal spillage must be assessed. In many cases, drainage and proximal diversion or tube drainage are more appropriate to control sepsis and to salvage the patient. When assessing the extent of surgical intervention, surgeons should keep in mind the potential need for subsequent chemotherapy and/or radiation therapy as well as the need for a speedy recovery for a patient with a limited life expectancy.

The perforation of a primary cancer is associated with a high risk of peritoneal spread of cancer cells in addition to the infectious complications. Colorectal cancer, in particular, may present in this manner. If the perforation is contained in the retroperitoneum or into the abdomen side wall, the affected area can be marked with radio-opaque clips for adjuvant postoperative radiation therapy. If the perforation occurs after a biopsy in the setting of prepared bowel, a formal resection in an otherwise stable patient would be most appropriate. If a large amount of spillage of bowel contents or delayed presentation has occurred, proximal diversion with limited resection may be appropriate, allowing a more elective formal resection and reanastomosis to be performed at a later date. These patients may also be candidates for an adjuvant hyperthermic intraperitoneal perfusion because of the risk of peritoneal spread. Decreased survival and increased morbidity are seen when patients undergo emergent colorectal cancer operations as a result of perforation as compared with elective resections. This survival decrement is also seen in acutely obstructed colorectal cancer patients.

Perforations of esophageal tumors are very poorly tolerated, but the same general surgical principles apply. Drainage alone is often not sufficient, because the cancerous tissue will not heal, and a persistent fistula will develop; therefore, resection is usually necessary. This may be performed transhiatally or transthoracically, depending on tumor location, local extension, and extent of inflammation. Reconstruction can be safely performed in stable patients; however, cervical esophagostomy, gastrostomy tube placement, and mediastinal drainage with or without primary tumor resection may be needed, with elective anastomosis at a later date.

Fistulas

As in other general surgery patients, fistulas can develop in cancer patients for a number of reasons. They can be postoperative from anastomotic leaks or bowel injury, or they can be the end result of percutaneous drainage for a perforation. In addition, fistulas can result from tumor involvement and invasion between hollow viscus, such as small-bowel loop to small-bowel loop, bowel to bladder, or bowel to vagina, skin, or other organ. General principles of drainage and sepsis control are followed. Some fistulas may heal with time but distal obstruction, irradiation, malnutrition, and the presence of tumor at the fistula site all contribute to the nonhealing of a fistula in a cancer patient as in other fistula patients.

Medical treatment initially with proximal nasogastric decompression, skin care, antibiotics (if associated with infection/sepsis), rehydration, electrolyte correction, and associated abscess drainage is almost always appropriate to allow for time for full cancer staging, for discussions with the patient and family, and for

BOX 27-4 REASONS THAT GASTROINTESTINAL FISTULAS FAIL TO HEAL

- Significant bowel integrity disruption
- Cancer at the fistula site
- Irradiation
- Foreign body
- Distal obstruction
- Inflammatory bowel disease
- Malnutrition
- Immunosuppression
- Abscess/sepsis
- Epithelization of the fistula tract

the formation of an overall treatment plan for the cancer and for fistula repair management within that plan. Treatment may involve resection of the fistula's tract and involved organs; bypass or diversion of intestinal flow away from the fistula; hyperbaric oxygen therapy; prolonged nutritional support; and possibly chemotherapy to treat the cancer if it is the underlying cause. In some patients, simple palliation of any fistula-related symptoms and skin care is all that is necessary, because the treatment may be worse than leaving the fistula alone. Fistulograms, bowel contrast studies, and CT scans can all be particularly helpful during treatment planning.

Tracheal esophageal fistulas usually result from esophageal cancer penetration and perforation into the respiratory tract. Overall prognosis is usually poor because of the locally advanced nature of these cancers. However, short-term palliation is achievable with covered metal stents placed in both the trachea and the esophagus.

Bleeding

Bleeding can be a particularly emergent situation in the cancer patient. In the majority of instances, bleeding is from non–cancer related causes, such as gastritis or diverticulosis. However, it may be exacerbated by cancer-related treatments (e.g., the exacerbation occurring with chemotherapy-induced thrombocytopenia or anticoagulation instituted for other cancer-related conditions). Non–cancer-related causes are typically treated as they are in non-cancer patients, with consideration of the overall prognosis of the patient. The specific source of the bleeding should be determined so that treatment can be effected to prevent recurrent bleeding with additional cancer treatments. Occasionally, bleeding can be the sole manifestation of recurrent cancer (e.g., a colon cancer local recurrence, a melanoma small-bowel metastasis).

Portal hypertensive bleeding can be particularly difficult to manage when it is induced by cancer-related portal vein thrombosis. Therapy is directed at the bleeding source, with variceal banding or sclerosis and pharmacologic control of portal hypertension. Bleeding gastric and esophageal varices caused by splenic vein thrombosis can be treated, if they are symptomatic, with splenectomy.

Bleeding can also occur directly from the tumor bed, either from the primary or from a distant metastasis. This can be immediately life-threatening (e.g., in the brain or a very fast GI hemorrhage), or it can be asymptomatic (e.g., a slow hemorrhage in the GI tract or one that slowly tamponades itself in the retroperitoneum). Supportive care is necessary, with the correction of underlying coagulopathies and quantitative or qualitative platelet defects. Operative resection may be required for resectable lesions in the stomach or bowel. Selected patients may benefit from angiographic embolization with or without eventual elective resection. This is particularly useful if the source is a liver metastasis bleeding into the biliary system. Radiation therapy is also effective for slowly bleeding lesions, but it requires several days to weeks for the therapy to take effect.

Pain

Pain control—although not typically emergent—deserves mention. Acute cancer-related fractures require orthopedic attention and fixation, whereas radiation therapy can be helpful for pain control. Most sources of pain can be relieved through a combination of oral and/or transdermal routes of narcotic and nonnarcotic pain medications. Excess sedation and other narcotic side effects can become particularly problematic. Surgical or percutaneous celiac plexus blockade can also be helpful for controlling abdominal pain, and so can other regional blocks. Thoracic sympathetectomy can be useful, and it can be performed minimally invasively. Implantable epidural pumps and subcutaneous continuous infusion devices are also useful in selective circumstances.

Consultation with pain management specialists can often be very helpful. Other adjuvant treatments—such as nonsteroidal antiinflammatory medications, visual imaging, exercise, massage, biofeedback, acupuncture, and other alternative medicine practices—may be extremely useful. In selected patients, resection of the tumor in an otherwise noncurative fashion can sometimes result in pain relief. For example, decompression of distended bowel loops, which could cause extreme pain, may be helpful, even if noncurative. However, as a rule, the part of the tumor that can be resected is not usually the area of the tumor that is invading the nerves and causing the pain.

Neutropenic Enterocolitis

Neutropenic enterocolitis goes by many other names, including *typhlitis* (from the Greek word for *cecum*), *agranulocytic colitis, neutropenic enteropathy,* and *ileocecal syndrome*. All of these terms refer to an inflammatory condition of the right colon and particularly the cecum in a setting of neutropenia. Presentation is often characterized by fever, right lower-quadrant pain, decreased neutrophil count, abdominal distention, diarrhea, nausea, vomiting, and bloody stools. Mortality is as high as 20%. Differential diagnosis includes other causes of inflammation, including *Clostridium difficile* colitis, diverticulitis, inflammatory bowel disease, appendicitis, intussusception, bowel ischemia, cholecystitis, diffuse peritonitis, mesenteric adenitis, and constipation. Physical examination is usually consistent with localized peritonitis, and a CT scan of the abdomen is often characterized by right colonic and cecal bowel-wall thickening, with occasional air within the bowel wall and pericecal fat stranding. The absolute neutrophil count is usually less than 500 per μL. Barium enema is usually contraindicated in this situation. The pathophysiology is not completely understood. However, because the cecum is often the most dilated portion of the large colon, per Laplace's law, it is often this area that becomes most distended with increased intraluminal pressure within the colon. This leads to localized ischemia, increased stasis, low-grade sepsis, and bacterial translocation. Concomitant steroid medication use, dehydration, decreased blood supply, malnutrition, and change in bowel flora may also contribute. Susceptibility of the right colon may also relate to a decrease in normal lymphoid tissue in this region with chemotherapy.

Treatment involves broad-spectrum antibiotic use and bowel rest, colony-stimulating factors to increase neutrophil count, and supportive care. In the majority of instances, medical management is sufficient. Surgical intervention is reserved for cases in which there is a lack of improvement or suspected perforation, bleeding, or uncontrolled sepsis. CT imaging is often helpful. Most often, surgical intervention requires the resection of the right colon, with diversion. Some authors have recommended surgical intervention even after a successful medically treated episode of neutropenic enterocolitis to prevent recurrences with subsequent chemotherapy cycles. This is not, however, widely practiced because of the delays incurred in chemotherapy administration by the intervening surgery and recovery time.

BOX 27–5 INDICATIONS FOR SURGERY IN NEUTROPENIC ENTEROCOLITIS

1. Evidence of free intraperitoneal perforation
2. Ongoing sepsis/acidosis, despite initial resuscitative therapy
3. Ongoing bleeding after correction of platelet and coagulation defects
4. Failure to improve after reversal of neutropenia
5. Uncertainty of diagnosis
6. Selectively, to prevent future episodes with additionally planned chemotherapy

Conclusions

In summary, the management of general surgical complications in the cancer patient is not that dissimilar from the management of complications in the non-cancer patient. In cancer patients, however, not only must the particular complication be addressed, but it must also be determined how that particular complication fits into the overall treatment plan for and prognosis of the patient. Risks and benefits to the patient must be addressed in the context of the potential need for subsequent radiation and/or chemotherapy or additional surgical interventions related to the cancer diagnosis. The treatment must consider the nonhealing and progressive nature of any residual cancer left behind after surgical intervention and the overall patient prognosis. Although very challenging, there is great opportunity for helping cancer patients with surgical interventions, and great personal satisfaction comes from dealing with cancer patients and their families at this particularly stressful time in their lives.

Key Selected Readings

Bavaro MF. Neutropenic enterocolitis. *Curr Gastroenterol Rep* 2002;4:297–301.

Smothers L, Hynan L, Fleming J, *et al.* Emergency surgery for colon carcinoma. *Dis Colon Rectum* 2003;46:24–30.

Selected Readings

Adam A, Ellul J, Watkinson AF, *et al.* Palliation of inoperable esophageal carcinoma: a prospective randomized trial of laser therapy and stent placement. *Radiology* 1997;202:344–348.

August DA, Kearney T, Schwarz RE. Surgical emergencies. In: Chang AE, Ganz PA, Hayes DF, *et al*, editors. *Oncology: an evidence-based approach.* New York: Springer, 2006.

Chen HS, Sheen-Chen SM. Obstruction and perforation in colorectal adenocarcinoma: an analysis of prognosis and current trends. *Surgery* 2000;127:370–376.

Cuffy M, Abir F, Audisio RA, Longo WE. Colorectal cancer presenting as surgical emergencies. *Surg Oncol* 2004;13:149–157.

De Palma GD, di Matteo E, Romano G, *et al.* Plastic prosthesis versus expandable metal stents for palliation of inoperable esophageal thoracic carcinoma: a controlled prospective study. *Gastrointest Endosc* 1996;43:478–482.

Feuer DJ, Broadley KE, Shepherd JH, *et al.* Systematic review of surgery in malignant bowel obstruction in advanced gynecological and gastrointestinal cancer. The Systematic Review Steering Committee. *Gynecol Oncol* 1999;75:313–322.

Glehen O, Kwiatkowski F, Sugarbaker PH, *et al.* Cytoreductive surgery combined with perioperative intraperitoneal chemotherapy for the management of peritoneal carcinomatosis from colorectal cancer: a multi-institutional study. *J Clin Oncol* 2004;22: 3284–3292.

Gouma DJ, van Geenen R, van Gulik T, *et al.* Surgical palliative treatment in bilio-pancreatic malignancy. *Ann Oncol* 1999;10 Suppl 4:269–272.

Kawamata M, Ishitani K, Ishikawa K, *et al.* Comparison between celiac plexus block and morphine treatment on quality of life in patients with pancreatic cancer pain. *Pain* 1996;64:597–602.

Keidan RD, Fanning J, Gatenby RA, *et al.* Recurrent typhlitis. A disease resulting from aggressive chemotherapy. *Dis Colon Rectum* 1989;32:206–209.

Lillemoe KD, Cameron JL, Kaufman HS, *et al.* Chemical splanchnicectomy in patients with unresectable pancreatic cancer. A prospective randomized trial. *Ann Surg* 1993;217:447–455; discussion 456–457.

Mercadante S. Celiac plexus block versus analgesics in pancreatic cancer pain. *Pain* 1993;52:187–192.

Moir CR, Scudamore CH, Benny WB. Typhlitis: selective surgical management. *Am J Surg* 1986;151: 563–566.

Polati E, Finco G, Gottin L, *et al.* Prospective randomized double-blind trial of neurolytic coeliac plexus block in patients with pancreatic cancer. *Br J Surg* 1998;85:199–201.

Ponec RJ, Saunders MD, Kimmey MB. Neostigmine for the treatment of acute colonic pseudo-obstruction. *N Engl J Med* 1999;341:137–141.

Segalin A, Bonavina L, Carazzone A, *et al.* Improving results of esophageal stenting: a study on 160 consecutive unselected patients. *Endoscopy* 1997;29: 701–709.

Siersema PD, Hop WC, Dees J, *et al.* Coated self-expanding metal stents versus latex prostheses for esophagogastric cancer with special reference to prior radiation and chemotherapy: a controlled, prospective study. *Gastrointest Endosc* 1998;47: 113–120.

Tamim WZ, Ghellai A, Counihan TC, *et al.* Experience with endoluminal colonic wall stents for the management of large bowel obstruction for benign and malignant disease. *Arch Surg* 2000;135:434–438.

Index